Textbook on
Clinical Ocular Pharmacology and Therapeutics

Textbook on
Clinical Ocular Pharmacology and Therapeutics

Editors

SK Gupta
PhD DSc FIPS FIACS
Head, Clinical Research
Delhi Institute of Pharmaceutical Sciences and Research (DIPSAR)
University of Delhi
New Delhi, India

Renu Agarwal PhD
Faculty of Medicine
Universiti Teknologi MARA
Selangor, Darul Ehsan, Malaysia

Sushma Srivastava PhD
Department of Pharmacology
Delhi Institute of Pharmaceutical Sciences and Research (DIPSAR)
University of Delhi
New Delhi, India

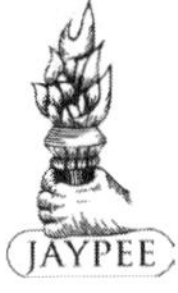

The Health Sciences Publishers

New Delhi | London | Philadelphia | Panama

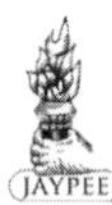 **Jaypee Brothers Medical Publishers (P) Ltd**

Headquarters

Jaypee Brothers Medical Publishers (P) Ltd
4838/24, Ansari Road, Daryaganj
New Delhi 110 002, India
Phone: +91-11-43574357
Fax: +91-11-43574314
Email: jaypee@jaypeebrothers.com

Overseas Offices

J.P. Medical Ltd
83 Victoria Street, London
SW1H 0HW (UK)
Phone: +44 20 3170 8910
Fax: +44 (0)20 3008 6180
Email: info@jpmedpub.com

Jaypee Medical Inc
The Bourse
111 South Independence Mall East
Suite 835, Philadelphia, PA 19106, USA
Phone: +1 267-519-9789
Email: jpmed.us@gmail.com

Jaypee-Highlights Medical Publishers Inc
City of Knowledge, Bld. 237, Clayton
Panama City, Panama
Phone: +1 507-301-0496
Fax: +1 507-301-0499
Email: cservice@jphmedical.com

Jaypee Brothers Medical Publishers (P) Ltd
17/1-B Babar Road, Block-B, Shaymali
Mohammadpur, Dhaka-1207
Bangladesh
Mobile: +08801912003485
Email: jaypeedhaka@gmail.com

Jaypee Brothers Medical Publishers (P) Ltd
Bhotahity, Kathmandu, Nepal
Phone: +977-9741283608
Email: kathmandu@jaypeebrothers.com

Website: www.jaypeebrothers.com
Website: www.jaypeedigital.com

© 2014, Jaypee Brothers Medical Publishers

The views and opinions expressed in this book are solely those of the original contributor(s)/author(s) and do not necessarily represent those of editor(s) of the book.

All rights reserved. No part of this publication may be reproduced, stored or transmitted in any form or by any means, electronic, mechanical, photocopying, recording or otherwise, without the prior permission in writing of the publishers.

All brand names and product names used in this book are trade names, service marks, trademarks or registered trademarks of their respective owners. The publisher is not associated with any product or vendor mentioned in this book.

Medical knowledge and practice change constantly. This book is designed to provide accurate, authoritative information about the subject matter in question. However, readers are advised to check the most current information available on procedures included and check information from the manufacturer of each product to be administered, to verify the recommended dose, formula, method and duration of administration, adverse effects and contraindications. It is the responsibility of the practitioner to take all appropriate safety precautions. Neither the publisher nor the author(s)/editor(s) assume any liability for any injury and/or damage to persons or property arising from or related to use of material in this book.

This book is sold on the understanding that the publisher is not engaged in providing professional medical services. If such advice or services are required, the services of a competent medical professional should be sought.

Every effort has been made where necessary to contact holders of copyright to obtain permission to reproduce copyright material. If any have been inadvertently overlooked, the publisher will be pleased to make the necessary arrangements at the first opportunity.

Inquiries for bulk sales may be solicited at: jaypee@jaypeebrothers.com

Textbook on Clinical Ocular Pharmacology and Therapeutics

First Edition: **2014**

ISBN 978-93-5152-341-3

Printed at Rajkamal Electric Press, Plot No. 2, Phase-IV, Kundli, Haryana.

Contributors

Anna Krasilnikova PhD
Faculty of Medicine
Universiti Teknologi MARA
Selangor, Darul Ehsan, Malaysia

Azida Juana Wan Abdul Kadir MD
University Malaya Medical Center
Faculty of Medicine
University of Malaya, Malaysia

Binit Kumar PhD
Department of Pharmacology
Delhi Institute of Pharmaceutical Sciences and
Research (DIPSAR), University of Delhi
New Delhi, India
Kresge Eye Institute
School of Medicine
Wayne State University
MI, USA

Brandie R Morgan PhD
Harry S Truman Memorial Veterans' Hospital
Columbia, Missouri, USA
Department of Ophthalmology
School of Medicine and College of Veterinary Medicine
University of Missouri
Columbia, Missouri, USA

Brinnell Annette Caszo PhD
Department of Physiology
Faculty of Medicine and Defence Health
National Defence University
Kuala Lumpur, Malaysia

Igor N Iezhitsa PhD
Faculty of Medicine
Universiti Teknologi MARA
Selangor, Darul Ehsan, Malaysia
Department of Pharmacology
Volgograd State Medical University, Russia

Lwin Lwin Nyein MD
Faculty of Medicine
Universiti Teknologi MARA
Selangor, Darul Ehsan, Malaysia

Meenakshi Kanwar Chauhan PhD
Department of Pharmaceutics
Delhi Institute of Pharmaceutical Sciences and
Research (DIPSAR), University of Delhi
New Delhi, India

Miswan Muiz Mahyudin MD
Faculty of Medicine
Universiti Teknologi MARA
Selangor, Darul Ehsan, Malaysia

Mustafa Ahmed Jirjees FIBMS
Faculty of Medicine
MAHSA University College
Kuala Lumpur, Malaysia

Nabanita Halder PhD
Department of Ocular Pharmacology
Dr Rajendra Prasad Center for Ophthalmic Sciences
All India Institute of Medical Sciences
New Delhi, India

Nafeeza Mohd Ismail PhD
Faculty of Medicine
Universiti Teknologi MARA
Selangor, Darul Ehsan, Malaysia

Preeti Sankaran MD
Dr Rajendra Prasad Center for Ophthalmic Sciences
All India Institute of Medical Sciences
New Delhi, India

Puneet Agarwal MD
Department of Ophthalmology
IMU Clinical School
International Medical University
Seremban, Malaysia

Rajani Mathur PhD
Department of Pharmacology
Delhi Institute of Pharmaceutical Sciences and
Research (DIPSAR), University of Delhi
New Delhi, India

Rajiv R Mohan PhD
Harry S Truman Memorial Veterans' Hospital
Columbia, Missouri, USA
Department of Ophthalmology
School of Medicine and College of Veterinary Medicine
University of Missouri
Columbia, Missouri, USA

Renu Agarwal PhD
Faculty of Medicine
Universiti Teknologi MARA
Selangor, Darul Ehsan, Malaysia

Rohit Saxena MD
Department of Ophthalmology
Dr Rajendra Prasad Center for Ophthalmic Sciences
All India Institute of Medical Sciences
New Delhi, India

SK Gupta PhD DSc FIPS FIACS
Head, Clinical Research
Delhi Institute of Pharmaceutical Sciences and
Research (DIPSAR), University of Delhi
New Delhi, India

Shrikant Gaur BSc BAMS (DU)
Head, Medical Research
Promed Research Center
Gurgaon, Haryana, India

Sujaya Singh MD
Faculty of Medicine
Universiti Teknologi MARA
Selangor, Darul Ehsan, Malaysia

Sunil Gurtu MD
Monash University, Sunway Campus
Jeffrey Cheah School of Medicine and
Health Sciences
Selangor, Darul Ehsan, Malaysia

Sushil Vasudevan MD
Faculty of Medicine
Universiti Teknologi MARA
Selangor, Darul Ehsan, Malaysia

Sushma Srivastava PhD
Department of Pharmacology
Delhi Institute of Pharmaceutical Sciences and
Research (DIPSAR), University of Delhi
New Delhi, India

T Velpandian PhD
Department of Ocular Pharmacology
Dr Rajendra Prasad Center for Ophthalmic Sciences
All India Institute of Medical Sciences
New Delhi, India

Vijay Kumar MPharm
Department of Ocular Pharmacology
Dr Rajendra Prasad Center for Ophthalmic Sciences
All India Institute of Medical Sciences
New Delhi, India

Vinay Gupta MD
Department of Ophthalmology
Dr Rajendra Prasad Center for Ophthalmic Sciences
All India Institute of Medical Sciences
New Delhi, India

Preface

The eye and the drugs used to treat ophthalmic ailments, although have been the attractive areas for scientific investigations since the ancient time; 21st century has witnessed explosive growth and development in this field. The students and practitioners are now confronted with the dilemma of how to consolidate basic concepts of pharmacology and knowledge about the newly developed drugs. This book aims to provide essential knowledge of the basic concepts of pharmacology, their application in ocular pharmacology and basic pharmacology of commonly used drugs in ophthalmology. The book also discusses the possible adverse drug reactions of systemically administered drugs. The ophthalmologists and postgraduates will find the book very useful in understanding basic pharmacology concepts, which can be utilized in therapeutics. The contents of the book are formatted in a way to provide quick to the point and easy access to the relevant matter. We believe that the subject matter in this book will be very useful for practicing ophthalmologist as a guide to answer questions that commonly arise during patient care. At the same time students find it useful to prepare for various board and certificate examinations. Although, this book can be used as quick reference, it provides enough subject matter to be used as stand-alone text without reference to larger volumes. Contents of the book have been organized with great caution; however, the feedback from the students and clinicians would be invaluable in improving the format as well as the contents of the book in future editions.

We sincerely thank all authors who have contributed immensely in putting the subject matter of this book in its current form. Without their expertise and time, this book would not be complete.

We shall feel highly rewarded if the objectives of presenting this book are fulfilled and students and practitioners can use it to their advantage in understanding the subject.

SK Gupta
Renu Agarwal
Sushma Srivastava

Acknowledgments

I acknowledge the financial support from Department of Science and Technology (DST), New Delhi, for the financial assistance received under USERS project. My sincere thanks to Dr SS Kohli, Scientist F/Director, SERC Division, DST, for his constant support and encouragement.

I thank all the contributors for their outstanding contributions. Despite their busy schedule and pressing commitments, they have put their best effort to give shape to this textbook.

My special thanks to my colleagues and students at Delhi Institute of Pharmaceutical Sciences and Research, for their valuable help in editorial assistance, without which this task would have been meaningless.

SK Gupta

DRUGS USED IN OCULAR THERAPEUTICS AT A GLANCE

Ocular therapeutics in recent years has undergone tremendous changes not only in terms of introduction of new drugs and new drug classes but also in terms of development of novel drug delivery systems. This introductory section presents a summary for quick reference to currently used drugs from different therapeutic classes. The chapters that follow this section will discuss the basic and clinical pharmacology of each of these drug classes and drugs.

Drug (generic)	Drug class	Clinical use	Trade name	Formulation	Route of administration
MYDRIATICS AND CYCLOPLEGICS					
Atropine sulfate	Anticholinergic	Pupillary dilatation and cycloplegia	Atropine-care	Solution 1% Ointment 1%	Topical
			Isopto atropine		
			Generic		
Homatropine hydrobromide	Anticholinergic	Pupillary dilatation and cycloplegia	Isopto homatropine	Solution 2%, 5%	Topical
			Generic		
Cyclopentolate hydrochloride	Anticholinergic	Pupillary dilatation and cycloplegia	Cyclogyl	Solution 0.5%, 1%, 2%	Topical
			AK-Pentolate	Solution 1%, 2%	
			Generic	Solution 1%	
Tropicamide	Anticholinergic	Pupillary dilatation and cycloplegia	Tropicacyl	Solution 0.5%, 1%,	Topical
			Mydriacyl		
			Generic		
Scopolamine hydrobromide	Anticholinergic	Pupillary dilatation and cycloplegia	Isopto hyoscine	Solution 0.25%	Topical
Phenylephrine hydrochloride	Sympathomimetic	Pupillary dilatation	Mydfrin	Solution 2.5%	Topical
			Neo-Synephrine	Solution 2.5%	
			AK-Dilate	Solution 2.5%, 10%	
			Generic	Solution 2.5%, 10%	
Hydroxyamphetamine hydrobromide/ tropicamide	Sympathomimetic/ anticholinergic	Pupillary dilatation and cycloplegia	Paremyd	Solution 1%/0.25%,	Topical

Following combinations are also available in India:

Atropine sulphate 1% w/v, chloramphenicol 0.5%, dexamethasone sodium phosphate 0.1%.

Atropine sulphate 1%, prednisolone 0.25%, chlorobutanol 0.5%.

Atropine sulphate 10 mg, tetracycline 10 mg.

Cyclopentolate 1%, dexamethasone sodium phosphate 0.1%.

Cyclopentolate hydrochloride 1%, phenylephrine hydrochloride 5%.

Phenylephrine hydrochloride 5%, tropicamide 0.8%.

Homatropine hydrobromide 2%, chlorbutol 0.5%.

Tropicamide 0.8%, phenylephrine 5%.

Tropicamide 0.8%, phenylephrine hydrochloride 0.5%.

Tropicamide 0.8% w/v, phenylephrine hydrochloride 5%.

Tropicamide 1%, chlorbutol 0.5%

Contd...

Contd...

ANESTHETIC AGENTS				
Lidocaine hydrochloride	Amide type of local anesthetic	Ocular surface anesthesia	Akten	Solution 3.5%
Proparacaine hydrochloride	Ester type of local anesthetic	Ocular surface anesthesia	Alcaine	Solution 0.5%
			Ocu-caine	
			Ophthetic	
			Paracaine	
			Generic	
Tetracaine hydrochloride	Ester type of local anesthetic	Ocular surface anesthesia	Generic	Solution 0.5%

Following injectable anesthetic agents are available for regional anesthesia:
1. Bupivacaine (Amide type): 0.25–0.75%
2. Lidocaine (Amide type): 1–2%/500 mg
3. Mepivacaine: (Amide type): 1–2%/500 mg
4. Prilocaine (Amide type): 1–2%/600 mg
5. Etidocaine (Amide type): 1%
6. Procaine (Ester type): 1–2%/500 mg
7. Tetracaine (Ester type): 0.25%

ANTI-INFLAMMATORY AGENTS				
Diclofenac sodium	NSAID	Ocular inflammation	Voltaren	Solution 0.1%
			Generic	
Flurbiprofen sodium	NSAID	Ocular inflammation	Ocufen	Solution 0.03%
			Generic	
Bromfenac	NSAID	Ocular inflammation	Bromday	Solution 0.09%
Nepafenac	NSAID	Ocular inflammation	Nevanac	Solution 0.1%
Ketorolac tromethamine	NSAID	Ocular inflammation, seasonal allergic conjunctivitis	Acular®	Solution 0.5%
			Acular LS	Solution 0.4%
			Acular PF (Preservative free)	Solution 0.5%
			Generic	Solution 0.5%

ANTI-HISTAMINICS, DECONGESTANTS, ASTRINGENT					
Olopatadine hydrochloride	Histamine H1-antagonist, Mast cell inhibitor	Seasonal allergic conjunctivitis	Patanol	Solution 0.1%	Topical
			Pataday	Solution 0.2%	
Epinastine hydrochloride	Histamine H1-, H2-antagonist, Mast cell inhibitor	Seasonal allergic conjunctivitis	Elestat	Solution 0.05%	Topical
			Generic		
Azelastin hydrochloride	Histamine H1-antagonist, Mast cell inhibitor	Seasonal allergic conjunctivitis	Optivar®	Solution 0.05%	Topical
			Generic		
Emedastine difumarate	Histamine H1-antagonist	Seasonal allergic conjunctivitis	Emadine®	Solution 0.05%	Topical

Contd...

Contd...

ANTI-HISTAMINICS, DECONGESTANTS, ASTRINGENT					
Alcaftadine	Histamine H1-antagonist, Mast cell inhibitor	Seasonal allergic conjunctivitis	Lastacaft	Solution 0.25%	Topical
Ketotifen fumarate	Histamine H1-antagonist, Mast cell inhibitor	Seasonal allergic conjunctivitis	Alaway	Solution 0.025%	Topical
			Zaditor		
			Generic		
Naphazoline hydrochloride + antazoline phospahte	Sympathomimetic + Histamine H1-antagonist	Seasonal allergic conjunctivitis	Albalon	Solution 0.05% + 0.5%	Topical
			Vasocon-A		
Naphazoline hydrochloride + pheniramine maleate	Sympathomimetic + Histamine H1-antagonist	Seasonal allergic conjunctivitis, decongestant, astringent	Naphcon-A	Solution 0.025% + 0.3%	Topical
			Visine-A		
			Opcon-A		
Cromolyn sodium	Mast cell inhibitor	Seasonal allergic conjunctivitis	Crolom	Solution 4%	Topical
			Generic		
Nedocromil sodium	Mast cell inhibitor	Seasonal allergic conjunctivitis	Alocril	Solution 2%	Topical
Lodoxamide tromethamine	Mast cell inhibitor	Seasonal allergic conjunctivitis	Alomide	Solution 0.1%	Topical
Pemirolast potassium	Mast cell inhibitor	Seasonal allergic conjunctivitis	Alamast	Solution 0.1%	Topical
Naphazoline hydrochloride	Sympathomimetic	Decongestant	AK-Con	Solution 0.1%	Topical
			Albalon	Solution 0.1%	
			All clear	Solution 0.012%	
			All clear AR	Solution 0.03%	
			Clear Eyes	Solution 0.012%	
			Generic		
Phenylephrine hydrochloride	Sympathomimetic	Decongestant	AK-Nefrin	Solution 0.12%	Topical
			Generic		
Oxymetazoline hydrochloride	Sympathomimetic	Decongestant	Visine LR	Solution 0.025%	Topical
Tetrahydrozoline hydrochloride	Sympathomimetic	Decongestant	Murine Tear Drops	0.05%	Topical
			Visine		
			Visine Advanced Relief		
			Generic		
Naphazoline hydrochloride + zinc sulfate	Sympathomimetic	Decongestant, astringent	Clear Eyes ACR	0.0125%	Topical

Contd...

Contd...

ANTI-HISTAMINICS, DECONGESTANTS, ASTRINGENT					
Naphazoline hydrochloride + polysorbate 80	Sympathomimetic	Decongestant, astringent	VIVA Lubricating Redness Relief		Topical
Tetrahydrozoline + zinc sulfate	Sympathomimetic	Decongestant, astringent	Visine AC	0.05%	Topical

Following combinations are available in India:
Sodium chloride 0.05%, boric acid 1.25%, chlorpheniramine maleate 0.01%, naphazoline hydrochloride 0.056%, zinc sulfate 0.012%
Diclofenac sodium 1 mg, gentamicin sulfate 3 mg/mL.
Ketorolac tromethamine 4 mg, ofloxacin 3 mg/mL.
Naphazoline 0.15%, methylcellulose 0.2%, chlorpheniramine maleate 0.01%.
Ketorolac 0.5 %, fluorometholone 0.1%.
Triamcinolone acetonide 1 mg, gramicidin 0.25 mg, neomycin sulphate 2.5 mg/g.
Ketorolac trometamol, ofloxacin.
Ketorolac trometamol 0.5%, chlorpheniramine maleate 0.2%, phenylephrine hydrochloride 0.12%.
Phenylephrine hydrochloride 0.12%, naphazoline hydrochloride 0.05%, menthol 0.005%, camphor 0.01%.

STEROIDS					
Dexamethasone sodium phosphate	Glucocorticoid	Anti-inflammatory	Ocu-Dex	Solution, Ointment 0.1%, 0.5%	Topical
			Maxidex	Suspension 0.1%, Ointment 0.1%, 0.5%	
Fluorometholone	Glucocorticoid	Anti-inflammatory	FML SOP	Ointment 0.1%	Topical
			Fluor-Op FML FML Forte Generic	Suspension 0.1% Suspension 0.1% Suspension 0.25% Suspension 0.1%	
			Flarex	Suspension 0.1%	
Loteprednol etabonate	Glucocorticoid	Anti-inflammatory	Lotemax	Ointment 0.5% Suspension 0.5%	Topical
			Alrex	Suspension 0.2%	
Prednisolone acetate	Glucocorticoid	Anti-inflammatory	Ecocnopred	Suspension 1%	Topical
			Omnipred		
			Generic		
			Pred Forte		
			Pred Mild	Suspension 0.12%	
Prednisolone sodium phosphate	Glucocorticoid	Anti-inflammatory	AK-Pred	Solution 1%	Topical
			Generic	Solution 0.125% and 1%	
Difluprednate	Glucocorticoid	Anti-inflammatory	Durezol	Emulsion 0.05%	Topical
Medrysone	Glucocorticoid	Anti-inflammatory	HMS	Suspension 1%	Topical

Contd...

Contd...

STEROIDS					
Rimexolone	Glucocorticoid	Anti-inflammatory	Vexol	Suspension 1%	Topical
Fluocinolone acetonide	Glucocorticoid	Anti-inflammatory	Retisert	0.59 mg	Intraocular
Ozurdex	Glucocorticoid	Anti-inflammatory	Dexamethasone	0.70 mg	Intraocular
Triamcinolone acetonide	Glucocorticoid	Anti-inflammatory	Triesence	40 mg/mL	Intraocular
			Trivaris	80 mg/mL	
ANTIGLAUCOMA AGENTS					
Apraclonidine hydrochloride	Sympathomimetic	Oculohypotensive	Iopidine	Solution 0.5%, 1%	Topical
			Generic	Solution 0.5%	
Brimonidine tartrate	Sympathomimetic	Oculohypotensive	Alphagan P	Solution 0.1%, 0.15%	Topical
			Generic	Solution 0.15%, 0.2%	
Dipivefrin hydrochloride	Sympathomimetic	Oculohypotensive	Propine	Solution 0.1%	Topical
			Generic		
Epinephrine hydrochloride	Sympathomimetic	Oculohypotensive	Generic	Solution 0.5%, 1%, 2%	Topical
Betaxolol hydrochloride	Beta-blocker	Oculohypotensive	Betoptic-S	Solution 0.25%	Topical
			Generic	Solution 0.5%	
Levobunolol hydrochloride	Beta-blocker	Oculohypotensive	Betagan	Solution 0.25%, 0.5%	Topical
			Generic		
Carteolol hydrochloride	Beta-blocker	Oculohypotensive	Generic	Solution 1%	Topical
Metipranolol	Beta-blocker	Oculohypotensive	OptiPranolol	Solution 0.3%	Topical
			Generic		
Timolol hemihydrate	Beta-blocker	Oculohypotensive	Betimol	Solution 0.25%, 0.5%	Topical
Timolol maleate	Beta-blocker	Oculohypotensive	Timoptic	Solution 0.25%, 0.5%	Topical
			Timoptic-XE	Gel 0.25%, 0.5%	
			Generic	Solution and Gel 0.25%, 0.5%	
Pilocarpine hydrochloride	Cholinomimetic	Oculohypotensive	Isopto carpine	Solution 1%, 2%, 4%	Topical
			Pilopine-HS	Gel 4%	
			Generic	Solution 0.5%, 1%, 2%, 3%, 4%, 6%	

Contd...

Contd...

ANTIGLAUCOMA AGENTS

Carbachol	Cholinomimetic	Oculohypotensive	Isopto carbachol	Solution 1.5%, 3%	Topical
			Miostat	Solution 0.01%	
Latanoprost	Prostaglandin analog	Oculohypotensive	Xalatan	Solution 0.005%	Topical
			Generic		
Bimatoprost	Prostaglandin analog	Oculohypotensive	Lumigan	Solution 0.01%, 0.03%	Topical
Travoprost	Prostaglandin analog	Oculohypotensive	Travatan	Solution 0.004%	Topical
			Travatan-Z		
Dorzolamide hydrochloride	Carbonic anhydrase inhibitor	Oculohypotensive	Trusopt	Solution 2%	Topical
			Generic		
Brinzolamide	Carbonic anhydrase inhibitor	Oculohypotensive	Azopt	Solution 1%	Topical
Methazolamide	Carbonic anhydrase inhibitor	Oculohypotensive	Generic	Tablets 25 mg, 50 mg	Oral
Acetazolamide	Carbonic anhydrase inhibitor	Oculohypotensive	Diamox	Tablets 125 mg, 250 mg, Capsules extended release 500 mg	Oral
Glycerine	Hyperosmotic agent	Oculohypotensive	Osmoglyn	Solution 50%	Oral
Mannitol	Hyperosmotic agent	Oculohypotensive	Osmitrol	Solution 5–20%	Intravenous
Urea	Hyperosmotic agent	Oculohypotensive	Ureaphil	Powder (4 g) to be reconstituted to 30% solution	Intravenous

Following combinations are available in India:
Brimonidine tartrate, timolol maleate.
Brimonidine tartrate 2 mg, timolol maleate 5 mg.
Timolol, bimatoprost.
Dorzolamide 2%, timolol 0.5%.
Bimatoprost 0.03%, timolol 0.5%.
Timolol maleate 0.5%, pilocarpine 2%.
Latanoprost 0.005%, timolol maleate 0.5%.

ANTIBACTERIAL AGENTS

Ciprofloxacin	Fluoroquinolone	Extraocular and intraocular infections	Ciloxan	Solution and Ointment 0.3%	Topical Intravenous: 500 mg/8 hours
Gatifloxacin	Fluoroquinolone	Extraocular and intraocular infections	Zymaxid	Solution 0.5%	Topical
			Zymar	Solution 0.3%	
Levofloxacin	Fluoroquinolone	Extraocular and intraocular infections	Iquix	Solution 1.5%	Topical Intravenous: 500 mg/24 hours
			Quixin	Solution 0.5%	
Moxifloxacin	Fluoroquinolone	Extraocular and intraocular infections	Moxeza	Solution 0.5%	Topical Intravenous: 400 mg/24 hours
			Vigamox		

Contd...

Contd...

		ANTIBACTERIAL AGENTS			
Besifloxacin	Fluoroquinolone	Extraocular and intraocular infections	Besivance	Solution 0.6%	Topical
Ofloxacin	Fluoroquinolone	Extraocular and intraocular infections	Ocuflox	Solution 0.3%	Topical
Sulfacetamide	Sulfonamide	Extraocular infections	Bleph-10	Solution 10%	Topical
			Sulf-10	Solution 10%	
			Sulf-10 preservative free	Ointment 10%	
Gentamicin sulfate	Aminoglycoside	Extraocular and intraocular infections	Genoptic	Solution 0.3%	Topical
			Genoptic SOP	Ointment 0.3%	Subconjunctival: 10–20 mg Intravitreal:
			Gentak	Solution 0.3% Ointment 0.3%	100–200 μg Intravenous: 3–5 mg/kg daily in 2–3 divided doses
Tobramycin sulfate	Aminoglycoside	Extraocular and intraocular infections	AK-Tob	Solution 0.3%	Topical
			Tobrex	Solution 0.3%, Ointment 0.3%	Subconjunctival: 10–20 mg Intravitreal:
			Tobrasol	Solution 0.3%	100–200 μg Intravenous: 3–5 mg/kg daily in 2–3 divided doses
Neomycin sulfate	Aminoglycoside	Extraocular and intraocular infections	Neomycin sulfate	Solution 0.5%	Topical
					Subconjunctival: 125–250 mg
Amikacin sulfate	Aminoglycoside	Extraocular and intraocular infections	Amikin	Solution 0.3%	Topical
					Subconjunctival: 25 mg Intravitreal: 400 μg Intravenous: 3–15 mg/kg daily in 2–3 divided doses
Kanamycin sulfate	Aminoglycoside	Extraocular and intraocular infections	Kanamycin sulfate	Solution 0.5%	Topical
					Subconjunctival: 30 mg Intravitreal: 500 μg
Ampicillin sodium	Penicillin	Intraocular infections	Topical: 50 mg/mL Subconjunctival: 50–150 mg Intravitreal: 5 mg Intravenous: 4–12 g daily in 2–3 divided doses		

Contd...

Contd...

ANTIBACTERIAL AGENTS				
Penicillin G	Penicillin	Intraocular infections	Topical: 100,000 units/mL Subconjunctival: 0.5–1 million units Intravitreal: 300 units Intravenous: 12–24 million units daily in 4–6 divided doses	
Piperacillin	Penicillin	Intraocular infections	Topical: 12.5 mg/mL Subconjunctival: 100 mg	
Ticarcillin disodium	Penicillin	Intraocular infections	Topical: 6 mg/mL Subconjunctival: 100 mg	
Cefazolin sodium	Cephalosporin	Intraocular infections	Topical: 50 mg/mL Subconjunctival: 100 mg Intravitreal: 2250 μg Intravenous: 2–4 g daily in 3–4 divided doses	
Ceftazidime	Cephalosporin	Intraocular infections	Topical: 50 mg/mL Subconjunctival: 100 mg Intravitreal: 2000 μg Intravenous: 1 g daily in 2–3 divided doses	
Ceftriaxone	Cephalosporin	Intraocular infections	Topical: 50 mg/mL Intravenous: 1–4 g daily in 1–2 divided doses	
Erythromycin	Macrolide	Extraocular and intraocular infections	Topical: Ointment 0.5%, solution 50 mg/mL Subconjunctival: 100 mg Intravitreal: 500 μg	
Azithromycin	Macrolide	Extraocular and intraocular infections	Azasite	Topical solution 1% Intravenous: 500 mg
Clarithromycin	Macrolide	Extraocular and intraocular infections	Topical: 10 mg/mL	
Bacitracin zinc	Bacitracin	Extraocular and intraocular infections	Topical: 10,000 units/mL, Ointment 500 units/g Subconjunctival: 5000 units	
Polymyxin B sulfate	Polymyxin	Extraocular and intraocular infections	Topical: 10,000 units/mL, Subconjunctival: 10,000 units	
Vancomycin hydrochloride	Glycopeptide	Extraocular and intraocular infections	Topical: 12.5–25 mg/mL Subconjunctival: 25 mg Intravitreal: 1000 μg Intravenous: 15–30 mg/kg daily in 1–2 divided doses	
Imipenem/ Cilastatin sodium	Carbapenem	Extraocular and intraocular infections	Topical: 5 mg/mL Intravenous: 2 g daily in 3–4 divided doses	
Combinations of antibacterial agents				

Combination	Trade name	Formulation
Bacitracin/hydrocortisone/neomycin/ polymyxin	Generic	Suspension, Ointment: 400 units—1%
Polymyxin B/bacitracin Zinc	AK-Poly-Bac Generic	Ointment: 10,000–500 units/g

Contd...

Contd...

ANTIBACTERIAL AGENTS		
Polymyxin B/neomycin/bacitracin	Neosporin Generic	Solution: 10,000 units—1.75–0.025 mg/mL Ointment: 10,000 units—3.5 mg–400 units/g
Polymyxin B/neomycin/gramicidin	Neosporin Generic	Solution: 10,000 units—1.75–0.025 mg/mL Ointment: 10,000 units—3.5 mg–400 units/g
Polymyxin B/trimethoprim	Polytrim Generic	Solution: 10,000 units—1 mg/mL
Dexamethasone/neomycin/ polymyxin B	Poly-Dex	Suspension and ointment: 0.1%—3.5 mg/mL–10,000 units/mL
	Maxitrol	Suspension and ointment: 0.1%—3.5 mg/mL–10,000 units/mL
	Dexasporin	Suspension: 0.1%—3.5 mg/mL–10,000 units/mL
	AK- Trol	Ointment: 0.1%—3.5 mg/mL–10,000 units/mL
Dexamethasone/tobramycin	Tobradex Generic	Suspension and ointment: 0.1–0.3%
Fluoromethalone-sulfacetamide	FML-S	Suspension: 0.1–10%
Gentamicin–prednisolone acetate	Pred-G	Suspension: 0.3–1.0%
	Pred-G SOP	Ointment: 0.3–0.6%
Loteprednol etabonate–tobramycin	Zylet	Suspension: 0.5–0.3%
Prednisolone acetate – Neomycin – Polymyxin B	Poly-Pred Generic	Suspension: 0.5–0.35%–10,000 units/mL
Prednisolone acetate – Sulfacetamide	Blephamide	Suspension: 0.2–10%
	Blephamide SOP	Ointment: 0.2–10%
Prednisolone sodium phosphate – Sulfacetamide	Vasocidin Generic	Solution: 0.23–10%

Following combinations are also available in India:
Moxifloxacin hydrochloride 5 mg, dexamethasone phosphate 1 mg.
Chloramphenicol 5%, beclometasone dipropionate 0.025%, clotrimazole 1%, lignocaine hydrochloride 2%.
Bacitracin 500 u and polymyxin B sulfate 10,000 u.
Trimethoprim 1 mg, polymyxin B sulfate 10000 IU, polyvinyl alcohol 0.25%.
Ciprofloxacin 0.3%, dexamethasone 0.01%.
Chloramphenicol 0.2%, prednisolone acetate 0.5%.
Chloramphenicol 0.5%, dexamethasone sodium phosphate 0.1%.
Chloramphenicol 0.5 % dexamethasone 0.01 %.
Chloramphenicol 0.5%, atropine 1%, dexamethasone 0.01%,.
Neomycin 0.5%, dexamethasone 0.01%.
Neomycin sulfate 0.5%, dexamethasone sodium phosphate 0.1%.
Moxifloxacin hydrochloride 0.5%, ketorolac 0.5%
Gatifloxacin 0.3%, dexamethasone 0.1%.
Polymyxin B 5000 IU, chloramphenicol 10 mg, betamethasone 1 mg.
Ofloxacin 0.3%, prednisolone acetate 1%, benzalkonium chloride 0.05%.
Polymyxin B sulfate 5000 IU, chloramphenicol 10 mg.
Ofloxacin 0.3%, betamethasone 0.01%.
Ofloxacin 0.3%, dexamethasone 0.01%.
Chloramphenicol 0.5%, flurbiprofen sodium 0.03%.
Gatifloxacin 0.3%, dexamethasone 0.01%.
Gatifloxacin 0.3%, prednisolone acetate 1%.
Gentamycin 0.3%, dexamethasone 0.01%.
Gentamycin sulfate 0.3%, hydrocortisone acetate 1%.
Gentamicin sulfate 0.3%, betamethasone sodium phosphate 0.1%
Ofloxacin 0.3%, dexamethasone 0.1%.
Ketorolac tromethamine 5 mg, ofloxacin 3 mg/1 mL.
Tobramycin sulfate 0.3%, fluorometholone 1%.

Contd...

Contd...

ANTIFUNGAL AGENTS		
Amphotericin B	Ambisome (intravenous)	Topical: 0.1–0.5% solution Subconjunctival: 0.8–1.0 mg Intravitreal: 5 µg Intravenous: 3–5 mg/kg/day
Natamycin	Natacyn	Topical: 5% suspension
Fluconazole	Diflucan	Oral: 150 mg single dose; 200 mg on day 1 followed by 100 mg daily; 400 mg on day 1 followed by 200 mg daily. Intravenous: 100–400 mg daily
Itraconazole	Sporanox	Oral: 200–400 mg daily Intravenous: 200 mg twice a day for 2 days followed by 200 mg daily for 14 days
Voriconazole	Vfend	Topical: 1% solution prepared from IV formulation. Oral: 200 mg twice a day Intravenous: 3–6 mg/kg every 12 hours
Clotrimazole		Oral: One troche 5 times a day
Ketoconazole	Nizrol	Oral: 200–400 mg/day
Posaconazole	Noxafil	Oral: 200 mg thrice daily; 100 mg twice on day 1 followed by 100 mg/day for 13 days; 400 mg twice a day
Anidulafungin	Eraxis	Intravenous: 100 mg/day
Caspofungin	Cancidas	Intravenous: 50 mg/day
Mycafungin	Mycamine	Intravenous: 100 mg/day
Flucytosine	Ancobon	Oral: 50–150 mg/kg daily in 4 divided doses
Griseofulvin		Oral: 500 mg/day Oral (Ultramicrosize): 375–750 mg/day
Terbinafine	Lamisil	Oral: 250 mg/day
ANTIVIRAL AGENTS		
Acyclovir sodium	Zovirax Generic	Herpes simplex keratitis (Acute infection): Oral: 400 mg 5 times/day for 1–2 weeks Herpes simplex keratitis (Prophylaxis): Oral: 400 mg twice/day Herpes zoster ophthalmicus: Oral: 800 mg 5 times/day for 7–10 days
Famcyclovir	Famvir	Herpes zoster ophthalmicus: Oral: 500 mg 3 times/day for 7 days
Gencyclovir sodium	Zirgan	Herpes dendritis keratitis: Topical 0.15% gel, 5 times/day until the ulcer heals followed by 3 times a day for 7 days
	Cytovene	Intravitreal: 200 µg Intravenous: Induction—5 mg/kg administered over 1 hours, every 12 hours for 2–3 weeks; Maintenance: 5 mg/kg/day for 7 days/week or 6 mg/kg/day for 5 days/week
	Vitrasert	Intravitreal insert: 4.5 mg-releases drug over 5–8 months

Contd...

Contd...

<table>
<tr><td colspan="3" align="center">ANTIVIRAL AGENTS</td></tr>
<tr><td>Valacyclovir</td><td>Valtrex</td><td>Herpes zoster ophthalmicus: Oral: 1 g thrice/day for 7 days</td></tr>
<tr><td>Valganciclovir</td><td>valcyte</td><td>CMV retinitis: Oral: Induction: 900 mg/12 hours for 21 days.
Maintenance: 900 mg/day</td></tr>
<tr><td>Cidofovir</td><td>Vistide</td><td>Intravenous: Induction—5 mg/kg administered over 1 hours once a week for 2 weeks.
Maintenance: 5 mg/kg infusion over 1 hours once every 2 weeks</td></tr>
<tr><td>Foscarnate sodium</td><td>Foscavir</td><td>Intravenous: Induction—60 mg/kg (adjusted to renal function) over 1 hour/8 hours for 2–3 weeks.
Maintenance: 90–120 mg/kg over 2 hours once daily</td></tr>
<tr><td colspan="3" align="center">OFF-LABEL DRUGS USED IN OPHTHALMOLOGY</td></tr>
<tr><td>DRUGS</td><td>COMMON USES</td><td>ACTION AND DOSE</td></tr>
<tr><td>Acetylcysteine</td><td>Used in corneal conditions like burns, filamentary keratitis, keratoconjunctivitis sicca, corneal melts</td><td>Acts by inhibiting collagenase, which delays the corneal healing

Dose: Hourly in acute cases, up to 4 times/day for maintenance</td></tr>
<tr><td>Alteplase (tissue plasminogen activator)</td><td>Intraocular injection in postvitrectomy patients to treat fibrin formation, to remove fibrin membranes occluding intraocular portions of shunts</td><td>Acts as a thrombolytic agent. There is significant risk of hyphema formation

Dose: 3–6 µg postvitrectomy, 6–12 µg to remove fibrin membranes</td></tr>
<tr><td>5-Fluorouracil</td><td>Post-glaucoma filtering surgery (indicated in patients with high risk of surgical failure)</td><td>It is an antimetabolite acts by inhibiting fibroblast proliferation. Associated with risk of conjunctival wound leak, corneal epithelial defects, keratitis, hypotony, reduced visual acuity

Dose: Postoperative: Subconjunctival 5 g twice/day for 7 days followed by once daily for 7 more days
Intraoperative: 50 mg/mL solution soaked in murocell sponge for 3–5 minutes</td></tr>
<tr><td>Mitomycin C</td><td>Same as 5-Fluorouracil

Additionally has ben used to prevent recurrence after pterygium surgery and to reduced scarring after corneal surgery such as excimer laser</td><td>Its action and complications are same as 5-Fluorouracil

Dose: Intraoperative: Applied once 0.02–0.04% on a small piece of Gelfilm or Weck cell sponge</td></tr>
</table>

Contd...

Contd...

OFF-LABEL DRUGS USE IN OPHTHALMOLOGY		
Bevacizumab (Avastin)	Used in age-related macular degeneration, macular edema due to retinal vein occlusion or diabetic retinopathy. Also used as surgical adjunct in procedures for treatment of neovascular glaucoma	Humanized monoclonal antibody. Acts by inhibiting vascular endothelial growth factor-A Dose: 1.25 mg intravitreal
Cyclosporin (Sandimmune)	Used to prevent transplant rejection after keratoplasty Also used to treat severe vernal conjunctivitis, ligneous conjunctivitis and noninfectious peripheral ulcerative keratitis associated with systemic autoimmune disorders	Acts as an immunosuppressant with high selectivity of T lymphocytes Dose: 0.5–2% topical
Doxycycline and Minocycline	Used to treat ocular rosacea meibomianitis and some conditions involving corneal melting.	Tetracyclines act by inhibiting bacterial protein synthesis Dose: 100 mg 1–2 times per day for 2–12 weeks

Source: PDR for Ophthalmic Medicines; 40th Edition, 2012; MIMS, India.

Contents

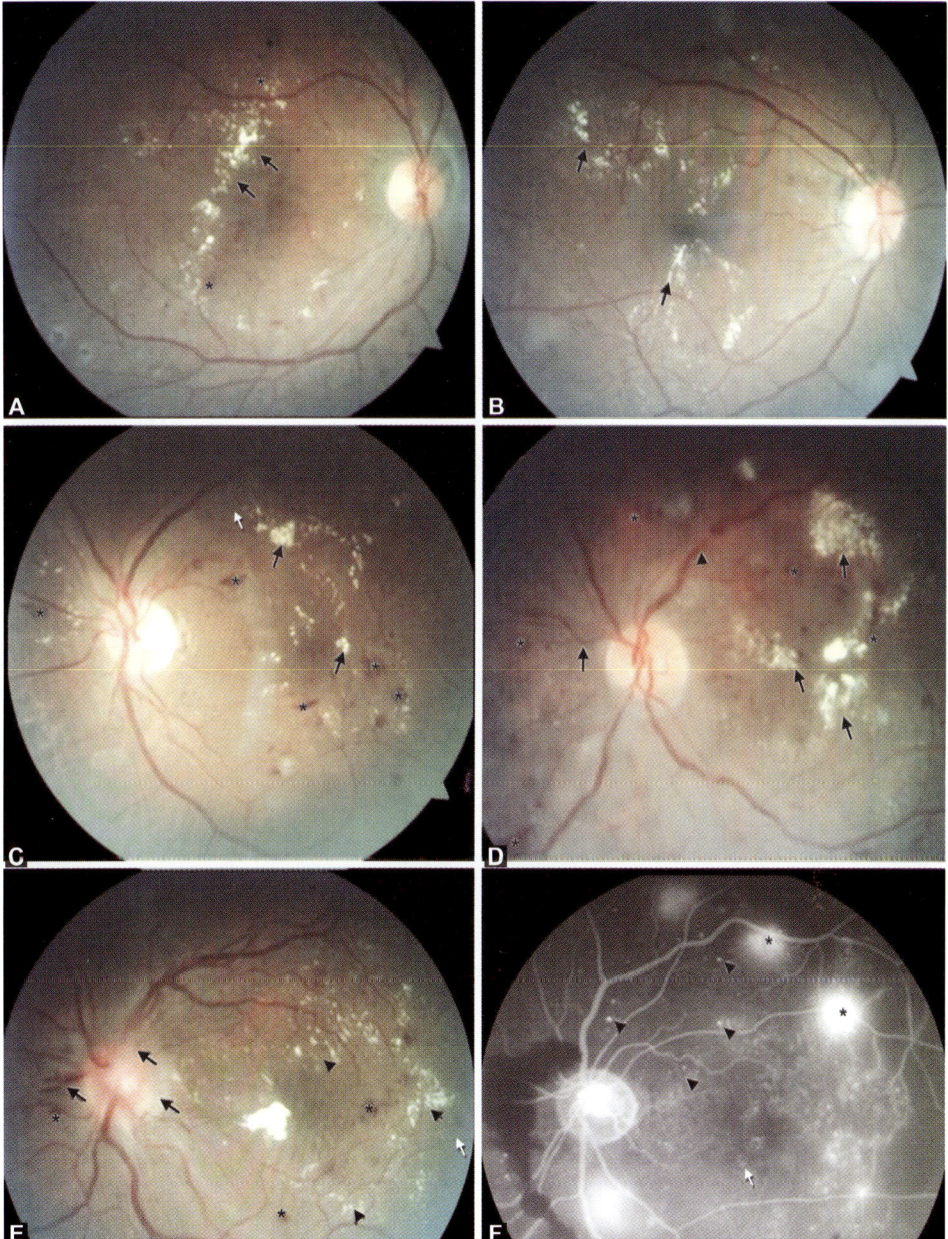

PLATE 1

Figures 17.1A to F (A and B) Representative fundus photographs from patient with moderate NPDR showing significant accumulation of hard exudates (arrow), microaneurysms and leakages at some areas (asterisk); (C) Fundus photograph from patient with severe NPDR showing significantly high leakage at multiple areas (star) and appearance of hard exudates; (D) Fundus photograph from patient with severe NPDR showing tortuous blood vessels (arrow head), large deposits of hard exudates (arrow) and leakages in the fundus (star); (E) A representative image from patient with PDR as evident from neovascularization of the optic disc (arrow), tortuous vessel, appearance of hard exudates (arrow head) and retinal hemorrhage (star); (F) A fluorescein fundus angiogram from a patient with PDR showing significant leakage of sodium fluorescein (star) and appearance of microaneurysms in the form of hyperfluorescent dots (arrow heads)

CHAPTER 1

Anatomical and Physiological Basis of Ocular Pharmacotherapy

OVERVIEW

The principles of therapeutics in the treatment of ophthalmic diseases require a comprehensive knowledge of ocular anatomy and physiology. The understanding of drug interactions at molecular, cellular and tissue level leading to pharmacological responses require special consideration due to the unique anatomical and physiological characteristics of eye. This chapter provides a basic account of the ocular anatomy and physiology as a basis of ocular pharmacotherapy.

The eye and orbit contain smooth and striated muscle, epithelial tissues, blood vessels, nerves both autonomic and sensorimotor, connective tissues and the neuronal tissue, i.e. retina. They are arranged in order to provide an optimum path for the transmittance of light to the light sensitive cells of the retina. Supporting tissues aid and enable this function, and also provide nutrition, blood supply and an excretory pathway.

EYELIDS

Structure

The eyelids or palpebrae cover the anterior surface of the eye protecting it from injury and exposure. The space between the upper and lower lids is called the palpebral fissure, the angle between the lids are called the medial and lateral canthi (Fig. 1.1).

The tarsal plate is the main supporting structure of the lids and is present in both the

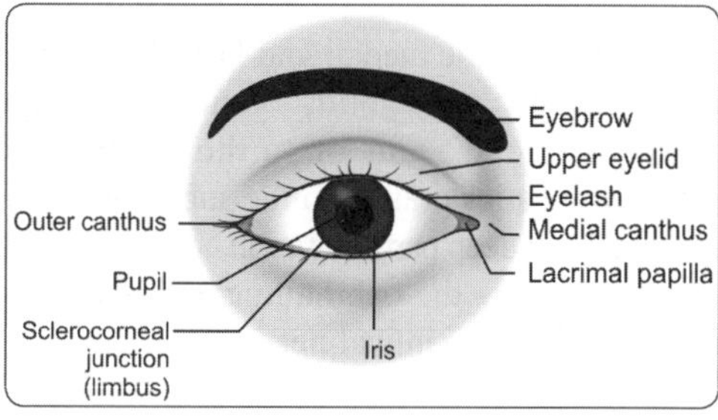

Figure 1.1 The eye

upper and lower lids. The plate is attached to the orbital septum, which is a thin membranous sheet attached to the rim and continuous with the periosteum of the bony orbit.

The layers of the upper eyelid from the facial aspect inwards include—skin, subcutaneous connective tissue, orbicularis oculi, connective tissue, tarsal plate, meibomian glands, connective tissue and conjunctiva. Meibomian glands are the tarsal glands that open at the lid margins behind the mucocutaneous junction. The tarsal plate also receives the insertion of the levator palpebrae muscle. The layers of the lower eyelid consist of skin, orbicularis oculi muscle, connective tissue, orbital septum and fat, retractors of the lower eyelid and palpebral conjunctiva.[1] The retractors of the lower eyelid are extensions of the fascia covering the inferior oblique muscle and passing forward to be inserted into the tarsal plate of the lower lid. It may be referred to as the inferior tarsal muscle though it has not been completely characterized yet.

Meibomian glands secrete lipids, mainly wax and steryl ester that are hydrophobic.

They contribute to the layers of the tear film and its stability. They are expressed from the gland during blinking.

> **MEIBOMIAN GLAND DYSFUNCTION**
>
> Meibomian gland dysfunction is a common cause of eye discomfort especially among users of VIDEO DISPLAY TERMINALS. Blockage of meibomian gland ducts is quite common and may affect a single or multiple glands.

Blood Supply, Lymphatic Drainage and Sensory Nerve Supply of Eyelids

Anastomoses of the medial and lateral palpebral arteries supply the eyelids. Venous drainage is into the facial veins or to the ophthalmic veins. Lymphatics drain into the submandibular, superficial and deep parotid lymph nodes. Sensory innervation is by the ophthalmic and maxillary divisions of the trigeminal nerves.

Motor Nerve Supply and Movements of the Eyelids

Movements of the eyelids are brought about by 2 muscles, the orbicularis oculi, for closure of the lids and the levator palpebrae superioris for opening of the eyelids. Firm closure of the eyelid is achieved by the action of the orbicularis oculi muscle, supplied by the facial nerve. Closure of the eyelid for example in the instance of a blink occurs by inhibition of the levator palpebrae superioris muscle, supplied by the oculomotor nerve and the elastic recoil of the supporting connective tissues.[3] The levator palpebrae superioris is responsible for the opening of the eyelid. Maximal eyelid opening is achieved by the added action of the frontalis muscle. Muller's muscle or the superior tarsal muscle arises from the distal part of the levator palpebrae superioris and inserts into the upper margin of the tarsus.[3] It is composed of smooth muscle fibers and connective tissue. It is supplied by sympathetic nerves. It is mainly responsible for the width of the palpebral fissure. The motor supply is through the oculomotor nerve, while the motor neurons arise from a single central caudal nucleus of the oculomotor nerve. Thus lesions affecting the nucleus often affect both eyelids.[3]

> **EFFECT OF DRUGS ON PALPEBRAL FISSURE**
>
> Cholinomimetic drugs with nicotinic action affect the skeletal muscle fibers of levator palpebrae superioris and may cause lid twitching. Adrenergic drugs cause contraction of Muller's muscle leading to widening of palpebral fissure. Adrenergic blockers such as guanethidine cause Muller's muscle paralysis and ptosis.

Eyelid movements occur in coordination with the movements of the globe in a way that on upward gaze vision may not be disturbed and on downward gaze the eyeball is protected. It appears that the interstitial nucleus of Cajal and the rostral interstitial nucleus of the medial longitudinal fasciculus are the main centers for coordinating eyelid and eye movement.[3]

> **DISORDERS OF EYELID POSITION**
>
> Ptosis is drooping of the upper eyelid. It may be bilateral due to midbrain lesions involving the 3rd nerve nucleus. When sympathetic fibers supplying Muller's muscle are affected, a slight depression of the upper eyelid may be present (Horners syndrome). Unilateral ptosis may occur with a 3rd nerve palsy, or a large hemispheric lesion, which may affect the corticobulbar fibers.
>
> Blepharospasm is an involuntary spasm of the orbicularis occuli muscle as well as the levator muscle. It is characterized by frequent prolonged blinks and the eyelids are pulled below the superior orbital margins. It may occur in association with hemifacial spasm caused by irritation of the 7th cranial nerve roots and also along with lesions of the thalamus and brainstem. Blepharocolysis is characterized by drooping eyes due to an involuntary inhibition of the levator palpebrae superioris and no active contribution from the orbicularis muscle. It is often associated with Parkinson's disease, putamenal and subthalamic lesions.[3]

Conjunctiva

Mucous membranes that cover the sclera up to the limbus and the palpebral portions of the eyelids are called conjunctiva. Their main function is protection of the anterior surface of the eye by secreting the mucous layer of the tear film, antibacterial and antiviral substances and providing immune defense. The three main regions of the conjunctiva include the palpebral portions covering the inner side of the eyelids, fornicial conjunctiva located at the fornices and the bulbar conjunctiva covering the white of the eyeball up to the limbus.

DEGENERATIVE DISEASES OF CONJUNCTIVA

Degenerative conditions of the conjunctiva are commonly seen with aging. They have minimal effect on vision and are seen frequently, and correlate with light exposure. Pinguecula is a thickening of the conjunctiva near limbus in the palpebral fissure characterized by elastotic degeneration, hyalinization and granular deposits. Pterygium is a fibrovascular growth arising from the conjunctiva and spreading onto the cornea. It occurs more frequently on the nasal aspect of the palpebral conjunctiva. They may require to be treated as they encroach onto the transparent cornea and affect the field of vision.

The conjunctival epithelium, which is non-keratinized squamous epithelium contains goblet cells secreting mucous and has been shown to be capable of phagocytosis.[4] Below this layer lies the conjunctival substantia propria. It is composed of loose connective tissue and is highly vascularized, and contains a large number of white blood cells.

TRANSCONJUNCTIVAL DRUG ABSORPTION

The cells in the superficial layer of conjunctival epithelium have tight junctions similar to cornea and form a barrier to drug absorption by transconjunctival route. However, the intercellular spaces in conjunctiva are larger than those in cornea and therefore hydrophilic drugs are absorbed better through conjunctiva as compared to cornea. Due to high vascularity conjunctiva is also a site for systemic absorption of topically applied drugs.

NASOLACRIMAL APPARATUS AND THE TEAR FILM

Structure

The lacrimal gland and accessory lacrimal glands are the main tear-producing structures. The lacrimal gland consists of an orbital part located within the orbital margin in the lacrimal fossa of the zygomatic process of the frontal bone. The palpebral part is located below the palpebral conjunctiva. Numerous accessory glands are located in the upper eyelid and the fornices and probably account for lacrimal secretions after removal of the lacrimal gland. Accessory glands of Krause are located in the superior and inferior fornix, while accessory glands of Wolfring are located on the margin of the superior tarsal plate of the upper eyelid.[5] The lacrimal gland is supplied by the lacrimal branch of the ophthalmic artery and drains into the superior ophthalmic vein. It is supplied by parasympathetic fibers from the pterygopalatine ganglion, which are secretomotor to the gland. Acini of the gland are surrounded by myoepithelial cells, which contract to help glandular secretions exit the acini and ductules.

Tears produced by the lacrimal gland bathe the eye and drain through to lacrimal canaliculi (Fig. 1.2). The canaliculi are located in the medial portion of each eyelid near the medial canthus. Each canaliculus begins as a punctum in the lacrimal papilla and drains into the lacrimal sac, which has a closed upper end and in turn drains into the nasolacrimal duct. The duct opens into inferior meatus of the nasal cavity. Secretions from the tarsal meibomian glands also contribute to the tear film by preventing the rapid evaporation of the fluid (Fig. 1.3).

Tear Film

The tear film is composed of three layers (Fig. 1.4). The outermost layer consists of lipids from the secretions of tarsal glands. It floats on a middle aqueous layer, contributed by the main and accessory lacrimal glands. An inner mucous

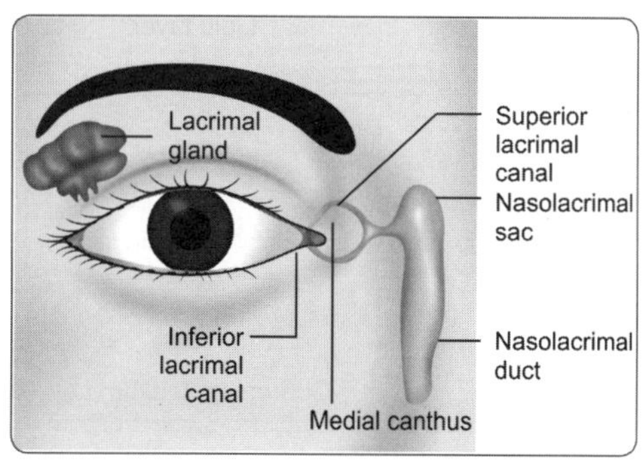

Figure 1.2 Nasolacrimal apparatus

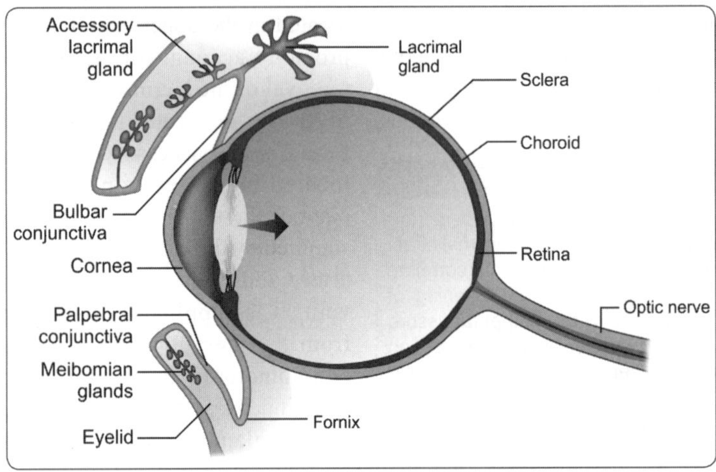

Figure 1.3 Glands secreting the tear film

layer secreted by goblet cells is in contact with the surface of the conjunctiva and cornea. The mucous layer is hydrophilic and traps particulate matter. The aqueous layer makes up more than 97% of the volume of secretions, and contains most of the proteins, immunoglobulins, lactoferrin and enzymes.

THE EFFECT OF RATE OF TEAR FLOW ON DRUG ABSORPTION

The flow of tears normally is about 0.5–2.2 μL/min. Ocular irritation results in increased secretion. An increased rate of tear flow will dilute drug concentrations and result in lower rates of absorption. Absorption may be increased by reducing drainage of tears from the eye. Blocking the nasolacrimal duct or tilting the head back may increase time for drug absorption through the cornea.

DRY EYES AND EFFECT OF DRUGS ON TEAR SECRETION

Osmolarity of the tear film is one of its most important properties. Increased osmolarity due to low rate of secretion or increased evaporation leads to inflammation of the cornea and conjunctiva and a further reduction in the rate of tear film secretion. Over a prolonged period of time the surface of the cornea and conjunctiva may be damaged by these changes.[6]

The drugs can affect the quality as well as quantity of tear secretion. Cholinomimetics stimulate the lacrimal gland and increase secretion of both the aqueous and mucous components of tears. Antimuscarinic agents produce the opposite effect and reduce the tear secretion. Sympathetic stimulation causes vasoconstriction leading to viscous secretion.

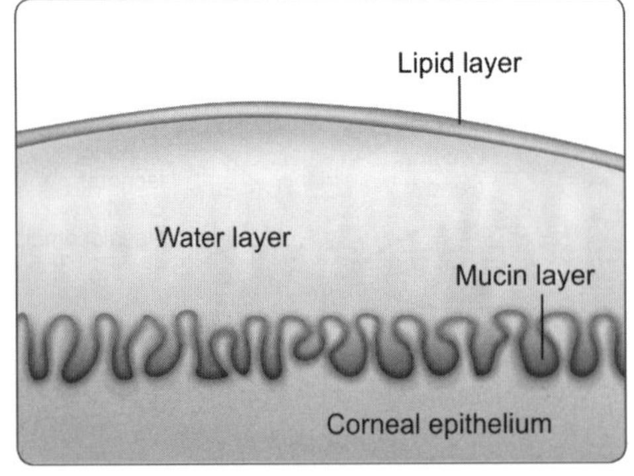

Figure 1.4 Tear film

THE BONY ORBIT

The orbit or the "sockets" of the eye are bony cavities that protect the eye and its supporting structures. The orbit also serves as a passage to connect the eye with its blood supply and nerves and also conduct the vessels and nerves that supply other parts of the face. The bony boundaries of the orbit are described below. It is a crowded space filled with numerous vessels, nerves, connective tissue and muscles apart from the eyeball. Anesthetic agents are administered into this space by the retro- and peribulbar route.

Orbital Margins

Superiorly, the orbital margin is formed by the orbital arch of the frontal bone. Laterally, it is formed by the zygomatic bone and the zygomatic process of the frontal bone. The zygomatic bone and the maxilla form the inferior border of the orbital margin. It is slightly raised above the floor of the orbit. Medially, it is formed by the maxilla and lacrimal bone.

EYEBALL INJURIES

The orbital margins are not easily damaged but may fracture due to severe injury. Frequently, the medial margins along with the nose are affected. The trochlea may be damaged or displaced leading to symptoms consistent with the paralysis of the superior oblique. Zygoma fractures may involve the lateral margins and also the lower margin of the orbit.

The orbital margin in general provides better protection when large objects strike the eye. Smaller objects such as a golf ball for example may strike the eye. The eyeball is most vulnerable to traumatic rupture when struck by a blow directed lateral to medial and upwards.

The outer limits of the orbit are formed by bony boundaries. They form a roughly quadrilateral pyramidal shape and accommodate the globe of the eye, the extra-ocular muscles attached to it, surrounding fat, blood vessels and nerves. The orbit is oriented with its apex directed postereo-medially and the base at the front of the skull. The medial walls are almost parallel with each other and to the sagittal plane. The lateral walls are roughly at an angle of 90° to each other. Dimensions of the orbit are shown in Table 1.1.

LOCAL ANESTHESIA IN PERIORBITAL SPACE

Awareness regarding the size and volume of the globe is required while administering local anesthesia (peribulbar or retrobulbar blocks) in order to lessen the danger of perforation especially if the axial length of the eyeball is expected to be increased (e.g. high myopia, staphyloma). Retrobulbar hemorrhage, proptosis and increased intraocular pressure may result with puncture of the ophthalmic veins. Puncture of the meningeal coverings of the optic nerve may result in the anesthetic agent entering the subarachnoid space and may cause respiratory depression.[8] Use of a semi-sharp needle and a 5/8-inch needle for peribulbar anesthesia may reduce the frequency of such complications directed away from the eyeball.

Table 1.1 Dimensions of the orbit[7]

Depth	50–70 mm
Volume	30 mL
Volume of extraocular muscles and eyeball	7 mL

Wall of the Orbit

The orbit has a superior, medial and lateral wall and a floor composed of a number of different bones. They are briefly summarized in the Figures 1.5 to 1.7 and Table 1.2.[9]

The superior wall is concave anteriorly, where the maximum diameter of the orbit is about 1.5 cm from the orbital margin and more or less flattened posteriorly. It contains the fossa for the lacrimal gland in the anterolateral aspect of the frontal bone. The trochlear fossa lies anteromedially, and contains the trochlea through which the tendon of the superior oblique passes. Anteriorly it is related to the air sinuses of the frontal bone. It separates the orbit from the anterior cranial fossa and the frontal lobes of the brain.

The medial wall contains the lacrimal fossa for the lacrimal sac anteriorly. It is thin and runs almost parallel with medial wall of the other orbit. It separates the orbit from the anterior, middle posterior and sphenoid air cells.

The floor of the orbit separates it from the maxillary sinus. It contains the infraorbital sulcus, which is continuous with the infraorbital fissure.

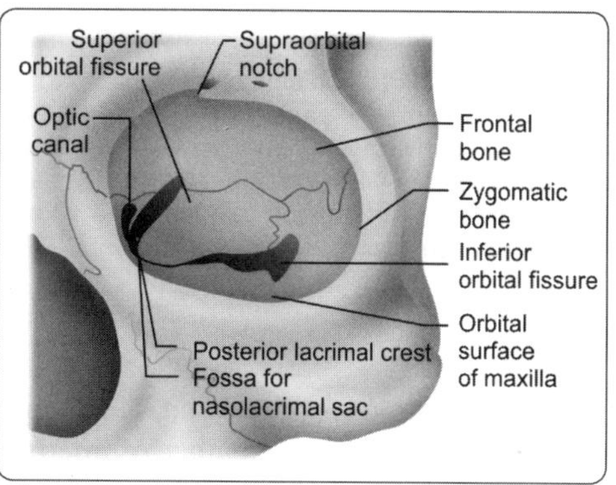

Figure 1.5 Left bony orbit

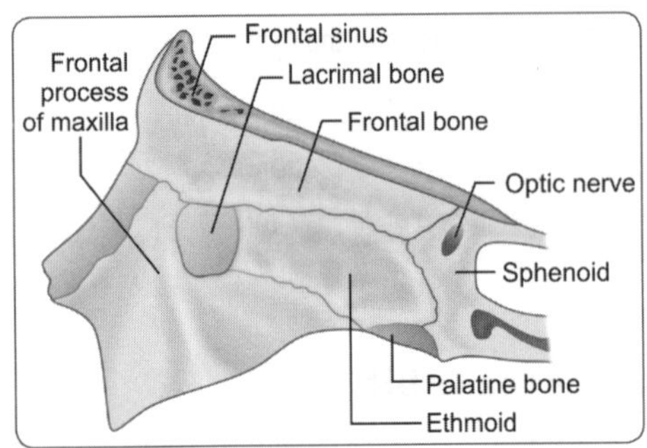

Figure 1.6 Medial wall of the orbit

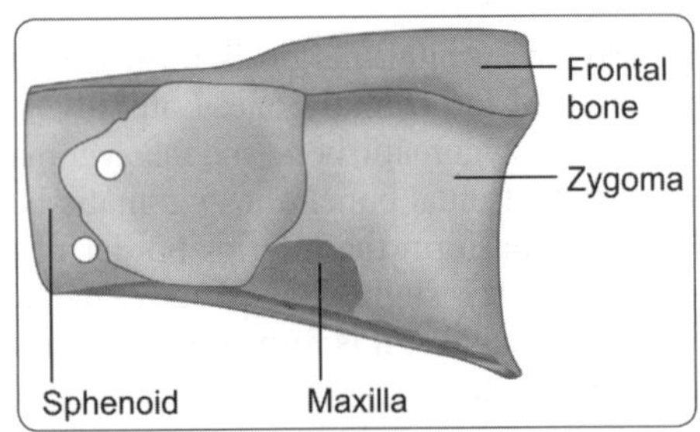

Figure 1.7 Lateral wall of the orbit

Table 1.2 Walls of the orbit

Orbit	Composing structures	Relations
Superior wall	Orbital plate of the frontal bone, sphenoid bone (lesser wing)	Frontal air sinuses and frontal lobes of the brain
Inferior wall	Orbital plate of maxilla, orbital surface of the zygomatic, orbital process of palatine bone	Maxillary air sinus
Medial wall	Maxilla(frontal process), lacrimal bone, ethmoid (orbital plate) and sphenoid body	Sphenoid air sinuses
Lateral wall	Zygomatic and sphenoid greater wing	-

It runs forward and passes below the surface as the infraorbital canal to open below the orbital margin as the infraorbital foramen.

The lateral walls are composed of the zygomatic anteriorly and the greater wing of the sphenoid posteriorly. They are triangular in shape with base present anteriorly and lie at an approximate angle of 90° with each other.[10]

> **SPREAD OF INFECTION AND MALIGNANCY INTO THE ORBIT AND ORBITAL WALL FRACTURES**
>
> The medial wall may often be the route through which infections spread from the ethmoidal sinuses into the orbit since it is thin as paper, though it is the floor of the orbit that is most often involved in traumatic blow-out fractures. Maxillary sinus tumors may also spread into the orbit through the floor. The floor of the orbit is often involved in blowout fractures.

Apertures

The pyramidal structure of the orbit is incomplete due to the presence of a number of apertures (Fig. 1.8).[12] These limited spaces are crowed with a number of blood vessels and nerves passing through. Thus lesions often present as a syndrome called "orbital apex syndrome" (Tables 1.3 and 1.4). [10]

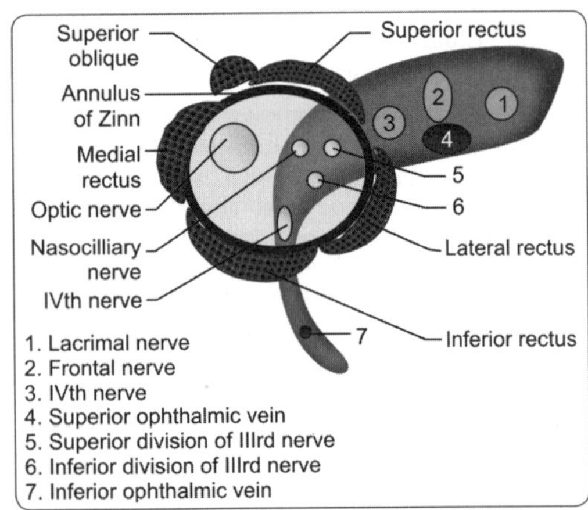

Figure 1.8 Apertures in the orbit

Table 1.3 Apertures in the bony orbit

Aperture	Location	Boundaries	Contents	Surgical Importance
Superior orbital fissure	Between the roof and lateral wall of the orbit	Greater and lesser wings of the sphenoid and closed off laterally by the frontal bone	Superior and inferior divisions of the IIIrd, IVth, VIth cranial nerve, the lacrimal, frontal and nasociliary branches of the Vth cranial nerve, superior and inferior branch of ophthalmic vein and sympathetic fibers of the cavernous plexus	Lesions that frequently present with multiple cranial nerve palsies along with loss of vision are called the **orbital apex syndrome** (OAS) The cavernous sinus syndrome may include features of OAS, and also Vth nerve involvement with also involvement of sympathetic fibers. They may occur in association with injuries to the facial bones, skull fractures, inflammatory conditions and orbital apical tumors The **Superior Oblique fissure or Rochon-Duvigneaud syndrome** involves lesions anterior to the apex, including the annulus of Zinn. However, the optic nerve and vision is left intact The optic nerve may also be damaged in its intra canalicular portion of the optic canal Ethmoid sinus surgery may cause optic nerve damage in cases where ethmoid air cells form the canal wall
Inferior orbital fissure	Lateral wall and the floor of the orbit and ending about 2 cm from the anterior margin of the orbit	Maxilla, the palatine bone and the greater wing of the sphenoid		
Optical canal	Apex of the pyramidal orbit structure, directed forwards, downwards and laterally	Roots of the lesser wings of the sphenoid and medially the body of the sphenoid. Posterior ethmoid air cells (Onodi cells) may form the medical wall in certain instances	The optic nerve along with its sheathings of dura, arachno and pia mater, the ophthalmic artery and a few fibers of sympathetic nerves that pass along with the artery	
Anterior Ethmoidal Canal	Between the roof and medial walls of the orbit	Frontoethmoidal suture between the medial and superior orbital walls	Anterior ethmoidal vessels and nerves	
Posterior Ethmoidal Canal	Between the roof and medial walls of the orbit	Frontoethmoidal suture between the medial and superior orbital walls	Posterior ethmoidal vessels and nerves	Vessels may bleed during extraperiosteal medial wall dissection and thus need to be clipped or cauterized

Table 1.4 Causes of orbital apex syndrome

Inflammatory	Infectious **	Neoplastic	Traumatic/ Iatrogenic	Vascular
1. Sarcoidosis 2. Systemic lupus erythematosus 3. Churg-Strauss syndrome 4. Wegener granulomatosis 5. Tolosa-Hunt syndrome (THS)* 6. Giant cell arteritis 7. Orbital inflammatory pseudotumor 8. Thyroid orbitopathy	**Fungi:** Aspergillosis, Mucormycosis **Bacteria:** *Streptococcus* species, *Staphylococcus* species, *Actinomyces* species, Gram-negative bacilli, anaerobes, *Mycobacterium tuberculosis* **Spirochetes:** *Treponema pallidum* **Viruses:** Herpes zoster	**Head and neck tumors:** Nasopharyngeal carcinoma, adenoid cystic carcinoma, squamous cell carcinoma **Neural tumors:** Neurofibroma, meningioma, ciliary neurinoma, schwannoma **Metastatic lesions:** 1. Lung, breast, renal cell, malignant melanoma 2. Hematologic: Burkitt lymphoma, non-Hodgkin lymphoma, leukemia 3. Perineural invasion of cutaneous malignancy	**Traumatic** 1. Penetrating injury 2. Nonpenetrating injury 3. Orbital apex fracture 4. Retained foreign body **Iatrogenic** 1. Sinonasal surgery 2. Orbital/facial surgery	1. Carotid cavernous aneurysm 2. Carotid cavernous fistula 3. Cavernous sinus thrombosis 4. Sickle cell anemia

*THS is a syndrome characterized by painful ophtalmoplegia due to granulomatous inflammation of unknown etiology affecting the cavernous sinus or orbital apex.

** Infections may spread from the paranasal sinuses, periorbital structures of the CNS. Cavernous sinus thrombosis may occur by spread of bacterial infections from the paranasal sinuses, while fungal infections should be suspected in patients with immunosuppression, diabetes mellitus, and hematologic malignancies.

Malignancies may spread from a primary ocular or orbital source or from adjacent paranasal sinuses. Metastasis especially in the cavernous sinus may also occur. Local spread from head and neck tumors may also occur.

Surgical intervention in sinonasal and periorbital procedures have also on occasion produced orbital apex syndrome (OAS).

CONTENTS OF THE BONY ORBIT

The Globe

The globe is located within the bony orbit. It is roughly spherical in shape, being composed of the transparent cornea anteriorly and the opaque sclera posteriorly. It is 2.5 cm in diameter and has a volume of approximately 25 mL. The cornea has a greater curvature as compared to the sclera, and has a radius of about 7.8 mm. The sclera is the larger of the two components and is part of a sphere of radius about 11.5 cm.

HYPERMETROPIA AND MYOPIA

Small globe size may result in hypermetropia, a refractive error caused when the image of objects viewed falls beyond the retina. Large globe size may result in myopia, where the image of objects viewed falls in front of the retina.

The globe is composed of an external layer made up of the sclera, a middle choroid layer and an inner retina. The sclera consists of dense collagenous tissue mixed with a few elastic fibers. At the limbus or corneoscleral junction, it continues anteriorly as the transparent cornea.

The choroid or "middle" layer of the globe lies in close approximation to the sclera. Anteriorly, behind the transparent cornea, it is present as the iris and ciliary body.

The retina is the light sensitive layer of the eye, containing light receptors and neural tissue.

The globe contains the crystalline lens, the anterior chamber between the cornea and the iris, the posterior chamber between the iris and the ciliary body and the vitreous chamber between the lens and the retina.

The Cornea

The cornea is an avascular 50–60 micron-thick structure composed of 5 layers—corneal epithelium, anterior limiting lamina, substantia propria, posterior limiting lamina and endothelium (Fig. 1.9). Since it is an avascular structure it obtains nutrition by diffusion from neighboring aqueous humor. It is transparent, strong and relatively resistant to abrasions. A tear film covers the surface of the cornea. Corneal epithelial layer is composed of a basal columnar germinal layer, intermediate wing cells and an outer layer of squamous, non-nucleated cells. These cells form a continuous layer over the cornea due to the zona occludens type of tight junctions that they form. Interstices present between these cells communicate directly with the aqueous humor. Adhesion of the basal layer to the anterior limiting membrane or Bowman's membrane is facilitated by network of anchoring fibrils and plaques. Cells from the basal layer are able to regenerate and replace other cells. The rate of corneal epithelial turnover is approximately 5–7 days.[11]

The main bulk of the substantia propria is composed of type 1 collagen fibers arranged in bundles that help maintain the structure of the cornea. They also form a strong junction with the sclera and thus maintain intraocular pressure and alignment of the visual apparatus including the lens. A network of fibroblast cells called keratocytes, is found in the stroma, connected to each other by gap junctions. These cells have well developed rough endoplasmic reticulum and Golgi apparatus. Their main function is the secretion and maintenance of the stroma. Hydrophilic molecules pass easily through the stroma, whereas the epithelial layers are more permeable to lipophilic molecules. Corneal endothelium lines the inner surface of the cornea. It is composed of a single layer of flattened polygonal cells whose main function is to allow passage of large amount of water, solute and molecules of size 1000000 Da and below. It is also capable of pinocytosis. A fluid pump responsible for the rapid rates of fluid transport is thought to be a HCO_3^- based transport linked to the Na^+ K^+ ATPase. It is thought to maintain the amount of fluid in the stroma and prevent stromal edema from

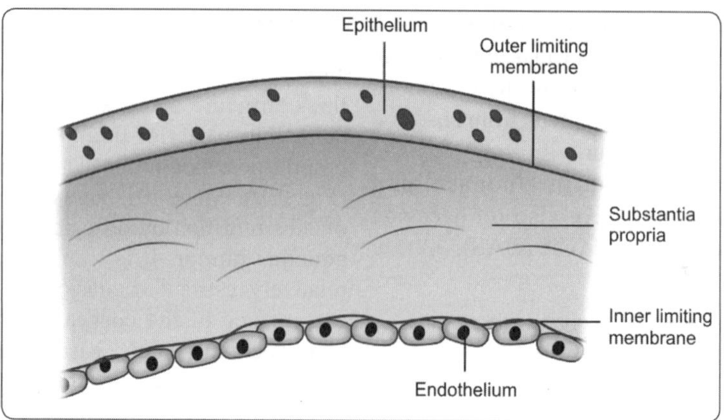

Figure 1.9 Cornea

occurring. Aquaporins (AQP1) have also been identified in the endothelium and thought to play a role in maintaining corneal thickness.

The absence of blood vessels and the particular arrangement of epithelial cells and the extracellular matrix are largely responsible for the smoothness and transparency of the cornea. Cornea also contributes most of the refractive power of the eye. Changes in its curvature may result in a refractive error called astigmatism.

Though it is avascular, the cornea is well supplied by sensory fibers from the trigeminal nerve. Fibers loose their sheaths near the limbus and run through the cornea radially. As they loose the sheaths there is no interference with the corneal transparency. Corneal epithelium has one of the densest nerve supplies of all epithelia. Loss of innervation of the cornea leads to neurotrophic keratitis and loss of corneal epithelium.

TRANSCORNEAL DRUG ABSORPTION

Transcorneal drug absorption is the main route of drug delivery to the intraocular tissue. It forms a lipid-water-lipid trilayer barrier to transcorneal drug absorption. The corneal epithelium provides easy entry to lipophilic drugs; stroma is more permeable to hydrophilic drugs while endothelium is more permeable to lipophilic drugs. Therefore, drugs must have both the lipophilic and hydrophilic properties to penetrate well through cornea.

Tenon's Capsule

A fascial membrane called Tenon's capsule surrounds the globe of the eye, separating it from the orbital fat (Fig. 1.10). It extends from the point where optic nerve exits the globe to the corneoscleral junction where it fuses with the conjunctiva. It is pierced by tendons of the extraocular muscles and it becomes continuous with their fascial coverings. It is divided into an anterior and posterior space by the tendons of the extraocular muscles and their fascia. A number of fascial septa arise from the eyeball and are fixed to the periosteum, separating the orbital fat into various compartments. They help in maintaining the position of the eye and the position of the orbital fat and hence assist in binocular vision.

SUB-TENON'S ROUTE OF DRUG ADMINISTRATION

A sub-Tenon's capsular approach may be used for delivery of anesthetic, steroid and antibiotic medications, by incising the conjunctiva and entering the episcleral space just inside the inferior border of the orbital margin. This route of administration carries a lower risk of penetration of the globe. The anesthetic agent acts directly on scleral nerves as well as spreads into the extraocular muscles and also through the thinner portions of the posterior capsule to block the extraocular muscles, the motor and sensory nerves.[12]

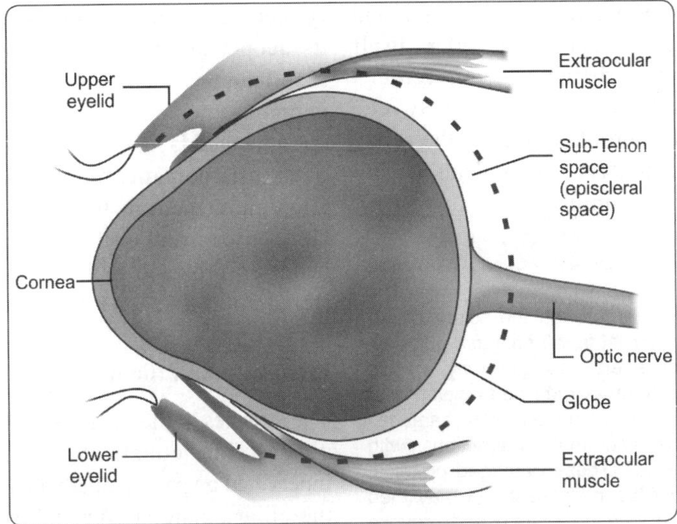

Figure 1.10 Tenon's capsule

The Sclera

The sclera is a tough, opaque fibrous structure, protecting the contents of the globe. It is continuous with the cornea at a junction known as the limbus. It permits a limited amount of drug absorption, due to its vascularity. It is covered by the conjuctival epithelium reflecting onto it from the inner surface of the eyelids. Posteriorly it is pierced by the optic nerve passing through a sieve like perforated plate. Anteriorly at the limbus, an endothelial canal called the canal of Schlemm is present. Externally, the sclera is covered by Tenon's capsule. Within this layer is present the episclera, followed by scleral stroma. The innermost layer is called lamina fusca, which is closely applied to the choroid. Sclera is composed of Type I and III collagen fibril with small amounts of type V and VI. These fibrils are surrounded by a matrix composed of decorin and biglycan. They are proteoglycans. Collagen fibers are interwoven and are also mixed with fibers from the insertions of the extraocular muscles. This particular arrangement of fibers gives the sclera its physical and mechanical properties. It is able to maintain shape while being subjected to the pull of extraocular muscles as well as accommodate minor changes in shape due to changing intraocular pressure. Interspersed between the collagen fibrils are scleral fibrocytes. They have long cytoplasmic processes that form gap junctions with other fibrocytes and are responsible for secretion and turn over of the extracellular matrix material. They are activated by injury.[13]

> **TRANSSCLERAL DRUG PERMEATION**
>
> The cellular structure of sclera provides an easier penetration to drugs as compared to cornea and conjunctiva. Therefore, subconjunctival and sub-Tenon's route of drug administration provide better intraocular bioavailability as compared to topical route of administration.

The scleral spur is formed by a ring of deep fibers of the sclera surrounding the limbus. It receives insertions of the trabecular tissue anteriorly, and posteriorly parts of the ciliary muscle are inserted into it. Thus, contraction of the ciliary muscle facilitates opening of the trabecular network. The optic nerve pierces the sclera posteriorly. Outer scleral fibers join the dural covering of the optic nerve. Lamina cribrosa is formed by the remaining fibers. They also form small canals through which fibers of the optic nerve exit the eye. A centrally located canal conveys the central retinal artery and vein.

Though the posterior ciliary blood vessels and nerve pass through the sclera, the sclera itself receives nutrition by diffusion from Tenon's capsule and episcleral blood vessel networks and also from the choroid. However, the sclera receives an abundant nerve supply. Thus, scleral inflammation is very painful.[13]

INFLAMMATION OF THE SCLERA

Inflammation of the sclera is known as scleritis. The slow rate of fluid fluxes through the sclera allows immune reaction to persist for a prolonged duration. Pathophysiology of scleral disease may involve antigen or immune complex mediated activation of scleral fibroblasts, which subsequently damages the collagen fibrils and their interactions with proteoglycan molecules. These damaged proteins, which have all along been sequestered may then be presented to the immune system and provoke localized or even systemic disease. They may also involve an element of vasculitis especially of the episcleral arterial anastomoses.[14]

Iris and its Muscles

The uveal tract is the pigmented middle layer of the eye. It is continuous with the pia-arachnoid coverings of the optic nerve. The iris and its muscles form the anterior part of the uveal tract. The iris acts as a diaphragm surrounding the pupil. It is composed of fibroblasts, melanocytes and loose collagenous material that contain its nerves and blood vessels. It lies between the cornea and lens, splitting the anterior segment of the eye into an anterior chamber between the cornea and iris and a posterior chamber between the iris and the lens. The main function of the iris is to control the aperture of the pupil. The larger the pupillary aperture is, the more the amount of light entering the eye and vice versa. The aperture is controlled by the sphincter pupillae and dilator pupillae. The sphincter pupillae is formed at the rim of the pupillary margin of the iris by a concentration of circularly arranged smooth muscle fibers. The pupillary aperture decreases upon contraction of these fibers. The dilator pupillae muscle fibers increase pupillary aperture when they contract as their fibers are arranged radially. The anterior surface of the iris has no epithelial covering. The epithelium of the posterior surface is bilayered, its deeper anterior layer being pigmented to absorb light. The more superficial posterior layer is non-pigmented and is in continuity with the unpigmented layer of the retina. The free surface of the iris contains numerous grooves, which allow movement of fluid from the posterior to the anterior chambers.[15] The iris is pigmented and hence absorbs and retains lipophilic drugs. The stored drugs are then released slowly.

Innervation of the iris

The muscles of the iris are supplied by autonomic nerves. The constrictor pupillae muscle is innervated by parasympathetic fibers arising from the ciliary ganglia. When stimulated the pupil constricts, reducing its diameter and causing a five-fold decrease in the amount of light entering the eye. The dilator pupillae muscle is supplied by sympathetic autonomic fibers that originate in the T1 segment of the spinal cord. Preganglionic fibers pass to the superior sympathetic cervical ganglion. Postganglionic fibers pass along with blood vessels and supply the muscle fibers. When stimulated, the radial fibers of the dilator pupillae constrict and the pupillary diameter increases.

Ciliary Body

The ciliary body is continuous with the choroid layer of the eye. Its main function is the suspension of the crystalline lens and the secretion of aqueous humor. It is attached to the scleral spur and passes around the eyeball in the iridiocorneal angle. Hence, anteriorly it is continuous with the tissues of the iris, while posteriorly it forms the ora serrata and continues as the choroid. It is brown in color due to the pigment contained in its epithelial layers. It has the following parts (Fig. 1.11)—pars plicata, present anteriorly, which is ruffled and pars plana present more posteriorly, which is smooth and continues with the ora serrata. Suspensory ligaments of the lens pass into the pars plana, anchoring the lens firmly. The ciliary body is covered by a bilayer of epithelial cells, a superficial unpigmented layer and an inner

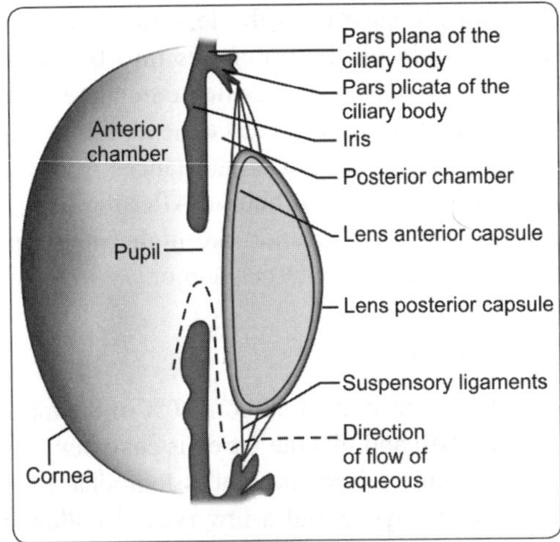

Figure 1.11 Lens and ciliary body

pigmented layer. Ciliary body stroma is composed of loose collagen bundles and the ciliary muscle. The ciliary muscle is a ring of muscle tissue. It contains circular, radial and meridional fibers. Nerve supply to the ciliary body and muscle is predominantly parasympathetic from the ciliary ganglion. Upon stimulation, it contracts towards the optical axis, relaxing the suspensory ligaments causing the lens to bulge and accommodate.[16]

PASSAGE OF DRUGS THROUGH IRIS AND CILIARY BODY

The iris and ciliary body have numerous capillaries that freely allow movement of particles through them. Drugs may enter systemic circulation following ocular administration and systemically administered drugs may enter into the aqueous through these sites. It also contains enzymes that are involved in the detoxifications of metabolites and drugs, which are rapidly removed by the high blood supply to the ciliary body.

Aqueous Humor

It is a fluid formed by the ciliary body and occupies the anterior and posterior chambers. It is secreted in the posterior chamber and flows through the pupil into the anterior chamber (Fig. 1.12). It drains through the canal of Schlemm into the episcleral veins. Some fluid may also leave the anterior segment through the surface of the iris. It provides nutrition to the avascular cornea, vitreous and lens. It also plays a major role in the regulation of intraocular pressure and the general shape of the eyeball. Any alteration to its drainage and/or secretion causes raised intraocular pressure.

Secretion of Aqueous Humor: It is secreted continuously by the epithelium of the ciliary processes of the pars plicata. They have a large surface area due to the presence of a number of folds, as well as an extensive capillary network. Fluid secretion is a result of active as well as passive processes. Fluid is essentially filtered out of the ciliary capillaries into the stroma and is then secreted by the pigmented and unpigmented epithelium of the ciliary processes into the posterior chamber of the eye. Here, the unpigmented epithelium actively secretes Na^+ ions into the lateral intracellular spaces. Cl^- and HCO_3^- ions follow the positively charged Na^+ ions. Water is drawn out due to the osmolar forces developed by these ions.

Fluid then flows into the posterior chamber and over the edge of the iris in the pupil to enter the anterior chamber. The rate of secretion of aqueous is influenced by intraocular pressure and blood pressure in the ciliary vessels.

Outflow of Aqueous Humor: Fluid exits the anterior chamber through outflow tracts in the iridiocorneal angle (Fig. 1.12). It passes through the trabecular meshwork and then enters the canal of Schlemm. From here, it drains into the extraocular veins. Though it is not a primary

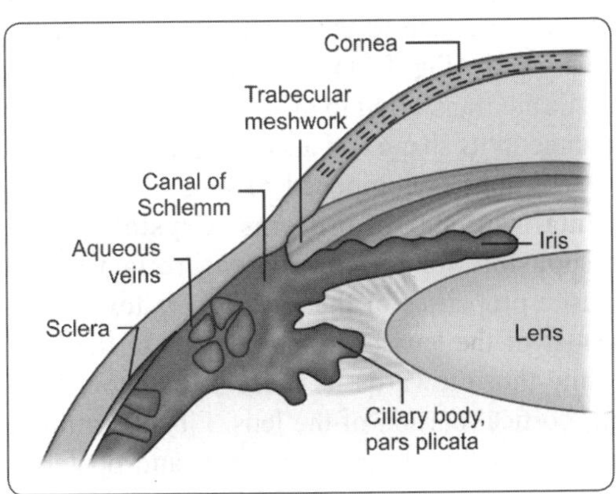

Figure 1.12 Outflow of aqueous

route, aqeuous also drains through uveoscleral outflow, which involves aqueous reabsorption by the ciliary body and iris and ultimately drains into the veins of the ciliary body, choroid and sclera.

Trabecular meshwork: It is the main site of resistance to the flow of aqueous and has a unique system to maintain its patency and prevent occlusion by debris. A population of phagocytic cells is found on the trabecular meshwork and also within the canal of Schlemm that removes debris and other molecules and keeps the drainage pathway clear.

GLAUCOMA

An imbalance in the rates of formation and outflow of aqueous humor leads to an increase in the intraocular pressure, a known risk factor for glaucoma. In a small subset of patients' intraocular pressure may remain normal. One of the common causes of increased intraocular pressure is an increased resistance to the outflow of aqueous humor through the canal of schlemm or open angle glaucoma. It may also occur if the iris obscures the outflow tract; in which case, it is called the angle closure glaucoma.

Crystalline Lens

The lens is a transparent biconvex structure, with a slightly flattened anterior surface and a more curved posterior surface that is in contact with the vitreous. It is devoid of any blood vessels or nerve fibers that may impede its transparency. Its refractive or diopteric power is less than that of the cornea and tears film. The importance of the lens is its ability to alter its shape and hence diopteric power. The lens is encircled by zonular fibers that attach to the ciliary processes of the ciliary body (Fig. 1.11). Changes in tension in this tissue are transferred to the lens, and result in the change in its shape and accommodative power.

The lens is composed of lens fibers which contain crystallin proteins. Crystallins are responsible for the transparent, refractile and elastic properties of the lens. Fibers toward the center of the lens form the nucleus of the lens, while those towards its margin (equator) form the cortical portion of the lens. Fibers terminate in sutures found on the anterior and posterior surfaces of the lens.

A capsule surrounds the lens that prevents entry of hydrophilic molecules into the lens, however, lipophilic molecules enter and pass through the lens slowly. Hence the lens acts as a barrier to the movement of substances from the aqueous to the vitreous humor. After the lens is removed, rates of transport are higher between the aqueous and the vitreous humor.[17]

Vitreous Humor

The vitreous accounts for about 80% of the mass of the eyeball and fills the vitreous chamber. It is composed of hyaluronan; that is long chains of glucosaminoglycan and a few type II collagen fibers. The fibers are anchored to the basal lamina of the ciliary body. It forms the suspensory ligaments of the lens. At the periphery, it is in a gel like state and towards the center it is in a more fluid state. Hyalocytes are found within the vitreous and they produce substance of the vitreous. The hyaloid canal occupies a central position in the vitreous and is the remnant of the hyaloids artery. It runs from the posterior surface of the lens to the optic disc. Rupture of the hyaloids artery may sometimes form structures called "floaters" that may interfere with vision.

INTRAVITREAL DRUG ADMINISTRATION

Due to poor bioavailability of drugs in the posterior segment of eye following systemic or other routes of ocular administration, drugs are often administered directly into the vitreous chamber to target posterior segment diseases. The vitreous may serve as a deposit for drugs injected or implanted intravitreally or administered by iontophoresis.

Retina and Optic Nerve

The retina is the sensory layer of the eyeball. It lies between the choroid and the vitreous. It is continuous with the optic nerve at the optic disc and continues anteriorly to cover the iris and ciliary body. It is composed of the pigment layer in opposition to the choroid, followed by the rods and cones, external limiting membrane, outer nuclear layer, outer plexiform layer, inner nuclear layer, inner plexiform layer, ganglion cell layer, nerve fiber layer and an inner limiting membrane, in contact with the vitreous.

The blood retinal barrier: Cells of the pigment layer form zona occludens type tight junction with each other and prevent movement of a number of particles between the vitreous and the choroid. This function is somewhat in continuation of the function of the blood–brain barrier as the retina may be considered to be part of the brain. The blood retinal barrier properties are also determined by the endothelial cells of its capillaries. They are of the continuous type and provide a barrier to the transport of metabolites and toxins in the blood. It is a barrier to hydrophilic drugs but lipophilic drugs cross easily. Therefore, orally administered drugs and other systemic agents may be present in the eye and sometimes cause retinal toxicity, e.g. digitalis, phenothiazines, methyl alcohol, quinoline derivaties, sildenafil.

Extraocular Muscles

There are 7 extraocular muscles in total (Fig. 1.13). There are 4 rectii (superior, inferior, medial and lateral), and 2 obliques (superior and inferior) that attach to the globe and allow its movements, while the seventh is the levator palpebrae superioris that attaches to the upper eyelid. Individual muscles and their actions are described below.

The Rectii

They arise from a common tendinous ring around the margins of the optic canal called the annulus of Zinn. Each muscle passes anteriorly in positions corresponding to their names and attach onto the sclera behind the corneoscleral junction. They receive their blood supply from the ophthalmic artery and its branches. The lateral rectus is supplied by the abducent nerve, while the oculomotor nerve supplies the others.

The Superior Oblique

Its origin is superomedial to the optic canal on the body of the sphenoid. It passes forward through the trochlea on the superior orbital margin. It passes posterior and laterally and inserts into the sclera between the insertions of the superior and lateral rectii. It is supplied by the trochlear nerve and ophthalmic artery and the maxillary artery.

The Inferior Oblique

It arises from the orbital surface of the maxilla, lateral to the nasolacrimal groove. It passes

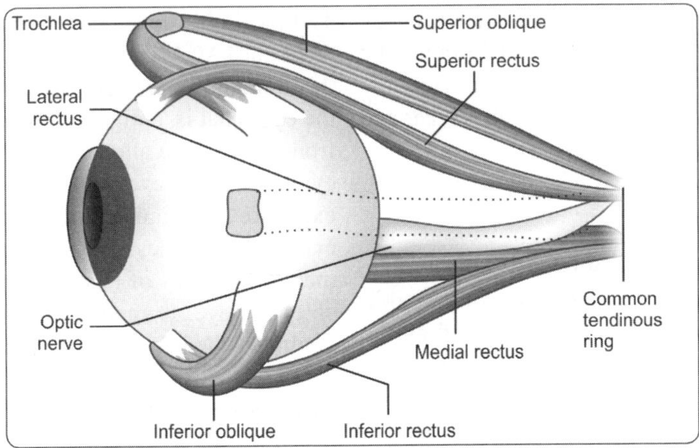

Figure 1.13 Extraocular muscles

posteriorly, laterally and upwards to insert between insertions of the inferior and lateral rectii.

The Levator Palpebrae Superioris

It arises above the optic canal, passes anteriorly and inserts into the skin and the tarsal plate of the upper eyelid. It has a component of smooth muscles, which receive sympathetic innervation (Muller's muscle). Its other fibers are supplied by the oculomotor nerve. It receives its blood supply from the ophthalmic artery.

Movements of the Globe

Together, the rectii and obliques are responsible for elevation, depression, adduction and abduction of the eyeball. Individual muscles may require to be tested to ensure that a particular nerve has been blocked by application of an anesthetic agent.

Blood Supply and Lymphatic Drainage

Arterial Supply

The ophthalmic artery, a branch of the internal carotid artery, and its branches supply blood to the orbit and its structures, along with branches of the maxillary artery. The important branches of the ophthalmic artery include the central retinal artery, branches to the muscles, the ciliary arteries (anterior and long and short posterior branches), the lacrimal artery, supraorbital branch, the anterior and posterior ethmoidal arteries, the meningeal, medial palpebral, supratrochlear and dorsal nasal artery.

Venous Drainage

Superior and inferior ophthalmic veins and the infraorbital vein are the main veins of the orbit. The superior ophthalmic vein is formed by the facial and the supraorbital vein. It also receives the central retinal vein and drains into the cavernous sinus. The inferior ophthalmic vein is formed on the floor of the orbit, anteriorly and receives tributaries from the inferior rectus and oblique, the nasolacrimal sac and eyelids, and also from the eyeball. It drains into the cavernous sinus, sometimes joining the superior ophthalmic vein. It also communicates with the pterygoid plexus and the facial vein.

Lymphatic Drainage and Immune Privilege of the Eye

Lymphatics draining the conjunctive only have been identified. Furthermore, the eye is a site of immune privilege. That is, potentially immunogenic tissues in the eye survive over prolonged intervals of time without provoking an immune reaction. It is believed that such a phenomenon occurs in order to protect an organ or tissue essential for the survival of the host, since loss of sight may have life-threatening consequences.

Factors that may explain this privilege is the presence of a relatively robust blood-ocular barrier that prevents mechanically entry of antigens and proteins from the blood stream. There is also a lack of lymphatic vessels within the eye, and aqueous humor drains directly into venous blood and not to regional lymph nodes. However, even though there is an absence of any defined anatomic lymphatic drainage pathway in the eye; there appears to be a functional pathway as has been recently shown. Aqueous humor is itself rich in inflammatory molecules such as TGF-β_2. Anterior chamber-associated immune deviation (ACAID) is also quoted to demonstrate that immunosuppressive environments operate in the eye. That is, antigen-presenting cells derived from the eye are altered by exposure to various cytokines in the eye and that suppress any future exposure to a similar antigen derived from the eye. Ocular tissues also express Fas ligands that induce apoptosis of Fas$^+$ immune cells that may enter the eye. It appears that neural input also facilitates the immune privilege of the eye.[14]

Innervation

The structures of the orbit receive motor inner vation from fibers that are somatic as well as autonomic. The optic nerves carry the sense of sight while other structures in the orbit are receiving somatic sensory innervation by the ophthalmic division of the trigeminal nerve. The ophthalmic nerve has three main branches; the lacrimal nerve, the frontal nerve and the nasociliary nerve. The conjunctiva and the skin covering the lateral part of the upper eyelid are supplied by the lacrimal nerve. The frontal nerve supplies the skin of the upper eyelid and conjunctiva. The skin of the lower eyelid is supplied by the infraorbital branch of the zygomatic nerve, which is a branch of the maxillary nerve. The cornea, sclera, iris and ciliary body are supplied by the nasociliary nerve.

Somatic motor innervation is provided by the oculomotor, abducent and trochlear nerves to the extraocular muscles. The lateral rectus muscle is supplied by the abducent nerve, the superior oblique by the trochlear nerve while all others are supplied by the oculomotor nerve.

The ciliary ganglion: The ciliary ganglion is located in the orbital fat near the apex. It has three main roots; they are the sensory, sympathetic and motor or parasympathetic. The sensory root arises as branches from the nasociliary nerve and passes through the ganglion to supply the sclera, cornea, iris and ciliary body. The sympathetic root arises from postganglionic neurons around the sympathetic plexus of the internal carotid arteries, and passes through the ganglion emerging as short ciliary nerves to supply the blood vessels of the eyeball and the dilator pupillae muscles of the iris. The parasympathetic root is derived from preganglionic fibers of the Edinger-Westphal nucleus and travels with the oculomotor nerve to the orbit. Here a branch separates and joins the ciliary ganglion. Postganglionic parasympathetic fibers arise from the ganglion and pass with the short ciliary nerves and supply the sphincter pupillae and the ciliary body.

Sympathetic stimulation causes pupillary dilation via α_1 adrenergic receptors in the dilator pupillae fibers of the iris. The pupillary aperture increases as also the amount of light entering the eye.

On the other hand, stimulation of the parasympathetics causes pupillary constriction via the action of the constrictor pupillae. This action is mediated via the muscarinic receptors. Parasympathetic stimulation also leads to accommodative changes in the lens. Stimulation of the parasympathetics to the eye causes contraction of the ciliary muscle. Contraction of the ciliary muscles provides a sphincter-like action, reducing its diameter around the suspensory ligaments of the lens. The ciliary ligaments then relax and the lens assumes a more spherical shape with a higher refractive power. The eye is thus able to adjust focal length and view near objects clearly. Since the ciliary body receives predominantly parasympathetic nerve supply, accommodation is controlled by parasympathetic autonomic nerves. A concomitant reduction in the pupillary size accompanies accommodative changes in the ciliary body and lens, due to stimulation of the constrictor pupillae.

> **EFFECT OF DRUGS ON PUPIL SIZE AND ACCOMMODATION**
>
> Cholinomimetic drugs cause miosis due to contraction of circular muscles of iris and spasm of accommodation due to ciliary muscle contraction. Cholinergic blockers have opposite effects, i.e. mydriasis and paralysis of accommodation. Sympathomimetics cause mydriasis due to radial muscle contraction but accommodation remains unaffected.

THE VISUAL PATHWAY

Impulses generated by the rods and cones of the retina leave each eye via the optic nerve. Fibers carrying impulses from the nasal halves of each retina cross over to the opposite sides at the optic chiasma, while fibers from the temporal halves of each retina pass on uncrossed. Thus fibers from the right halves of both the retinae pass in the right optic tract, while the fibers of the left halves both the retinae are carried in the left optic tract (Fig. 1.14). Fibers continue on in the optic tract, and relay at the lateral geniculate body of the thalamus. Fibers from this nucleus pass on to the occipital

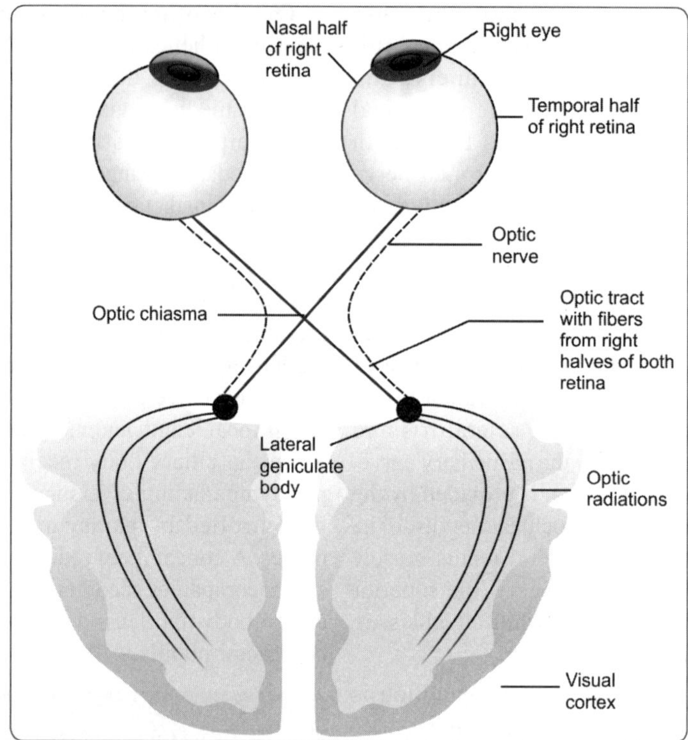

Figure 1.14 Visual pathway

cortex via the optic radiations (geniculocalcarine fibers) to the primary visual cortex. Impulses also enter various other pathways: fibers from the optic chiasma; pass on to the suprachiasmatic nucleus; the pretectal nucleus to coordinate the pupillary reflexes, superior colliculus for eye movements and also to the ventral lateral geniculate body.[18]

PUPILLARY LIGHT REFLEX

Direct reflex: When light is shone in one eye, the pupil constricts. The diagram representing the pupillary light reflex pathways is shown in Figure 1.15. Impulses travel to the pretectal nucleus, and from here to the Edinger-Westphal nucleus, parasympathetic fibers arise here and pass back to the constrictor pupillae muscle with the oculomotor nerve, and through the ciliary ganglion. Alteration of the pupillary diameter grossly affects the amount of light that enters the eye by a factor of about 1 to 30 and hence aids in dark adaptation. Dilator pupillae muscle fibers are supplied by sympathetic fibers originating from the intermediolateral gray horn of T1 thoracic segment, through the superior cervical ganglion. Postganglionic fibers pass along with blood vessels and supply the muscle (Fig. 1.15).

Indirect reflex: When light is shone in one eye, a pupillary reflex is observed in the unilluminated eye as well. It is called the consensual or indirect pupillary reflex. Fibers from the pretectal nucleus supply the Edinger-Westphal nucleus of both sides, hence leading to the consensual or indirect pupillary reflex.[19]

Accommodation and Pupillary Aperture

A high degree of visual acuity is permitted by the accommodation mechanism. This mechanism

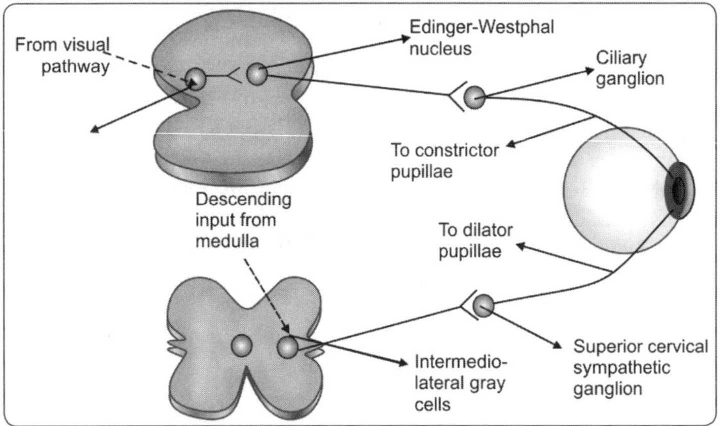

Figure 1.15 Pupillary and accommodation reflex pathways

involves the contraction or relaxation of the ciliary muscle, and adjustments in the focal length of the lens allowing the eye to maintain acuity of vision at all times. There appears to be a feedback mechanism related to chromatic aberration, where a difference in the ability of the lens to focus red and blue light acts as a signal to correctly adjust the focal power of the lens. Also, convergence of both eyes occurs at the same time. Pupillary diameter also adjusts along with the accommodation process.

REFERENCES

1. Helmchen C, Rambold H. The eyelid and its contribution to eye movements. Dev Ophthalmol. 2007;40:110–31.
2. Fenga C, Aragona P, Cacciola A, Spinella R, Nola CD, et al. Meibomian gland dysfunction and ocular discomfort in video display terminal workers. Eye. 2008;22(1):91–5
3. Kakizaki H, Malhotra R, Selva D. Upper eyelid anatomy: an update. Ann Plast Surg. 2009;63(3):336–43.
4. Kakizaki H, Malhotra R, Madge SN, Selva D. Lower eyelid anatomy: an update. Ann Plast Surg. 2009;63(3):344–51.
5. Burkat CN, Lucarelli MJ. Chapter 1, Anatomy of the lacrimal system. In: Cohen AJ, Mercandetti M, Brazzo BG (Eds). The Lacrimal System: Management, Diagnosis and Surgery. New York: Springer Science and Business Media, Inc. 2006; pp.11–6.
6. Lemp MA. Chapter 6, The tear- deficient patient. In: Cohen AJ, Mercandetti M, Brazzo BG (Eds). The Lacrimal System: Management, Diagnosis and Surgery. New York: Springer Science and Business Media, Inc. 2006. pp. 99–109.
7. Forrester JV, Dick AD, MacMenamim PG, Lee WR. Chapter 1, Anatomy of the eye and orbit. In: The Eye: Basic Science in Practice, 2nd (edn). Saunders; 2002. pp. 2–9.
8. Hamilton RC. Chapter 6, Complications of ophthalmic regional anaesthesia. In: Finucane BT (Ed). Complications of Regional Anaesthesia. Springer; 2007. pp. 87–101.
9. René C. Update on orbital anatomy. Eye. 2006; 20:1119–29.
10. Yeh S, Forzoozan R. Orbital apex syndrome. Curr Opin Ophthalmol. 2004;15(6):490–8.
11. Gipson IK, Joyce NC, Zieske JC. Chapter, 1, The anatomy and cell biology of the human cornea, limbus, conjunctiva and adnexa. In: Foster CS, Azar DT, Dohlman CH (Eds). Smolin and Thoft's The cornea: Scientific foundation and clinical practice, 4th edn. Philadelphia: Lippincott Williams & Wilkins. 2004. pp. 1-11.
12. Kavanan KS, Dark A, Garrioch MA. Sub-tenons administration of local anesthetic: a review of the technique. Br J Anaesth. 2003;90(6):787–93.

13. Watson PG, Young RD. Scleral structure, organisation and disease: A review. Exp Eye Res. 2004;78(3):609–23.

14. Masli S, Vega JL. Ocular immune privilege sites. Methods Mol Biol. 011;677:449–58.

15. Ruskell G. Chapter 42, The eye. In: Gray H, Standring H, Ellis H, Berkovitz BKB (Eds). Gray's Anatomy: The Anatomical Basis of Clinical Practice, 39th edn. Elsevier Churchill Livingston. 2005; pp. 708–10.

16. Ruskell GL. The eye. Standring S (Ed). Gray's Anatomy: The Anatomical Basis of Clinical Practice, 39th edn. Elsevier Churchill Livingston. 2005. Chapter 42, pp. 706–8.

17. Ruskell GL. The eye. Standring S (Ed). Gray's Anatomy: The orbit and its contents, 39th edn; Elsevier Churchill Livingston. 2005; pp. 691–6.

18. Barrett KE, Barman SM, Boitano S, Brooks HL. Ganong's Review of Medical Physiology, 23rd edn. McGraw-Hill. 2010, Chapter 12, Vision; pp. 184–5.

19. Barrett KE, Barman SM, Boitano S, Brooks HL. Ganong's Review of Medical Physiology, 23rd edn. McGraw-Hill; 2010. Chapter 12, pp. 189–95.

CHAPTER 2

Routes of Ocular Drug Administration

OVERVIEW

Routes of drug administration for the treatment of ophthalmic conditions are chosen with an objective of maximizing the amount of drug reaching its site of action in sufficient concentration. Drugs can be administered to ocular tissue by various routes, which include:

1. Topical
2. Periocular: Subconjunctival, Sub-Tenon's, Peribulbar, Retrobulbar
3. Intraocular: Intracameral, Intravitreal
4. Systemic

Topical

Topical application is the most favored route of ocular drug administration especially when targeting the ocular surface and anterior segment diseases. Drug solutions and suspensions are applied topically by instillation on the ocular surface. Gels and ointments are also popular dosage forms for topical drug administration. Inserts placed in the fornices and other drug impregnated devices such as contact lenses applied to ocular surface are also the means of topical drug delivery.

In order to maximize therapeutic benefit of topically applied drugs, it is important to practice an optimum method of drug instillation. Based on the tear flow patterns, Fraunfelder (1976) described the method for topical drug administration, which can maximize the duration of drug retention in the cul-de-sac.[1] Accordingly, with the patient's head tilted backwards, the lower eyelid is gently pulled away from the globe and a drop of medication is instilled in the cul-de-sac. Patient is asked to look down and gently close the eyes. Keeping the eyes closed for 1 minute after instillation prevents drainage into the nasolacrimal system. Additionally, pressure applied on the medial canthus with closed eyes, prevents quick outflow of drug into the lacrimal system. Care should be taken to avoid contamination during drug instillation.

Instillation of eye drops is the most convenient, least invasive and least expensive method of drug administration to the eye. Topical application also provides higher ocular drug concentration in the anterior segment as compared to that achieved after systemic administration. The topical application of 0.3% isotonic tacrolimus eye drops in rats was shown to provide significantly higher aqueous levels of the drug as compared to that achieved after its systemic administration at a dose of 0.1 mg/kg/day for 3 days. At the same time the serum levels were significantly high in orally treated animals compared to those treated topically.[2] Similarly, in human, topically applied gentamicin was shown to provide significantly higher drug concentration in cornea compared to that after systemic administration.[3] However, some drugs like ciprofloxacin have been shown to achieve comparable aqueous levels after oral and topical administration.[4]

Topical administration often provides inadequate drug concentration in the treatment of posterior segment diseases especially so in uninflamed eye. Vitreous concentration of gatifloxacin 0.5% and moxifloxacin 0.3%, after topical instillation in uninflamed human eye, was found to be lower than 90% minimum inhibitory concentration of most common bacterial pathogens causing acute postoperative endophthalmitis.[5] Although, dexamethasone-cyclodextrin eye drops were found to deliver significant amounts of dexamethasone to the retina in rabbit eye[6], repeated instillation of dexamethasone sodium phosphate failed to provide significant vitreous concentration in human.[7]

Topical administration carries the advantage of avoiding systemic exposure to high serum levels of drug and hence systemic adverse effects are minimized. For example, systemic use of genciclovir is associated with hematologic toxicity and, therefore, has limited use in the treatment of herpetic keratitis. However, topically applied gel provides high ocular tissue concentration and is highly effective against herpetic keratitis without significant risk of hematologic toxicity.[8] For some drugs like dexamethasone, systemic absorption after topical administration in rabbits has been shown to be comparable to that after systemic administration.[6] However, similar results were not observed after topical application in human eye.[7]

The drug penetration into the ocular tissue after topical application is affected by several factors, which are discussed in chapter 3.

Periocular

Periocular route of administration is used to inject drugs in the vicinity of globe without penetrating it. Periocluar routes of administration include subconjunctival, sub-Tenon's, peribulbar and retrobulbar. The anatomical details of the orbit and globe are important while injecting drugs in the periocular region. Relevant anatomical details are discussed in chapter 1.

Subconjunctival

Subconjunctival injections are used for ocular delivery of drugs that penetrate cornea poorly or are slowly absorbed. Under topical anesthesia, the drug solution is injected under the bulbar conjunctiva, adjacent to sclera. By injecting the drug subconjunctivally, conjunctival and corneal permeability barriers are bypassed. The sclera is highly permeable particularly for hydrophilic molecules and, therefore, required ocular tissue concentration of drug is quickly achieved with subconjunctival route. Moreover, high corneal drug concentration is also achieved by diffusion and leakage through the injection site.

Subconjunctival injections have been shown to produce high, transient and short lasting peak concentration as compared to topical administration, which produces moderate but sustained drug concentration over the period of treatment.[9] Clinical efficacy of antibiotics in the treatment of bacterial corneal ulcer has been shown to be comparable after subconjunctival and topical administration.[9,10] However, subconjunctival route of administration is indicated in patients with severe infection or impending corneal perforation to ensure drug delivery especially in non-compliant patients. Similar observations have also been made for other drugs like lidocaine. Subconjunctival as well as topical administration of lidocaine 2% provided equivalent pain relief in patients receiving intravitreal injection of triamcinolone.[11] In some cases, however, subconjunctival administration has been shown to provide better efficacy compared to topical administration. For example, anti-VEGF antibodies showed significantly higher efficacy in reducing neovascularization and corneal graft rejection in rats after subconjunctival injection compared to topical administration.[12] In other cases, combination therapy using subconjunctival along with topical administration has been shown to have higher efficacy as compared to topical alone. In patients with fungal keratitis, topical amphotericin with subconjunctival fluconazole provided better efficacy as compared to topical amphotericin alone.[13]

Subconjunctival injections provide significantly higher ocular tissue concentration as compared to systemic route of administration.

In one of the studies, 53 patients received 20 mg of vancomycin subconjunctivally and 47 received two doses of vancomycin intravenously (1 g twice a day). The peak aqueous humor levels of vancomycin were significantly higher and were achieved earlier after subconjunctival administration compared to intravenous.[14] Retinal delivery of drugs is also higher after subconjunctival injection as compared to systemic administration. For example, retinal concentration of celecoxib was significantly higher after subconjunctival injection compared to that achieved after intraperitoneal administration in rats.[15]

Although, subconjunctival administration of drugs is less invasive than intraocular drug administration, it is associated with several complications. Subconjunctival Injections cause irritation and pain at the site of injection. Subconjunctival injection can also cause subconjunctival hemorrhage, granuloma, necrosis and conjunctival scarring. Severity of conjunctival toxicity is also determined by the pH and osmolarity of the injected solution. Inadvertent globe penetration and intraocular administration is also a concern.

Sub-Tenon's

Sub-Tenon's route of administration is used to inject drugs under Tenon's capsule. Tenon's capsule is a thin membrane like fascia that surrounds the globe and separates it from the orbital fat. Between the inner surface of Tenon's capsule and outer surface of sclera lies a potentials space known as sub-Tenon's or episcleral space. Numerous delicate bands of connective tissue cross this space and attach the Tenon's capsule to sclera. Anteriorly, the fascia fuses with the sclera about 1.5 cm posterior to corneoscleral junction. Posteriorly, it fuses with the meningeal covering of the optic nerve. The posterior part of Tenon's capsule is thinner than the anterior part and may become fenestrated with advancing age.

Sub-Tenon's drug administration provides high intraocular drug levels by exploiting the permeability of sclera. The injection can be made in sub-Tenon's space in anterior, mid and posterior positions using cannulae with increasing length. Anterior sub-Tenon's injections do not offer much advantage over subconjunctival injections.

Sub-Tenon's is a commonly used route of administration of local anesthetics for ophthalmic surgery. For the administration of regional anesthesia for surgical procedures all three approaches, i.e. anterior, mid and posterior, have been described. Anterior, mid as well as posterior injections provide equivalent akinesia and intraoperative pain relief, however, the retention of lid closure is significantly higher with anterior and mid injection as compared to posterior. Posterior injection is more painful than anterior but the risk of chemosis and conjunctival hemorrhage is significantly higher with anterior than mid and posterior injections.[16] Sub-Tenon's block has shown higher efficacy as compared to topical anesthesia. In a double-blind randomized clinical trial involving 210 patients, the extent of patient discomfort and intraoperative complications after routine cataract surgery under sub-Tenon's or topical anesthesia were compared. All patients underwent phacoemulsification and intraocular lens implantation. Postoperative pain assessment immediately after surgery and 30 minutes later showed that sub-Tenon's block provided significantly greater pain relief at both time points. Intraopertaive complications, however, were the same in both groups.[17] In another randomized clinical trial involving 59 patients undergoing trabeculectomy, topically applied 2% lignocaine jelly was as effective in pain relief as lignocaine 2% administered by sub-Tenon's route.[18]

Sub-Tenon's block has also been found useful for vitreoretinal surgical procedures.[19] Sub-Tenon's route of administration is also widely used to administer drugs like triamcinolone acetonide when targeting posterior segment. Single sub-Tenon's injection of triamcinolone acetonide provides therapeutic concentrations in the posterior segment especially the retina and choroid for 30 days.[20] However, the drug concentration achieved in the retina is lower as compared to intravitreal administration and in patients with bilateral diffuse diabetic macular edema, intravitreal administration of triamcinolone acetonide provided better visual outcome as compared to sub-Tenon's injection.[21] Similarly, intravitreal triamcinolone acetonide was also found to be more effective than posterior sub-Tenon's injection in the treatment of branch retinal vein occlusion.[22]

The complications associated with sub-Tenon's injection include pain on injection, swelling, pseudoptosis and subconjunctival hemorrhage. Backflow of the injected drug through the incision has also been reported and this could lead to reduced efficacy and adverse effects.[23] The technique of administering sub-Tenon's injection is more difficult than other periocular injections as it requires accurate placement of the cannula in the potential sub-Tenon's space close to sclera. This increases the incidence of ocular penetration. Ocular penetration and inadvertent intraarterial injections can result in severe complications such as central retinal arterial occlusion and retinal and choroidal vascular occlusion.[24,25]

Peribulbar

Peribulbar route of administration is mainly used for injecting local anesthetic agents for surgical procedures. The 6 extraocular muscles form a muscle cone behind the globe and the injection is made behind the globe outside the muscle cone. The contents of the muscle cone include optic nerve, oculomotor nerves containing both superior and inferior branches, abducent nerve, nasociliary nerve, ciliary ganglion and vessels. The needle is inserted through the conjunctiva in the inferotemporal quadrant keeping it as far laterally as possible along the orbital floor. Often an additional medial injection is needed to achieve complete akinesia. The onset of action after peribulbar block is slower than retrobulbar block but the risk of damaging the structures inside the muscle cone is low. The risk of globe penetration is also low. As compared to sub-

Tenon's block, peribulbar block is more efficacious but is associated with more technique related complications because the sun-Tenon's route uses a blunt cannula and infiltration is superficial.[26,27]

Peribulbar route is also used for injecting drugs like triamcinolone acetonide in conditions such as diabetic macular edema and Graves ophthalmopathy.[28,29] Peribulbar injections can cause periorbital ecchymosis and conjunctival chemosis. The incidence of retrobulbar hemorrhage, optic nerve injury, and inadvertent intraocular or subdural injection is less as compared to retrobulbar injection.

Superficial peribulbar injection is a modified technique whereby the injection is made using a half-inch 25-gauge needle under the conjunctiva about 5 mm from the limbus inferiorly with needle directed towards the inferior wall of the orbit. The technique provides a quicker onset of action and higher efficacy as compared to conventional peribulbar block possibly due to spread of drug solution into the sub-Tenon's space. Subconjunctival hemorrhage is the main side-effect of this route of administration.[30]

Retrobulbar

Retrobulbar route of administration delivers drugs behind the globe inside the muscle cone. For retrobulbar injection, needle is inserted midway between the lateral canthus and lateral limbus through the inferior conjunctiva. The needle is at first directed backwards under the globe. After it passes the equator, it is directed upwards and medially so as to enter the muscle cone. Retrobulbar injections are painful and patients are often given sedation to prevent pain, anxiety and associated complications. The most common and serious complication of retrobulbar injection is retrobulbar hemorrhage. Optic atrophy can occur due to direct damage to optic nerve or nerve compression due to injection of drug solution inside the meningeal covering of the nerve. Other complications include stimulation of oculocardiac reflex, puncture of globe, inadvertent intravascular and subdural injection and brain stem anesthesia.

In a series of 6000 retrobulbar blocks, 16 cases of apparent central spread of local anesthesia were reported of which 8 developed respiratory arrest.[31] Retrobulbar block has also been shown to reduce blood flow in retrobulbar vessels and, therefore, is avoided in patients with poor ocular perfusion and glaucoma.[32] Other routes of administration such as peribulbar, sub-Tenon's and topical have now largely replaced retrobulbar route because of its potentially serious adverse effects.

Intraocular

Intraocular routes of drug administration, require drug administration inside the globe. The drugs can be injected in the anterior chamber, i.e. the intracameral route or into the vitreous chamber, i.e. the intravitreal route.

Intracameral

Several medications are administered by intracameral route such as for pupillary dilatation and anesthesia for surgical procedures, prevention of intraocular infection and inflammation. The method provides immediate and easy delivery of required concentration of drug into the aqueous humor and, therefore, provides high efficacy. Moreover, the need for repeated administration, as is necessary if using topical route, is avoided, which is especially a concern in non-compliant patients. The corneal surface toxicity associated with topical application is also avoided. Intracameral administration of medications, however, predisposes to toxic anterior segment syndrome (TASS). TASS is a general term that describes the sterile postoperative inflammation due to non-infectious causes such as intracameral medications. Presence of free radicals in the intracameral solutions seems to contribute to endothelial toxicity leading to corneal edema. In one of the studies, the free radical concentration equal to or higher than 0.5% hydrogen peroxide was detected in cefuroxime (0.61 mmol/L), 2% undiluted lidocaine (0.34 mmol/L) and bevacizumab (0.59 mmol/L).[33] The drug concentration, pH and osmolarity of the drug solution affect the possibility of endothelial cell toxicity. Solutions for intraocular injections are preservative free and, therefore, preservative-induced toxicity is not a concern.

Intravitreal

For intravitreal administration, drug solutions are injected directly into the vitreous humor. This route of drug administration provides high drug concentration in the posterior segment of eye and is used in the treatment of conditions like endophthalmitis, age-related macular edema and diabetic retinopathy. The medications can also be delivered intravitreally in the form of implants that provide sustained drug delivery over a prolonged period. This route of administration is especially useful for posterior segment drug delivery as other routes of administration provide insufficient drug concentration in posterior segment. Evaluation of an intravitreal fluocinolone acetonide implant versus standard systemic therapy in noninfectious posterior uveitis involving 140 patients showed that intravitreal implant provided better control of inflammation as compared to systemic therapy.[34] Similarly for the treatment of endophthalmitis, intravitreal administration of antibiotics is commonly practiced.

Systemic

Systemic routes of drug administration for intraocular drug delivery include oral and parenteral routes. Orally administered drugs require absorption from the gastrointestinal tract into general circulation before the drug is delivered to the ocular tissue. Although a convenient method for drug administration, this route suffers from several disadvantages such as slow onset of action, poor absorption of highly polar drugs from gastrointestinal mucosa, destruction by enzymes in gut, first-pass metabolism, uncooperative/unconscious patients or patients suffering from gastrointestinal conditions like vomiting, diarrhea or other pathologies. Even if the sufficient amount of drug is absorbed into the systemic circulation it may not be able to penetrate into the ocular tissue due to blood ocular barrier. Intramuscular injections are made into the deltoid or gluteus muscles while intravenous injections are given in the veins, mainly the anticubital vein. The parenteral injections require aseptic conditions, may be painful and besides causing local complications expose the body to high concentrations of drugs. Parenterally administered drugs have to pass through the blood-ocular barriers and, therefore, may not reach in sufficient concentration in the eye but the risk of systemic adverse effects increases.

REFERENCES

1. Fraunfelder FT. Extraocular fluid dynamics: how best to apply topical ocular medication. Trans Am Ophthalmol Soc. 1976;74:457–87.
2. Yalçındağ FN, Batıoğlu F, Arı N, Özdemir Ö. Aqueous humor and serum penetration of tacrolimus after topical and oral administration in rats: an absorption study. Clin Ophthalmol. 2007;1(1):61–4.
3. Insler MS, Helm CJ, George WJ. Topical vs systemic gentamicin penetration into the human cornea and aqueous humor. Arch Ophthalmol. 1987;105(7):922-4.
4. Çekiç O, Batman C, Yasar Ü, Başci NE , Bozkurt A, Kayaalp SO. Human aqueous and vitreous humour levels of ciprofloxacin following oral and topical administration. Eye. 1999;13(Pt 5):555–8.
5. Costello P, Bakri SJ, Beer PM, Singh RJ, Falk NS, Peters GB, et al. Vitreous penetration of topical moxifloxacin and gatifloxacin in humans. Retina. 2006;26(2):191–5.
6. Sigurdsson HH,1 Konráðsdóttir F, Loftsson T, Stefánsson E. Topical and systemic absorption in delivery of dexamethasone to the anterior and posterior segments of the eye. Acta Ophthalmol. Scand. 2007;85(6):598–602.
7. Weijtens O, Schoemaker RC, Romijn FP, Cohen AF, Lentjes EG, van Meurs JC. Intraocular penetration and systemic absorption after topical application of dexamethasone disodium phosphate. Ophthalmology. 2002;109(10):1887–91.
8. Tabbara KF, Al Balushi N. Topical ganciclovir in the treatment of acute herpetic keratitis. Clin Ophthalmol. 2010;4:905–12.
9. Baum J. Treatment of bacterial ulcers of cornea in the rabbit: a comparison of administration by eyedrops and subconjunctival injections. Trans Am Ophthalmol Soc. 1982;80:369–90.
10. Stern GA, Driebe. The effect of fortified antibiotic therapy on the visual outcome of severe bacterial corneal ulcer. Cornea. 1982;1:341.
11. Friedman SM, Margo CE. Topical gel vs subconjunctival lidocaine for intravitreous injection: a randomized clinical trial. Am J Ophthalmol. 2006;142(5):887–8.
12. Rocher N, Behar-Cohen F, Pournaras JAC, Naud MC, Jeanny JC, Jonet L, et al. Effects of rat anti-VEGF antibody in a rat model of corneal graft rejection by topical and subconjunctival routes. Mol Vis. 2011; 17:104–12.
13. Mahdy RA, Nada WM, Wageh MM. Topical amphotericin B and subconjunctival injection of fluconazole (combination therapy) versus topical amphotericin B (monotherapy) in treatment of keratomycosis. J Ocul Pharmacol Ther. 2010; 26(3):281–5.
14. Souli M, Kopsinis G, Kavouklis E, Gabriel L, Giamarellou H. Vancomycin levels in human aqueous humour after intravenous and subconjunctival administration. Int J Antimicrobial Agents. 2001;18(3):239–43.
15. Ayalasomayajula SP, Kompella UB. Retinal delivery of celecoxib is several-fold higher following subconjunctival administration compared to systemic administration. Pharm Res. 2004;21(10):1797–804.
16. Kumar CM, Dodds C, McLure H, Chabria R. A comparison of three sub-Tenon's cannulae. Eye. 2004;18(9):873–6.
17. Srinivasan S, Fern AI, Selvaraj S, Hasan S. Randomized double-blind clinical trial comparing topical and sub-Tenon's anaesthesia in routine cataract surgery. Br J Anaesth. 2004; 93(5):683–6.
18. Carrillo MM, Buys YM, Faingold D, Trope GE. Prospective study comparing lidocaine 2% jelly versus sub-Tenon's anaesthesia for trabeculectomy surgery. Br J Ophthalmol. 2004; 88(8):1004–7.
19. Kwok AKH, Van Newkirk MR, Lam DSC, Fan DSP. Sub-Tenon's anesthesia in vitreoretinal surgery: a needleless technique. Retina. 1999; 19(4):291–6.

20. Nan K, Sun S, Li Y, Qu J, Li G, Luo L, et al. Characterisation of systemic and ocular drug level of triamcinolone acetonide following a single sub-Tenon injection. Br J Ophthalmol. 2010; 94(5):654–8.

21. Cardillo JA, Melo LAS Jr, Costa RA, Skaf M, Belfort R Jr, Souza-Filho AA, et al. Comparison of intravitreal versus posterior sub-Tenon's capsule injection of triamcinolone acetonide for diffuse diabetic macular edema. Ophthalmology. 2005; 112(9):1557–63.

22. Ozdek S, Deren YT, Gurelik G, Hasanreisoglu B. Posterior sub-Tenon triamcinolone, intravitreal triamcinolone and grid laser photocoagulation for the treatment of macular edema in branch retinal vein occlusion.Ophthalmic Res. 2008; 40(1):26–31.

23. Shimura M, Yasuda K, Nakazawa T, Shiono T, Sakamoto T, Nishida K. Drug reflux during posterior sub-Tenon infusion of triamcinolone acetonide in diffuse diabetic macular edema not only brings insufficient reduction but also causes elevation of intraocular pressure. Graefes Arch Clin Exp Ophthalmol. 2009;247(7):907–12.

24. Shorr N, Seiff SR. Central retinal artery occlusion associated with periocular corticosteroid injection for juvenile hemangioma. Ophthalmic Surg. 1986;17(4):229–31.

25. Moshfeghi DM, Lowder CY, Roth DB, Kaiser PK. Retinal and choroidal vascular occlusion after posterior sub-Tenon triamcinolone injection. Am J Ophthalmol. 2002; 134(1):132–4.

26. Clarke JP, Plummer J. Adverse events associated with regional ophthalmic anaesthesia in an Australian teaching hospital. Anaesth Intensive Care. 2011;39(1):61–4.

27. Awan AH, Rauf A. Comparison of analgesia in subtenon and peribulbar anesthesia. Pak J Ophthalmol. 2007;23(3):126–9.

28. Chew EY, Glassman AR, Beck RW, Bressler NM, Fish GE, Ferris FL, et al. Ocular side effects associated with peribulbar injections of triamcinolone acetonide for diabetic macular edema. Retina–2011;31(2):284–9.

29. Bordaberry M, Marques DL, Pereira-Lima JC, Marcon IM, Schmid H. Repeated peribulbar injections of triamcinolone acetonide: a successful and safe treatment for moderate to severe Graves' ophthalmopathy. Acta Ophthalmol. 2009; 87(1):58–64.

30. Mahfouz AKM, Al Katheri HM. Randomized trial of superficial Peribulbar compared with conventional peribulbar anesthesia for cataract extraction. Clin Opthalmol. 2007:1(1) 55–60.

31. Nicoll JMV, Acharya PA, Ahlen K, Baguneid S, Edge KR. Central nervous system complications after 6000 retrobulbar blocks. Anesth Analg. 1987; 66(12):1298–302.

32. Huber KK, Remky A. Effect of retrobulbar versus subconjunctival anaesthesia on retrobulbar haemodynamics. Br J Ophthalmol. 2005; 89(6):719–23.

33. Lockington D, Macdonald EC, Young D, Stewart P, Caslake M, Ramaesh K. Presence of free radicals in intracameral agents commonly used during cataract surgery. Br J Ophthalmol. 2010; 94(12):1674–7.

34. Pavesio C, Zierhut M, Bairi K, Comstock TL, Usner DW, Fluocinolone Acetonide Study Group. Evaluation of an intravitreal fluocinolone acetonide implant versus standard systemic therapy in noninfectious posterior uveitis. Ophthalmology. 2010; 117(3):567–75.

CHAPTER 3

Ocular Pharmacokinetics

OVERVIEW

Pharmacokinetics refers to the process of the uptake of drug by the body, the distribution of drug to various tissues, its biotransformation and elimination from the body. The rate and extent to which the drug will reach its site of action and the duration for which it will be available for action is determined by the pharmacokinetic processes.

Ocular pharmacokinetics is the study of changes in drug concentration over time in the ocular tissue when the drug is administered in various dosage forms by various routes according to various regimens. Although the eye is an extremely accessible organ for topical drug administration, the ocular pharmacokinetic studies are extremely complex due to highly complex interplay of multiple anatomical and physiological ocular barriers and physicochemical properties of the drug. The pharmacological actions, efficacy and possible toxicities depend upon the rate and extent to which the drug enters the ocular tissue. Ocular pharmacokinetics involves the study of drug absorption, distribution, metabolism and excretion. The aim of the ocular pharmacokinetic studies is to understand the intraocular drug disposition and provide a basis for rational use of ophthalmic drugs.

DRUG BIOTRANSPORT

During the movement from the site of administration and from one body compartment to another, the drug molecules cross the biological barriers. The major transport mechanisms that help the drug molecules to pass across biological barriers include:

1. Passive diffusion
2. Carrier-mediated transport
   a. Facilitated diffusion
   c. Active transport
3. Endocytosis

Passive Diffusion

Passive diffusion refers to the process of movement of drug molecules across the biological barrier along its concentration gradient, i.e. from the site of higher concentration to the site of lower concentration (Fig. 3.1). The process does not require energy expenditure from biological system. Passive diffusion is the primary mode of drug transport across the biological membranes including the ocular surface. Instillation of ophthalmic solution into the cul-de-sac provides high drug concentration in the tear film creating a concentration gradient across the ocular surface. This facilitates the passive diffusion across the cornea and conjunctiva.

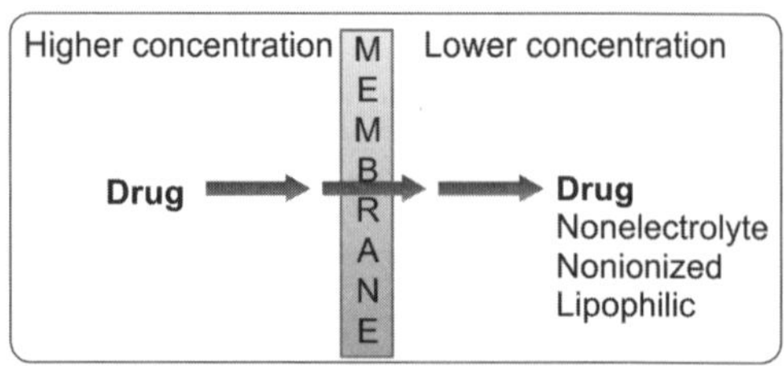

Figure 3.1 Passive diffusion through biological membrane

Besides concentration gradient, the passive diffusion of drug molecules also depends upon the ionization status and lipid solubility of the drug. The nonionized and highly lipid soluble drugs diffuse passively through the biological membranes at a rate that is proportional to their lipid:water partition coefficient, which means higher the lipid solubility, higher will be the rate of diffusion. Most of the drugs are either weak acids or weak bases. Passive diffusion of these drugs depends on their degree of ionization, which in turn depends on the pH of the surrounding medium. According to the Henderson-Hasselbalch equation:

$$\log \frac{(\text{Protonated})}{(\text{Unprotonated})} = pKa - pH$$

The pKa of a drug is equal to the pH of the medium at which half of the drug (50%) is ionized. According to above equation, smaller the pH relative to pKa, greater will be the protonated form of the drug. For acidic drugs the protonated form is neutral and lipid soluble but for basic drugs unprotonated form is neutral and lipid soluble. Thus, weakly acidic drugs will have better permeation at acidic pH and basic drugs will have better permeation at alkaline pH. Most of the non-steroidal anti-inflammatory drugs (NSAIDs) are weakly acidic and ionize at the pH of tears. Therefore, NSAIDs require formulation in an acidic solution so that the drug can be predominantly in nonionized form and can be better absorbed. Such acidic solutions can be irritant to ocular surface and are, therefore, formulated using exicipients that can reduce the irritating potential of the solution and stabilize the drug.[1]

Carrier-mediated Transport

The polar compounds like amino acids, sugars and some drug molecules are transported across the biological barriers by carrier mediated transport. The process utilizes a carrier molecule present on the surface of the membrane, which forms a complex with the drug molecule. The drug-carrier complex moves through the membrane, dissociates and delivers the drug molecule to the other side. Thereafter, the carrier molecule moves back to the surface for reuse.

Facilitated diffusion refers to carrier mediated diffusion of molecules along the concentration gradient, i.e. from higher to lower concentration (Fig. 3.2). The process does not require energy expenditure. It is a capacity-limited process and the rate of diffusion depends on the ability of drug molecules to bind with the carrier and the availability of carrier molecules. If two drugs utilize the same carrier molecule for transport, they will compete with each other for carrier binding and, therefore, will interfere with each others absorption. Transport of glucose across the corneal endothelium from aqueous humor to outer layers of cornea takes place by facilitated diffusion.[2]

Some drugs that are transported by facilitated diffusion include amino acids, antiviral drugs, anti-cancer drugs and vitamins like thiamine, riboflavin and B_{12}.

Active transport refers to carrier mediated transport of molecules against the concentration gradient and requires energy expenditure from biological system (Fig. 3.3). The required energy is generated by membrane ATPases and accordingly, the process of active transport can be inhibited by inhibiting cell metabolism and reducing ATP levels by agents like sodium cyanide. Like facilitated diffusion, it is a capacity-limited process and depends upon the ability of drug to bind with the carrier, availability

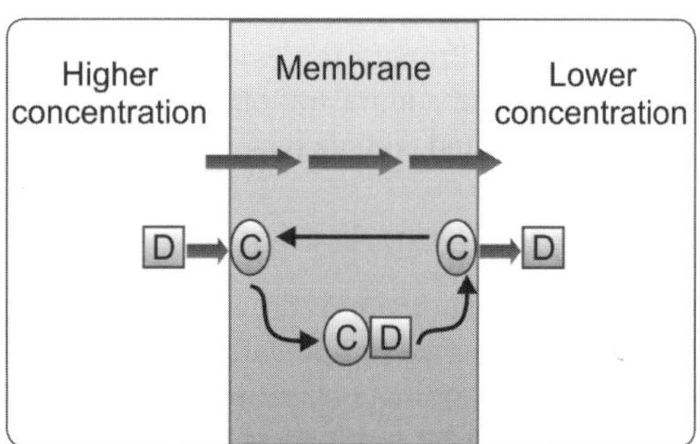

Figure 3.2 Facilitated diffusion through biological membrane

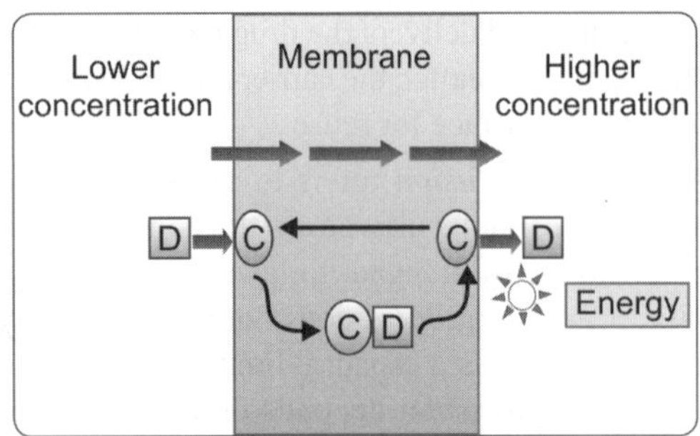

Figure 3.3 Active transport through biological membrane

of carrier molecules and presence of other substrates that utilize the same carrier. Presence of several transporter molecules involved in active transport such as amino acid transporters has been demonstrated in corneal epithelium.[3]

Endocytosis

The process of uptake of drug molecules by plasma membrane derived vesicles is known as the endocytosis. When the cell engulfs the fluid or drug in solution, the process is known as pinocytosis. If the material engulfed by the cell is a particulate matter the process is known as phagocytosis. The involvement of endocytosis for the transport of macromolecules has been demonstrated in cornea.[4]

DRUG ABSORPTION

Topical Route

Following topical administration, the process of drug absorption into the ocular tissue is quite complex. Primary routes of drug delivery following topical administration of ocular drugs include cornea and conjunctiva.

Transcorneal Drug Absorption

Cornea is the major site of drug absorption into the intraocular tissue for topically applied drugs. Cornea is a trilaminate structure consisting of an outer lipophilic epithelium and Bowman's membrane, middle hydrophilic stroma and

inner less lipophilic endothelium. The relative thicknesses of epithelium, stroma and endothelium are approximately 0.1:1.0:0.01. The corneal epithelium consists of a basal layer of columnar cells, 2–3 layers of wing cells and 1–2 outermost layers of squamous cells (Fig. 3.4).

Squamous cells in the outermost layer of corneal epithelium are surrounded by tight junctions (zonula occludens).The intercellular spaces between wing cells and basal cells are comparatively larger. The tight junctions in the most superficial layer of corneal epithelium serve as selective barrier for the small molecules and completely prevent the diffusion of macromolecules. The permeability of tight junctions depends not only on its structural integrity but also on the integrity of cytoskeleton of epithelial cells. High extracellular and low intracellular calcium levels are required for maintaining the normal permeability of tight junctions. Hypertonic solutions have been shown to increase the leakiness of tight junctions.[5] The pore size of the apical epithelium (< 3 nm) allows small hydrophilic molecules like glycerol (1.2 nm) to penetrate through the tight junctions but larger molecules like inulin (3 nm) fail to pass through the corneal epithelium.[6,7]

The stroma, which forms 90% of the corneal thickness, is hydrophilic in nature. It is relatively hypocellular and consists of large volume of tissue fluid. The cellular components of stroma are mainly the corneal fibroblast making about 2–3% of the total volume of stroma. The bundles of collagen fibrils in stroma have a regular arrangement. Because of the relatively open structure of stroma particles up to the molecular weight of 500,000 kd can pass through it.[8] It is a rate limiting barrier to small highly lipophilic molecules due to its hydrophilic nature but allows easy passage to the hydrophilic molecules. Because of the large fluid volume, the stroma also acts as a reservoir for drugs that gain entry through the epithelium (Fig. 3.5).

The endothelium, which forms the innermost layer of cornea is a single layer of hexagonal cells. It offers little resistance for the passage of drug molecules due to the presence of gap

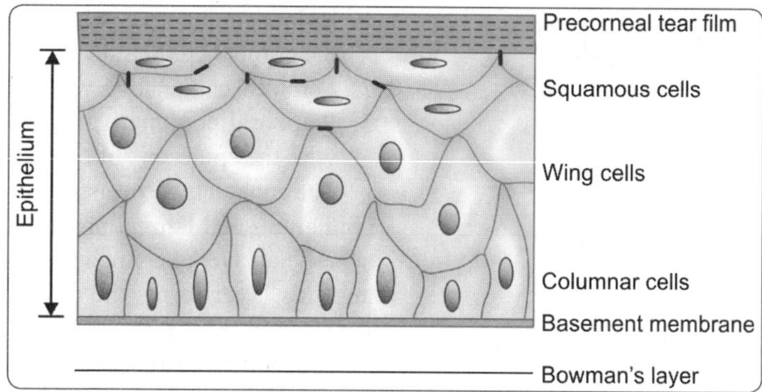

Figure 3.4 Corneal epithelium

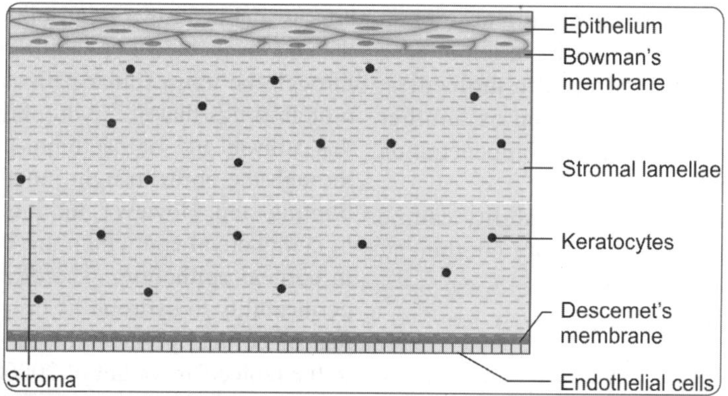

Figure 3.5 Corneal stroma and endothelium

junctions and easily pumps out the tissue fluid from stroma into the aqueous humor.

Due to its biphasic solubility characteristics, cornea functions as a barrier as well as depot for the topically applied drugs.[9] Most of the drugs diffuse through corneal epithelium through transcellular (intracellular) pathways but some through the paracellular (intercellular) pathway (Fig. 3.6). Lipophilic drugs traverse the corneal epithelium through transcellular pathway but great resistance is offered for the diffusion of hydrophilic molecules, which can diffuse only through tight junctions in paracellular pathways. Passive diffusion along the concentration gradient is the main permeation mechanism for most topically applied drugs by both the para- and transcellular routes. Although, small lipophilic drug molecules pass through the epithelium easily, they must possess adequate hydrophilicity as well, to facilitate passage through stroma. Accordingly, the drugs with very high lipophilicity have poor penetration through cornea as compared to those with intermediate lipophilicity.[3] For corneal absorption of drugs, optimal partition coefficient has been reported to be 10–100 (1–10 on log scale). As most of the drugs penetrate the cornea via transcellular pathway, along with other factors, lipophilicity, pKa of the drug and the molecular size and shape also affect the transcorneal drug absorption.

Besides the passive diffusion various active transport mechanisms have also been identified in corneal epithelium, which are important in maintaining the normal stromal hydration.

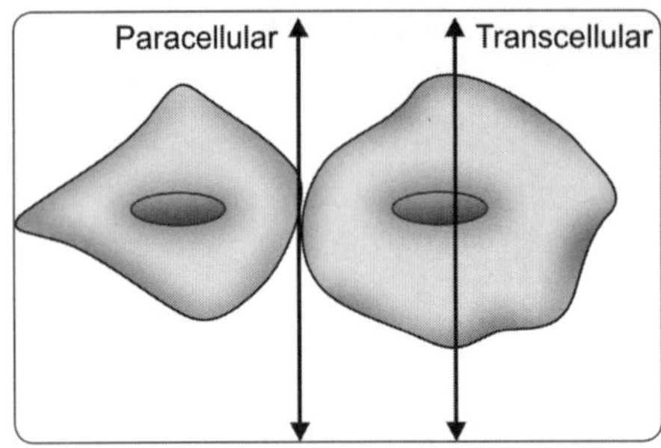

Figure 3.6 Paracellular and transcellular drug permeation

Although, evidence suggests that L-lysin and some peptides are actively transported by Na^+K^+-ATPase in corneal epithelium, significant role of active transport in transcorneal drug absorption has not been identified. It may be of importance for the transport of hypdrophilic molecules. Endocytosis has been suggested as another possible mechanism for intracellular penetration of large drug molecules.

The extent of corneal permeability can be estimated by corneal permeability coefficient, which is calculated as follows:

Corneal permeability coefficient (cm/sec) =

$$\frac{Corneal\ flux}{Initial\ drug\ concentration\ x\ corneal\ surface\ area}$$

The corneal flux can be calculated from the slope of regression line obtained from the linear part of the curve plotted between the amount permeated versus time.[10] For a large number of ophthalmic drugs the corneal permeability coefficient varies from 0.44×10^{-6} to 78.8×10^{-6} cm/sec. Value less than 10×10^{-6} cm/sec indicate poor corneal permeability. Corneal permeability of a drug can be modified by a number of factors, which are discussed in the following section.

Transconjunctival Absorption

Conjunctiva is a membrane of connective tissue that covers most of the ocular surface. It is a thin vascularised mucus membrane that plays an important role in the formation and maintenance of precorneal tear film. The conjunctiva is divided into three parts:

1. Bulbar conjunctiva, which is continuous with the corneal epithelium.
2. Forniceal conjunctiva, which lines the fornices.
3. Palpebral conjunctiva, which is continuous with the epidermis of eyelids.

The conjunctiva consists of stratified columnar epithelium and lamina propria. The cells in the superficial layer of epithelium have tight junctions and this layer forms the main barrier for drug penetration (Fig. 3.7).

Lipophilic drugs can diffuse through the transcellular pathway but hydrophilic drugs require passage through paracellular pathway. As the hydrophilic drugs have to pass through the tight junctions in the paracellular pathways, the surface area available for these drugs is significantly less than that available for lipophilic drugs, which pass through the transcellular pathway. Peptides and protein drugs that are hydrophilic pass through this pathway and for macromolecules the passage through the pores in tight junctions is the rate-limiting step. However, the intercellular spaces in conjunctival epithelium are larger than those in corneal epithelium. Therefore, conjunctival permeability to hydrophilic drugs is higher than that of corneal permeability and molecules up to the molecular weight of 20000–40000 kd can pass through the conjunctiva.[11-13] Accordingly, mannitol has 55 times higher conjunctival permeability as compared to corneal permeability. The ocular availability of peptide molecules through conjunctiva is limited not only due to large molecular size but also due to degradation by enzymes secreted by conjunctiva. Presence of carrier-mediated mechanisms in the conjunctival epithelium has also been suggested to play an important role in transferring drug molecules to the interior of the eye.

Due to its high vascularity, conjunctiva is also a major route for the entry of topically applied drugs into the systemic circulation. Some drugs such as timolol and nipradilol have significantly higher conjunctival permeability coefficient as compared to corneal permeability coefficient. Moreover, the surface area of conjunctiva (16–18 cm²) is significantly larger than that of cornea (1 cm²).[14] Therefore, due to higher permeability,

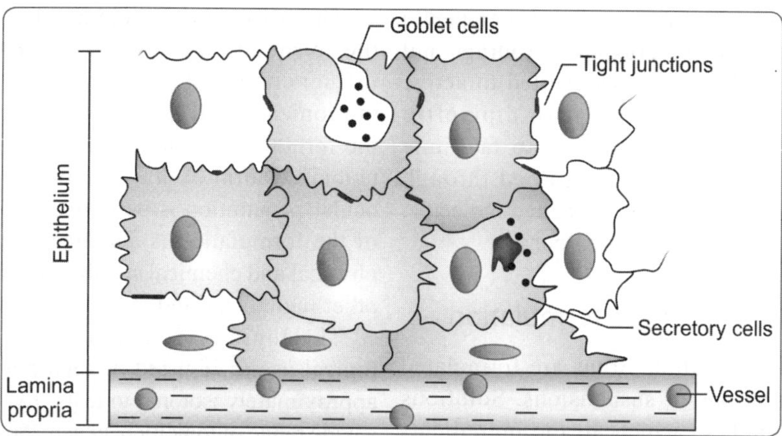

Figure 3.7 Conjunctival epithelium

high vascularity and large surface area, conjunctiva is a major route of systemic drug absorption following topical instillation.[15]

Transscleral Absorption

Sclera, the tissue lying immediately underneath the conjunctiva, is much more permeable to larger molecules than conjunctiva or cornea.[16] The sclera has three layers—episclera, stroma and lamina fusca. It consists of mucopolysaccharides and bundles of collagen fibrils. Topically applied drugs permeate easily through sclera by passing into perivascular spaces, through the gel-like mucopolysacchardises and through spaces between collagen network. For the subconjunctivally injected drugs, the physical and biological barrier of conjunctiva and cornea is circumvented and higher intraocular drug concentrations are achieved.

Factors Affecting Ocular Absorption of Topically Administered Drugs

1. Physicochemical characteristics of drug

The ionic characteristics of drug molecules in water greatly influence the drug absorption. The drug molecules with net positive or negative charge (ionized) at physiological pH and hence hydrophilic, penetrate poorly as compared to those with no net charge (non-ionized) and hence lipophilic. Lipophilicilty enhances drug permeation through transcellular route. The degree of ionization of weak acids and bases depends upon the pH of the medium. Timolol (weak base, pKa 9.2) is poorly ionized at higher pH of the instilled solution (6.2–7.5) and, therefore, has greater ocular tissue concentration at this pH as compared to lower pH solutions.[17] Flurbiprofen, an acidic drug, has shown reduced corneal permeability at higher pH.[18]

Besides the degree of ionization, the charge on the molecule also affects its corneal permeation. Above its isoelectric point (pI 3.2) the corneal epithelium is negatively charged.[19] Consequently, cations penetrate through cornea more easily as compared to anions. If the pH of the solution is below pI, cornea is more permeable to anions, however, at this pH the solution is too acidic for clinical use. Therefore, negatively charged drug molecules penetrate cornea poorly as compared to positively charged molecules.

The ocular tissue including cornea consists of significant levels of enzymes such as esterases, which metabolize drugs during and after absorption.[20] Presence of cytochrome P450 enzymes has also been demonstrated in cornea.[21] Consequently, drugs are likely to be destroyed by these enzymes causing reduced therapeutic efficacy. Some of the drugs are prodrugs and following metabolism are converted to active drug molecules. The drugs like dipivefrin (lipophilic) have been designed to facilitate corneal permeation. Once absorbed through the cornea it is metabolized to active molecule, epinephrine, which is more hydrophilic.

2. Composition of drug formulation

Most of the ophthalmic drugs are formulated either as solutions or suspensions. Solutions are clear liquids in which all the ingredients are completely soluble and there is minimal interference with vision. Although, the drug molecules in solutions are immediately available for absorption, there is equally rapid drainage out of cul-de-sac. Ophthalmic suspensions contain micronized drug molecules (< 10 μm in diameter) of relatively low aqueous solubility dispersed in liquid vehicle, such as prednisolone acetate. The small drug particles stay in cul-de-sac longer than those of solution, thus prolonging the drug's availability for absorption.[22] The drug delivery from suspension takes place in two phases. The first phase of rapid delivery and second phase of slow delivery from retained particles.

In general, small particle size favors faster dissolution and faster absorption. But in case of suspensions small particle size will favor the easier drainage out of the cul-de-sac thus reducing the retention time and consequently the net absorption. Suspensions require adequate shaking of the container before administration because of the sedimentation of particles. The rate of sedimentation depends on particle size. The larger the particles, faster the rate of sedimentation and lower the rate of resuspension. Larger particles in suspension cause more ocular irritation, tearing and drug loss by drainage. Particle size <10 μm generally minimizes ocular irritation, however, this is not a clear-cut limit because other factors such as particle shape, density and concentration can influence the degree of ocular irritation and drug loss.

The pH of the vehicle and buffers used in the formulation are other important factors influencing ocular absorption by affecting the ionization of drug molecules. The pH of the formulation is adjusted in such a way that unionized form of drug predominates and easy ocular penetration is permitted. An optimal pH of the formulation is also necessary to ensure physical and chemical stability of drug as well as other ingredients and for ocular comfort.

The tonicity of ophthalmic solution for topical use is adjusted in such a way that it is approximately isotonic to tears. Eye can tolerate a wide range of tonicity between 266–445 mOsm/kg without causing any pain or discomfort. Ophthalmic preparation with excessive tonicity cause stinging pain on instillation and induce reflex tearing. Tearing dilutes the drug solution and reduces its extent of absorption.

Increased viscosity of the solution allows the drug to stay in contact with ocular surface for a longer time, thereby increasing the drug absorption. This factor is further discussed in the next section.

Multi-dose containers of ophthalmic preparations usually contain a preservative to prevent growth of microorganisms. Preservatives in ophthalmic solutions such as benzalkonium chloride enhance the ocular absorption of drugs and can be toxic to ocular surface.[23]

3. Residence time on ocular surface

The capacity of conjunctival sac is approximately 15–30 μL and the natural tear film volume is 7–8 μL. At a normal blink rate of 15–20 blinks/min, tear turn over rate is approximately 16% per minute but is greatly influenced by environmental temperature and humidity. Most of the ophthalmic solution applicators deliver the solution in a volume of about 50–100 μL, therefore, a significant portion of the solution is lost due to overspill. The remaining is subjected to drainage through the nasolacrimal duct until the normal tear volume is restored. Once the normal tear volume is restored further tear turnover dilutes the drug solution and reduces the concentration gradient across the ocular surface. With spontaneous tear flow, the instilled drug completely disappears from cul-de-sac in about 5 minutes and 80% of the applied drug is lost through nasolacrimal drainage (Flowchart 3.1).

Following instillation of drug solution, lacrimation and blinking significantly influence the residence time of the drug on the ocular surface. Reflex tearing following instillation of an irritant drug causes increased rate of drug loss. Similarly, physical, psychological and emotional stress causes increased tearing and hence the higher drug loss. Lid closure, topical and general anesthesia reduce the rate of tear flow, thereby, reducing the drug loss. Blinking movements promote drainage of instilled drug through the nasolacrimal duct and each blinking movement removes about 2 µL of fluid from the cul-de-sac. Besides drug loss due to nasolacrimal drainage, a number of other factors such as tear evaporation, drug deposition on lid margins, drug binding to proteins in tears and drug metabolism by enzymes in tears also reduce the amount of drug absorption. Instillation of multiple drops of different medications in quick succession causes substantial loss by washout. If the second drop is applied about 5-minutes after the first, almost no washout effect occurs on the first drop.

Increasing the residence time of ophthalmic solution onto the ocular surface increases the amount of drug absorption. The measure that is commonly adopted for this purpose is by changing the vehicle of the solution to more viscous consistency by adding viscoelastic substances such as hydroxypropyl methylcellulose, polyvinyl alcohol or guar gum.[24-26] Optimal viscosity suggested for ophthalmic solution is 12–15 cp (centipoise). The preparations with higher viscosity do not allow easy mixing with aqueous phase in the eye, cause distortion of optical surface leading to blurred vision. High viscosity solutions cause ocular irritation, reflex blinking lacrimation and drug loss due to increased drainage. Formulations with viscosity higher than 30 cp are very sticky and uncomfortable for use.

4. Integrity of precorneal tear film and ocular surface

The topically applied ophthalmic drug mixes with the precorneal tear film before getting absorbed through the ocular surface. The pH of normal tear fluid ranges from 6.5 to 7.6. If the pH of instilled medication is not within physiological limits, increased tear turnover and to some extent the buffering system of tears brings its pH within physiological range. Any change in the pH of tear film will affect the ionization of drug and hence its capacity to diffuse and get absorbed through the ocular surface.

Precorneal tear film consists of an outer layer of mixed lipids, middle aqueous layer containing proteins and deeper mucin layer of glycoproteins. The deeper mucin layer is extremely important for the stability of tear film and promotes adherence of tear film to the lipophilic epithelium of cornea and conjunctiva. Any alteration in the composition of tear film causes instability of tear film and reduces drug's residence time on ocular surface.

Flow chart 3.1 Fate of topically administered drugs

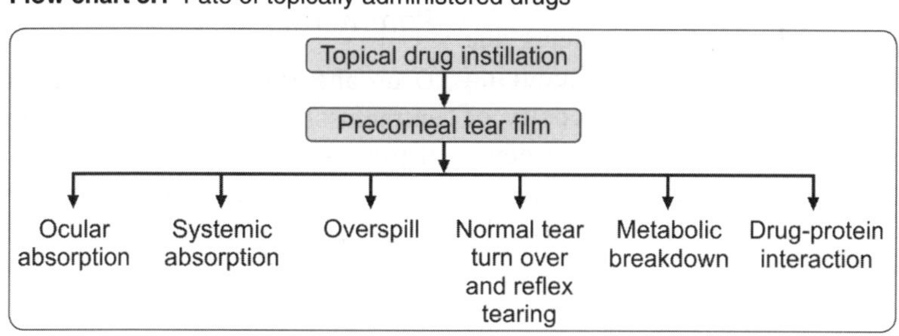

As discussed earlier an intact corneal and conjunctival epithelium form the most significant barrier to drug absorption from ocular surface. Any damage to corneal and conjunctival epithelium due to disease, trauma or toxins significantly damages this barrier causing enhanced absorption of drugs from the ocular surface.

5. Extent of systemic absorption

The drug remaining in contact with ocular surface is available for absorption through the ocular surface into the ocular tissue. However, following topical application, significant amount may get absorbed into the systemic circulation by

1. Getting absorbed through nasal and nasopharyngeal mucosa following drainage through nasolacrimal duct.
2. Getting absorbed through highly vascular conjunctiva and lid margins.

Normally, the topically administered formulations are rapidly drained through open punctum into the nasolacrimal duct, followed by absorption through the lining mucosa. Since, the punctal patency requires open lids, systemic absorption of the topically administered drugs can be restricted by gently closing the eyes for about 1 minute. The measure has been shown to greatly improve the efficacy of topically administered drugs. In the same way, applying gentle pressure over puncta for about 5 minutes also restricts drainage of drug into the nasolacrimal duct and increases ocular absorption.

Conjunctival vasculature is an important route for systemic absorption of topical drugs, which cannot be blocked by lid closure and punctual pressure. Instillation of multiple drops at a time does not increase the ocular bioavailability but increases the risk of adverse effects due to enhanced systemic absorption. Reducing the volume and increasing the viscosity of eyedrops, controlling drug release from depot preparations, prodrug-derivatization, and addition of vasoconstrictive agents can minimize the systemic drug absorption.[27]

Systemic Route

Drugs can also be administered systemically for the treatment of ophthalmic diseases. The systemic routes include the oral and parenteral routes.

Oral

Orally administered drugs are mainly absorbed through gastrointestinal mucosa by passive diffusion. The mucosa of gastrointestinal tract is more permeable to lipid soluble and nonionized forms of drug and less permeable to ionized and hydrophilic drugs. Sugars, amino acids and other nutrients are absorbed by active transport. Following absorption from gastrointestinal tract, drug molecules enter the portal circulation and reach liver prior to their entry into the systemic circulation. During the passage through the gut wall and liver drug may undergo metabolism and this will affect the amount of drug entering the systemic circulation in its unchanged form. Presence of efflux transporters such as P-glycoproteins in the enterocytes also interferes with the drug absorption. Inadequate drug absorption may sometimes be due to diseased condition of the gastrointestinal tract, vomiting or diarrhea.

The metabolism that the drug undergoes during its first passage through the gastrointestinal tract before entering the general circulation is termed as "first-pass metabolism" (Flowchart 3.2). Greater the extent of first-pass metabolism, lesser the amount of unchanged drug that enters the circulation.

Parenteral

Drug absorption following subcutaneous and intramuscular injection usually occurs by passive diffusion from the injection site to plasma or lymph. As the muscles are more vascular than subcutaneous tissue, drugs are more rapidly absorbed after intramuscular injections as

Flow chart 3.2 Systemic drug absorption by various routes

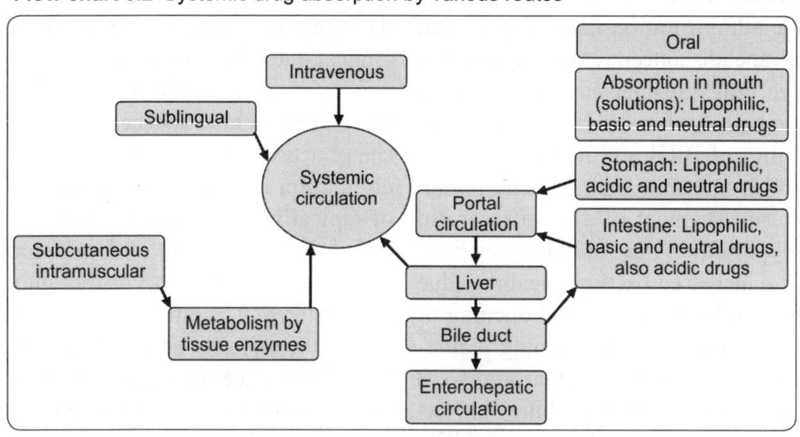

compared to subcutaneous. When administered by intravenous route, the total amount injected is immediately available in circulation.

Ocular Drug Absorption Following Systemic Administration

Following systemic drug administration, plasma concentration versus time profile usually translates into concentration versus time profile at the site of disease. But eye is a privileged site like brain where the concentration-time profile may differ significantly from that of plasma because of the existence of blood-ocular barriers. The blood ocular barriers that include blood-aqueous (BAB) and blood-retinal barriers (BRB) tightly control the chemical environment of the ocular tissue. These barriers also play an important role in eliminating the metabolic end products from the ocular tissue.

BAB is located in the anterior part of eye in the ciliary body and iris. The ciliary body plays more important role as it is located where the aqueous and vitreous meet. It has large surface area covered by ciliary processes and is equipped with multiple transport mechanisms. BAB is formed by capillary endothelial cells and nonpigmented ciliary epithelium. These layers do not allow passage of plasma proteins into the aqueous humor that would impair the osmotic and chemical equilibrium and hence the transparency of intraocular fluids. But the BAB is not absolutely impermeable to proteins and allows small amount of proteins to enter aqueous humor in normal eye, which contains soluble proteins equivalent to approximately 1% of plasma level. BAB has been shown to consist of several efflux and uptake transporters, which provide additional pathways for drug elimination from the aqueous humor and vice versa.[28,29]

BRB is located in the posterior part of eye and consists of an outer retinal pigment epithelium and endothelium of retinal capillaries. The endothelial cells in retinal capillaries have tight junctions made up of bands of zonula occludens. Because of the narrow tight junctions, passage to hydrophilic substances through paracellular pathways is highly restricted. There is absence of fenestrae and pinocytotic activity in the endothelial cells further contributing to the restricted permeability. The outer retinal pigment epithelium is the first barrier for the drugs that try to gain entry into the eye from systemic circulation. The adjacent pigmented epithelial cells are joined by extensive zonulae occludentes, which seal the intercellular spaces in pigment epithelium just like vascular endothelium. The cells in the BRB are known to consist of a variety of enzymes such as angiotensin converting enzyme, monoamine oxidase, pseudocholinesterase, dopa decarboxylase etc., which make up a metabolic barrier. Several efflux and uptake transporter molecules are expressed in BRB.[3,29] Penetration of drugs through BRB after systemic administration is often poor and to achieve therapeutic concentrations in posterior segment of eye, drugs are injected intravitreally. A number of methods have been described to alter the permeability of BRB and hence allow the penetration of drugs from systemic circulation into the posterior segment of eye. Intracarotid infusion of hypertonic saline solution has been shown to cause increased BRB permeability due to shrinkage of endothelial cells and opening of tight junctions.[30] However, this opening is non-specific and is associated with ocular and CNS side-effects. Exposure to white and blue light has been shown to increase the BRB permeability by promoting vesicular uptake.[31] Chemical modification of drug molecules to make them more lipophilic will allow better penetration through intracellular pathways. Drug molecules can also be modified in such a way that they resemble endogenous ligands and, therefore, can utilize the same carrier-mediated transport mechanisms for uptake into the ocular tissue. Liposome encapsulated drugs have also been used to enhance permeability through BRB. For targeted delivery of drugs into the retina another approach utilizes coupling of drugs with antibodies that are directed against epitopes present on endothelial cell surface. Such an approach allows selective transport through retina.[32]

BIOAVAILABILITY

Bioavailability is defined as the fraction of unchanged drug reaching the site of action following administration by any route. It is a measure of the rate as well as the extent to which the drug is available at the site of action after administration. Bioavailability of a drug after administration by a particular route is commonly measured by calculating the area under the concentration versus time curve. The peak concentration (C_{max}) and the time required to reach the C_{max} (t_{max}) are the indicators of the extent and rate of absorption respectively. Area under curve (AUC) indicates the drug's bioavailability. Both the rate and extent of absorption influence the clinical outcome (Fig. 3.8).

Ocular and systemic bioavailability refer to the rate and extent to which the drug is available at the site of action within the ocular tissue or systemic circulation respectively. Ocular bioavailability of topically administered drugs is generally an estimate of the amount of drug absorbed into the ocular tissue compared to the amount of drug administered. It is estimated that generally 5% or less of the topically administered drug penetrates the ocular surface and reaches the interior of the eye.

The total volume of the anterior and posterior chamber of the eye containing 200–300 µL of aqueous humor, is generally considered the central chamber into which the instilled drug enters following absorption through ocular surface barriers. The aqueous humor drug concentration versus time curve is often used to estimate the ocular bioavailability of topically administered drugs. However, the bioavailability can also be estimated in other parts of eye such as cornea, uvea, vitreous, retina by measuring drug concentrations in the corresponding tissue over time and calculating the AUC.

The ocular bioavailability increases with increased drug diffusion across cornea such as in cases of corneal ulcer when the epithelial barrier is destroyed. Increased partition coefficient also increases the ocular bioavailability and this can be achieved by increasing the drug's lipophilicity. Increased rate of drug elimination from tears and aqueous humor decreases aqueous drug

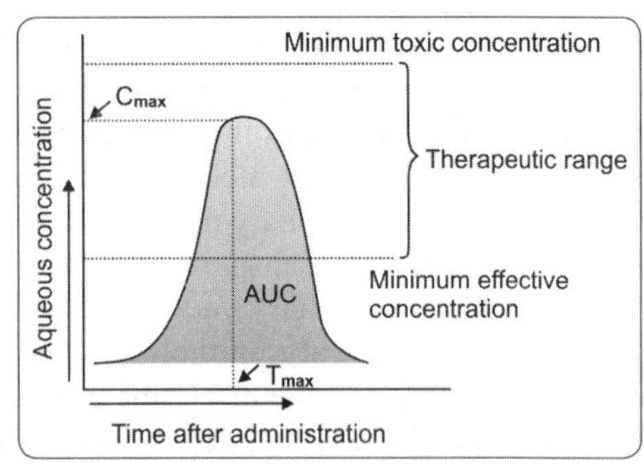

Figure 3.8 Concentration versus time curve

concentration. The drug elimination from tear film can be reduced by increasing the solution's residence time on ocular surface. The drug elimination from aqueous humor depends upon the aqueous turnover, which can be affected by the drugs like antiglaucoma medications.

Systemic bioavailability is determined by the AUC of the plasma concentration versus time curve. Since the bioavailability of intravenously administered drugs is 100%, the bioavailability by other routes of administration is calculated by a comparison with AUC after intravenous administration. However, for the drugs administered systemically for ophthalmic diseases, the plasma drug concentration may not be a true representation of ocular bioavailability due to the presence of blood ocular barriers. The bioavailability of systemically administered drugs is affected by physicochemical properties of the drug, route and site of administration, gastric emptying and intestinal motility, coadministration with food and other drugs, diseases of gastrointestinal tract, extent of first-pass metabolism and genetic polymorphism.

OCULAR DRUG DISTRIBUTION

For topically administered drugs, absorption of hydrophilic drugs is better through conjunctival-scleral route. The hydrophilic drugs absorbed through this route are deposited in the ciliary body whereas the lipophilic drugs are absorbed through cornea, diffuse through pupil and pass against the aqueous flow into the posterior chamber. Diffusion of drugs from aqueous humor to lens, vitreous and retina is slow and, therefore, immediately following absorption the aqueous humor levels of drug may be high. However, as the drug distributes to other parts of ocular tissue, the aqueous levels reduce. Usually following topical instillation, high drug concentration is achieved in anterior compartments, i.e. cornea, conjunctiva, sclera, uvea and aqueous. Distribution to the posterior ocular compartments is often poor after topical application as the drug diffuses slowly through lens and vitreous and at the same time undergoes elimination with aqueous humor turnover, metabolism and systemic absorption. Therefore, to achieve therapeutic concentrations in the posterior parts of eye, subconjunctival and intravitreal injections are used. Drugs injected intravitreally, provide high drug concentration in the posterior segment and diffuse predominantly to the posterior aqueous chamber due to the absence of a limiting membrane anteriorly. From the vitreous drugs can also diffuse through lens or retina-choroid-scleral membrane.

Systemically administered drugs enter the ocular tissue after passing through blood ocular barriers and follow the similar distribution pathway as described above. Generally, after systemic administration, lipophilic drugs penetrate better into the ocular tissue. Extensive plasma protein binding of drugs limits their penetration through the blood-ocular barriers.

Volume of Distribution (V_d)

After absorption into the central ocular compartment, the drugs are distributed to various parts of ocular tissue. In the simplest form, the eye can be considered as a single compartment into which the total quantity of absorbed drug gets distributed. The apparent volume of distribution (V_d) is the parameter used to indicate the extent of drug distribution. It is defined as the apparent volume required to distribute a known amount of drug at the concentration observed in central ocular compartment (anterior chamber). For drugs injected intravitreally, the vitreous humor forms the central compartment. Accordingly, V_d can be represented as follows:

Apparent volume of distribution (V_d) =

$$\frac{\text{Total amount of drug adsorbed}}{\text{Aqueous humor drug concentration}}$$

Figure 3.9 illustrates the relationship of drug concentration, V_d and the extent of drug distribution.

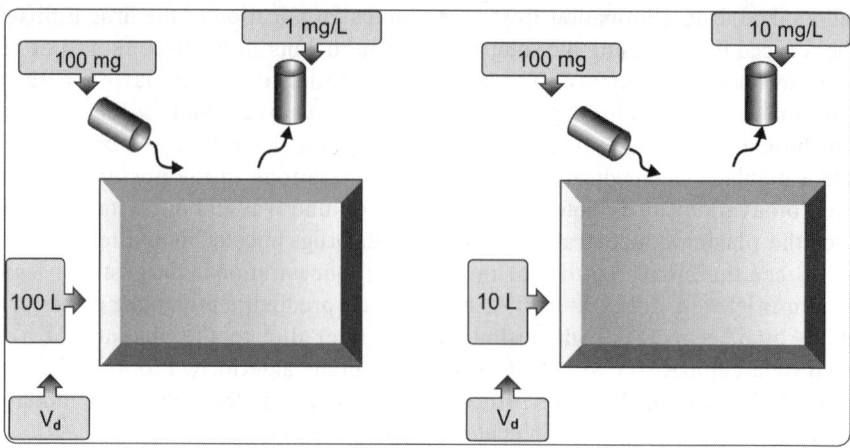

Figure 3.9 Apparent volume of distribution

Accordingly, considering the eye as a single compartment following absorption of equal amount of drug, smaller aqueous humor drug concentration indicates a larger tissue distribution of drug. But a relatively larger aqueous humor drug concentration indicates smaller tissue distribution of drug.

The eye, however, is not a single compartment and consists of multiple sub-compartments such as tear film, cornea, conjunctiva, sclera, uvea, aqueous, lens, vitreous and retina. Although, the volume of aqueous humor is approximately 0.3 mL but the apparent volume of ocular drug distribution (V_d) is usually larger due to multi-compartment distribution. The values of V_d typically vary from 0.24–0.64 mL, however, some drugs like ketorolac tromethamine (V_d = 1.93 mL) and levobunolol (V_d = 1.65 mL) have high values.

Effect of Protein and Pigment Binding on Drug Distribution

Extensive binding of drugs to proteins in aqueous humor reduces their distribution to other parts of eye. Binding of drugs with proteins is reversible and is in dynamic equilibrium, i.e.

Free drug (unbound) + protein ↔ Drug-protein complex (bound)

Drug when complexed with proteins is inactive and only the free form of the drug is pharmacologically active. It is the free form of the drug that can diffuse from one to another compartment to maintain equilibrium and can get metabolized and excreted. As the unbound drug is metabolized and excreted, more is released from bound form to replace the lost amount. Extensive protein binding increases the availability of drug over a prolonged period of time thus prolonging its duration of action.

Binding to uveal pigment also affects the drug distribution especially for drugs that have the site of action in ciliary body. For example, timolol will be required in comparatively higher doses to reduce intraocular pressure in people with heavily pigmented iris due to significant binding to uveal pigment. Some of the ocular compartments like uvea, lens and vitreous also act as drug reservoir. This may be responsible for increasing the aqueous humor half-life of drugs by allowing diffusion of drug when its level in aqueous humor is decreasing due to drug elimination. Drug accumulation in ciliary body

Flowchart 3.3 Ocular drug distribution and elimination

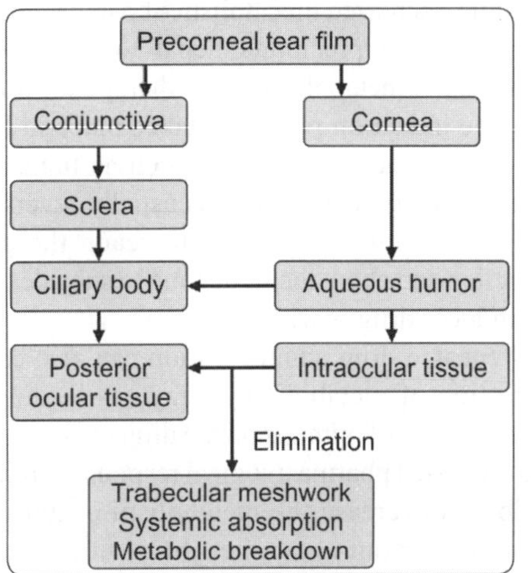

following repeated topical instillation may also be a cause of ocular toxicity (Flowchart 3.3).[33]

OCULAR DRUG ELIMINATION

Elimination of drugs to terminate their action involves both the drug metabolism or drug biotransformation and excretion. Drug biotransformation refers to the enzyme catalyzed chemical transformation of drugs within the biological system. For elimination of drugs from ocular tissue the three main pathways include: aqueous humor turnover, drug metabolism in ocular tissue and metabolism and excretion following systemic drug absorption.

Ocular Drug Metabolism and Elimination

Several enzymes that play important role in ocular drug metabolism include esterases, ketone reductase, catechol-O-methyl transferase, monoamine oxidase, acid phosphatase, β-hydroxylase, oxidoreductase, aminopeptidase, UDP-glucoronyl transferase, aryl amine acetyltransferase and aryl sulfatase.[20,34,35] These enzymes metabolize the drugs and either inactivate them or convert them into an active drug if the parent drug was a prodrug. For example, ketone reductase metabolizes the antiglaucoma β-blocker, levobunolol, into an active metabolite.[35] Similarly, latanoprost is a prodrug of $PGF_{2\alpha}$ and dipivefrin for epinephrine. Esterases are predominantly present in the iris-ciliary body followed by cornea and aqueous humor. The esterase activity in pigmented rabbits was found to be higher than in albino rabbits. Aminopeptidase activity is high in corneal epithelium and iris-ciliary body.[20] The activity of ketone reductase was shown to be highest in corneal epithelium followed by iris-ciliary body, conjunctiva and lens.

Besides the metabolic breakdown, drug elimination from ocular tissue also takes place by aqueous humor turn over and systemic absorption. Aqueous humor turn over is about 2–5 μL/min and amounts to 1–1.5% of the chamber volume/min.[36,37] Intravitreally injected drugs are primarily eliminated with aqueous humor turn over after diffusing anteriorly or through the retina-choroid-scleral membrane.

Systemic Drug Metabolism and Excretion

Absorption into the systemic circulation is the major route of drug elimination from the ocular tissue. For drugs administered by ocular routes that enter the systemic circulation or systemically administered drugs, liver is the primary site of metabolism. Other sites of drug biotransformation include intestine, kidney, lungs, placenta, adrenal cortex and skin. Biotransformation leads to conversion of a lipid soluble compound into water soluble compound, thus facilitating its excretion in urine. Drug biotransformation reactions are grouped into two types:

Phase I reactions take place in microsomes, involve microsomal enzymes and include oxidation, reduction or hydrolysis. Microsomal enzymes involved are associated with smooth surfaced endoplasmic reticulum and include mixed function oxidases and cytochrome P-450. These enzymes are non-specific and can be stimulated or inhibited by a number of drugs.

They metabolize only lipid soluble drugs. Resultant metabolites are small polar or non-polar molecules, which may be active or inactive.

Phase II reactions are synthetic or conjugation reactions in which parent drugs or their phase I metabolites conjugate with one of the endogenous compounds leading to formation of the polar compounds such as glucuronide, acetate, sulfate, riboside phosphates and methyl or glutathione derivatives. Except for the glucuronide conjugation, all other conjugation reactions require non-microsomal enzymes. Non-microsomal enzymes are present in the mitochondria and cytoplasm of hepatic cells, and in plasma. Metabolites are water soluble and inactive with the exception of morphine glucuronide, which is more potent than morphine. Some drugs can directly undergo phase II reactions without undergoing phase I reactions.

Various factors can affect the rate of hepatic drug metabolism. Neonates and premature babies due to their immature hepatic enzyme system may metabolize drugs at a slower rate. Elderly above the age of 60 also metabolize drugs slower than the young adults due to reduced hepatic blood flow. Enzyme expression may differ due to genetic polymorphism. Starvation leads to enzyme inhibition and a diet rich in proteins enhances the rate of metabolism. Dietary deficiency of vitamins and micronutrients can alter the rate of metabolism. Enzyme activity also gets altered in diseases like hepatitis, cardiac diseases, thyroid diseases, etc.

Enzyme Induction and Inhibition

Repeated drug administration may lead to growth of smooth endoplasmic reticulum and enhanced microsomal enzyme activity. As a result, the inducer drug is metabolized at a faster rate causing its reduced pharmacological effect. Enzyme induction increases the metabolism of not only the inducer drug but also other drugs that utilize the same enzymes when administered concurrently. However, if the metabolite of inducer or the concurrently administered drug is an active compound the pharmacological response

will increase and may lead to toxicity. For example, increased metabolism of paracetamol in alcoholics may precipitate hepatotoxicity due to paracetamol metabolite even at therapeutic doses. Enzyme induction primarily takes place in liver but may occur at other sites such as lungs and placenta. Enzyme induction is usually reversible and takes about 1–2 weeks to reach the peak induction and about the same time to subside once the inducer drug is withdrawn.

Repeated drug administration can also cause inhibition of metabolizing enzymes leading to accumulation of unmetabolized drug in circulation and increased pharmacological response. Enzyme inhibitors decrease the metabolism of not only the inhibitor but also other drugs utilizing the same enzyme, when co-administered. Enzyme inhibition is usually reversible but occurs rapidly. Enzyme inhibition may involve non-specific mixed function oxidases or specific enzymes like monoamine oxidase, xanthine oxidase, etc.

Drug Excretion

Drugs from systemic circulation are excreted either unchanged or in the form of their water soluble metabolites. Kidney is the major route of drug excretion.

Renal excretion of drugs involves three processes: glomerular filtration, tubular reabsorption and tubular secretion. Drugs that have molecular size of less than 20,000 kd and are not extensively bound to plasma proteins, undergo glomerular filtration. Rate of glomerular filtration is also affected by renal perfusion. Higher the renal perfusion, greater is filtration. Glomerular filtration can remove about 20% of the drug from circulation. The rest reaches proximal tubules from where it is actively secreted in the tubular lumen utilizing energy dependent carrier systems. High protein binding does not interfere with the tubular secretion but helps in delivering the drug molecules at the sites of secretion. As the plasma concentration falls, more drug dissociates from protein binding sites and becomes available for secretion. There are two independent carrier systems, one for acidic drugs like aspirin and penicillin and other for basic drugs like morphine. Both are nonspecific and, therefore, drugs utilizing same carrier molecule may compete with each other for tubular secretion causing drug interactions. Clinically significant drug interactions mainly involve acidic drugs. For example, probenecid increases efficacy of penicillin by competing for tubular secretion and delaying its excretion. The combination is used in the treatment of various infections. Following glomerular filtration and tubular secretion drugs may get reabsorbed from tubular lumen. Reabsorption is largely by passive diffusion and, therefore, depends upon the lipid solubility, degree of ionization of drug and the pH of urine. Excretion of weakly acidic drugs may be enhanced by making the urine pH alkaline and excretion of weakly basic drugs increases in acidic urine. Strongly acidic and basic drugs remain ionized at all pH ranges and hence will be excreted.

Clearance

Clearance is one of the basic pharmacokinetic parameter that indicates body's ability to eliminate the drug. It is defined as the theoretical volume of tissue/tissue fluid from which the drug is completely removed per unit time. Clearance of the drug predicts the rate of drug elimination in relation to its concentration as shown below:

$$\text{Clearance (Cl)} = \frac{\text{Rate of elimination}}{\text{Concentration}}$$

Clearance can be calculated for individual organ such as eye by dividing the rate of elimination from eye by the concentration of drug reaching the eye. Total systemic clearance is equal to the sum total of clearance by all organs.

Elimination Half-life

Elimination half-life ($t_{1/2}$) is defined as the time required to change the amount of drug in the tissue by half. It is expressed as follows:

Plasma half life ($t_{1/2}$) $= 0.693/k$

The constant $0.693 = \log$ of 2. (As the drug elimination can be described by an exponential process, the time taken for a twofold decrease can be shown to be proportional to log 2)

k = elimination rate constant = fraction of the total amount of drug removed from the tissue per unit time and is expressed as

$$k = Cl/V_d$$
$$t_{1/2} = 0.693 \times V_d/Cl$$

For the single compartment model of the eye, the half-life is directly proportional to V_d and indirectly proportional to clearance. Half-life is not an exact index of drug elimination, because it depends on Cl and V_d, both of which may change independently. Half-life can not predict the duration of action after single dose, which is related more to distribution rather than clearance/elimination. But it can predict the rate and extent of accumulation after repeated dose as well as the rate of wash out after the termination of treatment. Half-life predicts the time required to reach the steady state concentration following multiple dose administration.

Kinetics of Elimination

First Order Kinetics

Majority of ophthalmic drugs follow first order kinetic of elimination. For such drugs, a constant fraction of drug is eliminated per unit time, i.e.

$$200 \, (\mu g/mL) \xrightarrow{1 \text{ hour}} 100 \, (\mu g/mL) \xrightarrow{1 \text{ hour}} 50 \, (\mu g/mL)$$
$$[50\% \text{ is excreted per unit time}]$$

If the drug concentration increases such as due to increased dose, the amount of drug excreted also increases per unit time as is shown below:

$$200 \, (\mu g/mL) \xrightarrow{1 \text{ hour}} 100 \, (\mu g/mL) \xrightarrow{1 \text{ hour}} 50 \, (g/mL)$$
$$[50\% \text{ is excreted per unit time}]$$

$\downarrow$

$$400 \, (\mu g/mL) \xrightarrow{1 \text{ hour}} 200 \, (\mu g/mL) \xrightarrow{1 \text{ hour}} 100 \, (\mu g/mL)$$
$$[50\% \text{ is excreted per unit time}]$$

As is clear from the above example, increase in drug concentration from 200 µg/mL to 400 µg/mL does not change $t_{1/2}$ (50% of drug is excreted in 1 hour at both concentrations). Therefore, for the drugs following 1st order kinetics – $t_{1/2}$ remains constant because V_d and Cl do not change with the dose. The ocular drug clearance for the drugs following first order kinetics can be expressed as follows:

Ocular drug clearance (µL/min) = elimination rate constant × ocular V_d.

Elimination rate constant is the fraction of the total amount of drug removed from the ocular tissue.

Concentration versus time curve for drugs following first order kinetics is curvilinear but when plotted using log dose concentration it is a linear curve. First order elimination will allow excretion of 97% of drug in 5 half-lives following single dose administration as is shown below (Fig. 3.10):

Doubling the dose will allow increase in the duration of action by one $t_{1/2}$. In the above example if the efficacy of drug lasts until the concentration falls to 25 µg/mL, the duration of action at a dose, which gives 100 µg/mL will last for 2 hours. If the dose is doubled so that the initial concentration is 200 µg/mL the duration of action will last for 3 hours, i.e. increase by one $t_{1/2}$.

Following repeated fixed dose administration at an interval equal to $t_{1/2}$, it takes five $t_{1/2}$ to achieve 97% of its steady state concentration as is shown in Figure 3.11. At steady state, rate of drug absorption equals the rate of drug elimination, thereby, maintains a constant drug concentration.

At steady state following fixed dose administration at an interval of one $t_{1/2}$, the drug concentration fluctuates between peak and trough concentrations as is shown in the Figure 3.11 (Table 3.1).

Zero-order Kinetics

Some drugs undergo zero-order kinetics of elimination due to saturation of elimination processes and for such drugs a constant amount (not constant fraction) of drug is eliminated per unit time. Therefore, these drugs get eliminated at a rate independent of their concentration meaning, thereby, an increase in concentration will not proportionately increase the rate of elimination.

$$200 \text{ (µg/mL)} \xrightarrow{1 \text{ hour}} 100 \text{ (µg/mL)} \xrightarrow{1 \text{ hour}} \text{Nil}$$
[100 µg is excreted per unit time].

$$400 \text{ (µg/mL)} \rightarrow 300 \text{ (µg/mL)} \rightarrow 200 \text{ (µg/mL)}$$
[100 µg is excreted per unit time].

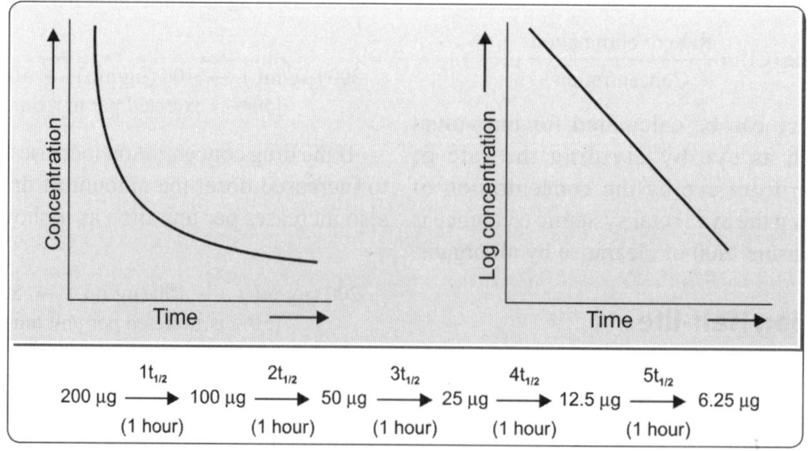

Figure 3.10 Concentration versus time profile for drugs following first order kinetics

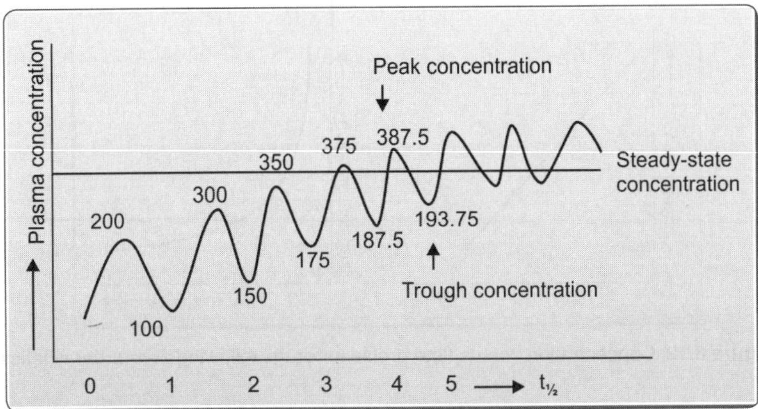

Figure 3.11 Steady-state concentration is achieved in 4–5 $t_{1/2}$

Table 3.1 First versus zero order kinetics

First order kinetics	Zero-order kinetics
• Elimination processes are not saturated	• Elimination processes are saturated
• A constant fraction of drug is eliminated per unit time	• A constant amount of drug is eliminated per unit time
• Amount of drug excreted per unit time increases with increase in drug concentration	• Clearance decreases with increase in drug concentration
• Clearance remains constant with increase in drug concentration	• Amount of drug excreted per unit time remains unchanged with increase in drug concentration
• Rise in drug concentration is linearly related to dose	• Rise in drug concentration is non-linearly related to dose
• Elimination half-life does not change with increase in dose	• Elimination half-life increases with increase in dose

As is clear from the above example, at drug concentration of 200 µg/mL, 50% of the drug is excreted in 1 $t_{1/2}$ but at drug concentration of 400 µg/mL it takes double the time for 50% elimination. Therefore, the Cl decreases as the dose increases. Hence, the $t_{1/2}$ of drugs following zero-order kinetics increases with increase in dose. For such drugs increase in dose can cause rapid increase in drug concentration to toxic levels especially so for drugs with narrow therapeutic index.

For drugs following zero-order kinetics clearance is expressed as follows:

$$Cl = V_m/(k_m+C)$$

V_m: maximal rate of elimination

K_m: concentration at which half the maximal rate of elimination is reached.

After single dose administration, concentration verses time curve for drugs following zero-order kinetics is a steep straight line but is curvilinear if log of concentration is used (Fig. 3.12).

Mixed Order Kinetics

Some drugs like aspirin follow mixed order kinetics. The elimination is dose-dependent. At low doses with low drug concentration, elimination follows first order kinetics but at higher drug concentration elimination follows zero order kinetics as the metabolizing enzymes

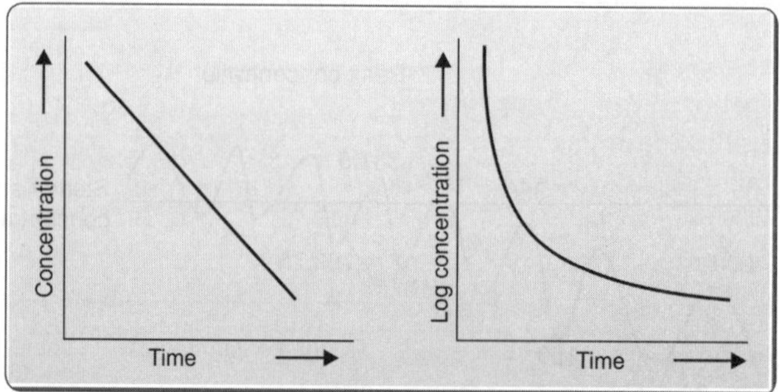

Figure 3.12 Concentration versus time profile for drugs following zero-order kinetics

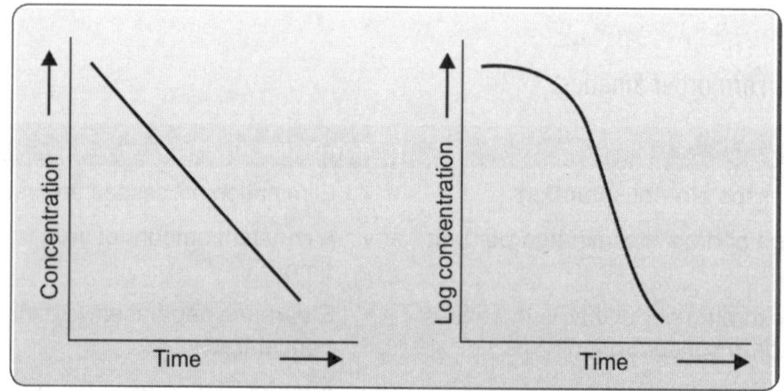

Figure 3.13 Concentration versus time profile of drugs following mixed kinetics

get saturated. Consequently, after single dose administration, drug concentration versus time curve is a steep line at higher concentration but curvilinear at lower concentration. If log of concentration is used for plotting the curve, it is curvilinear at higher plasma concentration and linear at low plasma concentration (Fig. 3.13).

For drugs following mixed order kinetics, increase in dose can rapidly change the elimination kinetics from first to zero order causing rapid increase in drug concentration and toxicity.

MULTIPLE DOSE ADMINISTRATION AND DOSING SCHEDULE

In therapeutics, multiple dose administration is done to maintain a steady state concentration. As discussed earlier, steady sate can be achieved in a time period equal to 5 $t_{1/2}$, if repeated doses are administered at an interval equal to 1 $t_{1/2}$. Drugs that have very short $t_{1/2}$ require administration by continuous infusion. For drugs that have $t_{1/2}$ between 30 minutes and 2 hours, it is practically difficult to administer the drug at every $t_{1/2}$. Such drugs, if have high margin of safety and follow first order kinetics, can be administered at high doses at an interval of 6–8 hours. Increase in dose will increase the duration of action and sustained therapeutic effect can be obtained with less frequent administration. Drugs that have $t_{1/2}$ between 4–12 hours, are administered at an interval equal to their $t_{1/2}$. Drugs that have a $t_{1/2}$ of about 24 hours are given in half of the therapeutic dose every 12 hours. Drugs that have very long $t_{1/2}$ take very long time to reach steady state concentration (5 $t_{1/2}$ is required to achieve steady state concentration). In clinical situations where immediate response is required such drugs are administered in loading dose so as to quickly achieve the target steady state concentration and then this is followed by maintenance doses so as to maintain steady state (Fig. 3.14).

Loading dose = Target drug concentration × V_d
Maintenance dose = Steady state concentration × Cl

Loading dose is often large and is associated with the risk of toxic effects. To reduce the risk of toxicity, loading dose can be divided into multiple small doses administered over a period of time.

Intermittent administration of multiple doses results in fluctuating plasma drug concentration, which varies between a peak and a trough concentration. At steady state this variation is repeated identically during each interdose interval. Reduction in dose and dosing interval reduces the amplitude of fluctuations. Mean steady state concentration does not depend on V_d. It is not determined by loading dose but is directly proportional to maintenance dose and indirectly proportional to clearance. Mathematically, steady state concentration can be calculated as follows:

$$C_{ss}av = \frac{F \times Dose}{Clearance \times T}$$

$C_{ss}av$ = average steady state concentration, F = bioavailability, T = dosing interval.

RATIONAL FIXED DOSE COMBINATIONS

Fixed dose combinations are the pharmaceutical preparations containing two or more drugs. Rational fixed dose combinations consist of drugs with approximately equal half-life. The ratio of the dose of each component depends upon the desired plasma concentration for optimal efficacy, which in turn depends upon the drug's V_d. For example, cotrimoxazole is a synergistic combination of sulfamethoxazole and trimethoprim in a ratio of 1:5. The half life of two drugs is similar and 1:5 ratio gives a required optimal serum concentration of 1:20 (trimethoprim: sulfamethoxazole) due to larger V_d of trimethoprim.

Fixed dose combinations provide a convenient dosing schedule and may allow reduction in the dose of individual component drugs, thereby, reducing the risk of adverse effects. Although the fixed dose combinations provide better patient compliance but if required, doses of individual components cannot be altered. Moreover, the component primarily responsible for benefits or adverse effects cannot be determined. Therefore,

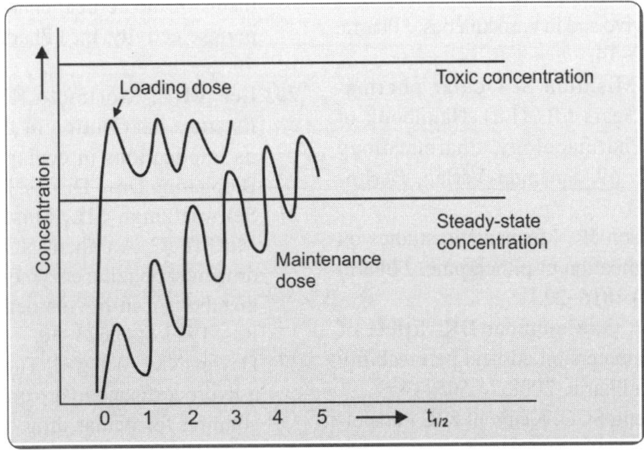

Figure 3.14 Steady-state achieved after loading and maintenance dose

fixed dose combinations are useful only when the component drugs have matching pharmacokinetic and pharmacodynamic features and patient requires all the component drugs in the formulation.

REFERENCES

1. Ahuja M, Dhake AS, Sharma SK, Majumdar DK. Topical Ocular Delivery of NSAIDs. AAPS. 2008;10(2):229–41.
2. Bildin VN, Iserovich P, Fischbarg J, Reinach PS. Differential expression of Na:K:2C1 cotransporter, glucose transporter 1, and aquaporin 1 in freshly isolated and cultured bovine corneal tissues. Exp Bio Med. 2001;226:919–26.
3. Mannermaa E, Vellonen KS, Urtti A. Drug transport in corneal epithelium and blood-retina barrier: Emerging role of transporters in ocular pharmacokinetics. Adv Drug Deliv Rev. 2006; 58(11):1136–63.
4. Gordon SR, Marchand DCMJ, Marchand J, Shuffett R. Endocytosis by the corneal endothelium. I. Regulation of binding and transport of hemeproteins and peroxidase-conjugated lectins across the tissue. Histochem Cell Biol. 1998; 110(3):251–62.
5. Jarvinen K, JarvinenT, Urtti A. Ocular absorption following topical delivery. Adv Drug Deliv Rev. 1995;16(1):3–19.
6. Lee VHL, Carson LW, Takemoto KA. Macromolecular drug absorption in the albino rabbit eye. Int J Pharm. 1986;29(1):43–51.
7. Grass GM, Robinson JR. Mechanisms of corneal penetration I: In vivo and in vitro kinetics. J Pharm. Sci. 1988;77(1):3–14.
8. Maurice DM, Mishima S. Ocular pharmacokinetics. In: Sears MC (Ed). Handbook of Experimental Pharmacology, Pharmacology of the Eye. Vol. 69, Springer-Verlag, Berlin-Heidelberg, 1984.
9. Sieg JW, Robinson JR. Mechanistic studies on transcorneal permeation of pilocarpine. J Pharm Sci. 1976;65(12):1816–22.
10. Ahuja M, Singh G, Majumdar DK. Effect of formulation parameters on corneal permeability of ofloxacin. Sci Pharm. 2008;76:505–14.
11. Huang AJW, Tseng SCG, Kenyont KR. Paracellular permeability of corneal and conjunctival epithelia. Invest Ophthalmol Vis Sci. 1989; 30(4):684–9.
12. Prausnitz MR, Noonan JS. Permeability of cornea, sclera, and conjunctiva: a literature analysis for drug delivery to the eye. J Pharm Sci. 1998;87:1479–88.
13. Geroski DH, Edelhauser HF. Transscleral drug delivery for posterior segment disease. Adv Drug Deliv Rev. 2001;52(1):37–48.
14. Hämäläinen KM, Kontturi K, Murtomäki L, Auriola S, Urtti A. Estimation of pore size and porosity of biomembranes from permeability measurements of polyethylene glycols using an effusion-like approach. J Control Release. 1997; 49(2-3):97–104.
15. Urtti A, Salminen L, Miinalainen O. Systemic absorption of ocular pilocarpine is modified by polymer matrices. Int J Pharm. 1985;23(2): 147–61.
16. Ambati J, Gragoudas ES, Miller JW, You TT, Miyamoto K, Delori FC, et al. Transscleral delivery of bioactive protein to the choroid and retina. Invest Ophthalmol Vis Sci. 2000;41(5): 1186–91.
17. Kyyrönen K, Urtti A. Effects of epinephrine pretreatment and solution pH on ocular and systemic absorption of ocularly applied timolol in rabbits. J Pharm Sci. 1990;79(8):688–91.
18. Chandran S, Archna R, Saha RN. Effect of pH and formulation variables on in vitro transcorneal permeability of flurbiprofen: A technical note. AAPS Pharm Sci Tech. 2008;9(3):1031–7.
19. Rojanasakul Y, Robinson JR. Transport mechanisms of the cornea: characterization of barrier permselectivity. Int J Pharm. 1989;55(2-3):237–46.
20. Lee VHL, Morimoto KW, Stratford RE Jr. Esterase distribution in the rabbit cornea and its implications in ocular drug bioavailability. Biopharma Drug Dispos. 1982;3(4):291–300.
21. Schwartzman ML, Masferrer J, Dunn MW, McGiff JC, Abraham NG. Cytochrome P450, drug metabolizing enzymes and arachidonic acid metabolism in bovine ocular tissues. Curr Eye Res. 1987;6(4):623–30.
22. Davies NM, Wang G, Tucker G. Evaluation of a hydrocortisone/hydroxypropyl-β-cyclodextrin solution for ocular drug delivery. Int J Pharm. 1997;156(2):201–9.

23. Acheampong AA, Small D, Baumgarten V, Welty D, Tang-Liu D. Formulation effects on ocular absorption of brimonidine in rabbit eyes. J Ocul Pharmacol Ther. 2002;18(4):325–37.

24. Trueblood JH, Rossomondo RM, Carlton WH, Wilson LA. Corneal contact times of ophthalmic vehicles. Evaluation by microscintigraphy. Arch Ophthalmol. 1975;93(2):127–30.

25. Saettone MF, Giannaccini B, Teneggi A, Savigni P, Tellini N. Vehicle effects on ophthalmic bioavailability: the influence of different polymers on the activity of pilocarpine in rabbit and man. J Pharm Pharmacol. 1982;34(7):464– 6.

26. Saettone MF, Giannaccini B, Ravecca S, La Marca F, Tota G. Polymer effects on ocularbioavailability—the influence of different liquid vehicles on the mydriatic response of tropicamide in humans and rabbits. Int J Pharm. 1984;20:187–202.

27. Urtti A, Salminen L. Minimizing systemic absorption of topically administered ophthalmic drugs. Sur Ophthalmol. 1993;37(6):435–56.

28. Hornof M, Toropainen E, Urtti A. Cell culture models of the ocular barriers. Eur J Pharm Biopharm. 2005;60:207–25.

29. Zhang T, Xiang CD, Gale D, Carreiro S, Wu EY, Zhang EY. Drug transporter and cytochrome p450 mRNA expression in human ocular barriers: implications for ocular drug disposition. Drug Met Dispos. 2008;36(7):1300–7.

30. Törnquist P, Ring A. The influence of hyperosmotic stress on the blood-retinal barrier effects on the electroretinogram. Acta Ophthalmol. 1980;58(5):707–11.

31. Putting BJ, Zweypfenning RC, Vrensen GF, Oosterhuis JA, van Best JA. Blood-retinal barrier dysfunction at the pigment epithelium induced by blue light. Invest Ophthalmol Vis Sci. 1992; 33(12):3385–93.

32. Cunha-Vaz JG. The blood-ocular barriers: past, present, and future. Documenta Ophthalmologica. 1997;93(1-2):149–57.

33. Abrahamsson T, Boström S, Bräutigam J, Lagerström PO, Regårdh CG, Vauqelin G. Binding of β-blockers timolol and H 216/44 to ocular melanin. Exp Eye Res. 1988;47:565–77.

34. Lee VHL, Robinson JR. Topical ocular drug delivery: Recent developments and future challenges. J Ocul Pharmacol. 1986;2:67–108.

35. Lee VHL, Chien DS, Sasaki H. Ocular ketone reductase distribution and its role in the metabolism of ocularly applied levobunolol in the pigmented rabbit. J Pharmacol Exp Ther. 1988;246:871–8.

36. Jones RF, Maurice DM. New methods of measuring the rate of aqueous flow in man with fluorescein. Exp Eye Res. 1966;5(3):208–20.

37. Conrad JM, Robinson JR. Aqueous chamber drug distribution volume measurement in rabbits. J Pharm Sci. 1977;66(2):219–24.

CHAPTER 4

Pharmacodynamics

OVERVIEW

Pharmacodynamics is the study of biochemical and physiological changes that the body undergoes after drug administration. It includes the study of the site and mechanisms of drug action and describes the relationship of drug's plasma concentration with its response.

The site of action of drug can be on the cell surface such as via receptors or intracellular such as interference with cellular metabolic pathways or gene transcription. The mechanisms by which drugs bring about biochemical and physiological changes can be receptor mediated or non-receptor mediated. Both the receptor and non-receptor mediated mechanisms can occur on the cell surface or intracellularly.

RECEPTOR-MEDIATED MECHANISMS OF DRUG ACTION

Most of the drugs produce their actions by interaction with macromolecular proteins known as receptors that can be present either on the cell surface or inside the cell. The receptors interact with the functional groups on drug molecules or endogenous substances. The three dimensional structure of receptors and drugs fits into each other just like a key in the lock resulting in the formation of a drug-receptor complex. Formation of drug-receptor complex triggers reactions leading to biological response. This interaction of drug with receptors is usually specific and reversible, but it can be irreversible if the drug forms a covalent bond with the receptor such as the organophosphate compounds.

Drugs acting through receptor mediated mechanisms are classified in four groups depending upon their two properties:

1. *Affinity,* which refers to the ability of the drug to bind the receptor.
2. *Intrinsic activity,* which refers to the ability of the drug to trigger the pharmacological response after binding.

Agonists are the drugs that have both the affinity and intrinsic activity (IA = 1), i.e. they bind with the receptor and initiate the pharmacological response. In other words they fit into the lock and open it (Fig. 4.1). Pilocarpine is an agonist and its interaction with cholinergic muscarinic receptors in the circular muscle of iris and ciliary body produces pupillary constriction and cyclospasm.

Antagonists are the drugs that have the affinity for the receptor but no intrinsic activity (IA = 0). They bind with the receptor, do not activate the pharmacological response and at the same time do not allow interaction of receptor with the agonist. Antagonists, that have structural similarity with agonist, compete with agonist for the same receptor site. Receptor-antagonist binding is usually by means of hydrogen bonds, which are weak linkages and allow easy separation of antagonist from receptor. Such competitive antagonism is, therefore, reversible. Atropine

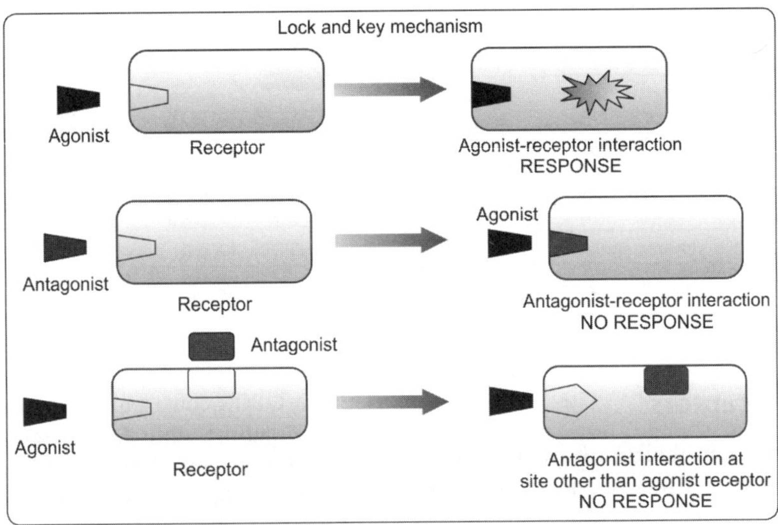

Figure 4.1 Drug-receptor interactions

is a competitive antagonist and its binding with muscarinic receptors prevents the binding of acetylcholine (agonist) at muscarinic receptors in the circular muscle of iris and ciliary body producing pupillary dilation and cycloplegia.

However, if the receptor antagonist interaction is by means of strong covalent bonds, the antagonism is irreversible. Antagonists can also interact with receptor at sites other than the agonist-binding site, i.e. non-competitive antagonism. Such an interaction induces change in the configuration of agonist binding site of the receptor and, therefore, interferes with agonist-receptor binding (Fig. 4.1).

Partial agonists are the drugs that have both the affinity and intrinsic activity but their intrinsic activity is less than the agonist (IA = zero to 1). Therefore, the pharmacological response produced is less than that of an agonist. (Fig. 4.1). Carteolol, a beta adrenoreceptor blocker, used in the treatment of glaucoma is a partial agonist. It occupies the beta receptors, prevents stimulation of these receptors by beta agonists and has some stimulant activity of its own.[1]

Inverse agonists are the drugs that have affinity for the receptor but the response produced is opposite to that of an agonist [IA = zero to (−1)] (Fig. 4.1). The 11-*cis* retinal is an inverse agonist

at G-protein coupled rhodopsin in the outer segments of rods.[2]

Two State Model of Receptor-mediated Drug Action

The difference in the response (agonist or antagonist) to two drugs binding the same receptor with same affinity can be explained on the basis of "the concept of dual nature of the receptors".[3] According to this model receptors exist in two conformations: active and inactive; and the two states exist in equilibrium. The drugs alter this state of equilibrium depending upon their relative affinity for the two types of receptor conformations.

Agonists have high affinity for activated receptor conformation, therefore, shifting the equilibrium in favor of activated form of the receptors whereas antagonists have equal affinity for activated and inactivated receptors, thereby maintain the equilibrium without a shift in any direction. Partial agonists have higher affinity for activated form of the receptors and shift the equilibrium towards activated form but to a lesser degree as compared to agonist. Inverse agonists have higher affinity for inactivated form and shift the equilibrium towards the inactivated form of the receptor (Fig. 4.2).

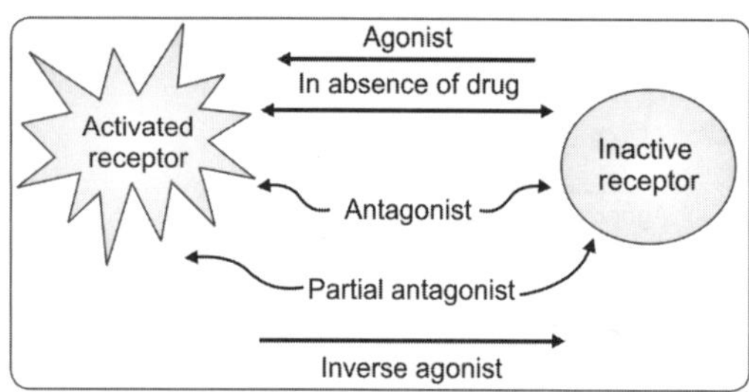

Figure 4.2 Drug actions based on dual nature of receptors

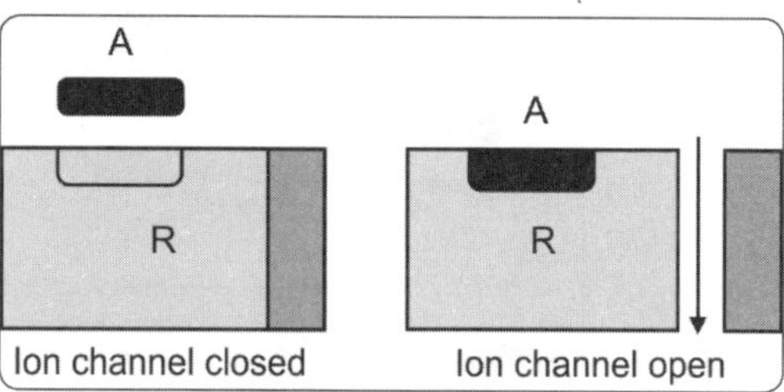

Figure 4.3 Ionotropic receptor

Types of Receptors

Receptors differ in their molecular structure and the post-receptor transduction mechanisms leading to differences in cellular responses. Accordingly, they are grouped into four receptor families:

1. Ionotropic receptors (Type I receptors): This family of receptors incorporates an ion channel within it. Binding with the agonist, opens the ion channel causing membrane depolarization or hyperpolarization (Fig. 4.3). The receptors for excitatory neurotransmitter glutamate in retina are ionotropic receptors. Their activation by glutamate increases the flow of calcium into the cells initiating the excitatory functions. For inhibitory neurotransmitter GABA, two subtypes $GABA_A$ and $GABA_C$, are ionotropic receptors. $GABA_C$ receptors are highly expressed in retina, mainly localized at the axon terminals of bipolar cells.[4] Both the receptor types incorporate a chloride channel. Opening of these channels in response to interaction with GABA causes inward flow of chloride ions causing membrane hyperpolarization. Some drugs allosterically enhance the effect of endogenous substance on channel opening such as benzodiazepines facilitate action of GABA on $GABA_A$ receptors. Ascorbic acid has been shown to potentiate the effects of GABA by allosteric modulation of the ionotropic GABA receptors.

2. Metabotropic receptors (Type II receptors): These receptors are present on the cell surface and are also known as G-protein coupled receptors (GPCR). GPCR consist of seven transmembrane helical domains with their N-terminal placed extracellularly and C-terminal intracellularly. The intracellular terminal of GPCR is coupled with trimeric G-proteins.[5] The three subunits of G-proteins include α, β and γ. When the receptor is in inactivated state the subunits are coupled with GDP. Interaction of agonist with receptor causes conformational change in the receptor triggering the exchange of GDP with GTP. Following the inclusion of GTP into the agonist-receptor-G protein complex, GTP-α and β-γ subunits dissociate from the complex. GTP-α subunit interacts with target molecule (effector system) and in the process GTP gets hydrolyzed to GDP. GDP-α complex so formed dissociates from the target molecule, reunites with β-γ subunit and returns the receptor to inactivated state (Fig. 4.4).

G-proteins act via one of the three effector systems, which form the second messenger systems for post receptor signal transduction:

1. Adenylyl cyclase: Cyclic AMP system
2. Phospholipase C: Inositol phosphate system
3. Ion channel regulation

Distinctive properties of α subunit determine its binding specificity with the type of effector system and accordingly, G-proteins can be of three types: G_s, G_i and G_q. G_s and G_i stimulate and inhibit adenylyl cyclase respectively. G_q affects the phospholipase C activity.

Adenylyl cyclase-cAMP system: The enzyme adenylyl cyclase may be the target following interaction of agonist with the receptors and

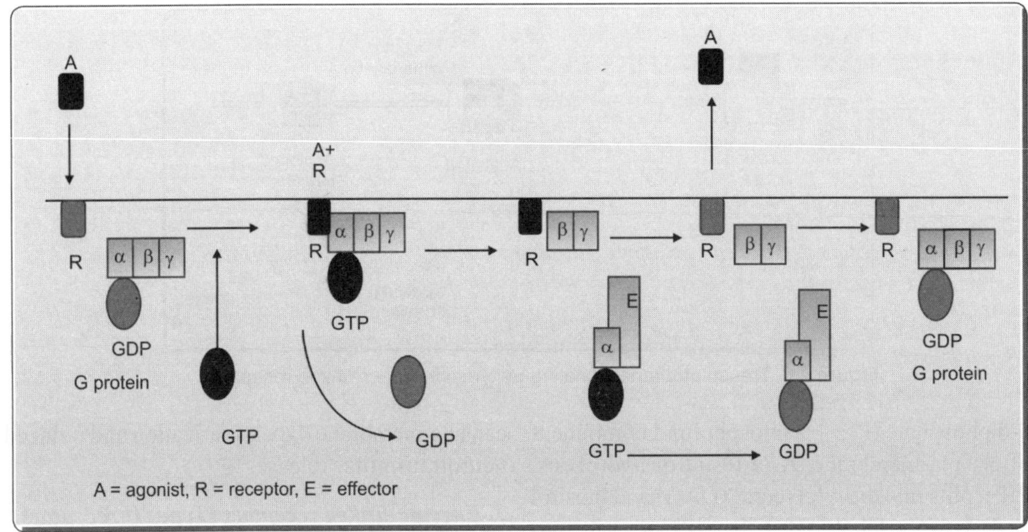

Figure 4.4 G-protein linked metabotropic receptor activation

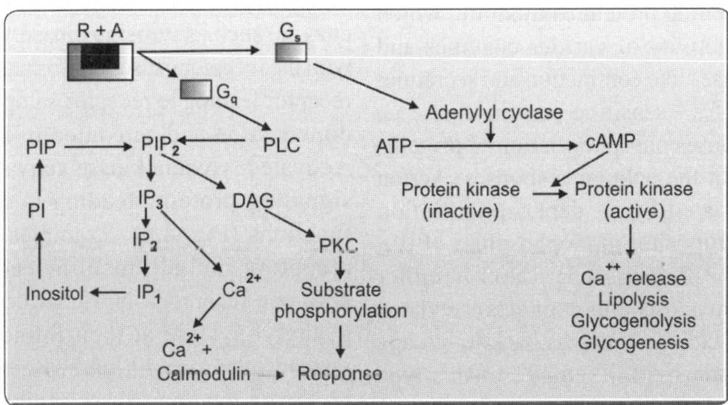

Figure 4.5 Second messenger system activation by G-proteins

activation of G-protein. As a result the enzymatic activity may get stimulated or inhibited leading to increase or decrease in the cellular levels of cAMP. Increased cAMP causes activation of protein kinase A, which in turn phosphorylates various proteins, thereby altering the cellular function (Fig. 4.5). For example: The non-pigmented ciliary epithelium has rich distribution of β2 adrenergic receptors, which are GPCR. Stimulation of these receptors causes activation of adenylyl cyclase leading to increased cellular cyclic AMP levels, which stimulates protein kinase A. Stimulated protein kinase A causes sustained stimulation of Na^+ K^+ Cl^- cotransport leading to increased aqueous humor formation.[6,7] Stimulation of prejunctional α2 adrenergic receptors in iris-ciliary body is negatively coupled with adenylyl cyclase and, therefore, reduces cellular cAMP level.[7-9]

Phospholipase C-Inositol phosphate system: Activation of G_q proteins in response to interaction of agonist with receptor causes activation of membrane-bound phospholipase C (PLC). Activated PLC causes hydrolysis of inositol 4,

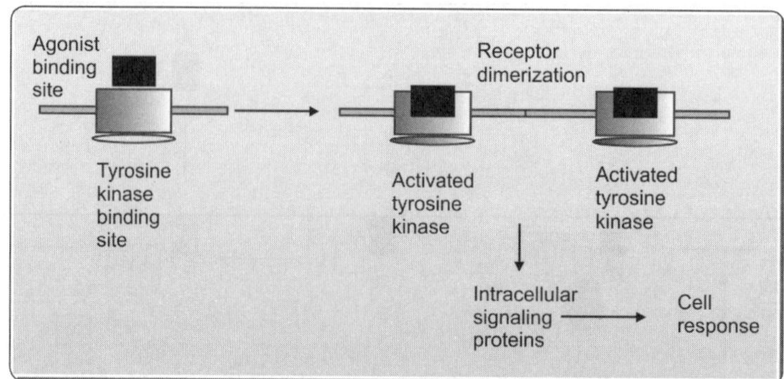

Figure 4.6 Transmembrane signaling by tyrosine kinase linked receptors

5-diphosphate (PIP_2), a phospholipid component of plasma membrane. As a result of hydrolysis, PIP_2 splits into diacylglycerol (DAG) and inositol 1, 4, 5-triphosphate (IP_3). IP_3 diffuses out into the cytoplasm and causes release of Ca^{2+} from intracellular storage sites. The released Ca^{2+} binds to Ca^{2+} binding protein calmodulin, which then regulates activity of various enzymes and produces responses like contraction and secretion. DAG activates Ca^{2+} sensitive protein kinase C, which in turn causes phosphorylation of proteins and brings about the cellular responses. Action of IP_3 is terminated by its dephosphorylation to phosphotidyl inositol monophosphate (PIP), a precursor of PIP_2 (Fig. 4.5). DAG is either converted back to phospholipids or gets acetylated to arachidonic acid. Ca^{2+} returns back to storage sites by active transport. Examples of this type of receptors include muscarinic receptors, α1 adrenergic receptors.[10]

Ion channel regulation: Some of the GPCR regulate opening or closure of ion channels in response to interaction with agonists without intervening second messengers. For example: rhodopsin located in the disc membrane of the outer segment of rods is a GPCR. Upon activation by light, the covalently attached chromophore 11-*cis* retinal isomerizes to all-*trans* retinal. Isomerization causes G-protein activation and dissociation of α subunit and activation of phosphodiesterase that hydrolyzes cyclic GMP. Reduced cellular cyclic GMP causes closure of cGMP-sensitive sodium channels causing membrane hyperpolarization and reduced neurotransmitter release.[11]

3. Enzyme-linked receptors (Type III receptors): These transmembrane receptors have an extracellular domain for binding with the ligand (agonist) and an intracellular domain linked to an enzyme such as tyrosine kinase. Agonist binding with the receptor causes conformational changes in receptor leading to receptor autophosphorylation, dimerization and activation of tyrosine kinase. Activated tyrosine kinase activates intracellular signaling proteins leading to altered cellular functions (Fig. 4.6). Examples of this type of receptors include insulin receptors, growth hormone receptors. Nitric oxide receptors have guanylyl cyclase at their intracellular domain instead of tyrosine kinase. Receptor activation by ligand binding causes synthesis of a second messenger, cyclic GMP, that brings about cellular responses.

4. Cytoplasmic receptors (Type IV receptors): The cytoplasmic receptors are precisely nuclear receptors. Interaction with ligand at their ligand binding domain unmasks their DNA-binding domain. The unmasked DNA-binding domain now binds with the DNA of specific genes and activates RNA polymerase. Activated RNA polymerase leads to synthesis of a specific m-RNA, which directs synthesis of specific proteins and produces cellular responses (Fig. 4.7). Examples of this type of receptors include steroid hormone receptors, thyroid hormone receptors.

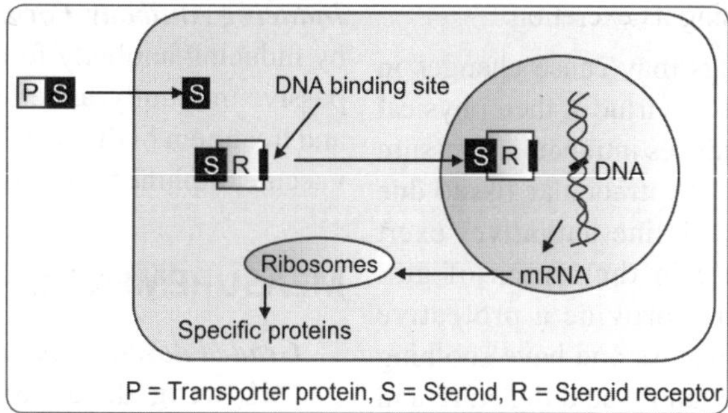

Figure 4.7 Regulation of DNA transcription by steroids through intracellular receptors

Modified Receptor Actions

Desensitization refers to reversible reduction of receptor mediated response upon continued exposure to agonist. Continued exposure to agonist causes conformational changes in receptor leading to tight binding with agonist without producing the effect such as channel opening at nicotinic neuromuscular junction receptors or inability to activate adenylyl cyclase at adrenoreceptors.

Supersensitivity, upregulation and down-regulation of receptors refer to increased or decreased receptor sensitivity/expression on prolonged exposure to antagonist or agonist, respectively. Continued exposure to antagonist causes increased number of receptors due to externalization of more receptors (upregulation). Moreover, the sensitivity of receptors to available agonists increases (supersensitivity). On the other hand, continued exposure to agonist causes receptor internalization leading to decreased number of receptors and decreased sensitivity. Prolonged treatment of bronchial asthma with β_2 agonist causes reduction in response over a period of time. This is because of receptor downregulation. Receptor upregulation may be responsible for excessive rebound agonist action after sudden withdrawal of a drug following long-term exposure leading to serious consequences. For example prolonged treatment of hypertension with non-selective β-blockers causes receptor upregulation as well as supersensitivity. If the β-blockers are suddenly withdrawn, increased number of receptors respond excessively to endogenous catecholamines leading to rebound hypertension. Therefore, in such cases the drugs should be withdrawn by gradually tapering the dose with close clinical monitoring.

Spare receptors refer to receptor reserve of the tissue. To achieve the peak effect it is not necessary that all the receptors are occupied by the drug molecules. Higher is the proportion of spare receptors for a drug in a tissue, higher is the tissue sensitivity to that drug. For example: myocardium requires only 10% of its receptors to be occupied by catecholamines for peak effect and accordingly even if 80–90% of the catecholamine receptors are blocked, peak effect to catecholamines can still be elicited. This indicates high sensitivity of myocardium to catecholamines.

NON-RECEPTOR MEDIATED MECHANISMS OF DRUG ACTION

Drugs may act by mechanisms other than receptor mediated. Some of the non-receptor mediated mechanisms of drug action are as follows:

Chemical Reactions: Drugs may react chemically with endogenous substances to bring about changes in physiological functions. For example: antacids react with hydrochloric acid in stomach to neutralize it and, thereby reduce hyperacidity, deferoxamine chelates with iron and facilitates excretion of excessive iron stored following repeated blood transfusions, cholestyramine lowers cholesterol level by exchanging with chloride ions in bile salts and increasing its excretion.

Physical Actions: Drugs may cause changes in physiological functions by virtue of their physical properties. Mannitol reduces intraocular pressure by drawing water out of intraocular tissue due to its hyperosmolarity. Saline purgatives exert high osmotic pressure in the lumen of gut. Demulcents like pectin provide a protective covering to inflamed mucosa and have soothing effect. Astringents like tannic acid denature and precipitate mucosal proteins and, thereby protect mucosa by firming it up. Adsorbants like kaolin adsorb bacterial toxins and are useful as anti-diarrheal agents.

Targeting Enzymes: Some drugs act by inhibiting the enzyme action, thereby altering the endogenous chemical reactions. For example: allopurinol, inhibits the enzyme xanthine oxidase, thereby reduces the synthesis of uric acid and is effective in the treatment of gout. Physostigmine inhibits acetylcholinesterase at neuromuscular junctions, thereby increases the availability of acetylcholine and causes pupillary constriction and reduced intraocular pressure. Sulfonamides act as antibacterial agents by competing with *p*-amino benzoic acid and replacing it in the synthesis of folic acid in bacteria; resultant compounds are nonfunctional.

Protoplasmic Poisons: Antiseptics like formaldehyde act as non-specific protoplasmic poison and kill the microorganism.

Inducing Antibody Formation: Vaccines, either by inducing antibody formation or by providing passive immunity, are effective in the prevention and treatment of diseases. For example: smallpox vaccine, diphtheria antitoxin.

MEASUREMENT OF DRUG EFFECTS

1. ***Graded dose-response curve*** : The responses following drug administration require quantitative assessment in order to evaluate its safety and efficacy. Quantitative assessment of the magnitude of response as a function of dose can be done using graded dose-response curve. It provides assessment of the relationship of the different doses (graded dose) with the corresponding responses in a single individual/animal/isolated tissue. The horizontal axis represents the dose while the vertical axis represents the response. The dose on the horizontal axis is commonly plotted in 'log' scale. This helps in accommodating wider dose range on a small graph paper and converts the hyperbolic curve (if arithmetic dose scale is used) into a sigmoid shape (if log dose scale is used). (Fig. 4.8)

Graded dose-response curve is useful for the assessment of the:

1. ED_{50} from its linear segment. ED_{50} is the dose that produces 50% of the maximum response.

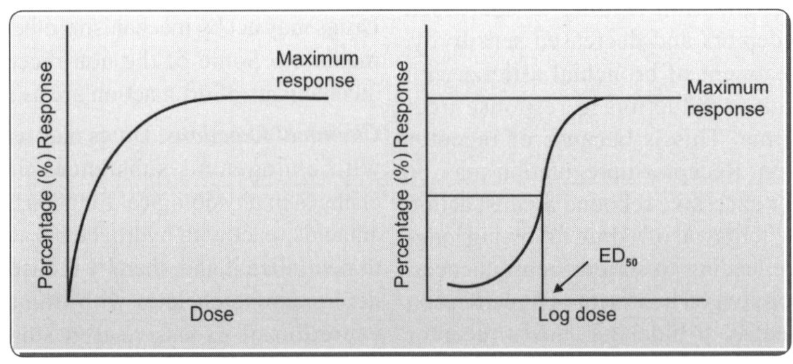

Figure 4.8 Graded dose-response curve

2. Potency of the drug. Potency refers to the amount of drug needed to produce a particular response. The relative potency of drugs can be assessed by comparing the placement of the curve in relation to each other on horizontal axis (Fig. 4.9).
3. Efficacy of the drug. Efficacy refers to the maximal response that the drug can produce. Relative efficacy of drugs can be assessed by comparing the height of the curves (Fig. 4.9).

Quantal dose-response curve: This curve provides an assessment of the relationship of the different doses with the percentage (%) of people showing a particular response. Here the response is prefixed such as 20% fall in blood pressure from baseline. The response can also be prefixed as 'all or none' response such as death or no death. It is a frequency distribution curve, which shows frequency distribution of the doses of drugs required to produce a specified effect, i.e. the percentage (%) of people that require a particular dose to exhibit specified effect. A cumulative frequency distribution curve derived from quantal dose response curve is a sigmoid curve (Fig. 4.10).

Quantal dose-response curve

1. Does not tell about the magnitude of the response as the response is "prefixed".

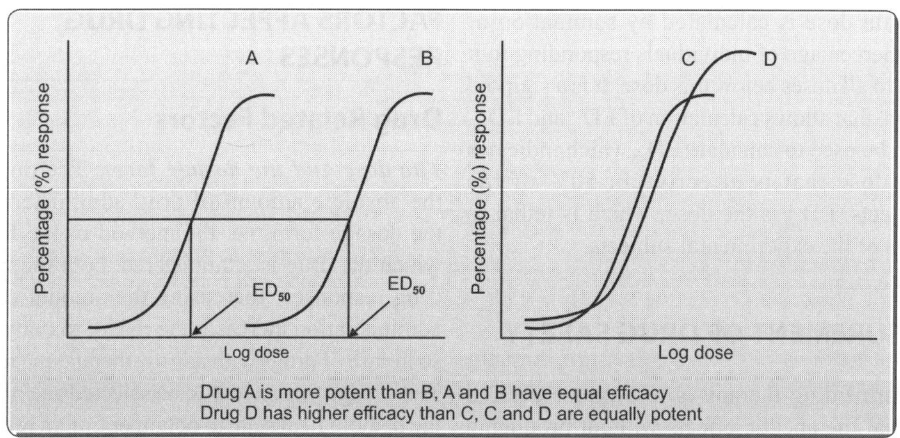

Figure 4.9 Potency and efficacy

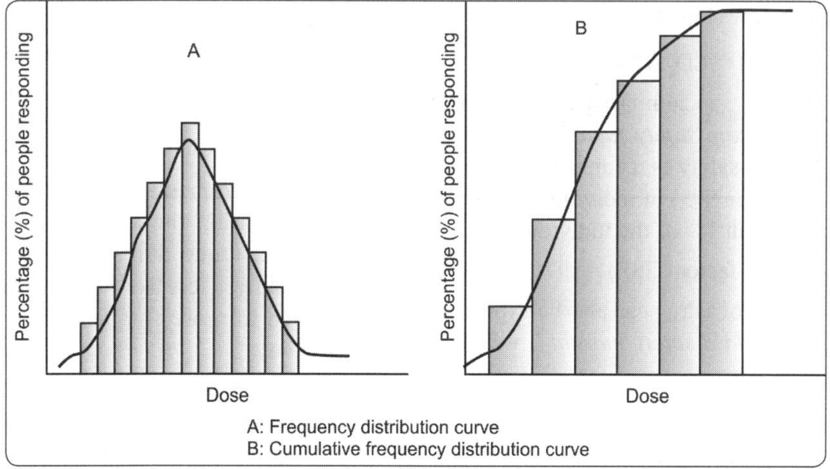

Figure 4.10 Quantal dose response curve

2. Is a frequency distribution curve and indicates the number of subjects (frequency) showing a "prefixed" response to a certain dose.
3. Provides information about the individual variations within a group.
4. Provides information about the optimal therapeutic dose range to which most of the patients show the desired response. The corresponding range of plasma concentrations of the drug is called its *"therapeutic window"*.
5. Can be converted to a cumulative frequency curve by plotting the doses on the horizontal axis and the cumulative percentage of individuals showing prefixed response on vertical axis. Cumulative percentage for a certain dose is calculated by summation of the percentage of individuals responding to it and to all doses below this dose. It is a sigmoid curve that allows calculation of ED_{50} and LD_{50}.
6. Can be used to calculate ED_{50} which indicates the dose that is effective in 50% of the subjects. LD_{50} is the dose, which is lethal to 50% of the experimental subjects.

MEASUREMENT OF DRUG SAFETY

The aim of drug therapy is to produce desired beneficial therapeutic effects without producing hazardous effects. *"Therapeutic index"* is an indicator of relative safety of drug and is calculated as below (Fig. 4.11):

$$TI = LD_{50}/ED_{50}$$

Larger the LD_{50} as compared to ED_{50}, safer is the drug. *"Certain safety factor"* is a better indicator of drug's safety as it compares the dose, which is effective in 99% of individuals with the dose that is lethal in 1% of the individuals.

$$\text{Certain safety factor (CSF)} = LD_1/ED_{99}$$

Relative safety of a drug can also be expressed in terms of *"standard safety margin"*, which is calculated as below:

$$\text{Standard safety margin} = [(LD_1 - ED_{99})/ED_{99}] \times 100$$

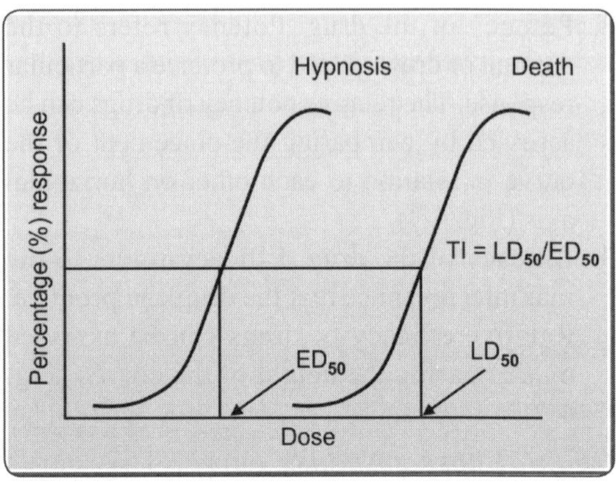

Figure 4.11 Therapeutic index

FACTORS AFFECTING DRUG RESPONSES

Drug Related Factors

The dose and the dosage form: The dose, i.e. the absolute amount of drug administered and the dosage form, i.e. the method or the form in which the drug is administered, both modify the drug responses. Increasing the amount of drug administration increases the risk of toxicity, more so in case of drugs with narrow therapeutic margin. The dosage form needs to be selected according to the pathological state to obtain optimum response. For example, sustained release preparations provide a longer duration of action.

The route of administration: The drug responses vary according to the chosen route of administration. For example, inhaled salbutamol more quickly relieves the bronchospasm as compared to orally administered salbutamol.

The dosing interval: The dosing interval may greatly affect the therapeutic outcome. For example: Once daily administration of aminoglycosides is less likely to cause ototoxicity as compared to more frequent administration during the day.

The duration of drug administration: The total duration of therapy influences the therapeutic outcome. For example, long-term glucocorticoid therapy is likely to be associated with more adverse effects as compared to short-term therapy.

The time of drug administration: The time of administration during the day can affect the response to drugs. For example: Sedatives produce sedation with smaller doses if given at night as compared to when given during the day.

Patient Related Factors

Age: The drug responses vary in relation to age and the doses required for children are different from the adult doses. In children, body surface to mass ratio is considerably higher than that of adults and accordingly doses for children are calculated on the basis of body surface area. As it may be cumbersome to calculate body surface area for all patients, nomograms can be used that provide information about body surface area based on height and weight.

Body weight: Average adult dose is calculated, based on the efficacy in 50% of adults, 18–65 years of age, and weighing about 70 kg. Therefore, abnormally lean or obese individuals require dose adjustment. This is because the proportion of body water is higher in lean as compared to obese individuals.

Sex: Drug responses may be different in males and females. For example: Barbiturates can produce excitation in females before sedation. Beta-blockers reduce libido only in males. Pregnancy and lactation may also require alteration in doses due to alterations in drug disposition. During pregnancy, plasma albumin levels reduce but plasma $\alpha 1$-acid glycoprotein levels increase. Therefore, the fraction of unbound form of the acidic drug increases but that of basic drug decreases.

Genetic variations: Some individuals may have a drug response different from the normally observed response due to genetic variations. For example, deficiency of the enzyme glucose-6-phosphate dehydrogenase predisposes to hemolytic anemia, deficient activity of pseudo-cholinesterase predisposes to apnoea in response to very small doses of succinylcholine.

Pathological state: The drug responses are modified by individual's metabolic, biochemical and pathological status usually due to changes in drug disposition. For example, patients with impaired renal functions are more likely to experience ototoxic adverse effects of aminoglycosides; patients with malabsorption show decreased absorption of amoxicillin but higher absorption of cotrimoxazole; hyperthyroid individuals are relatively less sensitive to morphine but highly sensitive to sympathomimetics.

Emotional and psychological state: Some individuals show therapeutic response to placebo (pharmacologically inactive constituents) whereas others may collapse while entering the operation theater and may show altered response to drugs due to altered emotional and psychological state.

MODIFIED DRUG RESPONSES

Drug tolerance: Tolerance refers to the inability to produce the response of same magnitude following repeated administration of a drug and an increase in dose is, therefore, required to produce the same effect. Development of tolerance causes the dose-response curve to shift parallel to the right. Intermittent dosing of some drugs like cocaine causes increased responsiveness over a period of time and this phenomenon is known as sensitization. Sensitization causes the drug-response curve to shift to left.

Development of tolerance is a relatively common phenomenon, often observed with drugs acting on the central nervous system. The tolerance may not develop to all pharmacological actions of a drug. For example, repeated use of morphine results into development of tolerance to its most pharmacological effects but not for miosis and constipation. Tolerance to a drug can be natural, acquired or cross tolerance.

Natural tolerance is genetically determined and is observed after the administration of first dose. For example, rabbits are tolerant to atropine, Blacks are tolerant to mydriatic action of sympathomimetics.

Acquired tolerance develops following repeated administration of a drug in an individual who was initially responsive to the drug. This type of tolerance can develop either due to alterations in drug disposition (known as pharmacokinetic tolerance) or due to adaptive changes in the target tissue (known as pharmacodynamic tolerance). Tolerance to some drugs results from both the pharmacokinetic and pharmacodynamic alterations.

Pharmacokinetic tolerance results when the drug reduces its own absorption, induces its own metabolism or increases its own excretion, thereby requiring larger doses to produce similar pharmacological effects after repeated administration. For example, alcohol reduces its own absorption after repeated consumption due to thickened gastric mucosa, barbiturates induce the metabolizing enzymes and increase their own metabolism, amphetamine promotes its own excretion after repeated administration as a result of acidification of urine due to reduced food intake and development of ketosis. The log plasma concentration-response curve after development of pharmacokinetic tolerance remains unchanged as the increased dose compensates of the losses in the process of drug disposition, while the relationship between plasma drug concentration and response remains unchanged.

Pharmacodynamic tolerance develops due to altered reactivity of the target tissue. After repeated administration, the response of the target tissue is less despite the same plasma level. Hence, to obtain the same degree of response higher plasma concentration is required as compared to initial plasma concentration. This is reflected by the shift of log plasma concentration-response curve to right. Some of the drugs that cause pharmacodynamic tolerance include morphine, nicotine, caffeine.

Acute tolerance or tachyphylaxis refers to development of the acute tolerance following rapid, repetitive administration of a drug at short intervals. Tachyphylaxis appears quickly after repetitive doses and the original drug response

can not be obtained even after increasing the dose. Drugs like ephedrine and amphetamine act by releasing catecholamines from storage sites. However, repeated administration of these drugs causes depletion of catecholamines from storage sites without a chance of replenishment. Therefore, following repeated administration, these drugs fail to produce the same pharmacological response. Prolonged exposure to nitrates also causes development of tolerance as is the case in workers exposed to nitroglycerine. These workers develop headache at the beginning of the week due to exposure to nitroglycerine but as the exposure continues during the week, headache disappears by Friday due to tachyphylaxis. However, when the workers return to work on Monday after staying away from nitroglycerine during the weekend, the headache reappears. Tachyphylaxis is rarely seen in clinical practice as the repetitive administration over a short period of time is not customary.

Cross tolerance can develop among the drugs belonging to the same category. For example, people tolerant to morphine are also tolerant to heroin.

Drug interactions: Concurrent administration of two or more drugs may lead to modified drug response. The modified drug response may appear as a summative effect, additive effect, synergistic effect or antagonistic effect.

Summation of the drug responses is observed when two drugs administered concurrently produce same effect by acting through two different mechanisms. Aspirin and codeine both produce analgesia but act through different mechanisms. Therefore, the degree of analgesia produced by concurrent administration of aspirin and codeine is equal to the sum of analgesic effects produced by each of them when administered individually.

Additive effect is also the sum total of the individual responses when two drugs are administered concurrently. However, the two component drugs produce the same effect by acting through same mechanism. For example, aspirin and paracetamol.

Synergistic effect is observed when the response following concurrent administration of two drugs is more than the sum total of their individual effects. The outcome of the synergistic effect may be in the form of potentiation of activity, prolongation of the duration of action or both. For example: combination of sulfamethoxazole and trimethoprim is bactericidal although each of these drugs is bacteriostatic when administered individually. This synergism is attributed to sequential action of the two drugs on two different steps in the same metabolic pathway for bacterial folic acid synthesis. Hypertensive crisis observed after co-administration of tyramine and monoamine oxidase inhibitors (MAOI) is also an example of synergistic effect. MAOIs inhibit metabolism of tyramine, which is then available in large quantities to release catecholamines causing hypertensive crisis.

Antagonism is observed when the response following concurrent administration of two drugs is less than the sum total of their individual effects. Antagonistic effects may be due to chemical antagonism, physiological antagonism, pharmacokinetic antagonism or pharmacodynamic antagonism.

Chemical antagonism appears due to chemical interaction between two drugs. For example, tetracyclines are chelated by divalent cations in antacids, thereby reducing the absorption of tetracycline. Negatively charged heparin is antagonized by positively charged protamine, which is used to terminate the action of heparin. Antacids act simply by neutralizing the acid in stomach. Deferoxamine facilitates excretion of iron by chelating with it.

Physiological antagonism refers to counter-balancing the opposite actions of two drugs on the same physiological system. This antagonism results from opposite responses and the ability of each drug to produce its own effect is uninhibited. For example: Effect of CNS depressants is antagonized by stimulants. Vasoconstrictors antagonize the effects of vasodilators.

Pharmacokinetic antagonism is observed when one drug alters the absorption, metabolism or excretion of other drug, if coadministered. Phenytoin reduces the efficacy of warfarin by inducing cytochrome enzymes and enhancing its metabolism.

Pharmacodynamic antagonism between two drugs is receptor mediated. As defined earlier, antagonists have affinity for the receptor but no intrinsic activity. They occupy the receptor and do not allow agonist to interact with it, thereby blocking the action of agonist. The receptor mediated antagonism may be of the following types:

1. Reversible (competitive or equilibrium type) antagonism: The antagonist competes with the agonist for the same receptor type and binds with it reversibly. However, if the concentration of agonist is increased the antagonism may be overcome and maximal effect can be achieved, i.e. the antagonism is surmountable. This is because the binding of antagonist is reversible and it dissociates easily from the receptors, which gradually become occupied by increasing concentration of agonist along with the spare receptors. This establishes a new equilibrium and hence is also known as equilibrium type of antagonism. As a higher quantity of agonist is required to produce the same effect in the presence of antagonist, ED_{50} increases. Presence of reversible antagonist causes the agonist dose-response curve to shift in parallel to right (Fig. 4.12). For example, atropine acts as a competitive antagonist of acetylcholine at muscarinic receptors.

2. Irreversible (non-equilibrium type) antagonism: Irreversible antagonism is observed when the antagonist binds with the same receptor as the agonist but this binding with receptor is irreversible due to covalent bonds. The strong covalent bonds make

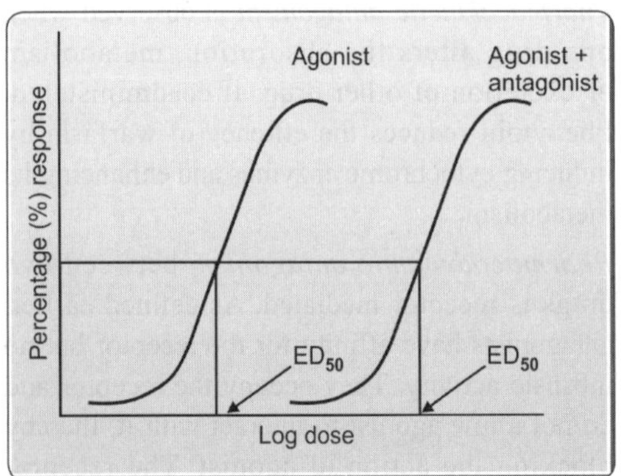

Figure 4.12 Shifting of agonist dose-response curve in presence of reversible antagonist

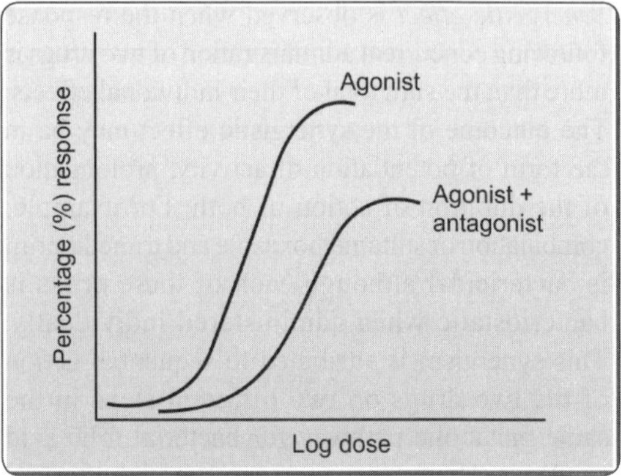

Figure 4.13 Shifting of agonist dose-response curve in presence of irreversible antagonist

the antagonist dissociate very slowly or not at all from the receptors. Therefore, by increasing the concentration of agonist, antagonist occupancy does not change to establish a new equilibrium (non-equilibrium type) and hence the antagonism can not be surmounted (insurmountable). As the higher concentration of agonist fails to overcome the antagonism, maximal effect can not be achieved and the agonist dose-response curve shifts down and to the right in the presence of irreversible antagonist (Fig. 4.13). Example; irreversible inhibition of acetylcholinesterase by organophosphate compounds. Some antagonists like phenoxybenzamine may not exhibit typical feature of irreversible antagonism initially due to smaller receptor occupancy by the antagonist and availability of spare receptors to agonist. However, eventually with increasing concentration of antagonist, typical features of irreversibility are observed.

3. Non-competitive antagonism: This type of antagonism is observed when the antagonist binds at a site other than the receptor for agonist. This binding alters the receptor configuration so that it can no longer bind with the agonist. Alternatively, the antagonist may block a particular step in the chain of events leading to agonist response. For example,

verapamil blocks Ca^{++} channels and, therefore, blocks norepinphrine-induced myocardial contraction without interacting with the β receptors.

4. Negative antagonism: These antagonists occupy the receptors and produce effects opposite to that of agonists. For example, negative antagonism of β-carbolins at benzodiazepine receptors.

OUTCOMES OF MULTIPLE DRUG THERAPY

Multiple drugs are often administered in clinical practice. This can be done either as concurrent administration of more than one drug or as a fixed dose combination of more than one drug in a single dosage form. The outcome of the multiple drug therapy may be in the form of:

i.   An adverse effect due to reduced efficacy or increased toxicity of one of the drug due to the presence of another. This type of effect is further discussed in the next section.

ii. A beneficial effect due to enhanced efficacy or reduced toxicity of one of the drug due to the presence of another. For example, combination of levodopa with carbidopa increase the availability of dopamine in brain.

iii. Interference with the diagnostic laboratory tests. For example, salicylates give a positive test for urine sugar, estrogens cause a false positive rise in serum thyroxin values.

Adverse Effects due to Drug-Drug Interactions

The drug-drug interactions manifesting in the form of reduced efficacy or enhanced toxicity may be observed in vitro or in vivo.

In vitro drug-drug interactions occur due to mixing of incompatible drugs prior to administration. For example, mixing penicillin and aminoglycosides in the same syringe.

In vivo drug-drug interactions occur due to pharmacokinetic or pharmacodynamic interaction.

Pharmacokinetic drug-drug interaction leading to adverse effects can be due to:

i. Altered absorption: Reduced tetracycline action due to chelation with antacids.
ii. Altered distribution: Excessive warfarin action due to displacement form protein binding sites by sulfonamides.
iii. Altered metabolism: Reduced efficacy of oral contraceptives due to metabolizing enzyme stimulation by rifampicin.
iv. Altered excretion: Enhanced excretion of barbiturates in alkaline urine and amphetamine in acidic urine.

Pharmacodynamic drug-drug interactions leading to adverse effects can be due to:

i. Additive or summative action: Digitalis + propranolol cause severe bradycardia.
ii. Altered ionic balance: Diuretics increase digitalis toxicity by causing hypokalemia.
iii. Altered neuronal uptake of neurotransmitters: Imipramine blocks action of clonidine by inhibiting neuronal norepinephrine uptake.

ADVERSE DRUG REACTIONS

Undesirable, untoward or adverse drug reactions can be classified into expected adverse drug reaction or unexpected adverse drug reaction.

Expected Adverse Drug Reactions (Type A–ADRs)

These are predictable adverse drug reactions that are related to pharmacological actions of the drug and are dose-related.

Side-effects are undesirable but unavoidable adverse effects observed with the therapeutic doses of drugs and are mild and dose-related. For example, promethazine when used for anti-allergic action also causes sedation, dicyclomine relieves abdominal pain but also causes dry mouth.

Secondary effects are due to major pharmacological action of drug and are predictable. For example, baclomethasone inhalation causes oral candidiasis due to reduced local immunity, broad spectrum antibiotics predispose to superinfection by suppressing the intestinal bacterial flora.

Toxicity can occur due to exaggerated pharmacological action such as due to overdoses or prolonged use and is predictable. For example, bleeding due to high doses of heparin, nephrotoxicity to aminoglycosides.

Unexpected Adverse Drug Reactions (Type B – ADRs)

These are unpredictable adverse drug reactions that are not related to pharmacological actions of the drug and are not dose-related.

Allergy or Immunologically mediated adverse drug reactions occur due to prior exposure to drug that initiates an immunological response. It can be a type I immune reaction such as anaphylaxis; type II immune reaction such as drug-induced hemolysis; type III immune reaction such as drug-induced glomerulonephritis or type IV immune reaction such as drug-induced contact dermatitis. Drugs within the same group often exhibit cross allergy.

Genetically determined adverse drug reactions are observed due to single gene mutation leading to qualitatively different drug response. For example, presence of atypical pseudocholinesterase causes excessive response to succinylcholine; isoniazid causes neurotoxicity in slow acetylators due to accumulation; deficiency of glucose-6-phosphate dehydrogenase predisposes to hemolysis by drugs with oxidizing properties like primaquine and sulfonamides; individuals deficient in uroporphyrinogen synthetase are at risk of developing attacks of intermittent porphyria when administered wit h drugs like barbiturates or phenytoin.

Idiosyncratic reactions occur in minority of individuals and can be fatal at times. Their cause is undetermined. For example, malignant hyperpyrexia in response to succinylcholine, aplastic anemia in response to single dose of chloramphenicol.

Carcinogenicity, i.e. ability of the drug to cause malignancy, is a known adverse effect with some drugs like estrogen, radio-isotopes.

Teratogenicity refers to drug-induced birth defects. Drugs like thalidomide, penicillamine, warfarin, phenytoin, valproate and many others are associated with teratogenic adverse effects.

REFERENCES

1. Frishman WH, Covey S. Penbutolol and carteolol: two new beta-adrinergic blockers with partial agonism. J Clin Pharmacol. 1990;30(5):412–21.
2. Milligan G. Constitutive activity and inverse agonists of G protein-coupled receptors: a current perspective. Mol Pharmacol. 2003;64(6): 1271–6.
3. Vauquelin G, Van Liefde I. G protein-coupled receptors: a count of 1001 conformations. Fund Clin Pharmacol. 2005;19(1):45–56.
4. Cecilia I, Calero CI, Vickers E, Cid GM, Aguayo LG, von Gersdorff H, et al. Allosteric modulation of retinal GABA receptors by ascorbic acid. J Neurosci. 2011;31(26):9672–82.
5. Zong H, Neubig RR. Regulator of G protein signaling proteins: novel multifunctional drug targets. J Pharmacol Exp Ther. 2001;297(3): 837–45.
6. Caprioli J, Sears M. The adenylate cyclase receptor complex and aqueous humor formation. Yale J Biol Med. 1984;57(3):283–300.
7. Crook RB, Riese K. Beta-adrenergic stimulation of Na+, K+, Cl- cotransport in fetal nonpigmented ciliary epithelial cells. Invest Ophthalmol Vis Sci. 1996;37(6):1047–57.
8. Jumblatt JE. Prejunctional alpha 2-adrenoceptors and adenylyl cyclase regulation in the rabbit iris-ciliary body. J Ocul Pharmacol. 1994;10(4): 617–21.
9. Bausher LP, Gregory DS, Sears ML. Alpha 2-adrenergic and VIP receptors in rabbit ciliary processes interact. Curr Eye Res. 1989;8(1): 47–54.
10. Caulfield MP, Birdsall NJM. International union of pharmacology. XVII. Classification of muscarinic acetylycholine receptors. Pharmacol Rev. 1998;50(2):279–90.
11. Alberts B, Johnson A, Lewis J, Raff M, Roberts K, Walter P. Signaling through G-protein-linked cell-surface receptors. Molecular Biology of the Cell, 4th edn. Alberts B et al. (eds.) New York: Garland Science; 2002.pp 852–62.

CHAPTER 5

Ophthalmic Formulations and Ocular Drug Delivery

OVERVIEW

Eye has unique anatomical and physiological characteristics. Administration of ophthalmic medications on the ocular surface or inside the eye requires specially formulated preparations that are compatible with ocular tissue. Ophthalmic formulations are developed to optimally deliver the active pharmaceutical agent at the targeted site in eye. The composition of formulations is designed in a way that allows easy administration and effective drug bioavailability into the ocular tissue with least amount of ocular irritation and toxic effects. It is desirable that ophthalmic preparations are free from foreign particles and microorganisms, have suitable pH, tonicity and viscosity. Moreover, the preparations should be stable and must have adequate shelf-life.

To achieve these properties in an ophthalmic formulation, appropriate selection of ingredients other than the active pharmaceutical agent in appropriate quantities is of critical importance.[1] These ingredients, known as excipients, are inactive, biodegradable and non-irritant. The commonly used excipients in ophthalmic formulations include preservatives, vehicles, tonicity agents, buffers, antioxidants and surfactant (Table 5.1). The use of excipients to impart color, odor or flavor is prohibited.

Table 5.1 Function of excipients

1. To act as solvent for active ingredient
2. To adjust required concentration
3. To adjust tonicity
4. To adjust pH
5. To prevent microbial contamination
6. To increase viscosity
7. To promote corneal/conjunctival adherence of active ingredient
8. To increase corneal drug permeation
9. To increase solubility
10. To stabilize the active ingredient and prevent its decomposition

EXCIPIENTS IN OPHTHALMIC PREPARATIONS

Preservatives

Treatment of various ocular diseases often requires patients to use topical medication multiple times a day for short-term or at times for prolonged period. To ensure the protection against the risk of contamination with microorganisms, preservatives are added to all non-surgical, multiple use topical preparations. Antimicrobial preservative in a multi-dose ophthalmic product prevent the patient from administering microbiologically contaminated product in the eye. The main criteria for selecting a preservative are:

a. It should be effective at a low concentration against broad spectrum of organisms
b. It should be soluble in the formulation
c. It should be compatible with the drug packaging components
d. It should be effective over the shelf-life.

The US Pharmacopoeia Preservative Effectiveness Test (PET) requires inoculation of preservative containing solution with 10^6 colony forming units/mL (CFU/mL) of *Staphylococcus aureus, Pseudomonas aeruginosa, Escherichia coli, Aspergillus niger* and *Candida albicans*. Each organism is tested separately. Following inoculation on day 0, survivor count is done on day 7, 14 and 28. To pass the PET requirement, preservative should be able to produce 1-log reduction on day 7, 3-log reduction on day 14 and no increase in survivor count from day 14 to day 28. Fungi should show no increase in survivor count from day 0 to day 28.

Addition of preservatives also prevents biodegradation and prolongs the shelf-life of the preparations. Although addition of preservatives provides protection against microbial contamination, their repetitive use is associated with ocular irritation, dry eyes, damage to epithelial surface and other adverse effects. The severity of adverse effects due to preservatives depends upon the type of preservative used, its concentration, frequency of use during the day and total duration of use. Various types of preservatives used in ophthalmic preparations are listed in Table 5.2.

Detergent Preservatives

Detergents interact with the lipid components of the microbial cell membrane and alter its permeability. Due to membrane instability, cell contents leak out causing cell death. The preservatives in this group include quaternary ammonium compounds like benzalkonium chloride, alcoholic and phenolic compounds and centrimonium.

Benzalkonium chloride (BAK): It is the most commonly used preservative in ophthalmic medications. It is highly stable at wide range of pH and temperature. It has a wide range of antibacterial activity and is highly effective in combating the common microbes contaminating the ophthalmic solutions. In antiglaucoma medications it is used in a concentration range of 0.004–0.02%. BAK breaks the cell-cell junctions in corneal epithelium and enhances drug

Table 5.2 Classification of preservatives used in ophthalmic formulations

Preservative group	Chemical class	Examples
Detergent preservatives	Quaternary ammonium compounds	Benzalkonium chloride, Polyquaternium-1, Centrimonium
	Alcohols	Chlorobutanol
	Phenols	Methyl/propylparaben
Oxidizing preservatives	Mercurial	Thimerosal
	Carboxylic acid	Sorbic acid
	Amidines	Chlorhexidine
Transient preservatives (oxidizing agents)	Stabilized oxychloro complex (SOC), Sodium perborate	
Ionic buffered preservatives	Combination of boric acid, zinc, sorbitol and propylene glycol	
Chelating agents	EDTA	

penetration into the anterior chamber. However, the effects of BAK are cumulative and, therefore, repeated use over a prolonged period causes damage to corneal epithelium. The damaging effects of BAK on corneal epithelial cells are dose-dependent causing cellular apoptosis at concentration as low as 0.0001% and necrosis at higher concentration. On repeated use BAK also disrupts the lipid layer of tear film. Therefore, use of medication containing BAK should especially be avoided in patients with deficient tear film or corneal epithelial abnormalities. Long-term use in antiglaucoma medications can result in toxic inflammation of ocular surface. In patients with superficial inflammation or corneal abrasion, simple measure of stopping all topical medication can promote healing.

Polyquaternium-1 (Polyquad®) is a derivative of BAK and acts in the same way as BAK. Initially, it was used in contact lens solutions. The significant difference in the action of polyquad® as compared to BAK is that although, it affects bacterial cells but is repelled by corneal epithelial cells. Therefore, repeated use is less likely to damage the ocular surface than BAK. However, polyquad® reduces the density of conjunctival goblet cells and its long-term use decreases production of the aqueous layer of tear film.

Centrimonium: It has its antibacterial action similar to BAK. The toxicity of centrimonium to ocular surface is also similar to BAK and includes keratinization and inflammatory infiltrates at the limbus and within the conjunctival stroma and epithelium. Although, it is a component of some artificial tear solutions, it is primarily used as softener in hair treatment solutions due to its antiseptic and cationic surfactant properties. It is also used as a fermentation aid, a dispersant and as preservative in antifungal creams.

Chlorobutanol: It has a wide range of antibacterial action but is less effective than BAK. It does not have surfactant action like BAK but causes bacterial cell lysis by damaging the lipid component of cell wall. Similar to BAK, it causes corneal and conjunctival cell damage, however,

the time required to produce toxic effects is longer than that due to BAK. Chlorobutanol has only limited use because of its lower efficacy and instability when stored over extended period at room temperature. It permeates through polyolefin plastic containers.

Parabens: There are esters of *p*-aminobenzoic acid and are especially effective against yeast and moulds. They have a wide spectrum of antibacterial activity and are unstable at a high pH. Parabens have been used as preservative in ophthalmic solutions, suspensions and ointments. Propyl paraben is most commonly used. Their aqueous solubility is relatively low and they may cause ocular irritation. Parabens permeate through polyolefin plastic containers.

Oxidizing Preservatives

The oxidizing agents are small molecules that penetrate the microbial cell membrane and interfere with the cellular functions by reacting with proteins, lipids and DNA. Oxidizing agents are less toxic to ocular surface as compared to detergents. The examples include thimerosal, sorbic acid, chlorhexidine. Transient acting preservatives sodium perborate and stabilized oxychloro complex (SOC) are also oxidizing agents.

Thimerosal: It is a mercury containing preservative that was used extensively in topical preparations and vaccines. However, it was found to be a common cause of allergy and its use in vaccines was associated with high incidence of autism. Because of the safety concerns, use of thimerosal in over-the-counter drugs was banned in 1998.

Sorbic acid: It is a natural organic compound. Potassium sorbate has fungistatic and limited antimicrobial properties. It has been used in ophthalmic medications and contact lens solutions. Its antimicrobial efficacy is poor and it is used in combination with other preservative. At certain concentrations, the products of sorbic acid oxidation are known to discolor some hydrophilic contact lenses. It can also cause allergic reactions.

Chlorhexidine and ***polyhexamethylenebiguanide*** have a broad range of antibacterial action like BAK. Additionally they are effective against *Acanthamoeba*. They have poor fungicidal action. They have been used in contact lens solutions. Unlike BAK, they do not cause significant alteration in corneal permeability or the tear film stability.

Transient Preservatives

These are the newer oxidative preservative systems. These compounds do not accumulate and upon exposure to tears dissipate into constituents already present in the tear film such as Na^+, Cl^-, O_2, and H_2O. They have high antibacterial activity but significantly less cellular toxicity as compared to traditional preservatives.

Stabilized oxychloro complex (SOC): It is also known as purite, is a component of a wide variety of ophthalmic medications such as artificial tears and antiglaucoma drugs. It has a broad antibacterial, antiviral and antifungal action. Chemically it consists of chlorine dioxide, chlorite and chlorate. SOC dissociates into water, oxygen, sodium and chlorine free radicals when exposed to light. The chlorine free radicals cause glutathione oxidation and inhibit microorganism protein synthesis leading to microbial cell death.

Sodium perborate: It is used in artificial tear solutions. It alters protein synthesis within bacterial cells by oxidizing cell membranes and inhibiting membrane-bound enzymes. After instillation in eye, it converts into hydrogen peroxide and then to oxygen and water. Hydrogen peroxide effectively kills microorganisms.

Ionic Buffered Preservatives

This is a newer class of preservatives that acts in the same way as oxidizing preservatives. An example in this category is a combination of boric acid, zinc, sorbitol and propylene glycol. Following instillation, contact with cations of tears converts these components into inactive forms. It is a broad spectrum antimicrobial system. The ocular surface toxicity caused by these preservatives is significantly less than the traditional preservatives and is almost comparable to that caused by preservative-free artificial tears. This preservative system has been used in travoprost formulation.

Chelating Agents

Chelating agents like disodium EDTA have the ability to bind with divalent metallic ions. EDTA is added to ophthalmic preparations to enhance the antimicrobial action of other preservatives like BAK. It does not cause significant cellular toxicity, however, allergic dermatitis may occur.

Vehicles

Ophthalmic solutions are prepared by dissolving the active ingredient in an appropriate vehicle. Purified water is the vehicle of choice for this purpose in topical preparations as all the major therapeutic agents are water soluble salts. The commonly used salt forms include hydrochloride, nitrate, sulfate and phosphate. Salicylate, hydrobromide and bitartrate salts are also used. For acidic drugs like sulfonamides, sodium salts are used. Non-aqueous liquids are rarely used as they cause ocular irritation and poor patient acceptability.

Excipients to Enhance Ocular Bioavailability

Ingredients, other than those used to dissolve the active ingredient are added to ophthalmic formulations to enhance the ocular bioavailability of drugs. Such vehicles can enhance ocular bioavailability by:

i. Increasing the corneal residence time: Viscosity enhancers and mucoadhesives, phase transition vehicles (*in situ* gelling system).
ii. Increasing the corneal permeability of drugs: Penetration enhancers

Exicipients That Increase Corneal Residence Time

Viscosity Enhancers and Mucoadhesives

A large number of vehicles are used in ophthalmic formulations primarily to increase the drug's corneal contact time either by increasing the viscosity of solution and/or by promoting its adherence to corneal surface. Viscosity enhancers increase the thickness of tear film, reduce the tear drainage and allow the drug to stay on corneal surface for a longer period. This increases the drug's bioavailability as the time for which drug stays on corneal surface increases. Hydrophilic high-molecular weight polymers are used as viscosity enhancers in concentrations that produce a viscosity of 5–100 cps. Use of viscosity enhancers in suspensions prevents particle sedimentation between uses. However, initial resuspension becomes more difficult due to high viscosity. Mucoadhesives are the high-molecular weight electrically charged polymers. They bind with the conjunctival and corneal mucin layer, stabilize the tear film and prolong the stay of drug on corneal surface. Mucoadhesive performance of several polymers is summarized in Table 5.3.

Polymers depending upon their loading capacity deliver drugs in a controlled manner over a prolonged period. This helps to achieve steady state concentration at target sites without significant fluctuations as is the case with other formulations that provide pulsed drug delivery. The polymers in controlled drug delivery systems are used either in the reservoir form or the matrix form. In the reservoir form, the polymer forms a coat around the active drug containing nucleus. In the matrix type, active drug is homogenously mixed with polymer and forms covalent or hydrogen bond with polymer molecules.

The polymers generally used as inactive vehicles with the active ingredients in artificial tear solutions help to improve tear film stability in dry eye conditions. There are several disadvantages of adding the polymers especially in high-viscosity solutions such as blurred vision due to thick layer of medication on the cornea and deposits on eyelids. High viscosity also makes the sterilization by filtration more difficult. Physical properties of vehicle are determined by molecular size, molecular weight, viscosity and presence of salts, divalent cations and anions. Some of the commonly used polymers are discussed below.

Cellulose derivatives are hydrophilic polymers. The commonly used agents in ophthalmic preparations include carboxymethyl cellulose (CMC) and hydroxypropyl methylcellulose (HPMC). CMC is a viscosity enhancer but in addition, due to its anionic charge, it promotes mucoadhesion and stabilizes tear film. The mucoadhesive property of CMC is significantly higher than other vehicles. HPMC is also a viscosity enhancer like CMC. It increases the tear film wetting time and significantly increases ocular retention time.

Table 5.3 Mucoadhesive performance of several polymers

Adhesive substances	Performance
Carboxymethyl cellulose	Excellent
Carbopol	Excellent
Carbopol and hydroxypropyl cellulose	Good
Carbopol base with white petrolatum	Fair
Carbopol 934 and EX 55	Good
Poly (methyl methacrylate)	Excellent
Polyacrylamide	Good
Poly (acrylic acid)	Excellent
Polycarbophil	Excellent
Homopolymers and copolymers of acrylic	Good
Gelatin	Fair
Sodium alginate	Excellent
Dextran	Good
Pectin	Poor
Acacia	Poor
Povidone	Poor
Poly (acrylic acid) crosslinked with sucrose	Fair

Polyvinyl alcohol (PVA) is a water-soluble viscosity enhancer and is commonly used in a concentration of 1.4%. The increase in viscosity by 1.4% PVA is only half to that of 0.5% CMC. Besides its use in ophthalmic preparations to enhance viscosity and corneal residence time, it is also used for the treatment of corneal epithelial erosions. It is nonirritating and promotes healing of abrasions.

Polyvinylpyrrolidone (PVP) is a polymer having an average molecular weight in the range of about 25,000–40,000. It is a thickening agent that increases the corneal residence time of active drug. As a lubricating agent, it is used in the treatment of dry eyes. It helps in solubilizing some drugs like chloramphenicol. Ocular irritation due to drugs like oxymetazoline reduces in the presence of PVP. It is also used as stabilizer in some ophthalmic suspensions like mefenamic acid suspension.

Sodium hyaluronate is a high molecular weight polymer. When added to ophthalmic solution it increases viscosity. Due to its high viscosity, it stabilizes tear film. After instillation, repeated blinking reduces viscosity, an effect known as 'shear thinning'. This property of sodium hyaluronate is advantageous as thinning of the solution due to blinking prevents feeling of ocular irritation. Several studies have shown that addition of sodium hyaluronate to ophthalmic solution prolongs the corneal residence time of some drugs and improves their bioavailability.

Polyacrylic acids such as carbopol gels are used in ophthalmic solutions to enhance corneal residence time of the drug. Enhanced viscosity of polyacrylic acid containing solutions decreases by increased shear rate due to blinking and eye movement. Reduced viscosity reduces ocular irritation and provides better patient acceptability. Moreover, polyacrylic acids are good mucoadhesives at the ocular surface.

Polyionic vehicles like poloxamer 407 have been used to improve the delivery of lipophilic drugs like steroids. Poloxamer has a lipophilic nucleus, which helps to deliver the lipid soluble drug to corneal surface and hydrophilic end chains that stabilize the tear film.

Cyclodextrins are used to improve the solubility and drug delivery to corneal surface. They consist of a lipophilic center to incorporate the lipid soluble drugs and adhere to corneal surface. Outer surface is hydrophilic consisting of 6–8 glucose units, which help to stabilize the tear film.

White petrolatum (60%) and liquid mineral oil (40%) mixture is used as vehicle in ointments. This molecular complex melts at body temperature and releases the active drug. Water-miscible agent lanolin is added sometimes, which allows water-soluble drugs to be retained in the ointment. Ointments are retained for a longer period in the conjunctival sac as they are cleared very slowly by tear drainage. The nonpolar oil base of ointments is readily absorbed by precorneal and conjunctival tear film. This allows increased corneal contact time and prolonged drug delivery.

Phase Transition Vehicles

These are liquids that are converted to gel form when instilled into the cul-de-sac. The polymers like lutrol FC-127 and poloxamer 407 undergo gel formation in response to change in temperature, i.e. at 37°C on the ocular surface. Cellulose acetate phthalate is a polymer that forms gel when its native pH of 4.5 rises to 7.5 after instillation in eye. Gelrite is a polysaccharide, low-acetyl gellan gum. It gels in the presence of mono or divalent cations normally present in tears. These gel forming vehicles increase the corneal residence time of the drug and prolong the drug's duration of action. Xanthan gum, a heteropolysaccharide is also used as phase transition vehicle to prolong corneal residence time of drugs.

Excipients That Increase Corneal Permeability

Penetration Enhancers

Penetration enhancers act by temporarily increasing the corneal permeability for drugs. The alteration in corneal epithelial permeability occurs either due to changes in cell cytoskeleton and tight junctions to allow better paracellular absorption or due to interaction with lipid or protein components of cell membrane to allow better transcellular permeation. Chelating agents, preservatives, surfactants and bile salts exhibit these properties but are associated with corneal toxicity.

Tonicity Agents

The ophthalmic solutions require adjustment of tonicity close to that of natural tears. The tonicity of natural tears is equal to that of 0.9% saline. Generally, a range of 0.5 to 2% saline equivalent tonicity is well tolerated by eye. Most formulations aim to achieve 0.7 to 1.5% saline equivalent tonicity. Commonly used tonicity agents are NaCl, KCl, dextrose, buffer salts, glycerin, propylene glycol and mannitol. Hypertonic solutions induce lacrimation causing immediate dilution and enhanced drainage of the drug. Hypotonic solutions are sometimes used in the treatment of dry eyes when the tonicity of natural tears is abnormally high. Hypertonic solutions are used to relieve corneal edema.

Buffers

The adjustment of the pH of the ophthalmic formulation is necessary not only for patient comfort and safety but it also stabilizes the formulation, improves solubility, enhances preservative action and increases bioavailability. The pH of normal tears is 7.4. Therefore, it is desirable to have the same pH for ophthalmic formulations. However, this is often difficult and some drugs precipitate at this pH and many are unstable. The pH is, therefore, adjusted in a way that it is as close to 7.4 as possible without affecting the stability of solution. Majority of ophthalmic drugs are salts of weak bases and are stable at acidic pH. Instillation of acidic solution is generally without much stinging sensation if the induced tearing quickly restores the pH of instilled formulation equal to that of tears. The choice of buffer system to be used is of critical importance in this regard. Preferably the buffer system should be of low-capacity so that it can maintain the acidic pH of formulation for stability but upon instillation allows tears to neutralize it. High capacity buffers resist the pH adjustment by tears and cause stinging due to presence of acidic solution on ocular surface for a longer period. The corneal endothelium is much less resistant to damage by pH variations as compared to epithelium. Therefore, the pH adjustment of intraocular formulation is extremely important. The commonly used buffers include phosphate, borate and acetate.

Surfactants

Surfactants in low concentration are added to increase the dissolution and dispersion of substances like steroids in solution. They also improve the clarity of solution. Nonionic surfactants are preferred over ionic as they are less toxic. Polysorbate 80 (Tween 80) is used in ophthalmic suspensions. Polyoxol 40 stearate and propylene glycol are used to solubilize a drug in anhydrous ointment. Some agents prevent drug loss due to adsorption to container. Other examples of surfactants include polyoxol 40, hydrogenated castor oil and cremophore EL (Table 5.4).

Table 5.4 Wetting and solubilizing agents used in ophthalmic formulations

Benzalkonium chloride	Polyoxyl 50 stearate	Polysorbate 80
Benzethonium chloride	Polyoxyl 10 oleyl ether	Sodium lauryl sulfate
Cetylpyridinium chloride	Polyoxyl 20 cetostearyl ether	Sorbitan monolaurate
Docusate sodium	Polyoxyl 40 stearate	Sorbitan monooleate
Nonoxynol 10	Polysorbate 20	Sorbitan monopalmitate
Octoxynol 9	Polysorbate 40	Sorbitan monostearate
Poloxamer	Polysorbate 60	

Antioxidants

Antioxidants are added to ophthalmic formulations containing epinephrine and other oxidizing drugs. They stabilize the formulation and prevent its degradation. Sodium sulfite and metabisulfite are used in a concentration of 0.3% in epinephrine hydrochloride and bitartrate solutions. Other antioxidants used are sodium thiosulfate, ascorbic acid and acetylcysteine.

OPHTHALMIC DRUG DELIVERY SYSTEMS

Critical Barriers in Ocular Therapeutics

Topical instillation remains the first choice in ocular drug delivery. However, due to the innate protective structure of the eye the bioavailability of an instilled drug is generally low. The cornea forms a non-vascularized barrier, which is highly resistant to passive diffusion of ions and molecules. It has a smaller surface area compared to conjunctiva, which has a leakier epithelium than the cornea. The conjunctiva not only acts as a protective covering but also functions as a passive physical barrier.[2]

The unique features of anatomical structures and physiological barriers for permeation and distribution in ocular tissue for topically applied drugs are represented in Figures 5.1 and 5.2. Relevant details are discussed in Chapter 3. Despite all the inconveniences of topical administration, this non-invasive method continues to be a favored route of drug administration in clinical practice. Thus, the development of topical ocular drug delivery systems with advances to overcome these constraints currently represents a promising approach for the treatment of ocular diseases.[3]

Physicochemical properties of drugs, such as lipophilicity, solubility, molecular size and shape, drug charge and degree of ionization, affect the mechanisms and rate of transport. Lipophilic drugs are transported through the transcellular pathway, while hydrophilic drugs penetrate through the paracellular pathway. The optimum apparent partition coefficient in octanol/buffer (pH 7.4) for corneal drug penetration was found to be in the range of 100 to 1000. The stroma is a highly hydrophilic tissue, which mostly consists of water. Due to a relatively open structure, drugs with molecular size up to 500000 can diffuse through normal stroma. Tight junctions are present in corneal endothelium but they are not as tight as those in the epithelium. It was estimated that drugs with molecular dimension up to about 20 nm can diffuse through normal endothelium. In addition to the physical barriers, ocular tissues contain metabolic enzymes, such as esterases, aldehyde and keton reductases, which may degrade and reduce the efficacy of the drugs. As a result of these anatomical and physiological constraints, after topical application, a major fraction of the administered drug is lost by different mechanisms, resulting in very low ocular bioavailability (Fig. 5.2). Systemically administered drugs also fail to achieve adequate level in ocular tissue due to blood-ocular barriers.

For transconjuctival influx and efflux, transporters such as P-glycoprotein, are known to play an important role. There is a significant systemic absorption via lymphatic and blood vessels. The lacrymal film secreted by the goblet cells of the conjunctiva not only cleanses, hydrates, lubricates and serves as a defense against the pathogens; but also, it involves an additional obstacle to any drug penetration. The lacrymal film is a dynamic fluid and undergoes a constant renewal and, therefore, limits the time of residence of the drugs on the surface of the eye.

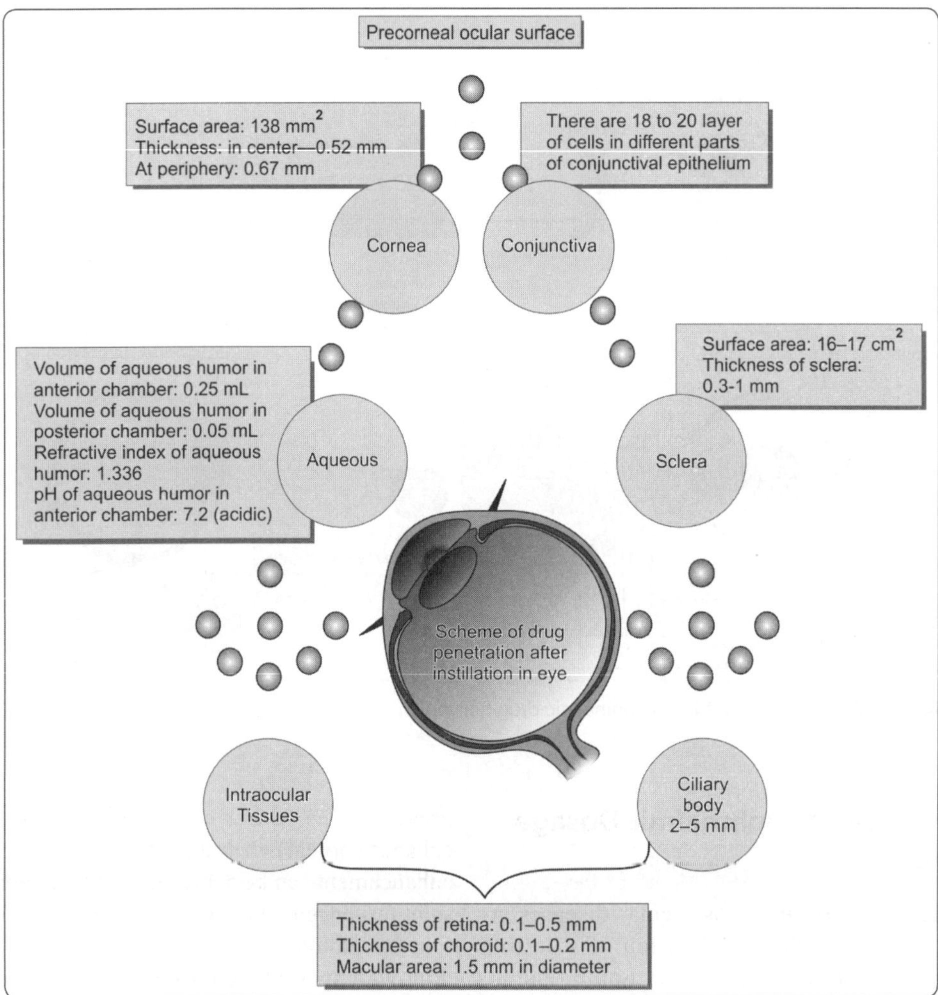

Figure 5.1 Compartmentalized scheme of drug penetration across human cornea, conjunctiva, and sclera into anterior and posterior segment of the eye

Topical Drug Delivery Systems

Ocular drug delivery systems represent an approach to control and optimize the drug delivery to target tissues in the eye. An optimum topical ocular drug delivery system would be one which can be delivered in eyedrop form without causing blurred vision or irritation and, which would need no more than one to two applications each day.[4]

The three major goals in developing topical ocular drug formulations are:

1. Enhance the drug permeation.
2. Control the release of drugs.
3. Achieve a targeted delivery.

Liquid and semiliquid forms are the most commonly used ophthalmic drug delivery systems. They are cheap, convenient to use and can be easily self-administered. However, these devices do not provide continuous drug delivery over a prolonged period, which is possible with solid drug delivery devices that are comparatively expensive and inconvenient at times. Patient acceptability in general is higher for liquid and semiliquid preparations.

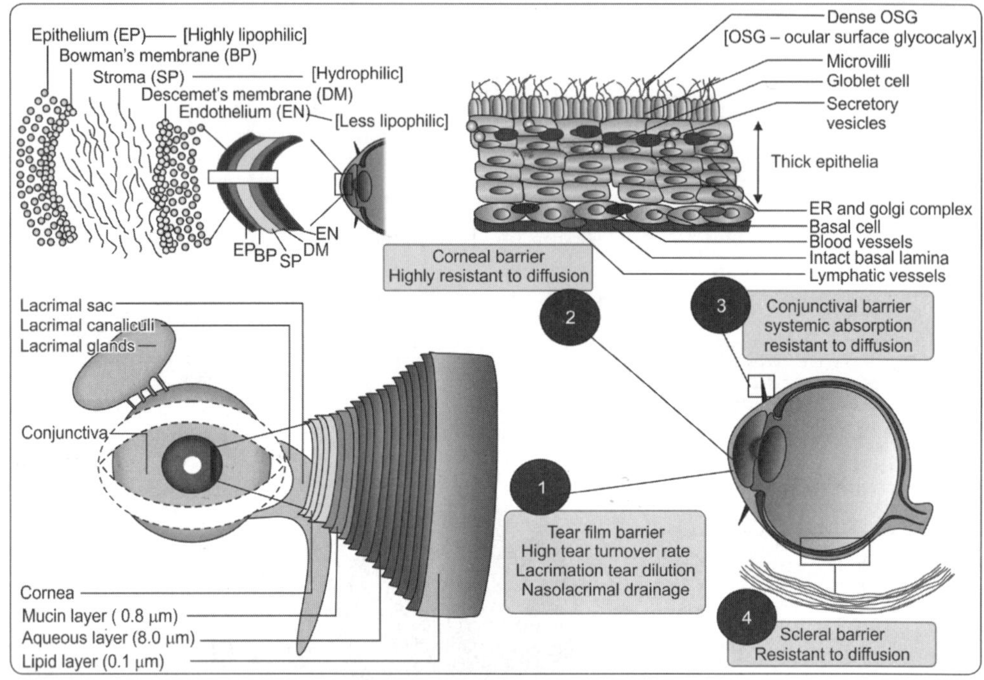

Figure 5.2 Constraints in topical ophthalmic drug delivery

Conventional Ophthalmic Dosage Forms[5]

Aqueous solutions: Most ocular diseases are treated with topical application of solutions administered as eyedrops. A homogeneous solution offers many advantages including the simplicity of large scale manufacture. The factors that must be taken into account while formulating aqueous solution include selection of appropriate salt of the drug substance, solubility, therapeutic concentration required, ocular toxicity, pKa, the effect of pH on the solubility and stability, tonicity, buffer capacity, viscosity, compatibility with other formulation ingredients, choice of preservative, ocular comfort and ease of manufacturing.

Generally aqueous ophthalmic solutions are manufactured by dissolution of the active ingredient and other inactive ingredients followed by heat sterilization or sterile filtration. Sterility of solution is further ensured by adding preservatives. Other excipients are added to enhance corneal penetration. Corneal penetration enhancement can be achieved best by increasing solution concentration, increasing corneal contact time by adding viscosity enhancers, selection of drug with appropriate pKa and offering optimal lipid solubility with the use of appropriate buffers.

The stability of ophthalmic solutions and other dosage forms determines the shelf-life and expiration dating of the product. The drug product is analyzed for physical (pH, osmolality, viscosity, color and appearance of the product), chemical (assays for the active and degradation product and preservative efficacy of the product and bioburden of all compounds) and microbiological parameters throughout the shelf-life.

Suspensions: Suspensions form an important part of the ophthalmic dosage forms and offer distinct advantages. Hydrophobic ophthalmic drugs have limited solubility in water. Formulation of a sterile, preserved, effective, stable and pharmaceutically elegant suspension is more complex and challenging compared to conventional ophthalmic solutions. Particle size of the active agent plays a key role in physical stability and bioavailability of the drug product. The rate of sedimentation, agglomeration and resuspendability are affected by particle size. Generally, the average particle size is less than 10 mm. The most efficient method of producing such particle size is by dry milling. Other methods of particle size reduction include micro-pulverization, grinding, and controlled precipitation. An ophthalmic suspension contains many excipients such as dispersing and wetting agents, suspending agents, buffers and preservatives. The selection of buffers and preservatives for suspension are similar to that of ophthalmic solutions in almost all aspects except that they must also be compatible with the flocculating systems.[6]

The formulation of ophthalmic suspension includes sterilization of the micronized active drug either by dry heat, exposure to gamma irradiation or ethylene oxide or in some cases steam sterilization of concentrated slurry followed by ball-milling. Major steps of formulating an ophthalmic suspension are:

a. Preparation of a dispersion of the drug
b. Preparation of the structured vehicle, followed by addition of the drug dispersion
c. Addition of the other adjuncts, and
d. Homogenization.

The advantages and disadvantages of using solutions and suspension are listed in Table 5.5.

Packaging and Storage

The packaging of solutions and suspensions in an appropriate container is important in determining the delivery of right amount of drug to the ocular surface. Conventional eyedroppers deliver the drops of the size ranging from 50–70 µL. Newer packages deliver antiglaucoma medications in the drops of the size 25–56 µL. Many ophthalmic medications are now dispensed in bottles with especially constructed dropper tip that allows control over the volume of each drop delivered. These dropper tips consist of an outer chamber that delivers the drop connected with an inner chamber through an aperture. The design allows only one drop to enter the outer chamber with each squeeze. A change in the outer diameter and platform width allows desired changes in the size of drops. Many ophthalmic solutions are now packaged in unit-dose dispensers to avoid toxicity due to added preservatives in multi-dose vials. The unit-dose dispensers contain about 0.1 to 0.6 mL of the solution and as there is no added preservative, they are for short-term use.

Various ophthalmic solutions and suspensions are packaged in containers that do not differ much in size and shape. Therefore, it is important to follow standardized labeling so as to facilitate clear identification of medications. Moreover, each time a medication is used the name on the label must be confirmed. The recommended color coding of various ophthalmic solutions and suspension is shown in Table 5.6. It is also important to look for the expiry date on the

Table 5.5 Advantages and disadvantages of solutions and suspensions

Formulation	Advantages	Disadvantages
Solutions	• Easy instillation • No interference with vision • Ocular irritation less than suspension/ointment	• Short corneal contact time • Contamination • Mechanical injury during instillation
Suspensions	• Easy instillation • No or minimal interference with vision • Corneal contact time longer than solution	• Require adequate shaking before use • Inconsistent drug delivery • May cause clogging of dropper tip • Ocular irritation • Contamination • Mechanical injury during instillation

label. The medications are not recommended for use after the expiry date as the ingredients may break down leading to loss of efficacy or toxicity. Eye drops if stored in refrigerator may have a prolonged shelf-life, although, the degree of ocular irritation is not affected by cold storage. Application of cold eye drops may help some patients to ensure proper instillation. Some ophthalmic preparations are better stored in inverted position. This allows air bubbles to escape on the top of the liquid and avoids interference by air bubbles while using the medication.

Ointments: Ointments are a common form of topical ocular drug delivery. They are applied to inferior fornix with patient looking up and lid retracted. Alternatively, especially in children, ointments can be applied with the help of a cotton bud to the lid margin, lashes, medial and lateral canthus. If the patient is required to use ointment in conjunction with solution, solution must be instilled first because once applied ointments do not allow the solutions to reach the precorneal tear film due to their waxy vehicle. Following application, ointments melt at body temperature and release the components, which spread over cornea. The spread of thick layer of medication over cornea may cause blurred vision. Therefore, ointments are preferably used at bed time to avoid the discomfort due to blurred vision. If a day-time application is required the amount instilled should be kept at minimum. Additionally, the ointment

can be applied to each eye on an alternating schedule. This helps to minimize discomfort due to blurred vision. The discomfort can also be avoided by applying the ointment to lid margins, lashes and canthi.

Use of ointments provides prolonged corneal contact time as compared to solutions because of two reasons.[1] After application to inferior fornix, ointments also spread over lid margin, lashes and surrounding skin depending upon the amount applied and extent of tearing due to irritation. The ointment that spreads over lid margin keeps on releasing the drug over cornea and thus enhances the drug-corneal contact time.[2] The nasolacrimal drainage of ointments is slower than that of solution, allowing drug to stay in contact with corneal surface for a longer period. Slower nasolacrimal drainage of ointments is also responsible for reduced systemic side-effects as compared to solutions.

The ointment can be applied postoperatively only if the corneal wound is tightly secured. The ointment can be used in the treatment of superficial corneal ulcers involving only the epithelial surface and with clean margins. Corneal ulcers with large flap-like overhanging margins, those with impending perforation and open conjunctival lacerations should not be treated with ointment due to the risk of entrapment of the ointment.

A typical formulation (Table 5.7) of an ophthalmic ointment includes micronization and sterilization of the active agent by dry heat, ethylene oxide irradiation or gamma irradiation. Antimicrobial preservatives like chlorobutanol or parabens are dissolved in a mixture of molten petrolatum and mineral oil and cooled to about 40°C with continuous mixing to assure homogeneity. Sterilized and micronized drug is then added aseptically to the warm sterilized petrolatum/mineral oil mixture with continuous mixing until the ointment is homogeneous. The ointment is then filled into presterilized ophthalmic tubes.

Gels: Ophthalmic gels consist of gelling-agent with high water binding affinity. Like ointments

Table 5.6 Standard colors for drug labeling and bottle caps

Drug Class	Standard Color
β-blockers	Yellow, blue, both
Mydriatics and cycloplegics	Red
Miotics	Green
Carbonic anhydrase inhibitors	Orange
Nonsteroidal anti-inflammatory drugs	Grey
Steroids	Pink
Anti-infective agents	Brown

Table 5.7 Formulation components for various dosage forms[7]

Component	Solution	Suspension	Ointment	Gel	Oral/injection	Insert
Drug	*	*	*	*	*	*
Drug carrier	#	#	#	#	#	#
Water	*	*	-	*	*	#
Buffer/acid and base	*	*	-	*	*	-
Preservative	*	*	#	*	*	-
Tonicity agent	#	#	-	#	#	-
Salts	#	#	-	#	#	-
Viscosifier	#	#	-	-	#	-
Bioadhesive agent	#	#	-	#	#	#
Phase modifier	-	-	-	*	#	-
Suspending agent	-	#	-		#	-
Solubilizer	#	-	-	#	#	-
Permeation enhancer	#	#	-	#	#	#
Wax/petrolatum/oil	-	-	-	-	-	#
Cross-linked polymer	-	-	*	-	-	*

* Component is included or generally included in the formulation, # Optional

they melt at body temperature to release the components. The blurred vision is much less as compared to ointments and they can be used during the day-time. Pilocarpine and some artificial tear preparations are available in gel form.

Nonconventional Ophthalmic Drug Delivery Systems

Polymeric Gels

Polymeric gels are classified into two distinct groups: preformed and *in situ* forming gels, both of which improve bioavailability and decrease the side-effects induced by the systemic absorption of topically applied ophthalmic drugs.

Bioadhesive Hydrogels: The efficacy of ophthalmic semisolid hydrogels is mostly based on an increase of ocular residence time, via enhanced viscosity and mucoadhesive properties.[8] Bioadhesive polymers are capable of forming strong non-covalent bonds with the mucin coating on the biological membranes and thus remain in place as long as the mucin is present. Bioadhesive polymers are usually macromolecular hydrocolloids with numerous hydrophilic functional groups. Most of the bioadhesives used in drug delivery systems are composed of synthetic mucoadhesives, including water-soluble polymers that are linear chains and water insoluble polymers that are swellable networks joined by cross-linking agents. Typically, these polymers have high molecular weight molecules (5000–10000 Da), which cannot cross biological membranes and include cellulosic components like sodium carboxymethyl cellulose (CMC), or polyanion bioadhesives like polyacrylic acid (PAA).

Hyaluronic acid (HA) is a high molecular weight biological polymer consisting of linear polysaccharides present in the extracellular matrix. In the eye, HA is present in the vitreous body and in low concentrations in the aqueous humor. HA has been shown to be a potent mucoadhesive polymer. Some investigations with the use of exogenous HA had led to the characterization of this compound as a topical pseudoplastic polymer that guarantees a better protection of the cornea.

With viscous Newtonian systems, the viscosity is independent of the shear rate. With increasing viscosity, beyond a limit, there is no further increase of the residence contact time and blinking becomes painful. On the other hand, non-Newtonian formulations that display pseudoplastic properties can acquire a viscosity decrease with increasing shear rate by blinking and ocular movement. Shear rates associated with normal blinking are quite important (ranges from 0 s^{-1} at rest to 10000 s^{-1} during blinking). Pseudoplasticity is thus interesting because it offers significantly less resistance to blinking and shows much greater acceptance than viscous Newtonian formulations. Moreover, it is widely accepted that such non-Newtonian vehicles as HA, and polyacrylic acids are more effective than Newtonian formulations containing polyvinyl alcohol or cellulose in a similar viscosity range. Furthermore, viscosity and rheological behavior are not the only factors to be considered. Mucoadhesive and wetting properties are also critical parameters to take into consideration during ophthalmic formulation.

In situ activated gel-forming systems: This can be described as viscous liquids that upon exposure to physiological conditions will shift to a gel phase. The principal advantage of this formulation is the possibility of administering accurate and reproducible quantities, in contrast to already gelled formulations and promoting precorneal retention. Three methods have been employed to cause phase transition on the eye surface: change in viscosity can be triggered by a change in temperature, pH, or electrolyte composition.[9-12] .

Sustained drug delivery can be achieved by use of a polymer that changes from sol to gel at the temperature of the eye. The poloxamers are polyols with thermal gelling properties. Their solution viscosity increases when temperature is raised to the eye temperature (33–34°C) from a critical temperature (16°C). Cellulose acetophtalate (CAP) is a polymer with potentially useful properties for sustained drug delivery to the eye. Latex is a free running solution at a pH of 4.4, which undergoes coagulation when the pH is raised by the tear fluid to pH 7.4. *In situ* activated gel-forming system has also been used with gellan gum, an anionic extracellular polysaccharide, secreted by *Pseudomonas elodea*. Gellan gum (Gelrite) formulated in aqueous solution, forms clear gels in the presence of mono or divalent cations typically found in the tear fluids.

To reduce polymer content, a combination of polymers, methylcellulose or HPMC and carbopol may also be used. The former polymers exhibit thermal gelation and the latter pH-dependent gelation. The formulation thus formed is an easy flowing formulation, which reversibly forms a gel in a sol-gel transition between 25 and 37°C, as well as with a pH increase from 4 to 7.4. A possible mechanism of the thermal effect could be a decrease in the degree of hydration of methylcellulose and a conformational change of the polymer structure with the increase in temperature. The acidic solution of polyacrylic acid can transform into a gel upon an increase in the pH by the buffering action of tear fluid.

Colloidal Systems

A liquid retention drug delivery system, can be represented by a colloidal system containing drug in carrier. Colloids consist of small particles ranging in size from 100–400 nm suspended in aqueous solution. Particle size above 10 μm gives a foreign body sensation. The particles consist of polymer complexed with the drug. Colloidal carriers act by increasing the specificity of the action of drugs towards a specific target, facilitate the bioavailability of drugs through biological membranes and protect a drug against enzyme inactivation. Corneal epithelial cells take up the particles by endocytosis and act as reservoir from which the drug is slowly released in the surrounding tissue. Thus the need to incorporate a viscous medium is eliminated. These preparations are easy to administer and require less frequent administration. Colloidal forms include liposomes, nanoparticles, niosomes, microemulsions, etc.

Liposomes: These are the more recent additions to drug delivery systems in ophthalmology. They offer a promising avenue to fulfill the need for an ophthalmic drug delivery system that has the convenience of a drop, but will localize and maintain drug activity at its site of action. Liposomes are microscopic vesicles composed of membrane-like lipid bilayers surrounding aqueous compartments. They can be multilamellar, small unilamellar and large unilamellar vesicles depending upon the number of lipid layers and size. The phospholipids used in lipid bilayer are phosphotidylcholine, phosphotidic acid, sphingomyeline, phosphotidylserine and cardiolipine. The drug, depending on its solubility characteristics, will be incorporated into either the aqueous compartment or the lipid layer. Thus, liposomes can entrap both hydrophilic and lipophilic compounds, so that it is possible to apply water-insoluble drugs in a liquid dosage form. Because of the nature of the components used for their preparation, liposomes are biocompatible and bioerodible vesicles. Liposomes are more suitable for lipophilic drugs because hydrophilic drugs tend to leak out quickly from the lipid enclosure. The storage stability of liposomes is poor. In some cases, liposomes have been shown to improve efficacy, reduce toxicity, prolong activity and provide site-specific delivery. Liposomes may not only offer a means to reformulate established drugs but also represent a novel dosage form, which can be used for new therapeutic entities unsuitable for traditional dosage form development.[13]

Biodisposition and pharmacological studies have demonstrated that vesicles carrying a positive surface charge often outperform vesicles with a neutral or negative charge. *In vitro* studies have shown that binding of liposomes to the cornea decreased in the order of positive, negative and neutral surface charge. Retention of liposomes on the corneal surface perhaps represents the major challenge for effective ocular drug delivery. Several studies, have shown that introducing a positive surface charge on vesicles can prolong precorneal retention time, enhance ocular bioavailability and ultimately increase the duration of pharmacological effect. This may be attributed to the ability of liposomes with a positive surface charge to have a more stable adsorption because corneal epithelium is thinly coated with negatively charged mucin.

Another strategy used to retard the precorneal drainage rate of liposomes has been to coat vesicles with mucoadhesive polymers. Liposomes dispersed in carbopol solutions demonstrated significantly enhanced precorneal retention compared to non-coated vesicles. This was only observed in preparations at pH 5.0 and not at pH 7.4. Decreasing the pH of the coated vesicles to 5.0 has been shown to change the initial and basal drainage rates such that there is significant increase in precorneal retention. The enhanced precorneal retention may result from the binding of polymer to the mucin. At pH 5 the adhesion is greater possibly due to protonation of the carboxyl groups, thereby permitting hydrogen-bonding between the polymer and the mucin layer.

Since the cornea has been shown to have poor endocytic activity, other proposed mechanisms by which liposomes interact with cells such as lipid exchange, contact release, adsorption and fusion, may predominate. Consequently, the rate and extent of drug release from the vesicles may be an important prerequisite for drug absorption at precorneal sites, particularly the corneal epithelium.

Nanoparticles: Nanoparticles are polymeric colloidal particles ranging in size from 10 to 1000 nm. They consist of macromolecular materials, in which the drug is dissolved, entrapped, encapsulated, and/or to which the drug is adsorbed or attached. They can be classified into two groups: nanospheres and nanocapsules. Nanospheres are small solid matricial spheres consisting of dense solid polymeric network. Drugs can either be incorporated in the matrix of the nanospheres or adsorbed onto the surface of the colloidal carrier. Nanocapsules are small capsules with a central cavity (oily droplet) surrounded by a polymeric membrane. Various polymers can be used to fabricate nanoparticles such as polyacrylamide, polymethylmethacrylate, polylactic-co-glycolic acid and E-caprolactone. All of these polymers are biodegradable and undergo hydrolysis in tears. The drug polymer binding depends upon the physicochemical characteristics of both and determines the rate of drug release. Nanoparticles are coated with bioadhesive polymers like chitosan. This prolongs the stay of particles in the cul-de-sac and corneal surface. Nanoparticles as drug carriers for ocular delivery have been found to be more efficient than liposomes and in addition to all positive features of liposomes, the nanoparticles are exceptionally stable and the sustained release of drug can be modulated.[14]

Niosomes: The niosomes are physically similar to liposomes but the vesicle membrane is made up of nonionic surfactant. Niosomes are chemically stable and entrap both the hydrophilic and lipophilic drugs. Niosomes contain nonionic surfactants, which are non-antigenic and non-toxic to the eye so they can be used over a longer period of time. The bioavailability of hydrophilic drugs is better than liposomes as the surfactant also acts as penetration enhancer. Niosomes provide site-specific drug delivery for prolonged period and are stable on storage.[15]

Discomes: The discomes are similar to niosomes but the particle size is larger (12–16 μm). Solulan C24 is the nonionic surfactant used. They are retained in the cul-de-sac and are poorly drained into the systemic circulation due to large particle size. They provide prolonged drug release of hydrophilic drugs.[16]

Microemulsions: Microemulsions are dispersions of water and oil that require surfactant and co-surfactant agents in order to stabilize the interfacial area. They have a transparent appearance, thermodynamic stability and a small droplet size in the dispersed phase (< 1.0 mm). Microemulsions are an interesting alternative to topical ocular drug delivery, because of their intrinsic properties and specific structures; they can be easily prepared through emulsification, can be easily sterilized, are stable and have a high capacity for dissolving drugs. The administration of oil-in-water microemulsions could be advantageous, because of the presence of surfactant and co-surfactant, which act as penetration enhancers. Moreover, microemulsions achieve sustained release of a drug applied to the cornea and higher penetration into the deeper layers of the ocular structure and the aqueous humor than the native drug. Additional advantages of these systems include: low viscosity, a greater ability as drug delivery vehicles and increased properties as absorption promoters. The possibility of prolonged release of drugs in microemulsions makes these vehicles very attractive for ocular administration and can greatly decrease the frequency of application of eye drops. Besides this, the low surface tension of microemulsions also guarantees a good spreading effect on the cornea and mixing with the precorneal film constituents, thus possibly improving the contact between the drug and the corneal epithelium. Some of the developed microemulsions also presented a viscosity value that allows sterile filtration and easy dispensing as eye drops.

Other Drug Delivery Systems

Cyclodextrins

The pharmaceutical use of cyclodextrins (CD) is confined mainly to the complexation of problematic drugs (poorly soluble, unstable, irritating, and difficult to formulate substances). CD complexation generally results in improved wettability, dissolution, solubility, stability and reduced side-effects.[17] CDs are a group of homologous cyclic oligosaccharides with a hydrophilic outer surface consisting of six, seven or eight glucose units. Although soluble in water, CDs have a lipophilic cavity in the center. They form inclusion complexes with many lipophilic drugs by taking up a drug molecule, or part of it, within the lumen, resulting in an increase in solubility. The first cyclodextrins studied, had relatively low aqueous solubility and were shown to cause hemolysis and nephrotoxicity, These cyclodextrins had only limited use. Among cyclodextrin derivatives, hydroxypropyl-fl-cyclo-dextrin has been shown to be the most favorable in the hemolysis study on human erythrocytes.

Inserts

Inserts can be erodible or non-erodible. They have proven long duration of release and ability to modify drug bioavailability when compared with their solution dosage forms. Although, inserts have shown therapeutic success, they are not well tolerated by patients, and considering their high cost per dose, are not perceived as desirable next-generation topical ocular drug delivery systems.[18]

Ocusert® (Alza Corporation) is an insoluble ophthalmic insert classified in the group of diffusional systems. It consists of a central reservoir of drug (e.g. pilocarpine) enclosed between two semipermeable membranes, which allow the drug to diffuse from the reservoir at a precise rate for a period of 7 days. Prolonged reduction in intraocular pressure was achieved with a single Ocusert® in patients with open-angle glaucoma. Because of the insolubility of the Ocusert® device, it must be removed after use. The inserts were well tolerated but after prolonged wear they tend to swell and partially fragment. Now it is recommended that they not be worn for more than 12 hours, despite the potential for prolonged release over several days.

Lacrisert is a solid artificial tear preparation measuring about 1 mm in width, 4 mm length and contains 5 mg of hydroxypropyl cellulose without preservative. It is packaged in dehydrated form and with the help of an applicator is inserted into the inferior fornix. After insertion it imbibes tear fluid, swells and is converted to a gelatinous mass. This gelatinous mass keeps on releasing the polymer over 24 hours. Lacrisert is useful in the treatment of moderate to severe dry eyes. Some amount of basal tear secretion is necessary for lacrisert to act and in eyes with absolute tear deficiency lacrisert fails to provide therapeutic benefit. Although, once a day application provides sufficient relief of symptoms, some patients may require twice a day insertion. Lacrisert is generally well tolerated and displacement of the device is uncommon. The most common problems encountered during its use are foreign body sensation and blurred vision due to spread of polymer over cornea.

A collagen shield is a soluble insert, which offers the advantage of being entirely soluble so that it does not need to be removed from its site of application, thus limiting the interventions to insertion only. Collagen shields are made up of porcine or bovine scleral collagen. They are thin membranes ranging in diameter from 14.5–16 mm. The water content varies from 63–85%. They are packaged as dehydrated shields. Before insertion they are soaked for about 3 minutes in saline, lubricant or drug solution. The rehydrated shield upon insertion takes the shape of cornea. Initial insertion may be uncomfortable and may require use of a local anesthetic. Following insertion, collagen shields undergo dissolution by the enzymes in tear film and release the drug on ocular surface. Dissolution time depends upon the amount of cross-linking in its material and varies from 12–72 hours for different preparations. The oxygen permeability of collagen shields is comparable to that of hydroxyethyl methacrylate lens of similar water content.

For conditions requiring prolonged drug delivery to ocular surface collagen shields are more effective, convenient and safe devices as compared to multiple daily eye drops, daily subconjunctival injections or soft contact lenses. However, collagen shields are expensive and are available in a limited number of base curves and diameters, which may not be suitable to fit on all corneas. They can cause foreign body sensation and allergy. Using collagen shields to deliver a combination of drugs may be problematic due to drug-drug interactions. They should be used with caution in patients with compromised corneal endothelium and cases of significant chemical burn.

Prodrug (Chemical Delivery System)

Use of prodrug molecules of some drugs allows better corneal drug permeation. It also gives selective and site-specific drug delivery. Some of the drugs used in prodrug forms include epinephrine, phenylephrine, albuterol. Soft-drugs, unlike prodrugs, are active drugs, which are designed to undergo a predictable and controllable deactivation *in vivo*. An example of ophthalmic application of the soft-drug approach is metoprolol. If the prodrug approach is applied to a soft-drug the resulting drug is known as a 'pro-soft drug'. A chemical delivery system (CDS) or site-specific CDS is an inactive drug derivative, which undergoes several predictable enzymatic transformations via inactive intermediates and finally delivers the active drug to the site of action. Ophthalmic applications of a CDS include adrenolone esters (CDS of adrenaline), propanoloneoxime (CDS of propanolol) and alprenoxime (CDS of alprenolol).

Prodrugs were introduced in ophthalmology about 30 years ago when ocular absorption of epinephrine was substantially improved by its prodrug, dipivefrine. Currently, it has replaced epinephrine in the treatment of elevated intraocular pressure associated with glaucoma. Since dipivefrine, numerous prodrugs have been designed to improve the efficacy of ophthalmic drugs, to prolong their duration of action and/ or to reduce the systemic side-effects. Prodrugs have been tested experimentally and clinically but stability and solubility problems as well as local irritation after topical application have limited their efficacy and clinical acceptability.[19] An ideal ocular prodrug should be stable and soluble in aqueous solutions to enable formulation, sufficiently lipophilic in order to penetrate through the cornea, non-irritant, and able to release the parent drug within the eye at a rate that meets therapeutic need.

POSTERIOR SEGMENT DRUG DELIVERY SYSTEMS

Iontophoretic Devices

Numerous iontophoretic devices with different capabilities are commercially available. The most basic of these units consist of two electrodes, a power source, timers, and an ampere meter for measuring current output. As iontophoresis is not entirely without risks, efforts are continuously made to develop systems that can substantially reduce, if not eliminate, any risk of injury caused by use of the device. The systems discussed below represent a small sampling of those available.

Coulomb Controlled Iontophoresis (CCI)

The amount of drug delivered by iontophoresis depends on the current density, duration of treatment, drug concentration, pH, and the permeability of the tissue for the drug molecule. As current is being applied, the damage to tissues caused by heat may affect the hydration level of the tissue. With time, the resistance may change in the damaged tissue, resulting in variable electrical fields. Thus, the iontophoretic character of the drug being applied changes with time. The CCI system was developed to avoid these problems.[20] The CCI iontophoretic system produces and maintains a constant electrical field across the conjunctival epithelium, allowing a constant drug flow (i.e. electrical current) during transscleral iontophoresis. The ability of the CCI system to automatically adjust to changes in resistance is a major advantage over other iontophoretic delivery methods. Poor probe contact or disruption of the circuit is indicated by an audio-visual alarm, and the instrument continuously records the total Coulombs delivered, thus ensuring a calibrated and controlled delivery of drug.

Mini-ion Iontophoretic Unit

The mini-ion device is portable and can be operated by battery or external electrical source. The mini-ion device applies a variable electrical current in the range of 0.1–1.0 mA for preset periods of 10–120 s. The device uses a disposable drug-loaded hydrogel probe to safely deliver doses of charged drugs to different segments of the eye following transscleral iontophoresis.[21]

EyeGate

The EyeGate iontophoresis device/applicator is made of medical grade, soft silicone rubber and is designed to closely fit the human eye contour and palpebral conjunctival opening. The applicator has an annular shape; the diameter of the proximal part is slightly larger than the limbus, while the distal part covers 2 mm of the anterior sclera behind the limbus. The annular well of the device (0.5 cm^3) contains a pure tungsten electrode immersed in the solution.[22] The drug solution is infused into the applicator *via* two silicone tubes, one of which is a drainage tube that generates a slight suction to maintain the applicator in perfect contact with the conjunctiva and ensures a constant flow of drug inside the cup. Vanes located between the walls prevent the electrode from touching the eye, but allow drug contact with the conjunctiva and sclera (fluidic surface of 0.5 cm^2). The drug solution does not cover the corneal surface and vision is not impaired during treatment, which makes treatment more comfortable for the patient.

Electrical Fields

The basis of electrophoresis, electroporation, or iontophoresis is the use of an electrical field to enhance delivery of substances into and/or across support media, cell membranes or tissues. The DNA and RNA, being hydrophilic and highly charged at neutral pH, would be ideal molecules for enhanced ocular drug delivery by electrical fields. It has been demonstrated that small RNA or DNA (up to 8 million Daltons) synthetic oligonucleotides could be driven across the human sclera by an electrical field.[23] The sclera has many microscopic to molecular-scale, water-filled pores. The pores in the sclera are large enough for nucleic acids to wander through under the influence of an electrical field.

Scleral Implants

Sustained release scleral implants provide controlled drug release that is achieved by a polyvinyl alcohol membrane. It has been observed that in terms of the drug release profile, an implant with a non-biodegradable polymer membrane is more controllable than one using a biodegradable polymer. Since non-biodegradable devices could release drugs over a longer period of time, these systems may be well suited for the treatment of chronic ocular diseases, such as age-related macular degeneration and diabetic retinopathy.[24] This system may be more useful than the intravitreal drug delivery systems in delivering the drug more effectively to the macular region without increasing drug concentration in the aqueous humor and site-specific treatment in the retina-choroid.

Transdermal Systems

Transdermal therapeutic systems (TTS) enable one to avoid the peaks and valleys in the drug plasma levels that occur with oral dosing. Large variations in the plasma levels of any drug may cause unwanted side-effects. A new TTS for delivery of ocular drugs has been reported for prednisolone.[25] The results suggested that the prednisolone-TTS was more effective than conventional topical or oral administration. Furthermore, the ocular bioavailability and tissue concentration profiles suggest that other ocular hydrophobic drugs similar to prednisolone may be amenable to TTS delivery. Thus, TTS delivery of ocular drugs may be a safe and effective method for treating chronic posterior segment diseases.

Photodynamic Therapy

Photodynamic therapy plays an important role in the treatment of neovascular age-related macular degeneration. The method requires intravenous administration of a photosensitive dye, verteporfin. The dye accumulates in the neovascular tissue and is activated by exposure to non-thermal light at 689 nm. This activation generates free radicals, which cause cell death and occlusion of abnormal new vessels. The method helps in destroying the neovascular tissue with minimal or no damage to normal vasculature.

MODES OF ADMINISTRATION OF TOPICAL OPHTHALMIC FORMULATIONS

The most common route of drug administration in ophthalmology is by topical application and, therefore, several modes of topical application are in use. Instillation of liquid ophthalmic formulations is the most commonly employed method. The method of topical instillation is described in Chapter 2. The modes of topical administration other than instillation are described here.

Sprays

Sprays are the alternative method of delivering ophthalmic solutions to eye. They are less irritating than solutions. The spray device is held at a distance of 5–10 cm from eye and the lid margins of gently closed eyes are sprayed. Subsequently, patient is asked to blink several times over 10–15 seconds. A stinging sensation is an indicator of the presence of drug in precorneal tear film. If no stinging sensation is experienced a second application is required.

Mydriatic and cycloplegic combinations such as phenylephrine-tropicamide or phenylephrine-tropicamide-cyclopentolate can be used in the form of spray. Their efficacy is as good as that of solutions and risk of contamination is negligible. Application with eyes closed allows only minimum quantity to reach the precorneal tear film. Ocular irritation is less and patient acceptability is high especially with pediatric patients.

Extraocular Irrigation

Extraocular irrigation with copious amount of fluid is required in the treatment of acute chemical burns, to remove foreign body, dye or viscous fluid used in gonioscopy. With patient in supine position and head tilted towards the side to be irrigated, extraocular irrigation fluid at room temperature is delivered to the surface of eye from a simple container. The fluid flowing out of the eye is removed or collected in tissue, towel or a collecting pan. The method is easy to use and cost-effective but requires an attendant to carry out the irrigation. For patients who require long-term irrigation and especially those who are not ambulatory, continuous irrigating system is used. This irrigation system consists of a polyethylene tube, which is inserted through the lid and is placed in lower fornix. The other end of tube is anchored to the skin by stitches or tapes and connected with an overhead reservoir, from which fluid flows into the eye. The flow can be controlled with the help of an adaptor attached to tubing. The system is usually well tolerated with no apparent discomfort. In cases where lid penetration by tubing is not desirable, other measures such as loops, rings, tubes and heptic contact lens shells are used.

Lid Scrubs

Lid scrubs consist of solutions and ointments applied directly to lid margins with the help of a cotton-tipped applicator. Baby shampoo or other eyelid cleansers are used to clean the lid margins in contact lens users or to remove oil, debris and desquamated skin in inflamed eye. Use of lid scrubs is especially helpful is cases of blepharitis and the efficacy is better as compared to instillation of drops or ointment in the inferior fornix. Antibiotics can also be used as scrubs. The commercial preparations available as lid scrubs should not be instilled directly into the eye.

Filter Paper Strips

Ophthalmic dyes such as fluorescein sodium, rose bengal and lissamine green are available as drug-impregnated filter paper strips. The strips are moistened with a drop of saline or extraocular irrigating solution and are touched with the superior or inferior bulbar conjunctiva or inferior fornix. The method allows easy administration of adequate amount of drug. Administration of excessive quantity of drug is avoided. Importantly, the methods helps in avoiding contamination due to use of solution especially the risk of contamination of sodium fluorescein with *Pseudomonas aeruginosa* is eliminated. Separate filter paper strips should be used for two eyes to avoid cross-contamination.

Cotton Pledgets

Cotton pledgets are thin and elongated cotton bodies. They are soaked in ophthalmic solution and placed in inferior fornix. Prolonged drug delivery and corneal contact time is achieved. They cause foreign body sensation and at present are used for prolonged delivery of mydriatics in cases with slow dilating pupil, to break posterior synechiae or for sector dilation in inferior pupillary quadrant.

Contact Lenses

Disposable soft contact lenses are used for topical drug delivery and this device is extremely useful in the treatment of conditions like dry eyes, bullous keratopathy and conditions requiring corneal protection. Drug-impregnated hydrogel lenses do not offer any significant advantage over topical application of solutions or suspensions but soft lenses presoaked in ophthalmic solution are efficient devices for topical drug delivery. The extent of drug permeation into the lens material depends upon the size of pores within the lens material, molecular size of drug, water content of lens, thickness of lens, concentration of drug in the soaking solution and soaking time. If the pore size of the lens material and the molecular size

of drug are complementary to each other, better drug permeation occurs. Lenses with high water content absorb higher amounts of water soluble drugs. Thicker lenses absorb and store greater amount of drug whereas thinner lenses allow greater amount of drug to enter precorneal tear film. Higher concentration of soaking solution and longer soaking time allows greater drug permeation into the lens. The efficacy of soft contact lenses as drug delivery devices has been found to be as good as subconjunctival injections. Use of hydrogel contact lenses in conjunction with ophthalmic solutions containing benzalkonium chloride has also been found to be clinically acceptable.

REFERENCES

1. Feldman EG. In: Handbook of Nonprescription Drugs/Nonprescription Products: Formulation and Features, 11th edn. Washington, DC, APhA, 1982; pp. 417–50.
2. Maurice DM, Mishima S. Ocular Pharmacokinetics. In: Sears ML (ed). Handbook of Experimental Pharmacology, vol. 69, Springer Verlag, Berlin-Heidelberg, 1984; pp. 116–9.
3. Fuente MDL, Ravina M, Paolicelli P, Sanchez A, Seijo B, Alonso MJ. Chitosan-based nanostructures: A delivery platform for ocular therapeutics. Adv. Drug Deliv Rev. 2010;62:100–17.
4. Ali Y, Lehmussaari K. Industrial perspective in ocular drug delivery. Adv Drug Deliv Rev. 2006;58:1258–68.
5. Olejnik O. Conventional systems in ophthalmic drug delivery. In: Mitra AS (ed). Ophthalmic Drug Delivery Systems, Marcel Dekker, Inc.; 1993. p. 177–98.
6. Bapatla KM, Hecht G. Ophthalmic ointments and suspensions. In: Lieberman HA, Rieger RM, Banker GS (Eds). Pharmaceutical Dosage Forms: Disperse Systems, vol. 2, Marcel Dekker, Inc., 1996. P. 357–97.
7. Lang JC. Ocular drug delivery conventional ocular formulations, Adv Drug Deliv Rev. 1995;16:39–43.

8. Kreuter J. Nanoparticles as bioadhesive Ocular drug delivery systems. In: Lenaerts V, Gurny R, (eds). Bioadhesive Drug Delivery Systems, Boca Raton, FL, CRC Press; 1990. pp. 203–12.

9. Miller SC, Donovan MD. Effect of poloxamer 407 gel on the miotic activity of pilocarpine nitrate in rabbits. Int J pharm. 1982;12:147–52.

10. Gurny R. Preliminary study of prolonged acting drug delivery. Pharm Acta Helvetica. 1981;56 (4-5):130–2.

11. Gurny R, Ibrahim H, Aebi A, Buri P, Wilson CG, Washington N, et al. Design and evaluation of controlled release systems for the eye. J Contr Rel. 1985;2:353–61.

12. Gurny R, Boye T, Ibrahim H. Ocular therapy with nanoparticulate systems for controlled drug delivery. J Contr Rel. 1987;6:367–73.

13. MeisnerD, Mezei, M. Liposome ocular delivery systems, Adv Drug Deliv Rev. 1995;16:75–93.

14. Zimmer A, Kreuter J. Microspheres and nanoparticles used in ocular delivery systems, Adv Drug Deliv Rev. 1995;16:61–73.

15. Mahale NB, Thakkar PD, Mali RG, Walunj DR, Chaudhari SR. Niosomes: Novel sustained release non-ionic stable vesicular systems- An Overview, Adv Colloid Interface Sci. 2012;183-184:46–54.

16. Vyas SP. Discoidal niosome based controlled ocular delivery of timolol maleate, Pharmazie. 1998;53:466–9.

17. Szejtli L. Medicinal applications of cyclodextrins. Med Res Rev. 1994;14(3):353–86.

18. Urquhart J. Development of the OCUSERT pilocarpine ocular therpeutic systems: a case history. In: Robinson J, (ed). Ophthalmic Delivery Systems. APhA Publishers, Washington, D.C. 1980. pp. 105–18.

19. Jarvinen T, Jarvinen K. Prodrugs for improved ocular drug delivery, Adv Drug Deliv Rev. 1995;19:203–24.

20. Behar-Cohen FF, El-Aouni A, Gautier S, David G, Davis J, Chapon P, et al. Transscreal coloumb-controlled iontophoresis of methylprednisolone into the rabbit eye: Influence of duration of treatment, current Intensity and drug concentration on ocular tissue and fluid levels, Exp Eye Res. 2002;74:51–9.

21. Eljarrat-Binstock E, Raiskup F, Frucht-Pery J, Domb AJ. Hydrogel probe for iontophoresis drug delivery to the eye, J Biomater Sci Polym. 2004;15:397–413.

22. Halhal M, Renard G, Courtois Y, Ben Ezra D, Behar-Cohen F. Iontophoresis: From lab to the bed side, Exp Eye Res. 2004;78:751–7.

23. Ambati J, Gragoudas ES, Miller JW, You TT, Miyamoto K, Delori FC, et al. Transcleral delivery of bioactive protein to the choroid and retina, investig. Ophthalmol Vis Sci. 2000;41:1186–91.

24. Yasukawa T, Ogura Y, Tabata Y, Kimura H, Wiedmann P, Honda Y. Drug delivery systems for viteroretinal diseases. Prog Retin Eye Res. 2004;23:253–81.

25. Isowaki A, Ohtori A, Matsuo Y, Tojo K. Drug delivery to the eye with a transdermal therapeutic System, Bio Pharm Bull. 2003;26:69–72.

CHAPTER 6

Mydriatics and Cycloplegics

OVERVIEW

Mydriatics and cycloplegic drugs, both dilate the pupil (mydriasis). Additionally, cycloplegics paralyze the ciliary muscle and cause loss of accommodation (cycloplegia), i.e. inability to focus on the near objects. Mydriatics and cycloplegics are widely used drugs in ophthalmology for diagnostic and therapeutic purposes.

MECHANISM OF ACTION

The diameter of pupil is controlled by two sets of muscles: dilator pupillae and sphincter pupillae. The dilator pupillae consists of radial fibers and is innervated by sympathetic nervous system. The adrenergic receptors in the dilator pupillae are mainly α and a few β (β_2-receptor subtype). Sympathetic control of ciliary muscle action is not well established. However, there is some evidence that sympathetic stimulation of ciliary muscle antagonizes accommodation in human eye.[1-2]

Sphincter pupillae consists of circular fibers and is innervated by parasympathetic (cholinergic) nerves. Parasympathetic nerves also innervate ciliary body and lacrimal glands. Therefore, parasympathetic activation causes not only the contraction of sphincter muscle leading to pupillary constriction but also causes ciliary muscle contraction leading to spasm of accommodation and stimulation of tear secretion.

Cholinergic receptors in sphincter and ciliary muscle are of muscarinic type with predominance of M_3 subtype.[3] Sympathetic input to eye is relatively small as compared to parasympathetic input and maintains a persistent tone in dilator muscle, aiding relaxation of the sphincter and pupillary dilatation. The time course of the sympathetic responses is slower as compared to parasympathetic responses and takes about 30–40 seconds to reach the peak effect. Parasympathetic responses reach the peak effect within 1–2 seconds.

Sympathomimetic drugs cause contraction of radial fibers of dilator pupillae and, thereby, cause mydriasis. Sympathomimetic drugs have little effect on accommodation and light reflex remains intact. Sympathomimetics also affect the width of palpebral fissure, diameter of ocular blood vessels and aqueous flow. Cholinergic antagonists act by blocking the muscarinic receptors, which are present on both the sphincter pupillae and ciliary muscle, thereby, producing pupillary dilatation and paralysis of accommodation. Sympathomimetics are comparatively weak mydriatic agents and in people with an iris difficult to dilate, such as diabetics or blacks, stronger antimuscarinic agents are used. Mydriatics can raise the intraocular pressure and can precipitate glaucoma in predisposed individuals.

USES: DIAGNOSTIC AND THERAPEUTIC

Mydriatics and cycloplegic drugs are primarily used to
1. Facilitate ophthalmoscopic examination of the lens periphery, vitreous and retina.
2. Paralyze the ciliary muscle in young patients as an aid for refraction.
3. Dilate the pupil and paralyze the ciliary muscle in uveitis; to prevent formation of synechia and relieve the symptoms of pain and photophobia.

When used for diagnostic purpose, mydriatics allow examination of small details, which are of great diagnostic importance such as diabetic microaneurysms, hypertensive arteriolar attenuation, small retinal holes and other peripheral lenticular and retinal lesions. A reasonably good examination of optic disc and retinal vessels can be performed through an undilated pupil especially in young adults with spontaneously large pupils but in elderly patients dilatation is frequently required. Moreover, the risk of missing an important diagnostic finding by failing to dilate is more than the risk of precipitating glaucoma by dilating the pupil. Therefore, it is important to perform mydriasis in appropriate cases and it is a moral and legal duty of the optometrists to refer the pathological conditions for medical attention. Some of the indications and contraindications for the use of mydriatics are listed in Table 6.1 and 6.2.

COMMONLY USED MYDRIATICS AND CYCLOPLEGICS

The mydriatics and cycloplegics commonly used in clinical practice are:
1. Sympathomimetics: Phenylephrine, hydroxyamphetamine.
2. Antimuscarinic: Atropine, homatropine, hyoscine, cyclopentolate, tropicamide.

Phenylephrine

Phenylephrine is an α-adrenergic agonist and is the only sympathomimetic mydriatic in clinical use.

Table 6.1 Indications for the use of mydriatics for diagnostic purposes

1. Sudden decrease in visual acuity
2. Unexplained loss of visual field
3. Diabetes mellitus
4. Symptoms of floaters, photopsia, metamorphopsia, spots, shadows
5. Ocular pain in the absence of elevated intraocular pressure (IOP)
6. Red eye that can not be attributed to infection, allergy of elevated IOP
7. Recent blunt ocular trauma (except when hyphema is present)
8. Myopia > 6D or when degenerative changes are present
9. Media opacities making posterior segment examination difficult
10. Retinal diseases, detachment, tears
11. Vitreous hemorrhage
12. Peripheral lenticular opacities

Table 6.2 Contraindications for the use of mydriatics

1. A known or suspected case of angle closure glaucoma
2. Abnormally narrow anterior chamber angle
3. Active corneal disease
4. Iris fixation lens pseudophakia
5. Hyphema
6. Suspected penetrating ocular injury
7. Conditions when pupil reactions need to be preserved such as head injury, recent neurological anomalies, iris trauma
8. Known hypersensitivity to a mydriatic drug

It causes contraction of dilator pupillae causing pupillary dilatation, constriction of conjunctival vessels causing blanching and contraction of Muller's muscle causing widening of palpebral aperture.[4,5] The effect of phenylephrine on accommodation is relatively weak . It is available in single-use units in concentrations of 2.5 and 10%. As a mydriatic agent, higher efficacy of 10% phenylephrine as compared to 2.5% is not established. However, higher concentration is more often associated with adverse effects. Following topical application, mydriasis begins in about 10 minutes and reaches peak in 45–60 minutes. The pupil returns to pre-instillation size in 6–7 hours. These times can vary significantly. Diabetics dilate slowly and less widely as compared to non-diabetics. Phenylephrine 10% has shown significantly higher efficacy as compared to 2.5% concentration in diabetics. People with dark iris tend to develop mydriasis slowly but for a longer duration as the drug binds to pigment in iris. It produces less effect on accommodation as compared to muscarinic antagonists.

In addition to its uses as mydriatic agent, phenylephrine is also used for other therapeutic purposes. Phenylephrine causes blanching of superficial conjunctival blood vessels (whitening of the eye) and in very low concentrations (0.125%), it is used as ocular decongestant. In a concentration of 10% phenylephrine is applied topically for breaking synechiae.[4] Topical 10% solution is also used for peripheral corneal vasoconstriction during LASIK surgery. Phenylephrine 2.5% in combination with ecothiophate can be used to prevent the formation of miotic cysts in the treatment of open-angle glaucoma or accommodative estropia.[6] The mechanism involved in prevention of cyst formation is not known. Phenylephrine also causes widening of palpebral fissure by stimulation of Mueller's muscle and ptosis resulting from sympathetic denervation such as in Horner's syndrome may respond favorably. Phenylephrine 1% is also used in the diagnosis of Horner's syndrome.[7] It causes marked pupillary dilatation in the eye with postganglionic sympathetic denervation but minimal or no dilatation in normal eye. If the lesion is central or preganglionic, the pupil behaves in the same way as in the normal eye.

Adverse Effects

Topical use of phenylephrine may give rise to local as well as systemic adverse effects.

Ocular adverse effects: Local adverse effects of phenylephrine include stinging, pain, lacrimation and keratitis. Phenylephrine can cause allergic dermatoconjunctivitis giving a scalded appearance around the eye. It can cause transient corneal edema. In elderly patients, phenylephrine causes rebound miosis and re-instillation at this time gives a slow response. Long-term repeated use results in slow and less intense mydriasis. In elderly patients, phenylephrine has been shown to cause release of pigment from iris, which appears as aqueous floater in about 30–40 minutes and disappears in 12–24 hours.[8] Long-term use of low concentrations as ocular decongestants also causes rebound conjunctival congestion.

Skin pallor due to cutaneous vasoconstriction caused by over spilling phenylephrine 2.5% eye drops was reported in premature neonates.[9] Blepharoconjunctivitis and dermatitis due to phenylephrine eyedrops has also been reported.[10]

Systemic adverse effects: Phenylephrine 10% has been shown to cause rise in mean arterial blood pressure in dogs.[11] Elderly patients especially those with cardiovascular disease are prone to develop acute rise in blood pressure following topical application of 10% phenylephrine.[12] Neonates and insulin-dependent diabetics with vascular disease and autonomic dysfunction also respond similarly to 10% phenylephrine.[13,14] Other systemic adverse effects of 10% phenylephrine include occipital headache, ventricular arrhythmias, tachycardia, reflex bradycardia, subarachnoid hemorrhage, ruptured aneurysm, skin blanching.

Cardiovascular adverse effects of topical 10% phenylephrine can be potentiated in patients receiving tricyclic antidepressants and monoamine oxidase inhibitors. Patients on reserpine, methyldopa and guanethidine also show excessive pressor response to phenylephrine due to denervation hypersensitivity. Phenylephrine 2.5% is rarely associated with systemic adverse effects and is recommended for routine clinical use. The guidelines for the use of 10% phenylephrine are outlined in Table 6.3.[12,14,15]

Table 6.3 Guidelines for the use of 10% phenylephrine

1. Use with caution in patients with cardiac disease, hypertension, insulin-dependent diabetes mellitus, aneurysm, advanced atherosclerosis, idiopathic orthostatic hypotension
2. Do not use more than one application per hour in each eye
3. Do not use in atropinized patients; this can cause tachycardia and hypertension
4. Do not use in patients receiving tricyclic antidepressants, monoamine oxidase inhibitors, reserpine, methyldopa and guanethidine
5. Use only 2.5% solution in infants and elderly
6. Prolonged irrigation/application and subconjunctival injection is not recommended

Hydroxyamphetamine

Hydroxyamphetamine is an indirect acting sympathomimetic. It acts by stimulating the release of norepinephrine from adrenergic nerve terminals. Topical instillation of 1% solution causes pupillary dilatation and also some vasoconstriction. It has no significant effect on accommodation and refractive state.[16] It is used only as a mydriatic agent. The time of onset of mydriasis and the time to reach the peak effect is comparable to phenylephrine 2.5%.[17] However, the maximal dilatation may not be adequate especially in diabetics to examine peripheral retinal abnormalities. To achieve greater pupillary dilatation, it is used in combination with a muscarinic antagonist such as tropicamide 0.25%. The mydriatic effect of this combination is independent of the effect of age or color of iris.

Hydroxyamphetamine is useful in differentiating preganglionic or central sympathetic lesions from postganglionic lesions in Horner's syndrome. In patients with preganglionic or central lesion hydroxyamphetamine causes pupillary dilatation by stimulating release of norepinephrine from intact postganglionic fibers. This effect is not observed if the lesion involves postganglionic fibers.

Adverse Effects

Topical use of hydroxyamphetamine for routine mydriasis causes little, if any, ocular irritation. Due to its indirect action it is considered a safer mydriatic in patients with shallow anterior chamber.[18] Systemic absorption of the hydroxyamphetamine can cause rise in blood pressure, however tachyphylaxis develops for this effect. It is also ineffective in patients with postganglionic denervation. Because of these reasons hydroxyamphetamine is safer than phenylephrine in patients with insulin-dependent diabetes, idiopathic orthostatic hypotension and patients receiving reserpine, methyldopa and guanethidine.

Atropine

Atropine is a naturally occurring alkaloid obtained from the plant *Atropa belladonna* (deadly nightshade). It was the first antimuscarinic used in medicine and is the most potent mydriatic-cycloplegic drug. It is a non-specific muscarinic antagonist that acts by competitively inhibiting the actions of acetylcholine. It acts both centrally and peripherally. It is available commercially as sulfate derivative in 1% solution or 1% ointment formulation.

Topical application results in persistent mydriasis unresponsive to light and cycloplegia. Following application of single drop of 1% solution, mydriasis begins in about 10 minutes and reaches peak in 25–30 minutes. It starts returning to normal size in 2 days and reaches pre-instillation size by the 10th day. Cycloplegia begins in about 15 minutes, reaches peak in about 100 minutes and disappears in 7–12 days.

Atropine allows measurement of refractive error without interference by the accommodative power of the eye and is, therefore, used for refraction in young children. However, shorter acting cycloplegics are now preferred. People above 40 years of age have decreased ability to accommodate and often refraction can be done without cycloplegia. Ocular pain in patients with uveitis and corneal ulcer due to ciliary muscle spasm is relieved by atropine, which causes ciliary muscle relaxation. Some studies have shown that prolonged use of atropine may prevent or delay the progression of myopia.[19]Atropine can also be used to provide pharmacological occlusion in the better eye for the treatment of amblyopia.[20]

Adverse Effects and Contraindications

Topical instillation causes transient stinging. Prolonged duration of mydriasis causes photophobia and blurred vision for many days. In patients with narrow angle, atropine can precipitate an acute attack and is, therefore, contraindicated in patients with angle closure glaucoma. Topical atropine exacerbates aqueous tear deficiency and is, therefore, contraindicated in patients with dry eyes. It is also contraindicated in patients with previous history of allergy. The pharmacological response to atropine may be potentiated if administered to patients on drugs with antimuscarinic action such as antihistaminics, tricyclic antidepressants and monoamine oxidase inhibitors.

Atropine if absorbed systemically in significant amount can cause

- Tachycardia, headache, flushing
- Dry mouth, heartburn
- Exacerbation of gut hypomotility, urinary retention in patients with enlarged prostate
- CNS toxicity in elderly patients.

Atropine should be used with caution in pediatric and elderly patients. It should be used in pregnant and lactating mothers only if clearly indicated. Measures should be taken to avoid excessive systemic absorption such as digital pressure for 2–3 minutes after topical administration.

Systemic atropine toxicity presents with dry and flushed skin, fever, blurred vision, rapid and irregular pulse, distended abdomen in infants, mental aberrations and loss of neuromuscular coordination. Atropine poisoning is usually self-limiting and is rarely fatal if further administration is discontinued. Treatment involves supportive measures such as maintaining the patent airways and symptomatic treatment such as for fever and CNS excitation. Physostigmine is used as antidote to quickly terminate the systemic toxicity of atropine and is specially useful in patients with hallucinations, seizures and cardiac toxicity.

Homatropine

Homatropine hydrobromide is a semi-synthetic derivative of atropine. It is available commercially in a concentration of 2% and 5%. The mydriatic effect appears in 10–20 minutes and reaches peak in 30–40 minutes. Both the light and accommodative reflexes are lost in 30 minutes. Pupil takes 1–3 days to recover to normal size. It is a less potent antimuscarinic agent than atropine and thus produces significantly less cycloplegia as compared to comparable doses of atropine and cyclopentolate. The duration of cycloplegia produced by homatropine is longer than that produced by cyclopentolate, especially in people with pigmented iris.[21]

Homatropine is primarily indicated for therapeutic use in the treatment of anterior uveitis as its effects are similar to atropine. It is not a preferred drug for fundus examination or cycloplegic refraction because of its prolonged duration of action and relatively weak cycloplegic action.

The adverse effects and contraindications of homatropine are same as those of atropine.

Scopolamine (Hyoscine)

The alkaloid scopolamine is obtained from the shrub *Hyoscyamus niger* and *Scopolia carnfolica*. It is a non-selective antimuscarinic agent and has effects similar to atropine, although, the duration of mydriatic and cycloplegic action is shorter. The maximal mydriatic effect of scopolamine hydrobromide 0.5% solution appears in 20–30 minutes and pupil recovers to normal size in 1–3 days. Cycloplegia appears in 30–60 minutes and persists for 3–7 days.[22]

Scopolamine even in low doses easily crosses blood brain barrier and produces CNS effects such as drowsiness and confusions. A high incidence of idiosyncratic reactions with scopolamine has been reported as compared to other anticholinergic drugs. Therefore, scopolamine is not a preferred drug for fundoscopy, cycloplegic refraction or treatment of anterior uveitis. Its use is reserved for patients showing allergy to atropine.

The adverse effects and contraindications of scopolamine are same as those of atropine; however, CNS toxicity is more common. Contraindications for scopolamine are same as for atropine.

Cyclopentolate

Cyclopentolate is a water soluble ester and is available commercially in concentrations of 0.5, 1 and 2% solutions. Instillation of two drops of 0.5% solution 5 minutes apart or one drop of 1% solution causes mydriasis in 20–30 minutes and cycloplegia in 30–40 minutes. Thus the onset of mydriasis and cycloplegia requires almost the same time but the time course of the two effects is not similar. Pupillary dilatation lags behind the cycloplegia. Adequate cycloplegia appears even before the pupil is fully dilated and refraction can be done early.

It is a less effective mydriatic in blacks and in people with black iris. In people with light iris, acceptable level of cycloplegia may appear within 10 minutes of instillation of 1% solution. In blacks and people with dark iris it may take up to 40 minutes for acceptable level of cycloplegia to appear. The cycloplegic effect lasts longer in blacks and in people with black iris as compared to people with light iris but in all eyes cycloplegia terminates within 24 hours.

Cyclopentolate is the cycloplegic agent of choice for routine cycloplegic refraction in all age groups especially in infants and young children. The cycloplegia obtained is superior to homatropine and parallels atropine. The onset of cycloplegia is faster and of shorter duration. Although complete recovery from cycloplegia takes about 24 hours, an acceptable level of recovery occurs in 12 hours. The light reflex is also lost so the pupils do not constrict on exposure to bright light such as during binocular indirect ophthalmoscopic examination or fundus photography. In patients who are sensitive to atropine, cyclopentolate is used for the treatment of anterior uveitis. However, if the inflammation is severe, more frequent instillation is required due to its short duration of action.

Adverse Effects and Contraindications

The most common adverse effect of cyclopentolate is stinging, burning and tearing on initial instillation. This effect is minimum at 0.5% concentration but increases as the concentration increases. In patients allergic to cyclopentolate, ocular irritation, redness, facial rash, lacrimation, white mucus discharge and blurred vision may appear within minutes or hours. Repeated use of high concentration solutions of cyclopentolate over prolonged period causes diffuse epithelial punctuate keratitis with marked conjunctival hyperemia. Cyclopentolate can increase the intraocular pressure in patients with primary open-angle glaucoma and can precipitate an attack of acute glaucoma in patients with narrow angle.

Systemic absorption of cyclopentolate causes adverse effects similar to atropine but the CNS effects are more common with cyclopentolate as compared to atropine. CNS toxicity of cyclopentolate is manifested as drowsiness, ataxia, disorientation, slurred speech, restlessness, tactile and visual hallucinations. The CNS symptoms are particularly common in children when higher concentrations (2% or multiple instillations of 1%) are used. CNS symptoms usually subside within 2 hours in adults and 4–6 hours in children without any permanent damage. A few cases of serious toxicity with epileptic seizures have been reported especially in children with neurological impairment.[23,24] As the infants and children especially those with neurological impairment are more susceptible to adverse effects of cyclopentolate, it should not be used in concentrations higher than 0.5% in this group of patients and systemic absorption should be minimized by nasolacrimal occlusion.

Other peripheral adverse effects of antimuscarinic agents due to systemic absorption such as flushed, dry skin and mucus membranes, fever and tachycardia are not observed with cyclopentolate. Treatment of cyclopentolate toxicity is the same as that of atropine toxicity.

Tropicamide

Tropicamide is a synthetic derivative of tropic acid. It is a non-selective antimuscarinic agent. Its penetration through corneal epithelium is better than atropine, homatropine and cyclopentolate and, therefore, it causes quick onset of mydriasis, which lasts for a short duration. It is available in two concentrations, 0.5 and 1%. Maximum mydriasis occurs in 20–40 minutes and pupil reaches pre-instillation size in 6 hours. Mydriatic effect of tropicamide is not dependent on concentration and 1% concentration produces only slightly larger pupil. Cycloplegia appears in 30–35 minutes and is dose-related. The mydriatic effect of tropicamide is stronger than its cycloplegic effect. The lower concentration is used for mydriatic effect and higher concentration for cycloplegia. It is not a drug of choice for cycloplegic refraction but 1% concentration has been found to be useful for measuring distance refractive error in school children with mild to moderate hyperopia.

Tropicaimde is free form vasopressor effects and is the safest mydriatic to use in neonates and patients with hypertension or other cardiovascular disease. Tropicamide 1% was also reported to cause greater mydriasis as compared to phenylephrine 2.5% and a combination of tropicamide 1% and phenylephrine 2.5% was more effective than either of them used alone.[25]

Tropicamide and cyclopentolate are often combined with phenylephrine and hydroxyamphetamine to overcome the constrictor effect of cholinergic stimulation, particularly on exposure to bright light. Phenylephrine 1% combined with cyclopentolate 0.2% is used for fundus examination in neonates. Hydroxyamphetamine 1% is combined with tropicamide 0.25%. The size of the pupil after the use of combination is larger than that produced by hydroxyamphetamine alone or tropicamide 0.5 and 1%.[26] The combination has an equivalent mydriatic efficacy and greater cycloplegic efficacy as compared to phenylephrine 2.5% followed by tropicamide 0.5% instilled separately for the first 45–60 minutes.[27] The mydriasis produced with the combination is sufficient to allow indirect ophthalmoscopy and fundus photography and does not vary with age or iris pigmentation. The combination is also more comfortable to use as compared to phenylephrine 2.5% or tropicamide 0.5%.

A combination of tropicamide 0.5% and phenylephrine 0.5%, injected intracamerally has been shown to be safe and effective in dilating pupils in cases with poor mydriasis after preoperative instillation.[28] Combination of tropicamide 1% and phenylephrine 2.5% has shown significantly greater efficacy as mydriatic in dark eyes subjects as compared to tropicamide 1% and cyclopentolate 1% combination.[29]

Adverse Effects and Contraindications

Adverse effects include stinging and burning sensation especially after instillation of 1% solution. In patients with narrow angle, intraocular pressure may rise. It is, therefore, contraindicated in patients with angle-closure glaucoma. Tropicamide is significantly absorbed in systemic circulation but it has poor affinity for systemic muscarinic receptors and, therefore, its systemic adverse effects are rare. Hypersensitivity to tropicamide has been reported.[30] Patients with hypersensitivity to belladonna also show cross-sensitivity to topical tropicamide.

REFERENCES

1. Cogan DG. Accommodation and the autonomic nervous system. Arch Ophthalmol. 1937;18(5):739–66.

2. Stephens KG. Effect of the sympathetic nervous system on accommodation. Am J Optom Physiol Opt. 1985;62(6):402–6.

3. Gil DW, Krauss HA, Bogardus AM, WoldeMussie E. Muscarinic receptor subtypes in human iris-ciliary body measured by immunoprecipitation. Invest Ophthalmol Vis Sci. 1997;38(7):1434–42.

4. Heath P, Geiter CW. Use of phenylephrine hydrochloride (Neosynephrine) in ophthalmology. Arch Ophthalmol. 1949;41(2):172–7.

5. Munden PM, Kardon RH, Denison CE, Carter KD. Palpebral fissure responses to topical adrenergic drugs. Am J Ophthalmol. 1991; 111(6):706–10.

6. Chiri NB, Gold AA, Breinin G. Iris cysts and miotics. Arch Ophthalmol. 1964;71:611–6.

7. Thompson HS, Menscher JH. Adrenergic mydriasis in Horner's syndrome; hydroxyamphetamine test for diagnosis of postganglionic defects. Am J Ophthalmol. 1971;72(2):472–80.

8. Fraunfelder FT, Meyer SM (eds). Drug-induced ocular side effects and drug Interactions. Philedelphia: Lea and Febiger, 1989; Chapter 6.

9. Alpay A, Ermis B, Ugurbas SC, Battal F, Sagdik HM. The local vasoconstriction of infant's skin following instillation of mydriatic eye drops. Eur J Clin Pharmacol. 2010;66(11):1161–4.

10. Raison-Peyron N, Du Thanh A, Demoly P, Guillot B. Long-lasting allergic contact blepharoconjunctivitis to phenylephrine eyedrops. Allergy. 2009;64(4):657–8.

11. Martin-Flores M, Mercure-McKenzie TM, Campoy L, Erb HN, Ludders JW, Gleed RD. Controlled retrospective study of the effects of eyedrops containing phenylephrine hydrochloride and scopolamine hydrobromide on mean arterial blood pressure in anesthetized dogs. Am J Vet Res. 2010;71(12):1407–12.

12. Fraunfelder FT, Scafidi AF. Possible adverse effects from topical ocular 10% phenylephrine. Am J Ophthalmol. 1978;85(4):447–53.

13. Calenda E, Richez F, Muraine M. Acute hypertension due to phenylephrine eyedrops in a newborn. Can J Ophthalmol. 2007; 42(3):486.

14. Kim JM, Stevenson CE, Mathewson HS. Hypertensive reaction to phenylephrine eye drops in patients with sympathetic denervation. Am J Ophthalmol. 1978;85(6):862–8.

15. Robertson D. Contraindication to the use of ocular phenylephrine in idiopathic orthostatic hypotension. Am J Ophthalmol. 1979;87(6):819–22.

16. Abbott WO, Henry CM. Paredrine (β-4-hydroxyphenylisopro-pylamine): A clinical investigation of a sympathomimetic drug. Am J Med Sci. 1937;193:661–73.

17. Semes LP, Bartlett JD. Mydriatic effectiveness of hydroxyamphetamine. J Am Optom Assoc. 1982;53(11):899-904.

18. Gartener S, Billet E. Mydriatic glaucoma. Am J Ophthalmol. 1957;43(6):975–6.

19. Brodstein RS, Brodstein DE, Olson RJ, Hunt SC, Williams RR. The treatment of myopia with atropine and bifocals. A log-term prospective study. Ophthalmology. 1984;91(11):1373–8.

20. Simons K, Stein L, Sener EC, Vitale S, Guyton DL. Full-time atropine, intermittent atropine, and optical penalization and binocular outcome in treatment of strabismic amblyopia. Ophthalmology. 1997;104(12):2141–55.

21. Emiru VP. Response to mydriatics in the African. Br J Ophthalmol. 1971;55(8):538–43.

22. Marron J. Cycloplegia and mydriasis by use of atropine, scopolamine and homatropine-paredrine. Arch Ophthalmol. 1940;23(2): 340–50.

23. Kennerdell JS, Wucher FP. Cyclopentolate associated with two cases of grand mal seizure. Arch Ophthalmol. 1972;87(6):634–5.

24. Fitzgerald DA, Hanson RM, West C, Martin F, Brown J, Kilham HA. Seizures associated with 1% cyclopentolate eyedrops. J Paediatr Child Health. 1990;26(2):106–7.

25. Park JH, Lee YC, Lee SY. The comparison of mydriatic effect between two drugs of different mechanism. Korean J Ophthalmol. 2009;23(1):40–2.

26. Cooper J, Feldman JM, Jaanus SD, et al. Pupillary dilation and fundoscopy with 1.0% hydroxyamphetamine plus 0.5% tropicamide (Paremyd) versus tropicamide (0.5% or 1%) as a function of iris and skin pigmentation and age. J Am Optom Assoc. 1996;67(11):669–75.

27. Zeise MM, McDougall BWJ, Bartlett JD et al. Comparison of efficacy and tolerance between 1.0% hydroxyamphetamine plus 0.5% tropicamide (Paremyd) and 0.5% tropicamide combined with 2.5% phenylephrine. J Am Optom Assoc. 1996;67(11):681–9.

28. Mori Y, Miyai T, Kagaya F, Nagai N, Osakabe Y, Miyata K, et al. Intraoperative mydriasis by intracameral injection of mydriatic eye drops: in vivo efficacy and in vitro safety studies. Clin Experiment Ophthalmol. 2011;39(5):456–61.

29. Anderson HA, Bertrand KC, Manny RE, Hu YS, Fern KD. Comparison of two drug combinations for dilating dark irides. Optom Vis Sci. 2010;87(2):120–4.

30. Wahl JW. Systemic reaction to tropicamide. Arch Ophthalmol. 1969;82(3):320–1.

CHAPTER 7

Ophthalmic Dyes

OVERVIEW

Dyes as a diagnostic tool are widely used in ophthalmic practice. Fluorescein, synthesized by Baeyer in 1871, was the first dye used for diagnostic purpose.[1,2] Several such dyes are currently in use for various diagnostic purposes such as to assess the integrity of corneal surface, patency of lacrimal system, anterior segment and retinal vascular functions and Goldmann tonometry.

Fluorescein Sodium

Fluorescein is a dye of xanthine series with a molecular weight of 376 kd and solubility of 50% in water at 15°C. It is an acidic dye and is formulated as sodium salt. When exposed to light, fluorescein absorbs certain wavelength and then emits light at longer wavelength. The wavelength of emitted light can be measured spectrophotofluorimetrically. Fluorescein does not stain tissues but shows characteristic green color due to its fluorescent properties. The fluorescence of fluorescein in solution is affected by several factors. An increase in the concentration increases the intensity of fluorescence and a maximum fluorescence is achieved at 0.001% concentration. The intensity of fluorescence is also affected by pH. As the fluorescein is an acidic dye, at pH less than 2, its cationic form predominates, which gives a blue-fluorescence. At physiological pH of 7, the anionic form predominates, which gives a brilliant yellow-green fluorescence. Thus, the maximum fluorescence is achieved at physiological pH and increase beyond 8 reduces the fluorescence. The wavelength of absorbed light also affects the intensity of fluorescence and a maximum intensity is produced at the wavelength of 530-nm.[3,4]

Fluorescein is available for topical use as solution and in the form of fluorescein-impregnated filter paper strips. Fluorescein solution is highly susceptible to bacterial contamination and especially by *Pseudomonas aeruginosa*.[5] To prevent the bacterial contamination of solutions, preservatives such as chlorobutanol and thimerosal have been used. Non-preserved preparations are used in sterile single-dose vials. Wet filter paper strips when applied to eye release dye and are used clinically for various diagnostic purposes. Use of filter paper strips helps to avoid the risk of bacterial contamination.

Clinical Uses

Topical: Fluorescein is widely used topically for a variety of diagnostic and other purposes:

1. Assessment of ocular surface integrity: Application of dye in the cul-de-sac allows detection of corneal and conjunctival lesions such as abrasion, ulcer, edema and presence of a foreign body. At physiological pH, dye is highly ionized and fails to penetrate intact corneal epithelium. However, if the corneal epithelium is not intact dye comes in contact with stroma and when observed with cobalt-blue filter of slit lamp, the epithelial defect

appears as green fluorescent spot. The reason for this color change from orange-yellow to green is not fully understood. According to some, penetration of dye into the stroma allows it to come in contact with interstitial fluid derived from aqueous humor leading to pH-dependent change in the color of the dye. According to other views, the dye enters the dead cells and staining appears due to the fluorescence of intracellular structures.[3,6]

2. Assessment of tear film stability: Tear break-up time (TBUT), which is measured as the time interval between the last complete blink and appearance of the first dry spot in the tear film, is commonly used to assess the dry eyes and efficacy of tear substitutes. The test requires application of dye to bulbar conjunctiva followed by observation with slit lamp until the dry spot appears in the tear film. TBUT of less than 10 seconds indicates tear film instability. A wide variation in TBUT have been reported and, therefore, the validity of this test is questionable.

3. Applanation tonometry: Fluorescein (0.25%) is used for measurement of intraocular pressure using Goldmann applanation tonometer. Dye stains the meniscus of tear fluid around the flattened corneal surface and allows clear visualization of the apex of the wedge-shaped meniscus. An anesthetic solution is first instilled and sufficient time is allowed for the anesthetic to get absorbed before the dye is applied. Instillation of dye together with anesthetic agent reduces fluorescence as the acidic pH of anesthetic solution ionizes fluorescein, which now has poor fluorescence. Although Goldmann applanation tonometry can be performed without using fluorescein, the IOP measurements are significantly lower.[7,8]

4. Detection of aqueous leakage: Fluorescein is used to detect leakage of aqueous humor such as during corneal transplant or from the surgical wounds. In cases of leakage, the dye stains the leaking aqueous, which appears as a bright green streak flowing over the cornea.[6]

5. Contact lens fitting: Staining of tear film with fluorescein helps in determining the fitting of rigid gas permeable contact lenses as the areas where the lens makes contact with cornea, minimal or no fluorescence is observed. Besides aiding in contact lens fitting, fluorescein staining also helps in assessing the integrity of corneal surface in contact lens wearers.

6. Assessment of the patency of lacrimal system: Fluorescein can be used to assess patency of the lacrimal system. The dye is instilled into the lower fornix. Following instillation, appearance of dye in nose or posterior pharynx, is an indicator of the patency of lacrimal apparatus.

Intravenous: Fluorescein is used by intravenous route to study vascular integrity and abnormalities in posterior and anterior chambers.

1. *Fluorescein angiography:* Intravenous injection of 10 mL of fluorescein (5%) makes the dye appear in central retinal vein in 10–15 seconds.[9] Fluorescein binds to plasma albumin and this protein binding prevents it from passing through the blood-ocular barrier. In the bloodstream, fluorescein is excited by a wavelength of 465 nm and emits a wavelength of 525 nm. Retinal blood vessels are visualized in high contrast. Nonvascularized areas are seen as dark areas against green fluorescing background whereas neovascularization produces enhanced fluorescence. Pathological lesions causing enhanced capillary permeability are visualized as leakage of the dye in extravascular space. Some retinal abnormalities allow greater visibility of choroidal fluorescence. Fluorescein angiography is, therefore, very useful in the diagnosis of a wide range of conditions like diabetic retinopathy, central serous choroidopathy, papilledema, disciform macular degeneration, choroidal hemangiomas and melanomas.

2. *Iris angiography:* Fluorescein after injection into the antecubital vein, appears in the radial vessels of iris in 9–20 seconds. Iris vessels

are better visualized in people with blue iris as compared to brown iris as the pigment distribution affects the visualization of iris vessels. Pathological conditions of iris such as tumor or infarct can be visualized in iris angiogram.

3. The rate of aqueous flow can be determined by measuring the time course of the changes in fluorescein concentration in anterior chamber with the help of a slit lamp fluorophotometer.

4. Vitreous fluorophotometry helps in detecting presence of dye in the vitreous. Normally the blood-retinal barrier does not allow dye to pass through and appear in the vitreous and, therefore, appearance of dye in vitreous is an indicator of the damage to blood-retinal barrier.

Oral: Fluorescein can be administered orally to study certain lesions in retina. For adults 1 or 2 gram powder or 3 vials of 10% fluorescein mixed in a citrus drink are used. For children 1mL of 10% fluorescein per 20 mL of fruit juice per 5 kg body weight is used.[10] Following oral administration, dye appears in the fundus in about 15 minutes and maximum fluorescence appears in 45–60 minutes.[11] The adverse effects are less likely after oral administration as compared to intravenous administration.

Adverse Effects

Topical fluorescein may cause transient ocular irritation. Topical fluorescein stains the soft contact lenses and, therefore, soft lenses should be reinserted after 1–2 hours or following thorough rinsing of upper and lower fornix with sterile saline or extraocular irrigating solutions. Intravenous injection of 10% fluorescein causes nausea in 10% of the patients with higher incidence among females. Incidence of nausea increases with increasing concentrations of fluorescein.[12] Slow intravenous injection also reduces the incidence of nausea.[13] Promethazine 50 mg orally can be used one hour before intravenous fluorescein to reduce the incidence of nausea in susceptible patients. Family and personal history of allergy must be obtained from all patients as intravenous fluorescein can also cause allergic reactions such as urticaria. Serious allergic reactions like anaphylaxis are rare. Intravenous fluorescein colors the urine and skin temporarily and appears in milk 76 hours after intravenous injection.[14] Other adverse effects include pain at the injection site, paraesthesias of tongue and lips, dizziness, and rarely fainting.

Fluorexon

Fluorexon is N,N-bis(carboxymethyl)-amino-ethylfluorescein tetrasodium salt. Its molecular weight is 710 kd and it has a pale yellow-brown color. It stains the epithelial defects and the devitalized tissue. Observation of fluorescence requires enhancement by yellow filter.

Clinical Uses

Fluorexon is used as an aid in contact lens fitting as it is less readily absorbed by the soft lens material. The use of this dye, therefore, allows visualization of tear film under the lens. Fluorexon is a useful aid in fitting hybrid lenses and fitting of lenses in cases like keratoconus where rigid lens is placed over a hydrogel lens. Fluorexon is not a widely used dye in clinical practice as the evaluation of contact lens fitting is as effective in the presence as in the absence of the tear film visualization.

Adverse Effects

Fluorexon is remarkably non-toxic to ocular tissue. Topical application can cause stinging sensation and conjunctival injection. If allowed to remain in contact with soft contact lenses, lenses can get stained. Repeated rinsing with saline helps to remove the dye from the lenses. Fluorexon is not recommended for use with high water content (60% or higher) lenses. Such lenses can absorb significant quantity of dye and will be discolored. Fluorexon solution allows easy bacterial contamination and is, therefore, dispensed in single-dose sterile pipettes.

Rose Bengal

Rose bengal is 4,5,6,7-tetra-chloro-$2^1,4^1,5^1,7^1$-tetraiodo derivative of fluorescein, which gives the stained tissue a pink or magenta color when viewed with white light. Although known as a vital dye that colors the dead, degenerated tissue and mucus strands, recent studies have shown that rose bengal also stains healthy cultured cells.[15,16] The nucleus of healthy cells has been shown to retain the dye. Rose bengal has also been shown to possess cytotoxic properties especially upon exposure to light.[15,17] Rose bengal is a photoreactive compound and in the presence of 55-nm wavelength and oxygen it generates singlet oxygen.[18,19] Singlet oxygen is highly reactive and damages cell proteins and DNA. Because of this action, rose bengal is effective against a wide range of micro-organisms like bacteria, viruses and protozoa. In vitro studies have shown that rose bengal due to its intrinsic toxicity damages unprotected epithelial cells. However, in the presence of albumin and mucus such toxicity does not occur. This indicates that the rose bengal staining of epithelial cells is not due to staining of dead cells but due to absence of protective tear film as is seen in keratoconjunctivitis sicca.

Clinical Uses

Topical: For topical use rose bengal is used as 1% solution or in the form of sterile impregnated filter paper strips. Its most frequent clinical use is in the evaluation of dry eye syndromes. The efficacy of rose bengal used alone in the differential diagnosis of dry eye is debatable. It has been recommended that rose bengal staining must be combined with other tests such as fluorescein stain or tear function tests for better efficacy. A grading system to quantify rose bengal staining described by George et al. can be used to assess the severity of dry eye.[20] Rose bengal staining has also been used to assess the treatment efficacy, however, its utility remains debatable. The evaluation of most types of conjunctival and corneal lesions such as abrasions, ulcers, foreign bodies, conjunctival dysplasia and metaplasia has also been done with rose bengal staining. This dye is particularly useful in identifying herpetic corneal ulcer as it gives characteristic staining to dendritic margins. However, because of its antiviral properties, subsequently performed culture test may provide a false negative result leading to inappropriate treatment.

Intravenous: In animal studies, intravenous injection of rose bengal has been shown to cause vascular occlusion by photothrombosis. It photochemically induces endothelial damage leading to platelet aggregation and vascular occlusion.[21,22] Since the thrombus can not be degraded by tissue plasminogen as it mainly consists of platelets and no fibrin, it is long lasting. The method has been used in rabbits to cause occlusion of corneal neovascularization. Animal studies done so far indicate potential use of rose bengal in the treatment of ocular surface disorders with overgrowth such as chemical burns, contact lens-induced vascularization, exudative keratopathy and vascularized cornea.[23]

Adverse Effects

Topical application of rose bengal causes stinging and smarting. Rose bengal stains skin, clothing and contact lenses. Intravenously administered rose bengal is non-toxic to human. The dye is metabolized in liver and, therefore, is contraindicated in patients with impaired liver function.

Lissamine Green

Lissamine green is a vital stain and just like rose bengal stains mucus and dead degenerated cells. It gives a bluish-green color to the stained tissue and its staining effect is longer lasting than rose bengal. It has a molecular weight of 576.6 kd and is also used as food colorant.

Clinical Uses

Lissamine green 1% as solution or filter paper strip is used for assessing dry eye conditions, recurrent corneal erosions and herpetic ulcers. Its staining effect is easier to see in red and inflamed eye and that is why it is especially useful when a red dye is not desirable or in combination with a red dye.

Adverse Effects

Lissamine green does not cause any ocular irritation on topical application. No other adverse effects are known. The dye, however, stains the soft lenses and should not be used in eyes with lenses in place.

Indocyanine Green

Indocyanine (ICG) is a water soluble tricarbocyanine dye. When injected intravenously, it is highly protein bound. Extensive protein binding does not allow dye to leak from the capillaries and, therefore, the details of choroidal and retinal vasculature can be studied. ICG is dissolved in aqueous solvent at a concentration of 12.5 mg/mL and a total dose of 50 mg is injected in anticubital vein at a rate of 1 mL/sec.[24] Following intravenous injection, photographs are taken at 1–2 second interval until full fluorescence is achieved. Subsequently, photographs are taken at increasing interval over 30–40 minutes until fluorescence disappears. ICG is taken up exclusively by liver and is a helpful index of liver functions.

Clinical Use

It is used as fluorescent dye for retinal and choroidal angiography. It shows peak absorption at 805 nm and maximum emission at 835 nm. This near infrared range, provides better viewing of angiograms in the presence of media opacities and subretinal exudation. Choroidal vasculature is better visualized with ICG than fluorescein. Rapid choroidal filling is also better visualized with ICG. Videoangiography using ICG is a useful tool in studying a variety of choroidal pathologies such as congenital, ischemic, inflammatory or degenerative. ICG angiography is commonly used to characterize choroidal neovascularization. Choroidal neovascularization is treated with laser photocoagulation and the success of this treatment depends on identification and accurate localization of the areas of neovascularization. ICG angiography has been shown to provide better localization and identification of these areas as compared to fluorescein. The dye stays in the areas of neovascularization long after it disappears from surrounding areas. Therefore, ICG is of particular value in visualizing poorly defined membranes overlying hemorrhage or lying close to previously treated areas. Use of infrared scanning laser ophthalmoscope further enhances the resolution in ICG videoangiography.

Adverse Effects

Intravenous use of ICG is generally safe without many adverse effects. It does not stain skin, mucous membranes or urine. Use of ICG is, however, associated with allergic reactions. ICG contains small amount of sodium iodide and should not be used in patients with allergy to iodine or shellfish.

Methylene Blue

Methylene blue is an aniline dye and just like Rose Bengal stains dead devitalized cells and mucus. It is used as 5% solution and also has bacteriostatic properties.

Clinical Uses

Methylene blue is mainly used to stain lacrimal sac before dacryocystorhinostomy. Before surgery the sac is irrigated with dye. The dye is allowed to remain in sac for several minutes and is washed out of the sac before starting surgery. Methylene blue is also used to visualize anterior lens capsule during cataract surgery and in gonioscopic ab interno laser sclerostomy. It can be used topically to stain corneal nerves.

Adverse Effects

Topical application of methylene blue causes ocular tissue irritation. It is also contraindicated for use in patients who are allergic to the dye.

REFERENCES

1. Baeyer A. Uber eine neue klasse von farbstofefn. Ber Deutsch Chem Ges. 1871;4(2):555–8.
2. Ehrlich P. Ueber provocirte fluorescenzerscheinungen am auge. Dtsch Med Wochenschr. 1882;8:35–6.
3. Romanchuk KG. Fluorescein: physiochemical factors affecting its fluorescence. Surv Ophthalmol. 1982;26(5):269–83.
4. Maurice DM. The use of fluorescein in ophthalmological research. Invest Ophthalmol. 1967;6(5):464–77.
5. Vaughan DG. The contamination of fluorescein solutions – with special reference to *Pseudomonas aeruginosa*. Am J Ophthalmol. 1955;39(1): 55–61.
6. Havener WH. Ocular Pharmacolo. St Louis: CV Mosby, 1983: Chapter 17.
7. Roper DL. Applanation tonometry with and without fluorescein. Am J Ophthalmol. 1980;90(5):668–71.
8. Bright DC, Potter JW, Allen DC, Spruance RD. Goldmann applanation tonometry without fluorescein. Am J Optom Physiol Optics. 1981;58(12):1120–6.
9. Smith JL, David NJ, Hart LM, Levenson DS, Tillett CW. Haemangioma of the choroid: fluorescein photography and photocoagulation. Arch Ophthalmol. 1963;69(1):51–4.
10. Morgan KS, Franklin RM. Oral fluorescein angioscopy in aphakic children. J Paedtr Ophthalmol Strabismus. 1984;21(1):33–6.
11. Kelly JS, Kincaid M. Retinal fluorography using oral fluorescein. Arch Ophthalmol. 1979;97(12):2331–2.
12. Willerson D, Tate GW, Baldwin HA, Hernsberger PL. Clinical evaluation of fluorescein 25%. Ann Ophthalmol. 1976;8(7):833–42.
13. Charzan BI, Balodimos ML, Konez L. Untowards effects of fluorescein angiography in diabetic patients. Ann Ophthalmol. 1971;3(1):42–9.
14. Maguire AM, Bennette J. Fluorescein elimination in human breast milk. Arch Ophthalmol. 1988;106(6):718–9.
15. Feenstra RGP, Tseng SCG. What is actually stained by rose bengal? Arch Ophthalmol. 1992;110(7):984–93.
16. Chodosh J, Banks MC, Stroop WG. Rose bengal inhibits herpes simplex virus replication in vivo and human corneal epithelial cells in vitro. Invest Ophthalmol Vis Sci. 1992;33(8):2520–7.
17. Norn MS. Vital staining of cornea and conjunctiva. Acta Ophthalmol. 1962;40(4):389–401.
18. Gandin E, Lion Y, Van der Vorst A. Quantum yield of singlet oxygen production by xanthine derivatives. Photochem Photobiol. 1983;37:271–8.
19. Paczkowski J, Lamberts JJM, Paczkowska B, Neckers DC. Photophysiological properties of rose bengal and its derivatives. J Free Rad Biol Med. 1985;1:341–51.
20. George MA, Abelson MB, Schaefer K, Mooshian M, Weintraub D. A precise method of using rose bengal in the evaluation of dry eye and the detection of changes in its severity. Adv Exp Med Biol. 1994;350:549–52.
21. Watson BD, Dietrich WD, Busto R, Wachtel MS, Ginsberg MD. Induction of a reproducible infarction by photochemically initiated thrombosis. Ann Neurol. 1985;17(5):497–504.
22. Nanda SK, Hatchel DL, Tiedeman JS, Dutton JJ, Hatchell MC, McAdoo T. A new method for vascular occlusion: photochemical initiation of thrombosis. Arch Ophthalmol. 1987;105(8):1121–4.
23. Huang AJW, Watson BD, Hernandez E, Tseng SCG. Photothrombosis of corneal neovascularization by intravenous rose bengal and argon laser irradiation. Arch Ophthalmol. 1988;106(5):680–5.
24. Yannuzzi LA, Slakter JS, Sorenson JA, Guyer DR, Orlock DA. Digital indocyanine green videoangiography and choroidal neovascularization. Retina. 1992;12(3):191–223.

CHAPTER 8

Antibacterial Agents

OVERVIEW

Anti-infective agents are drugs used to treat infections. A more common term, which carries a similar connotation and is used widely but not accurately is the "antibiotics". The term "antibiotic" is used loosely to refer to drugs, natural or synthetic, used to treat bacterial infections. The term "antibiotic" was coined by Selman Waksman, a professor of biochemistry and microbiology, who discovered numerous antibiotics, the first of which was streptomycin. He referred antibiotics as substances produced by microorganisms, which were able to either kill or inhibit the growth of other microbes. As such, the original definition excludes synthetic compounds.

A more precise term and closer to anti-infectives is antimicrobial drugs, which refers to drugs, natural or synthetic, for the treatment of infections caused by microorganisms, not limited to bacteria but also the fungi and protozoa. In practice, however, the term "antibiotics" is used interchangeably with "antimicrobials" or "anti-infectives".

Historical Perspectives

In the 1800, with acceptance of a theory, which linked microorganisms as etiological agents with variety of ailments, scientists began work on searching for compounds, which antagonised the survival of disease-causing microbes in humans. The aim was to find a compound that would be toxic to the microbes but not to humans who were infected by such microbes, hence, developed the idea of 'selective toxicity', which has remained not only a relevant feature but pertinent one.

In 1877, Louis Pasteur showed that soil bacteria could render *Bacillus anthracis* harmless and at about the same time, Rudolf Emmerich showed that *Vibrio cholera* could not survive in the presence of streptococci. Following this, German scientist E. de Freudenreich demonstrated that an isolated product from bacterium had antibacterial properties. In the early 1920s, the British scientist Alexander Fleming reported that human tears contained lysozyme that could lyse bacterial cells. It was the first example of an antibacterial agent found in humans but was devoid of selective toxicity. Later, Fleming discovered a connection between a fungus and a substance that had antibacterial properties, thus the antibiotic properties of penicillium were reported. This discovery changed the course of medicine.

Classification

There are several ways to classify antibiotics. Schemes for classification may be based on their origin (natural or synthetic), route of administration (injectable, oral, topical), antibacterial activity (bacteriostatic or bactericidal), spectrum of activity (broad and narrow spectrum) or the chemical structure, which is the most useful pharmacological classification. Antibiotics within a structural class will generally have similar patterns of effectiveness, toxicity, and allergic potential.

The commonly used types of antibiotics are penicillins, fluoroquinolones, cephalosporins, macrolides, and tetracyclines. While each class consists of several drugs, each drug has its own distinctive features.

BETA LACTAM ANTIBIOTICS

Beta lactam antibiotics are among the most commonly prescribed drugs. The first beta lactam antibiotic, penicillin, was discovered by Sir Alexander Fleming in 1928. The first successful clinical use of penicillin was in 1930 when Cecil George Paine attempted to use penicillin in the treatment of neonatal gonococcal infection, however, the wide clinical use of penicillin started only in 1941.[1]

The beta lactam antibiotics are grouped together based upon a shared structural feature, a thiozolidine ring and a beta lactam ring (Fig 8.1) connected to a side chain. Their structures are shown in Figure 8.2.

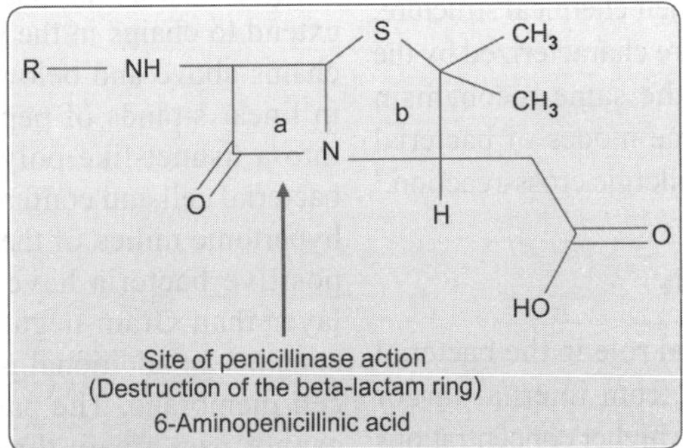

Figure 8.1 Penicillin structure; (a) The characteristic beta lactam ring; (b) Thiozolidine ring

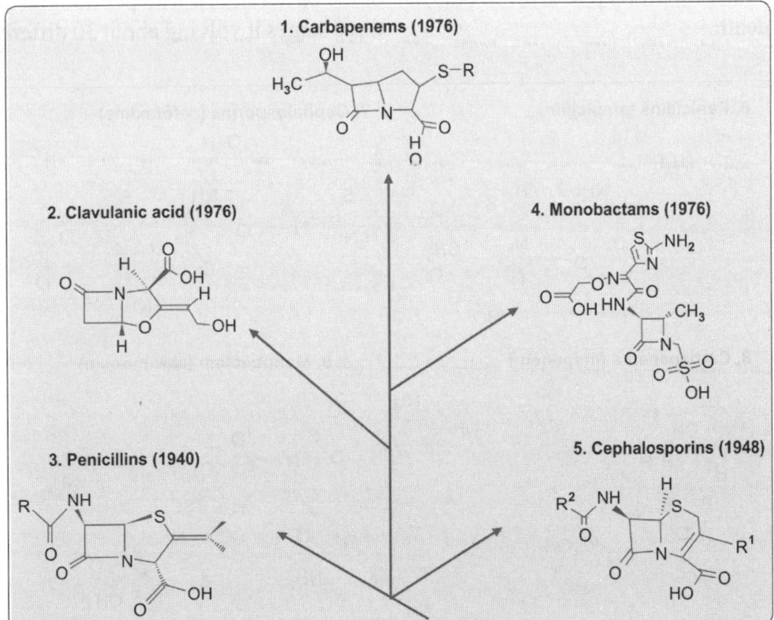

Figure 8.2 Chemical structure of the beta lactam family

Majority of the beta lactam antibiotics are semi-synthetic derivatives of the natural compounds with modifications of the 6 (7) beta-acylamido side chains of penicillins and cephalosporins (Fig. 8.3).

Synthetic beta lactam antibiotic are also available (Fig. 8.4). The beta lactam chain is essential for biological activity, whereas the side chains are primarily responsible for determining the antibacterial spectrum. Modification of these side chains has a profound influence on their antibacterial activity.

Due to the similarity in their chemical structure, all beta lactam antibiotics are characterized by the same properties such as the same mechanism of antibacterial action, same modes of bacterial resistance and presence of allergic cross-reaction.[2]

Mechanism of Action

The cell walls play a crucial role in the bacterial cell protection especially from internal turgor pressure caused by the much higher concentrations of proteins and other molecules inside the cell compared to its external environment. Loss or damage of this integral protective layer results in bacterial cell death.

The walls of bacteria are made of a complex material called peptidoglycan containing both amino acids and amino sugars. The two types of amino sugars it contains are N-acetylglucosamine (NAG) and N-acetylmuramic acid (NAM). So, essentially peptidoglycan is a linear polymer of NAG alternating with NAM linked by a glycosidic bond. A four or five amino acids peptide chain is attached to each NAM and these chains form covalent bonds with amino acids in adjacent chains. The bonds may be direct to the next chain or include additional peptide cross bridges such as the pentaglycine bridge, which extend to chains in the same plane as well as to chains above and below (Fig. 8.5). This results in linear strands of peptidoglycan cross-linked into a fishnet-like polymer that surrounds the bacterial cell and confers osmotic stability in the hypertonic milieu of the infected patient. Gram-positive bacteria have thicker peptidoglycan layer than Gram-negative, however, the later contains an additional phospholipid layer in the cell membrane. The particles larger than 2 nm cannot pass freely through the peptidoglycan meshwork of the cell wall of both the Gram-positive and Gram-negative bacteria.[3] Synthesis of the bacterial cell wall peptidoglycan consists of three stages involving about 30 different enzymes.

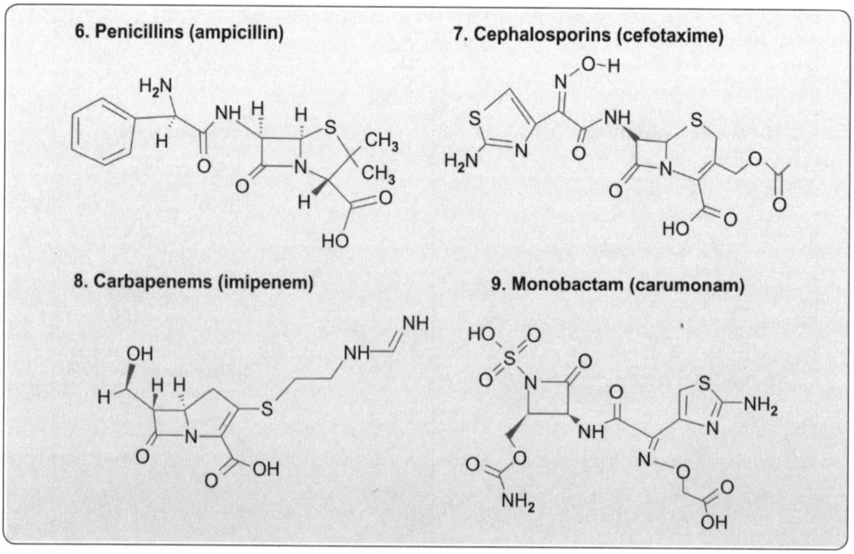

Figure 8.3 Semi-synthetic beta lactam antibiotics

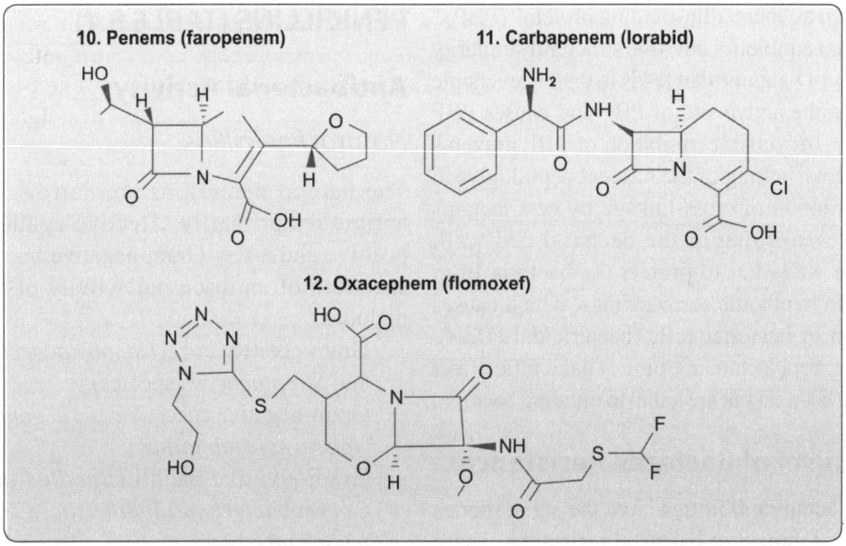

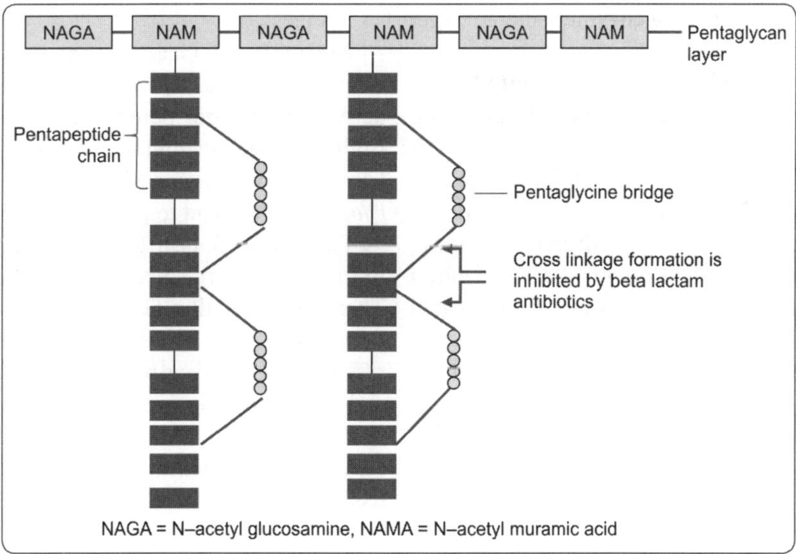

Figure 8.4 Synthetic beta lactam antibiotics

Figure 8.5 Peptidoglycan layer and the site of action of beta lactam antibiotics

During the first stage, the peptidoglycan monomers are synthesized in the cytoplasm. The first stage can be inhibited by fosfomycin and cycloserine. The second stage, which occurs in the cell membrane, is the construction of a linear polymer of a peptidoglycan chain. The second stage can be inhibited by antibiotics such as vancomycin and bacitracin. The third stage involves the formation of cross linkages between peptidoglycan layers and the attachment of nascent peptidoglycan to the cell wall. The enzyme essential for these cross linkages is the D-alanyl-D-alanine-transpeptidase also known as "penicillin-binding protein" (PBP).[4] Beta lactam antibiotics have the structural similarity to D-alanyl-D-alanine that leads to their irreversible binding to the active site of PBP and causes PBP inhibition. Irreversible inhibition of PBP prevents the final crosslinking of the nascent peptidoglycan layer. Inhibition of cross-linkage by beta lactams causes a weakening of the bacterial cell wall. Defective walls fail to protect the bacteria from bursting in hypotonic surroundings, which causes disruption of bacterial cells (bactericidal effect). Therefore, beta lactam antibiotics have little effect on resting bacteria but are lethal to dividing bacteria.

Mechanism of Bacterial Resistance

All beta lactam antibiotics have the same modes of the development of bacterial resistance. There are three important modes by which bacteria acquire resistance against beta lactam antibiotics: production of inactivating enzymes, altered target and altered permeability.

The first mechanism is associated with enzymatic hydrolysis of the beta lactam ring by the bacterial enzymes, beta lactamases or penicillinases. The beta lactamase family includes more than 300 different enzymes, that are classified according to their hydrolytic spectrum, susceptibility to inhibitors, genetic localization (plasmidic or chromosomal), gene or amino acid protein sequence.[5,6] This mechanism of beta lactam resistance is very common in Gram-negative bacteria such as *E. coli*, *Klebsiella* species, *Proteus* species, *Pseudomonas aeruginosa*.

Resistance to methicillin and other penicillinase resistant penicillins is associated with alteration of PBP structure. Such altered PBP does not allow for the binding to all beta lactams, including cephalosporins and carbapenems. This mode of penicillin resistance is often manifested in *Staphylococcus aureus* and such strains are labeled as methicillin-resistant *Staphylococcus aureus* (MRSA).

Lastly, another mechanism of resistance to beta lactam, decreased permeability through cell wall and membrane proteins, is more common among Gram-negative bacteria.

PENICILLINS (TABLE 8.1)

Antibacterial Activity

Natural Penicillins

The natural penicillins are narrow spectrum antibiotics primarily effective against Gram-positive and a few Gram-negative bacteria. The spectrum of antibacterial activity of penicillin includes:

- Gram-positive cocci (*Staphylococcus* species and *Streptococcus* species)
- Gram-negative cocci (*Neisseria gonorrhoeae*, *Neisseria meningitidis*)
- Gram-positive bacilli (*Bacillus anthracis*, *Corynebacterium diphtheriae*, *Clostridium tetani* and others)
- *Listeria* species
- Spirochetes (*Treponema pallidum*, *Leptospira* species)

Majority of Gram-negative bacilli are insensitive to natural penicillins. The antibacterial activity of natural penicillins is considerably limited by the secondary bacterial resistance. Currently, most strains of *S. aureus* and *N. gonorrhoeae* are resistant to penicillin.[7,8]

Penicillin G is highly acid-labile and is hydrolyzed in the presence of gastric acid. Therefore, penicillin G is administered parenterally. Penicillin V can be given orally as it is more resistant to hydrolysis by acidic gastric secretions and is absorbed to a greater extent than penicillin G. Procaine and benzathine penicillins are so called depot penicillins because they provide a tissue depot from which absorption takes place over several hours to several days. They should be given by deep intramuscular injections. Benzathine penicillin has longer action than procain penicillin.[9]

Penicillins penetrate well into all parts of the ocular tissue such as the lid margins, conjunctival sacs, corneae and lacrimal sacs but not the ocular muscles. Penicillins cross the placenta and are also distributed into breast milk. They are not metabolized and are excreted unchanged through the kidneys by filtration and active

Table 8.1 Classification of penicillins

A. Natural Penicillins	i. Short-acting	Penicillin G (Benzylpenicillin) Penicillin V (Phenoxymethylpenicillin)
	ii. Long-acting	Procaine penicillin Benzathine penicillin
B. Semi-synthetic Penicillins	i. Aminopenicillins	Ampicillin Amoxicillin Bacampicillin
	ii. Penicillinase resistant Penicillins (antistaphylococcal Penicillins)	Methicillin Oxacillin Cloxacillin Dicloxacillin Nafcillin
	iii. Extended-spectrum penicillins (Antipseudomonal penicillins)	**Ureidopenicillins** Azlocillin Mezlocillin Piperacillin **Carboxypenicillins** Carbenicillin Carbenicillin indanyl sodium Ticarcillin Piperacillin
	iv. Penicillins and beta lactamase inhibitor combinations	Ampicillin/sulbactam Amoxicillin/clavulanate Piperacillin/tazobactam Ticarcillin/clavulanate

tubular secretion. Renal excretion is rapid but concurrent administration with probenecid can slow the excretion rate. The plasma half-life is about 30 minutes, but in premature neonates and individuals with impaired kidney function, excretion is considerably delayed, requiring longer dosing intervals and dose reduction.[10]

Penicillinase-resistant Penicillins

Penicillinase resistant penicillins include methicillin, nafcillin, oxacillin, cloxacillin and dicloxacillin. Drugs in this group are structurally resistant to beta lactamase activity. They have a narrower spectrum of activity than the natural penicillins. This class is indicated for infection by beta lactamase producing strains of Staphylococcal species including *S. aureus*. Methicillin-resistant strains of Staphylococci are resistant.

These acid-stable penicillins are given orally and are reasonably well absorbed. However, food interferes with their absorption and they have to be taken at least an hour after meals. They can also be administered intravenously. Excretion for all is via kidneys, with the exception of nafcillin, which undergoes biliary excretion.

Aminopenicillins

In general, this class retains the spectrum of activity of penicillin G or the natural penicillins. They differ from the natural penicillins in that they have enhanced ability to penetrate Gram-negative organisms thus they have greater activity against

- Enterobacteriaceae *(E. coli, Shigella* species, *Salmonella spp., Proteus mirabilis)*
- *Haemophilus influenzae*
- *Helicobacter pylori*

Aminopenicillins are not active against *Klebsiella* species, *Enterobacter* species, *Pseudomonas aeruginosa*, *Citrobacter*, *Serratia*, indole-positive *Proteus* species, and other Gram-negative aerobes that are commonly encountered in hospital-acquired infections.

Like the natural penicillins, they are susceptible to hydrolysis by beta lactamase. They have a similar pharmacokinetic profile as natural penicillins. They are administered orally and, amoxicillin has better absorption compared to ampicillin and bacampicillin. Ampicillin can also be given intravenously.

Antipseudomonal Penicillins

As indicated by the name, antipseudomonal penicillins are active against *Pseudomonas aeruginosa* and other Gram-negative bacteria such as *Enterobacter* species, *Klebsiella* species, but they have no Gram-positive activity. Currently most strains of *Pseudomonas aeruginosa* produce different types of beta lactamase.[11] As such antipseudomonal penicillins are generally used in combination with beta lactamase inhibitors for the treatment of pseudomonal infections.[12]

Carbenicillin indanyl sodium is acid-stable and is administered orally. These drugs are widely distributed in most body fluids like all penicillins. High serum levels potentiate neurotoxicity manifested as lethargy, neuromuscular irritability, and seizures.

Beta Lactamase Inhibitors and Beta Lactamase Inhibitor Combinations

Beta lactamase inhibitors are clavulanic acid, sulbactam and tazobactam. These drugs are not antibiotics. Although their structures resemble beta lactam molecules, they have negligible antibacterial activity. They can inactivate many, but not all beta lactamases thus can protect hydrolysable beta lactam antibiotics from being destroyed by these enzymes. The addition of beta lactamase inhibitors extends the activity of penicillins to include beta lactamase-producing strains of *S.aureus* and some Gram-negative bacteria. The combination of clavulanic acid and ticarcillin is known as timentin. It is given parenterally. The combination increases the spectrum of activity of ticarcillin to include Gram-negative aerobic organisms, *Staphylococcus aureus* and *Bacteroides*. Clavulanic acid is also combined with amoxicillin, and the combination is known as augmentin. Augmentin is given orally and effectively treats infection by beta lactamase producing organisms that include *Haemophilus influenzae*, *Staphylococcus* species, *Escherichia coli* and *Neisseria gonorrhea*. The ampicillin-sulbactam combination (unasyn) is effective against beta lactamase producing *S. aureus* and *H. influenzae* but not *Serratia*, which produces beta lactamase that is not inhibited by sulbactam.

Administration and Dosage

Besides oral and parenteral routes, penicillins can be administered by topical, subconjunctival and intravitreal routes for the treatment of ophthalmic infections. Ampicillin sodium, penicillin G, piperacillin and ticarcillin disodium are available for ophthalmic use and their available concentrations are listed under "drugs used in ocular therapeutics". The dose of the penicillins depends on several factors including dosage form of the antibiotic, the type and severity of the infection. Parenteral doses are measured in units, with one unit equal to 0.6 mg of standard penicillin, USP.

Therapeutic Uses

Penicillins are useful in the treatment of many acute ophthalmic bacterial infections and are suited for surface application in the form of drops. Only small quantities are needed; doses in the order of 1,000 units are sufficient for effective treatment. Penicillins used in the form of sodium salt are well tolerated in the eyes, and can be used for subconjunctival injections as well intravenous or intramuscular injections.

As is the principle of anti-infective therapy, treatment with penicillins is successful only when the primary infecting organism is sensitive to the drug in therapeutic concentration. Organisms commonly found in ocular infections, which are susceptible to the action of penicillin are *Staphylococcus pyogenes*, the hemolytic *Streptococcus*, the *Gonococcus* and the *Pneumococcus*.

Types of Ocular Infection Suitable for Treatment by Penicillins

1. Acute conjunctivitis, blepharitis and canaliculitis. Penicillin G potassium ophthalmic solution has been used, however, currently not a favored choice in clinical practice due to its narrow spectrum and instability.
2. Chronic blepharitis due to *S. aureus*. Oxacillin subconjunctival injections.
3. Keratitis and corneal ulcers caused by *S. aureus*. Oxacillin subconjunctival injections.
4. Gonococcal conjunctivitis and gonococcal corneal ulcer.
5. Ocular syphilis. Acquired syphilis with ocular involvement should be treated as neurosyphilis with intravenous penicillin G. The dose is 18–24 million units (MU) daily for 10 to 14 days, followed by procaine penicillin, intramuscular, 2.4 MU weekly for three weeks.[13] Treatment failure may occur if the patients initially are treated with intramuscular penicillin, due to inadequate intraocular concentrations.[14]

Adverse Effects

Penicillins are among the least toxic drugs known. The most common side-effect of penicillins is diarrhea. Nausea, vomiting, and epigastric discomfort are also common. Penicillins can cause immediate and delayed allergic reactions - specifically, skin rashes, fever, and anaphylactic shock.

CEPHALOSPORINS

The cephalosporins are beta lactam antibiotics that have 7-aminocephalosporanic acid nucleus, which resembles the 6-aminopenicillinic acid of the penicillins (Fig. 8.6). The difference between penicillins and cephalosporins is that the beta lactam ring of cephalosporin bears the amino moiety at the 7th position whereas, in penicillins, this moiety is attached to the 6th position. This difference makes the cephalosporins more resistant to penicillinase compared to penicillins.

Classification

These drugs were first obtained from *Cephalosporium acremonium*, a fungus. The cephalosporins structures have now been modified to include various substitutions of their side chains (R_1 and R_2) and have proliferated to four "generations".[15] In general Gram positive activity decreases from first generation to the fourth and Gram negative activity increases in a reverse order. Stability to beta lactamase also increases from the first to fourth generations (Table 8.2.).

First Generation

First generation cephalosporins have the similar spectrums of activity as natural penicillins. They

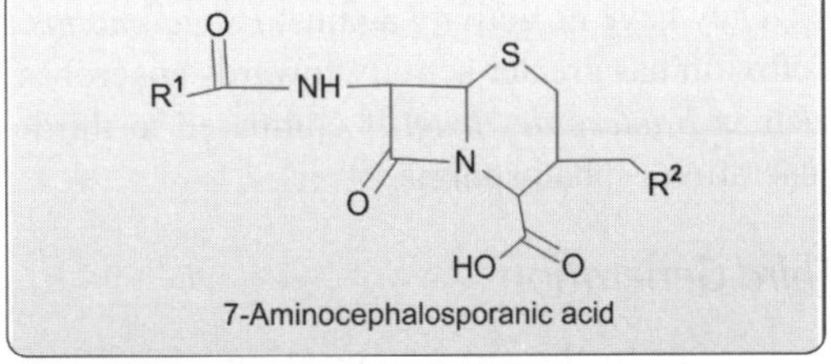

Figure 8.6 Cephalosporin structure showing: (a) Characteristic beta lactam ring; (b) Thiozolidine ring

Table 8.2 Classification of cephalosporins

Generation	Drugs
First generation	Cefalotin, cefazolin, cefapirin, cefacetrile, cefadroxil, cefalexin, cefradine, cefaloridine, cefrezole
Second generation	Cefaclor, cefuroxime, cefamandole, cefonicid, ceforanide, cefoxitin
Third generation Basic third generation cephalosporins:	Cefotaxime, ceftriaxone, cefixime, ceftizoxime, ceftibuten, cefpodoxime, cefteram
Third generation cephalosporins with antipseudomonal acivity:	Cefoperazone, ceftazidime
Fourth generation	Cefclidine, cefepime, cefluprenam, cefpirome, cefozopran, cefquinome.

possess excellent coverage against most Gram-positive pathogens but poor coverage against most Gram-negative pathogens. Sensitive Gram-positive bacteria include Group A streptococcal pyogenes, beta lactamase producing and non-producing *Staphylococcus aureus*, *Clostridium perfringens*, and many other strains of streptococci.

Second Generation

These agents are broad spectrum and are effective against Gram-positive and Gram-negative organisms. However, their activity against Gram-positive organisms is less than that of the first-generation agents and their activity against Gram-negative organisms is less than that of the third-generation agents. Examples of Gram-negative organisms that are susceptible include *Neisseria gonorrhoea*, *Neisseria meningitidis*, *Haemophilus influenzae*, *Proteus* and *Enterobacter*. They have no activity against *Pseudomonas*. Cefoxitin has greater activity towards anaerobes such as *Bacteroides fragilis* compared to third-generation cephalosporins.

Third Generation

Compared to the first generation, the third-generation cephalosporins have better activity against Gram-negative organisms but are less active against Gram-positive organisms with some of them having activity against *Pseudomonas*.

Fourth Generation

They are extended-spectrum agents with similar activity against Gram-positive organisms as the third-generation cephalosporins. They are highly effective against Gram-negative organisms such as *P. aeruginosa*, Enterobacteriaceae, *Haemophilus, Proteus* and *Neisseria*. They also have a greater resistance to beta lactamases than the third generation cephalosporins.

Pharmacokinetics

Besides oral and pareteral administration, cephalosporins can be administered by topical, subconjunctival and intravitreal route for the treatment of ophthalmic infections. The formulations of cefazolin sodium, ceftazidime and ceftriaxone available for ophthalmic use are listed under "drugs used in ocular therapeutics". These drugs are widely distributed to most body tissues and fluids including aqueous humor.

Overall, cephalosporins do not undergo metabolism and are excreted unchanged by glomerular filtration and tubular secretion in urine. Some cephalosporins do, however, undergo metabolism and their metabolites show less antibacterial activity. Cefoperazone and ceftriaxone undergo billiary secretion, which makes them both, the choice in patients with renal impairment.

Adverse Effects

Cephalosporins are generally a safe class of antibiotics. As in the case of penicillins, hypersensitivity can occur with cephalosporins, which may range from mild allergic reaction that manifest as an urticarial or a maculopapular rash to a life-threatening reaction like-anaphylaxis. Approximately, 20% of patients with hypersensitivity to penicillins will also have cross-reactivity with cephalosporins. Because this cross-reactivity is not absolute, with caution, cephalosporin can still be administered to patients with a history of hypersensitivity reactions to penicillins.

Therapeutic Uses

Types of Ocular Infection Suitable for Treatment by Cephalosporins

1. Acute conjunctivitis and blepharitis caused by Gram-positive flora (*S. aureus, Streptococcus* species): Topical first generation cephalosporins (cefazolin).
2. Gonococcal conjunctivitis and gonococcal corneal ulceration: Basic third generation cephalosporins (ceftriaxone, cefotaxime) intramuscularly or intravenously. In the only published study by Haimovici and Roussel, a single 1 gram intramuscular injection of ceftriaxone was used in the treatment of gonococcal conjunctivitis.[16]
3. Bacterial keratitis and corneal ulceration due to Gram-positive flora: First generation cephalosporins (cefazolin) by subconjunctival injections.
4. Pseudomonal keratitis and corneal ulceration: Third and fourth generation cephalosporins with antipseudomonal activity (ceftazidime, cefipime), subconjunctival injections or systemic (intramuscular and intravenous) injection in case of corneal perforation.
5. Dacryocystitis and dacryoadenitis: Second and third generation cephalosporins intravenously.[17]

6. Bacterial endophthalmitis: Usually combination therapy of ceftazidime and vancomycin intravitreal.[18]
7. Pre-operative prophylaxis of post-operative endophthalmitis: Second generation cephalosporins (cefuroxime) intracameral injection.[19]

CARBAPENEMS

This class of beta lactam antibiotics include imipinem/cilastatin, meropenem, etarpenem, doripenem, panipenem, biapenem, razupenem and are derived from thienamycin, naturally obtained from *Streptomyces cattleya*. The prototype drug is imepenem. The antibacterial activity of the carbepenems includes both, Gram-positive and Gram-negative organisms such as *Streptococcus, Staphylococcus, Listeria, Pseudomonas and Acinetobacter*. They are also effective against anaerobes, including *Clostridium difficile* and *Bacteroides fragillis*.[20] This drug class is resistant to most beta lactamases.

Pharmacokinetics

Carbapenems are administered intravenously and are not absorbed orally. They penetrate well into aqueous humor and vitreous.[21]

Imipenem is hydrolyzed by an enzyme found in renal tubules, dehydropeptidase and produces nephrotoxic metabolites. It is marketed in combination with cilastatin, a drug that inhibits dehydropeptidase. This combination does not increase the plasma levels of imipenem but significantly reduces the nephrotoxic metabolites. It has a half life of proximately 1 hour. Imipenem is largely excreted unchanged in urine and a small amount into the bile, which is insufficient to disturb the normal flora of the colon. Although cilastatin is also excreted by the kidneys, only imipenem is cleared by extra-renal mechanisms. Therefore, in patients with renal impairment, a dose adjustment may be necessary. Both drugs are cleared by hemodialysis and hemofiltration.

Adverse Effects

Imipenem causes thrombophlebitis on intravenous administration. It can also cause nausea and vomiting. Some metabolites of imipenem are neurotoxic with effects such as tremor, seizure and confusional state. It can also cause fits but this is usually seen in patients with pre-existing CNS disease or patients with renal failure and excessively high levels of imipenem metabolites.

Therapeutic Uses

Carbapenems are administred intravenously and are used in the treatment of severe ocular infections such as bacterial endophthalmitis. They also may be used as pre-operative prophylaxis of post-operative endophthalmitis and in the treatment of orbital cellulitis.[22]

MONOBACTAMS

These are the drugs with a monocyclic beta lactam ring. The prototype is aztreonam. Its mechanism of action is similar to other beta lactams. It is beta lactamase resistant and is highly effective against most Gram-negative aerobes, including *Pseudomonas aeruginosa, Escherichia coli, Klebsiella,* and *Enterobacter.* Due to its specific spectrum of activity, aztreonam does not disturb the normal Gram-positive and anaerobic intestinal flora.

Like imipenem, aztreonam is not absorbed orally. It is given either intramuscularly or intravenously. It is largely excreted unchanged by the kidneys. It is widely distributed throughout the body. The clinical uses of aztreonam include severe ocular infections such as bacterial endophthalmitis caused by Gram-nagative bacteria including *Pseudomonas aeruginosa* resistant to other beta lactam antibiotics. Aztreonam has a little allergic cross-reactivity with beta lactams (except ceftazidime) and may be used in case of a prior allergic reaction.[23]

OXACEPHEMS

Oxacephems are synthetic drugs and include moxalactam and flomoxef. They have a molecular structure similar to cephalosporin core and, therefore, they are usually grouped with cephalosporins. Their mechanism of action is the same as that of other beta lactams. Antibiotic spectrum and therapeutic uses are similar to the third generation cephalosporins and include both Gram-positive and Gram-nagative bacteria. Moxalactam can induce hemopoietic disturbances like hypoprothrombinemia, thrombocytopenia and platelet dysfunction, which may result in bleeding.

NON BETA LACTAM ANTIBIOTICS

Chloramphenicol

Chloramphenicol was introduced more than 50 years ago. It was derived from the bacterium *Streptomyces venezuelae,* though now it is produced synthetically. Chloramphenicol is a neutral and stable compound. The formal chemical name (IUPAC) is 2, 2-dichloro-N-((1R,2R)-1, 3-dihydroxy-1-(4-nitrophenyl) propan-2-yl) acetamide. The structure activity relationship of chloramphenicol mandates that not many changes can be made to the molecule. The aromatic ring is essential for the activity of the agent. The structure is as shown in Figure 8.7.

Mechanism of Action

Chloramphenicol is a bacteriostatic antibiotic. It inhibits bacterial protein synthesis. It binds to the 50S ribosomal subunit and inhibits the activity of the enzyme, peptidyl transferase. This results in inhibition of peptidyl tRNA at the donor site 'P' from "donating" the growing peptide chain to aminoacyl t-RNA at the acceptor site 'A', hence preventing elongation of peptide chain (Fig. 8.8). There is some evidence that chloramphenicol inhibits protein synthesis in rapidly proliferating mammalian cells, which may be the cause of reversible bone marrow suppression.

Antibacterial Spectrum

Chloramphenicol exerts bacteriostatic effect on a wide range of Gram-positive and Gram-negative organisms and is active against *Rickettsia* species, *Chlamydia* species and *Mycoplasma* species. It is particularly effective against *H. influenzae, S. pneumoniae, S. typhi, Neisseria meningitidis, Neisseria gonorrhoeae, Brucella* species and *Bordetella pertussis.*

Acquired resistance to chloramphenicol is very common. Usually it is caused by plasmid-mediated production of acetyltransferase. These inactivating enzymes decrease chloramphenicol's ability to bind to the bacterial ribosomes. Another mechanism of resistance is decreased permeability into the bacterial cell. Both natural and acquired resistance to chloramphenicol has been seen in strains of *P. aeruginosa, Staphylococccus,* and Enterobacteriaceae particularly *Shigella, Salmonella,* and *Escherichia.*

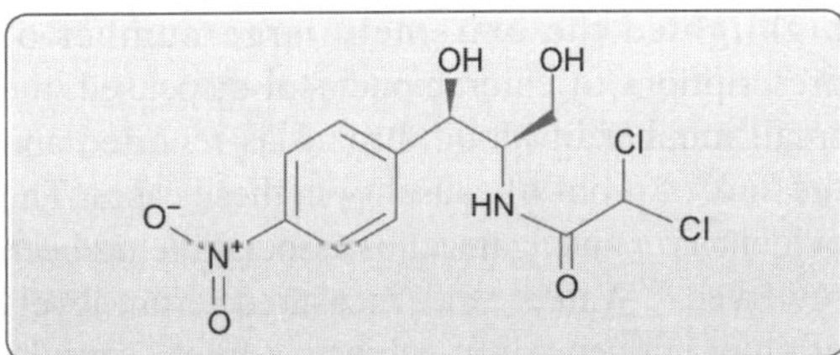

Figure 8.7 Structure of chloramphenicol $(C_{11}H_{12}C_{l2}N_2O_5)$

Pharmacokinetics

Chloramphenicol is uncharged and neutral. It is also relatively water soluble and is well absorbed. It penetrates well into the aqueous humor after topical application.[24] After oral administration of chloramphenicol palmitate, it is rapidly absorbed as free chloramphenicol. The peak serum level after an oral dose of chloramphenicol is acheived in 1 to 3 hours. Chloramphenicol sodium succinate is hydrolyzed to free chloramphenicol following intravenous administration, by esterases in the liver, kidneys and lungs. The rate and extent of hydrolysis and renal elimination of the succinate ester are subject to a high degree of interindividual variation. The palmitate and sodium succinate esters are inactive until hydrolyzed to free chloramphenicol, which occurs rapidly *in vivo.*

Chloramphenicol is approximately 60% protein bound. It is widely distributed in the body. An important aspect of chloramphenicol's distribution is that it is able to penetrate blood ocular barrier. The drug crosses the placenta and is distributed into the breast milk.

Chloramphenicol is metabolized in the liver, mainly by conjugation with glucuronic acid; only about 5 to 15% of an oral dose is excreted unchanged in the urine. The half-life of chloramphenicol is 1.5 to 4 hours in adults. The plasma half-life is increased in patients with markedly reduced hepatic function. In patients

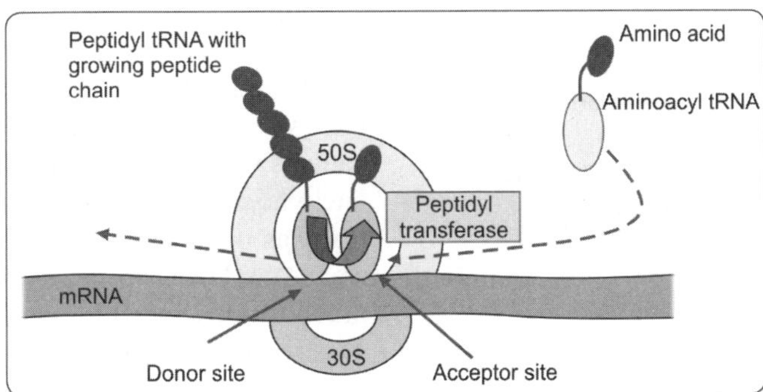

Figure 8.8 Mechanism of action of chloramphenicol

with impaired renal function, the half-life of chloramphenicol itself is not significantly altered although the half-life of the inactive metabolites may be prolonged. Since the processes for glucuronide conjugation and renal excretion in neonates may be immature, the half-life of the drug in neonates less than 3 days old may be in excess of 24 hours and about 10 hours for infants 10–16 days old. In these cases the dosage and administration interval should be adjusted using measured serum concentrations.

Therapeutic Uses

Chloramphenicol's spectrum of activity covers the majority of ocular pathogens. In a study of 738 patients with acute bacterial infections of the external eye, there was an overall resistance rate of only 6% to chloramphenicol, compared to 9% with tetracycline and around 20% to the aminoglycosides tested.[25]

Chloramphenicol is, in many ways, an ideal drug for topical use. It penetrates well into the aqueous humor after topical application and has low ocular surface toxicity. The use of systemic chloramphenicol is reserved for the treatment of serious infections caused by susceptible organisms when less toxic antimicrobials are ineffective or contraindicated.

Types of Ocular Infections Suitable for Treatment by Chloramphenicol

1. Acute bacterial conjunctivitis and blepharitis.
2. Gonococcal conjunctivitis and gonococcal corneal ulcer. Chloramphenicol is used as an alternate for the treatment of gonococcal infection when the cephalosporins or penicillin are not suitable.
3. Bacterial keratitis and corneal ulceration.
4. Dacryocystitis and dacryoadenitis.

Adverse Effects

Chloramphenicol can cause two types of hematological effects, a dose-dependent and a non-dose dependent one. Of the two, the more serious adverse effect is the non-dose dependent aplastic anemia, which can occur with systemic or topical therapy. Although rare (1:25,000 to 40,000), it is a serious adverse event as it is irreversible and may be fatal. It is probably an idiosyncracy that can occur anytime during treatment or weeks and even months after treatment. Although non-dose dependent, it occurs more with prolonged or repetitive treatment. It is more common with doses exceeding 4 g daily or a plasma concentration exceeding 25 mg/mL. Despite the risk of aplastic anemia, it is not contraindicated in patients with serious infections requiring chloramphenicol treatment. The drug should, however, be discontinued if reticulocytopenia, leukopenia, thrombocytopenia, anemia or other hematologic abnormalities occur.

Doona and Walsh recommended that the topical use of chloramphenicol should be restricted due to the possibility of systemic blood dyscrasias.[26] A large number of ophthalmologists and hematologists countered this view and highlighted the extremely large number of prescriptions of chloramphenicol dispensed, the small number of blood dyscrasias reported and the lack of proof of causality in these cases. The evidence for and against this association has been reviewed.[27] Walker et al. measured serum levels of chloramphenicol in subjects after 1–2 weeks of treatment with four times daily instillation. They found that serum levels did not accumulate to detectable levels of 1 mg/L and concluded that topical chloramphenicol did not present a risk of inducing dose-related bone marrow toxicity.[28]

Lancaster et al. used the general practice research database to describe prescribing patterns of chloramphenicol eyedrops and to estimate the risk of aplastic anemia after their use. Three patients with serious hematological toxicity and one who developed mild, transient leukopenia that was not considered serious were identified among the 442,543 patients who received 674,148 prescriptions for chloramphenicol eyedrops. The researchers concluded that, even in the unlikely event that all three cases were caused by chloramphenicol eyedrops, these data indicated that the risk of serious hematological toxicity after treatment with ocular chloramphenicol was small.[29] Wilholm et al. also concluded that data provided no support for the claim that chloramphenicol eyedrops increased the risk of aplastic anemia.[30]

Although, the risk of aplastic anemia due to topical application of chloramphenicol is not well founded, it is very important to monitor the blood count during the chloramphenicol treatment.

Nausea, vomiting and diarrhea occurring early in the course of treatment are commonly due to gastrointestinal tract mucosal irritation. However, if these symptoms are prolonged or if the onset occurs later in therapy, they must be investigated to rule out superinfection.

Optic and peripheral neuritis have been reported, usually following long-term therapy. If this occurs, the drug should be promptly discontinued.

Fever, macular and vesicular rashes, angio-edema and urticaria may occur, especially after topical use. A toxic reaction can occur in premature and newborn infants receiving large doses of chloramphenicol. It is characterized by abdominal distention, vomiting, blue-gray skin color, hypothermia, irregular breathing and cardiovascular collapse, followed by death in few hours or days. If chloramphenicol is stopped early after the onset of symptoms, the infant may recover completely.

Contraindications

Chloramphenicol is contraindicated in individuals with a history of previous hypersensitivity or toxic reaction to it. As chloramphenicol readily crosses the placenta, it should be used with caution in pregnant women although birth defects in humans have not been documented. However, it should not be used in pregnancy at term or during labor because of potential toxicity in premature or full-term infants, including gray baby syndrome. Chloramphenicol should not be used in premature and full-term infants for the same reasons. As chloramphenicol is excreted in human breast milk, it should not be used in nursing mothers because of the possibility of adverse effects in the infant.

Interactions

Chloramphenicol inhibits hepatic microsomal enzymes and may interfere with the metabolism of alfentanil, chlorpropamide, phenobarbital, phenytoin, tolbutamide, warfarin or other drugs metabolized by the microsomal system. Dosages of these drugs may need to be adjusted accordingly. Conversely, drugs such as rifampin or phenobarbital, which induce microsomal enzymes may increase the metabolism and reduce serum concentrations of chloramphenicol. Chloramphenicol may prolong the prothrombin time in patients receiving anticoagulant therapy by interfering with vitamin K production by intestinal bacteria.

Concurrent therapy with chloramphenicol may delay the clinical response to iron preparations, vitamin B_{12} or folic acid in the treatment of anemias. Concomitant administration of chloramphenicol in patients receiving radiation therapy or myelosuppressive drugs may result in additive bone marrow suppression.

Chloramphenicol has been reported to antagonize the bactericidal activity of penicillins and aminoglycosides *in vitro* and some clinicians recommend that these antibiotics not to be used concomitantly. However, *in vivo* antagonism has not been demonstrated and chloramphenicol has been used successfully with ampicillin, penicillin G or aminoglycosides with no apparent decrease in activity.

QUINOLONES AND FLUOROQUINOLONES

The first quinolone, nalidixic acid was introduced into the clinical practice in 1962 by Lescher and colleagues. The fluoroquinolones are a relatively new group of synthetic antibiotics, first introduced in 1986. They are derivatives of quinolones which have a fluorine atom attached to the central ring, typically at the C-6 or C-7 position (Fig. 8.9.)

Classification

Quinolones and fluoroquinolones are divided into four generations (Table 8.3).

First Generation

The first generation agents are the oldest and least often used quinolones. These drugs had poor systemic distribution and limited activity and were used primarily for Gram-negative urinary tract infections. Cinoxacin and nalidixic acid require more frequent dosing than the newer quinolones, and they are more susceptible to the development of bacterial resistance.

Second Generation

The second generation fluoroquinolones have increased Gram-negative activity, as well as some Gram-positive and atypical pathogen coverage. Compared with first generation quinolones, besides the use in ocular infections, these drugs have broader clinical applications in the treatment of complicated urinary tract infections and pyelonephritis, sexually transmitted diseases, selected pneumonias and skin infections. Ciprofloxacin is the most potent fluoroquinolone against *P. aeruginosa*. Ciprofloxacin and ofloxacin are the most widely used second generation quinolones because of their availability in oral, intravenous and topical formulations and their broad set of FDA-labeled indications.

Third Generation

The third generation fluoroquinolones have expanded activity against Gram-positive organisms, particularly penicillin-sensitive and penicillin-resistant *S. pneumoniae*, and atypical pathogens such as *Mycoplasma pneumoniae* and *Chlamydia pneumoniae*. Although the third-generation agents retain broad Gram-negative coverage, they are less active than ciprofloxacin against *Pseudomonas* species. Besides their extensive use in the treatment ocular infections in topical formulation, they are also useful in the treatment of community-acquired pneumonia, acute sinusitis and acute exacerbations of chronic bronchitis.

Fourth Generation

The fourth generation fluoroquinolones have significant antimicrobial activity against anaerobes while maintaining the Gram-positive and Gram-negative activity of the third generation drugs. They also retain activity against *Pseudomonas* species comparable to that of ciprofloxacin. They are available in topical formulation for the treatment of ocular infections.

Mechanism of Action

Fluoroquinolones are the only class of antimicrobial agents in clinical use that are direct inhibitors of bacterial DNA synthesis. Fluoroquinolones inhibit two bacterial

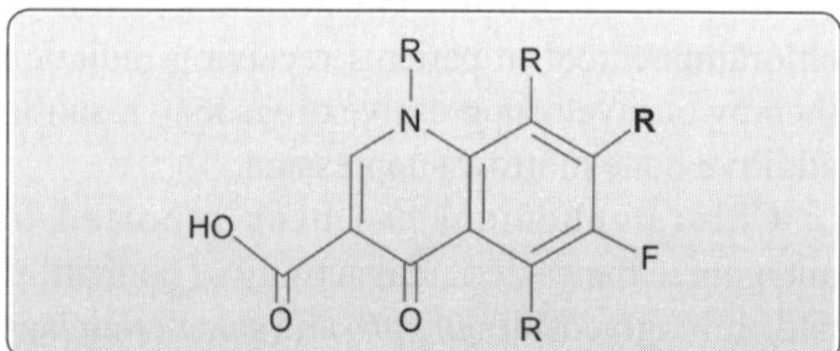

Figure 8.9 Essential structure of all quinolone antibiotics: The R shown in bold is usually piperazine; if the molecule contains fluorine, it is a fluoroquinolone.

Table 8.3 Classification of fluoroquinolones

Generation	Drugs
First generation	Nalidixic acid, cinoxacin, oxolinic acid, pipemidic acid
Second generation	Ciprofloxacin, ofloxacin, norfloxacin, pefloxacin, enoxacin, lomefloxacin
Third generation	Levofloxacin, sparfloxacin, gatifloxacin
Fourth generation	Moxifloxacin, gemifloxacin, trovafloxacin

enzymes, DNA gyrase (topoisomerase II) and topoisomerase IV. DNA gyrase is an essential enzyme involved in the replication, transcription and the repair of damaged DNA. Topoisomerase IV is involved in the separation of chromosomal DNA during cell division. Both enzymes, DNA gyrase and topoisomerase IV, have essential and distinct roles in DNA replication. Topoisomerase IV is the primary quinolone target in Gram-positive bacteria, while DNA gyrase is primarily inhibited by quinolones in Gram-negative microbes.[31]

The quinolones bind to the complex of each of these enzymes with DNA; the resulting complexes, including the drug, block progress of the DNA replication enzyme complex. Finally, this action results in damage to bacterial DNA and bacterial cell death. Thus, fluoroquinolones are bactericidal agents.

Pharmacokinetics

Fluoroquinolones available for treatment of ophthalmic infections are listed under "drugs used in ocular therapeutics". Oral absorption of fluoroquinolones is good but is diminished by coadministration of cations (aluminum, Mg, Ca, zinc, and iron preparations). After oral and parenteral administration, fluoroquinolones are widely distributed in most extracellular and intracellular fluids and are concentrated in the prostate, lungs, and bile.

Fluoroquinolones penetrate well into the aqueous humour after topical application.[32] Moxifloxacin 0.5% has better corneal penetration compared to gatifloxacin 0.3%. Moxifloxacin 0.5 % achieves highest level in aqueous humor followed by gatifloxacin 0.3% and ciprofloxacin 0.3%. Compared to ofloxacin 0.3%, levofloxacin 0.5% has better ocular penetration. Levofloxacin 1.5% better penetrates the corneal tissue and aqueous compared to gatifloxacin.[33] Most fluoroquinolones are metabolized in the liver and excreted in urine, reaching high levels in urine. Moxifloxacin is eliminated primarily in bile.

Therapeutic Uses

The newer fluoroquinolones have a wider clinical use and a broader spectrum of antibacterial activity including Gram-positive and Gram-negative aerobic and anaerobic organisms and have become available for ophthalmic use.

Types of Ocular Infection Suitable for Treatment by Fluoroquinolones

1. Acute bacterial conjunctivitis and blepharitis. Second generation fluoroquinolones are very effective in the treatment of acute bacterial conjunctivitis and blepharitis. Ciprofloxacin has been compared with chloramphenicol and tobramycin in the treatment of conjunctivitis and blepharitis. Power et al. investigated the efficacy of ciprofloxacin and chloramphenicol in 57 culture-positive patients and reported that the difference between the groups was not significant.[34] Safety was also similar, with only one patient from each treatment group suffering an adverse event. Liebowitz compared ciprofloxacin with tobramycin in a placebo controlled trial of 288 culture-positive patients with bacterial conjunctivitis. Both antibiotics were highly effective and significantly superior to placebo.[35]

2. Gonococcal conjunctivitis and gonococcal corneal ulcer. Second generation fluoro-quinolones (ciprofloxacin) are used topically and parenterally in the treatment of gonococcal conjunctivitis and keratitis.

3. Bacterial keratitis and corneal ulceration. The common pathogens causing bacterial keratitis are *Pseudomonas aeruginosa, Pneumococcus, Moraxella* species, and Staphylococci. Fluoroquinolones such as levofloxacin 0.5%, ofloxacin 0.3%, norfloxacin 0.3%, or ciprofloxacin 0.3% are commonly used as first-line agents to treat this condition as long as local prevalence of resistant organisms is low.[36] If the pathogen identified is *Mycobacteria*, the fourth-generation fluoroquinolones (moxifloxacin 0.5% and gatifloxacin 0.3%) are indicated. In a prospective, multicenter clinical

study, the clinical and antibacterial efficacy of ciprofloxacin 0.3% with that of standard dual therapy in 148 culture proven cases of bacterial keratitis was compared. Most patients in the standard dual therapy group received cefazolin 3.3% with gentamicin or tobramycin 1.4%. Success rates were similar at 92% for ciprofloxacin and 88% for the dual therapy.[35]

4. Bacterial endophthalmitis.
5. Pre-operative prophylaxis for post-operative endophthalmitis. Fluoroquinolones are the drug of choice in the prophylaxis of post-operative endophthalmitis. In contrast with cephalosporines, that are used as intracameral injection, fluoroquinolones are used as topical ophthalmic solution.[37]

Adverse Effects

The fluoroquinolones as a class are generally well tolerated. Most adverse effects are mild in severity, self-limited, and rarely result in treatment discontinuation. Some of the adverse effects are outlined below.

Local Adverse Reactions

Local adverse effects following ocular administration of fluoroquinolones include pain or discomfort in the eye, swelling, foreign body sensation, itching, conjunctival hyperemia and transient burning. The frequencies of occurrences with individual fluoroquinolone are as tabulated in Table 8.4.

One of the untoward ocular events associated with ciprofloxacin therapy was a white crystalline precipitate, commonly located in the superficial portion of the corneal defect (i.e. the area of inflammation). This problem was encountered in 16.6% of patients. A group of ophthalmologists involved in the multicenter study noted the appearance of the white precipitate as the only potential adverse effect in the ciprofloxacin group.[38] Although, the precipitate resolved in all patients and did not appear to cause any scarring, they saw it as a disadvantage because it caused a temporary decrease in vision and prevented adequate evaluation of the corneal infiltrate. Precipitation of ciprofloxacin occurs as a result of change in the pH of the eyedrop as it mixes with the tear film.[39]

Phototoxicity

Exposure to ultraviolet rays from direct or indirect sunlight should be avoided during treatment and for several days (5 days with sparfloxacin) after the use of the drug. The degree of phototoxic potential of fluoroquinolones is as follows: lomefloxacin > sparfloxacin > ciprofloxacin

Table 8.4 Prevalence of adverse effects of fluoroquinolones

Adverse effects / Drugs	Local Discomfort or pain	Local edema	Sensation of foreign body	Itching	Conjucntival hyperemia	Burning
Ciprofloxacin[29]	2%	< 1%	< 10%	< 10%	< 10%	Reported
Ofloxacin 0.3% (Ocuflox)[34]	Reported	Reported	Reported	Reported	Reported	Reported
Levofloxacin 0.5% (Quixin)[31]	1–3%	< 1%	1–3%	< 1%	Not reported	1–3%
Levofloxacin 1.5% (Iquix)[31]	1–2%	< 1%	Not reported	Not reported	Not reported	1–2%
Gatifloxacin 0.3% (Zymar)[30]	1–4%	1–4%	Not reported	1–4%	1–4%	1–4%
Moxifloxacin 0.5% (Vigamox)[31]	1–6%	Not reported	Not reported	1–6%	1–6%	1–6%

> norfloxacin = ofloxacin = levofloxacin = gatifloxacin = moxifloxacin.

Systemic Adverse Reactions

The most common adverse events experienced with oral fluoroquinolone administration are gastrointestinal such as nausea, vomiting, diarrhea, constipation, and abdominal pain, which occur in 1 to 5% of patients.

Headache, dizziness, and drowsiness have been reported with all fluoroquinolones. Insomnia was reported in 3–7% of patients with ofloxacin. Severe CNS effects, including seizures, have been reported in patients receiving trovafloxacin. Seizures may develop within 3 to 4 days of therapy but resolve with drug discontinuation. Although seizures are infrequent, fluoroquinolones should be avoided in patients with a history of convulsion, cerebral trauma, or anoxia. No seizures have been reported with levofloxacin, moxifloxacin, gatifloxacin, and gemifloxacin. With the older non-fluorinated quinolones neurotoxic symptoms such as dizziness occurred in about 50% of the patients.

Concern about the development of musculoskeletal effects, evident in animal studies, has led to the contraindication of fluoroquinolones for routine use in children and in women who are pregnant or lactating.

Although fluoroquinolone-related tendinitis generally resolves within one week of discontinuation of therapy, spontaneous ruptures have been reported as long as nine months after cessation of fluoroquinolone use. Potential risk factors for tendinopathy include age > 50 years, male gender, and concomitant use of corticosteroids.

Trovafloxacin use has been associated with rare liver damage, which prompted the withdrawal of the oral preparations from the US market. However, the IV preparation is still available for treatment of infections so serious that the benefits outweigh the risks.

The newer quinolones have been found to produce additional toxicities to the heart that were not found with the older compounds. Evidence suggests that sparfloxacin and grepafloxacin may have the most cardiotoxic potential.

Recently, rare cases of hypoglycemia have been reported with gatifloxacin and ciprofloxacin in patients also receiving oral antidiabetic medications, primarily sulfonylureas. Although hypoglycemia has also been reported with other fluoroquinolones (levofloxacin and moxifloxacin), the effects have been mild.

Hypersensitivity reactions occur only occasionally during quinolone therapy and are generally mild to moderate in severity, and usually resolve after treatment is stopped.

Contraindications

Contraindications include previous allergic reaction to ciprofloxacin or other quinolones and certain disorders that predispose to arrhythmias such as QT-interval prolongation, uncorrected hypokalemia or hypomagnesemia, significant bradycardia.

Fluoroquinolones are approved for use only in people older than 18 years of age. They are contraindicated in children and in pregnant women because they may cause cartilage lesions if growth plates are open. However, some experts, who challenge this view because evidence is weak, have recommended prescribing fluoroquinolones as a 2nd-line antibiotic and restricting use to a few specific situations with severe and life-threatening infections. The safety and efficacy of fluoroquinolone eyedrops in children under the age of one year has not been established.

Fluoroquinolones are assigned to pregnancy risk category C (FDA), indicating that these drugs have the potential to cause teratogenic or embryocidal effects. Giving fluoroquinolones during pregnancy is not recommended unless the benefits justify the potential risks to the fetus. These agents are also excreted in breast milk and should be avoided during breast-feeding.

Interactions

Ciprofloxacin is a potent inhibitor of cytochrome P450 and may interfere with the metabolism of chlorpropamide, phenytoin, tolbutamide, warfarin, theophylline and other drugs metabolized by the microsomal system. Dosages of these drugs may need to be adjusted accordingly. The use of fluoroquinolones with drugs known to prolong the QT interval or to cause bradycardia (e.g. metoclopramide, cisapride, erythromycin, clarithromycin, classes Ia and III antiarrhythmics, tricyclic antidepressants) will increase the risk or worsen their cardiovascular adverse effects.

TETRACYCLINES

Tetracyclines were discovered in the 1950s. Their antimicrobial spectrum was broader than any other antibiotic known at that time. The individual tetracyclines differ in pharmacokinetic properties such as absorption, tissue distribution and elimination. Presently, the name "tetracycline" refers to a group of antibiotics of either natural (derived from a species of *Streptomyces*), or semi-synthetic origin with a similar basic structure of four linearly annealed six-membered rings (Fig. 8.10).

Mechanism of Action

Tetracycline is a group of broad spectrum antibiotics that inhibit bacterial protein synthesis and are bacteriostatic. Tetracycline must first gain entry into the bacterial cell; either by passive diffusion through hydrophilic pores present on bacterial cellular membrane or by active uptake, requiring energy. Tetracyclines enter Gram-negative bacteria by passive diffusion through porin proteins in the outer membrane, followed by active (energy-dependent) transport across the inner cytoplasmic membrane. Uptake into Gram-positive bacteria, such as *Bacillus anthracis* (the causative agent of anthrax), occurs similarly via an energy-dependent transport system. In contrast, mammalian cells lack the active transport system found in susceptible bacteria.

Once in the cell, tetracycline binds reversibly to the 16S rRNA on the 30S ribosomal subunit and inhibits protein synthesis by blocking the binding of aminoacyl tRNA to the A-site on the mRNA-ribosome complex. This action prevents the addition of further amino acids to the nascent peptide. However, inhibition of protein synthesis does not account entirely for the high bacterial selectivity of tetracyclines, because these drugs can also halt eukaryotic protein synthesis *in vitro* at low concentrations. The active accumulation of these drugs in bacteria but not in mammalian cells allows for high selectivity of tetracyclines.

Classification (Table 8.5)

Antibacterial Activity

Tetracyclines are characterized by their exceptional chemotherapeutic efficacy against a wide range of Gram-positive and Gram-negative bacteria, *Rickettsia, Spirochetes*, and large viruses, such as members of the lymphogranuloma group. The list of antibacterial activity of tetracyclines includes:
- Gram-positive cocci (*Staphylococcus* species and *Streptococcus* species)
- Gram-negative cocci (*Neisseria gonorrhoeae*).
- Gram-positive bacilli (*Bacilus anthracis,*

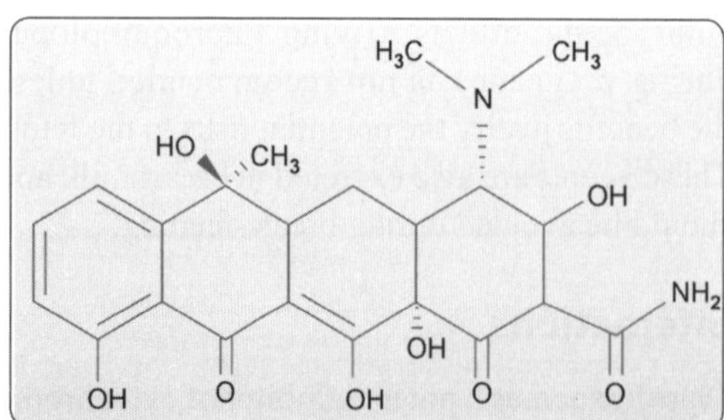

Figure 8.10 Basic structure of tetracycline consists of four rings

Table 8.5 Classification of tetracyclines

Naturally occurring	Semi-synthetic
Tetracycline	Doxycycline
Chlorotetracycline	Minocycline
Oxytetracycline	Methacycline
Demeclocycline	Rolitetracycline
	Tigecycline

Corynebacterium diphtheriae, Clostridia tetani and others)

- Gram-negative bacilli *(Haemophilus influenzae, Helicobacter pylori)*
- Atypical bacteria (*Chlamydia* species *Mycoplasma* species, *Legionella* species, *Ureaplasma)*
- Spirochetes (*Treponema pallidum, Borrelia recurrentis, Borrelia burgdorferi*)
- *Rickettsiae*
- *Listeria* species
- *Vibrio cholera*
- Anaerobes *(Bacteroides* species, *Propionibacterium, Peptococcus).*

Bacterial Resistance

Since the bacterial selectivity of tetracyclines results from drug-concentrating mechanisms, it follows that resistance can occur through increased drug efflux or decreased drug influx. In fact, plasmid-encoded efflux pumps represent the most widespread mechanism employed by tetracycline-resistant microbes. A second form of resistance arises through the production of proteins that interfere with the binding of tetracyclines to the ribosome. Yet a third mechanism is the enzymatic inactivation of tetracyclines.

Because of the development of strains of microorganisms resistant to the tetracyclines, these antibiotics have lost some of their usefulness. They are no longer the drugs of first choice for the treatment of staphylococcal, streptococcal, or pneumococcal infections.[40]

Pharmacokinetics

About 60 to 80% of tetracycline and $\geq$ 90% of doxycycline and minocycline are absorbed after oral use. Absorption is decreased by metallic cations (e.g. Al, Ca, Mg, Fe); thus, tetracyclines should not be taken with preparations containing these substances such as antacids, many vitamin and mineral supplements. Food decreases absorption of tetracycline but not of doxycycline or minocycline. Tetracyclines penetrate into most body tissues and fluids and tetracycline particularly penetrates well into the ocular

tissue. Tetracycline and minocycline are excreted primarily in the urine and doxycycline undergoes billiary excretion. Tetracycline is available as eyedrop and ointment.

Therapeutic Uses

Types of Ocular Infection Suitable for Treatment by Tetracyclines

1. Acute conjunctivitis and blepharitis.
2. Ophthalmia neonatorum. Tetracycline ointment 1% is used in prevention and treatment of gonococcal and chlamydial ophthalmia neonatorum (neonatal conjunctivitis).[41,42]
3. Trachoma. Doxycycline and tetracycline are the first line drugs in the treatment of trachoma.
4. Bacterial keratitis and corneal ulceration due to Gram-positive flora (*Staphylococcus* species). Tetracyclines are used as an alternative treatment, usually in cases of allergic reaction to other antibiotics.
5. Dacryocystitis and dacryoadenitis. Tetracycline is used as alternative to other antibiotics.
6. Bacterial endophthalmitis.

Adverse Effects

Common side-effects associated with tetracyclines include cramps or burning of the stomach, diarrhea, sore mouth or tongue. Tetracyclines should not be used in children under the age of 8 years, and specifically during periods of tooth development.

Tetracyclines are classed as pregnancy category D (there is evidence of human risk, but clinical benefits may outweigh risk). Tetracyclines cross the placenta, enter fetal circulation, accumulate in fetal bones, and, if used during the 2nd or 3rd trimester, may cause permanent discoloration of teeth and alterations in bone development. Tetracyclines enter breast milk, but usually in small amounts (particularly tetracycline). Use during breast feeding is usually discouraged.

Excessive blood levels due to use of high doses or renal insufficiency may lead to fatal acute fatty degeneration of the liver, especially during pregnancy. Minocycline commonly causes vestibular dysfunction, particularly in women, limiting its use. Use of minocycline has also been associated with development of autoimmune disorders such as SLE and polyarteritis nodosa, which may be reversible.

Tetracycline can exacerbate azotemia in patients with renal insufficiency. Expired tetracycline capsules can degenerate and, if ingested, cause Fanconi syndrome. Patients should be instructed to discard the expired drug.

Other side-effects include, candidiasis, *Clostridium difficile*-induced diarrhea (pseudomembranous colitis) and if not swallowed with water, tetracycline can cause esophageal erosions. Tetracyclines can cause skin photosensitivity, which increases the risk of sunburn upon exposure to UV light. Rarely, tetracyclines may cause allergic reactions. Very rarely severe headache and vision problems may be signs of dangerous secondary intracranial hypertension.

MACROLIDES

Macrolides are products of *Actinomycetes* (soil bacteria) or semi-synthetic derivatives of them. The prototype drug, erythromycin, which consists of two sugar moieties attached to a 14-atom lactone ring, was obtained in 1952 from *Streptomyces erythreus*. Clarithromycin and azithromycin are semi-synthetic derivatives of erythromycin (Fig. 8.11).

Classification

According to their chemical structure macrolides may be divided into 14-membered, 15-membered and 16-membered structures (Table 8.6).[43]

Mechanism of Action

Erythromycin and other macrolide antibiotics inhibit protein synthesis by binding reversibly to the 23S rRNA molecule on the 50S subunit of the bacterial ribosome. They inhibit the enzyme peptidyltransferase from forming the peptide

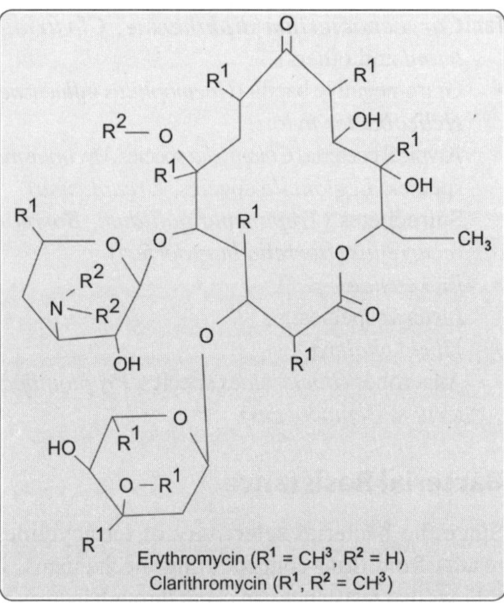

Figure 8.11 Chemical structure of macrolides

bonds between the amino acids. In addition to inhibition of peptide bond formation, macrolides also prevent the translocation of peptidyl tRNA from the A-site to the P-site thus blocking the elongation of growing peptide chain of sensitive microorganisms. Their binding site is either identical or in close proximity to that for clindamycin and chloramphenicol.

Antibacterial Spectrum

The macrolides have an antimicrobial spectrum similar to or slightly wider than that of penicillin, and are often used for patients allergic to penicillins. They are effective against Gram-positive organisms especially *Streptococcus* species *Staphylococcus* species (except MRSA), and *Corynebacteria diphtheriae*.

In contrast to beta lactams they are active against atypical organisms, such as *Mycoplasma* species, *Chlamydia* species (including *Chlamydia trachomatis, C. psittaci, C. pneumoniae), Legionella* species, *Listeria and Ureaplasma urealyticum*.[44] Certain mycobacteria (*Mycobacterium kansasii, M. scrofulaceum*) are

Table 8.6 Classification of macrolides

14-Membered	15-Membered (Azalides)	16-Membered
Naturally occurring	**Naturally occurring**	**Naturally occurring**
Erythromycin	—	Spiramycin Midecamycin Josamycin
Semi-synthetic	**Semi-synthetic**	**Semi-synthetic**
Clarithromycin Roxithromycin	Azithromycin	Midecamycin acetate

also susceptible. Gram-negative organisms such as *Neisseria, Bordetella pertussis, Bartonella henselae, B. quintana,* some *Rickettsiae* species, *Treponema pallidum*, and *Helicobacter pylori* are susceptible. However, *Haemophilus influenzae* is somewhat less susceptible.[45]

Bacterial Resistance

There are a few mechanisms by which microorganisms can become resistant to macrolides. The most common are altered binding site and active efflux of antibiotic.[46] The active efflux of antibiotic (plasmid-mediated) is mostly associated with Gram-positive bacteria and may be overcome by high doses of macrolides. Mutational changes of the 23S ribosomal RNA of the 50S ribosomal subunit, which may be chromosomal, plasmid or on a transposon can also result in failure of drug binding.

Pharmacokinetics

Macrolides are usually administered orally. Erythromycin is also available as ophthalmic ointment. Macrolides are highly liposoluble and, therefore, are well absorbed through conjunctiva and cornea. They can also be administered intravenously. Orally administered erythromycin is inactivated by gastric acid and thus given as an enteric coated formulation. Esters of erythromycin such as stearate or estolate are resistant to inactivation. Clarithromycin is less susceptible to acid but undergoes extensive first pass hepatic metabolism.[47]

After systemic administration, macrolides penetrate well into all tissues including ocular tissue. The tissue concentration of macrolide can be 10–200 times higher than in plasma. The ability for azithromycin to accumulate in tissues, which act as a reservoir, provides post antibiotic effect of azithromycin.[48] Macrolides tend to accumulate within leukocytes, and are, therefore, actually transported into the site of infection.[49] Gram-positive bacteria accumulate erythromycin about 100 times more than do the Gram-negative microorganisms. The non-ionized form of the drug is considerably more permeable to cells, and this probably explains the increased antimicrobial activity observed in alkaline pH.

Macrolides are metabolized by the cytochrome P450 in liver and their elimination is mainly through bile, although, some undergo renal excretion.

Therapeutic Uses

Types of Ocular Infection Suitable for Treatment by Macrolides

1. Bacterial conjunctivitis and blephritis. Macrolides can be used to treat conjunctivitis caused by bacteria sensitive to them. Chronic or recurrent conjunctivitis may be treated with erythromycin ointment 4 times a day for 7 to 10 days, more useful as a nocturnal agent. They are also indicated in the treatment of adult inclusion conjunctivitis (AIC) and neonatal inclusion conjunctivitis (NIC). For AIC, erythromycin 250 mg is administered orally 4 times a day for 21 days and for NIC, erythromycin 50 mg/kg/day divided in 4 daily doses for 14 days. Erythromycin ophthalmic ointment may be applied to newborn eyes

within 1 hour of delivery for prophylaxis against NIC.

2. Trachoma. Macrolides are used in the treatment of trachoma. In children, azithromycin 20 mg/kg orally may be given as a single dose due to its significant postantibiotic effect. [50]

Adverse Effects

The most frequent side-effects of oral erythromycin are gastrointestinal and are dose-related. They include nausea, vomiting, abdominal pain, diarrhea and anorexia. Onset of the symptoms of pseudomembranous colitis may occur during or after antibacterial treatment. Symptoms of hepatitis, hepatic dysfunction and/or abnormal liver function tests may occur. Erythromycin has been associated with QT prolongation and ventricular arrhythmias, including ventricular tachycardia and torsades de pointes. Allergic reactions with rash and eosinophilia can occur rarely. A less well-known but nonetheless significant adverse reaction to erythromycin, especially after intravenous administration, is ototoxicity, which manifests as tinnitus and/or deafness.

Azithromycin and clarithromycin have fewer gastrointestinal side-effects than erythromycin. The most frequent side-effects are diarrhea, nausea, abnormal taste, dyspepsia, abdominal discomfort, and headache. Most of these events are mild or moderate in severity. Overall, in clinical trials, the rate of premature discontinuation of therapy with azithromycin and clarithromycin has been less than with erythromycin.[51] Table 8.7 summarizes the key differences between erythromycin, clarithromycin and azithromycin.

Contraindications

Patients with severe liver disease should not be given macrolides due to increased risk of toxicity and altered handling. Macrolides should not be given to patients with previous history of an allergic reaction to them.

Interactions

Macrolides inhibit cytochrome P450 and can increase plasma concentration and toxic effects of some drugs. The degree of cytochrome inhibitory potency of macrolides is as follows: *Erythromycin > Clarithromycine > Josamycin = Roxithromycin > Midecamycin > Azithromycin > Spiramycin.* Therefore, azithromycin is unlikely to interact with drugs metabolized via the hepatic cytochrome P450 enzyme system, and few interactions have been reported clinically.[52] Earlier case reports on sudden death prompted a study on a large cohort that confirmed a link between erythromycin, ventricular tachycardia and sudden cardiac death in patients also taking drugs that prolong the metabolism of erythromycin (like verapamil or diltiazem) by interfering with CYP3A4.[53] Hence, erythromycin should not be administered in patients using these drugs, or drugs that also prolong the QT time. Other

Table 8.7 Key differences among macrolides

1. Azithromycin and clarithromycin have improved tolerability and fewer gastrointestinal side-effects than erythromycin.
2. Azithromycin is considered to have little potential for interactions than erythromycin and clarithromycin.
3. Azithromycin and clarithromycin have improved pharmacokinetic properties—better bioavailability, better tissue penetration, prolonged half-lives.
4. Clarithromycin and azithromycin have advantages over erythromycin in dosing regimen.
5. The Gram-positive activity of clarithromycin is superior to that of erythromycin and azithromycin.
6. Azithromycin offers increased Gram-negative coverage compared to erythromycin and clarithromycin.

examples include terfenadine, astemizole, cisapride (withdrawn in many countries for prolonging the QT time) and pimozide.

AMINOGLYCOSIDES

The aminoglycosides are a clinically important group of antibiotics that have bactericidal action. The family includes streptomycin, gentamicin, tobramycin, kanamycin, amikacin and netilmicin. Aminoglycosides that are derived from bacteria of the *Streptomyces* genus are named with the suffix-mycin, whereas those derived from *Micromonospora* are named with the suffix -micin.

The aminoglycosides consist of a centrally positioned hexose nucleus, which is linked by glycosidic bonds with 2 or more amino sugars. The aminoglycoside families differ from each other by having different amino sugars. Neomycin and paromomycin have 3 aminosugars while kanamycin and gentamicin have 2 amino sugars (Fig. 8.12).

Classification (TABLE 8.8)

Mechanism of Action

Aminoglycosides inhibit bacterial protein synthesis and lead to bacterial cell death. The uptake of aminoglycosides into the bacterial cell

Table 8.8 Classification of aminoglycosides

Generation	Drugs
First generation	Streptomycin
	Kanamycin
	Neomycin
	Framycetin
Second generation	Gentamicin
	Tobramycin
	Netilmicin
Third generation	Amikacin
	Sisomicin

is an active one, requiring energy and oxygen. Uptake specifically into Gram-positive organisms is enhanced by cell wall inhibitors such as beta lactams. Once in the cell, aminoglycosides inhibit the protein synthesis in the following ways:

1. Aminoglycosides interrupt the formation of the essential initiation complex and instead form abnormal and dysfunctional complexes.
2. Aminoglycosides induce misreading of the code leading to incorporation of the wrong amino acid into the peptide chain.
3. Aminoglycosides prevent the monosomal linkages, thereby, inhibit the formation of polyribosomes.[54]

It remains unclear how aminoglycosides cause bacterial cell death. Inhibition of protein synthesis provides inadequate explanation of its bactericidal effect as other protein inhibitors produce bacteriostatic effects.

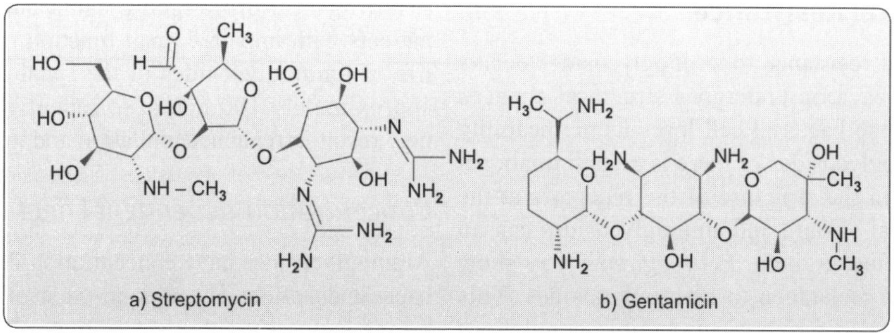

Figure 8.12 Structure of aminoglycoside: Streptomycin and gentamicin

Antibacterial Spectrum

Aminoglycoside antibiotics are primarily active against Gram-negative bacteria. They are the most useful group of antimicrobials for the treatment of Gram-negative infections. Aminoglycosides have no activity against anaerobic bacteria and little activity against Gram-positive bacteria.

The first generation aminoglycosides have more limited spectrum compared to second and third generations. They are effective against *M. tuberculosis* and streptomycin is still the first line drug in the treatment of tuberculosis.

The second generation aminoglycosides are effective against most aerobic Gram-negative bacilli, especially Enterobacteriaceae (*E. coli*, *Proteus* species, *Klebsiella* species, *Enterobacter* species, *Serratia* species), and nonfermentative Gram-negative bacilli (*P. aeruginosa*, *Acinetobacter* species), Tobramycin is more active by one or two MIC tube dilutions than gentamicin against *Pseudomonas aeruginosa* whereas gentamicin is usually more active against *Serratia*. Other aerobic Gram-negative bacilli (*Neisseria gonorrhoeae*, *Neisseria meningitidis*, *Haemophilus influenzae*) are susceptible but are rarely treated with aminoglycosides.

Amikacin according to its chemical structure is not inactivated by aminoglycoside-inactivating enzymes and has been successfully used against gentamicin-resistant strains. Enterococcal infections may be treated with a combination of aminoglycosides with penicillin, ampicillin, or vancomycin.

Bacterial Resistance

Bacterial resistance to aminoglycosides occurs when a bacteria undergoes structural changes such as the bacterial cell loses its permeability to aminoglycosides or there is a conformational change in the structure of the receptors at the ribosomal subunit and aminoglycosides can no longer bind to them. *P. aeruginosa* may show adaptive resistance to aminoglycosides. This occurs when formerly susceptible populations become less susceptible to the antibiotic as a result of decreased intracellular concentrations of the antibiotic.

Bacteria producing enzymes that can inactivate aminoglycoside are also resistant to aminoglycosides. Because of structural differences, amikacin is not inactivated by the common enzymes that inactivate gentamicin and tobramycin. Therefore, a large proportion of the Gram-negative aerobes that are resistant to gentamicin and tobramycin are sensitive to amikacin. In addition, with increased use of amikacin, a lower incidence of resistance has been observed compared with increased use of gentamicin and tobramycin.[55]

Pharmacokinetics

Topically applied aminoglycosides are primarily absorbed through conjunctiva due to their hydrophilic nature. Periocular injections (subconjunctival) provide significant ocular tissue concentration. Aminoglycosides are poorly absorbed from the gastrointestinal tract. After parenteral administration, aminoglycosides are primarily distributed within the extracellular fluid. They do not penetrate well into the aqueous humor and vitreous fluid of the eye. Penetration of biologic membranes is poor because of the drug's polar structure, and intracellular concentrations are usually low, with the exception of the proximal renal tubule.

Aminoglycosides are primarily eliminated unchanged by the kidney through glomerular filtration. This route accounts for elimination of approximately 85 to 95% of the dose administered resulting in a prolonged plasma half-life in patients with impaired renal function. The half-life of aminoglycosides in the renal cortex is approximately 100 hours, so repetitive dosing may result in renal accumulation and toxicity.

Concentration-dependent Effect

Aminoglycosides have concentration-dependent bactericidal effect. The rate and extent of bacterial killing increases with increase in concentration. It is suggested that the optimum antibacterial effect is observed at serum concentration to bacterial MIC ratio of > 10:1. The postantibiotic effect of aminoglycosides may not increase with concentration and Gram-negative bacteria may show reducing postantibiotic effect over time with multiple doses of aminoglycoside.

Administration and Dosage

The commercially available topical ocular aminoglycosides include gentamicin, neomycin, framycetin and tobramycin. The fortified 1.5% preparation, available from special order manufacturers, is used in combination with a cephalosporin for the treatment of bacterial keratitis. Gentamicin causes corneal toxicity at this strength. Neomycin is rarely used alone as an antibacterial agent but is widely used in combination with topical corticosteroids in preparations such as Betnesol-N and Maxitrol. Framycetin, which has a similar antibacterial spectrum to neomycin, previously available as a single agent in eyedrop and ointment form, is now only available with gramicidin and dexamethasone as Sofradex eye/ear drops for the short-term treatment of steroid responsive conditions of the eye when prophylactic antibiotic treatment is also required. Tobramycin, like framycetin, is only available as a combination product. Tobradex contains tobramycin and dexamethasone. Gentamicin is also administered subconjunctivally and intravitreally.

Therapeutic Uses

Gentamicin and tobramycin (in fortified form) has been a "go to" agent for the treatment of Gram-negative ocular infections, especially *Pseudomonas aeruginosa*. Gentamicin is the aminoglycoside used most often because of its low cost and reliable activity against Gram-negative aerobes. However, local resistance patterns should influence the choice of therapy. In general, gentamicin, tobramycin and amikacin are used in similar circumstances, often interchangeably.

Types of Ocular Infection Suitable for Treatment by Aminoglycosides

1. Acute conjunctivitis, blepharitis and blepharo-conjunctivitis.
2. Bacterial keratitis and corneal ulceration.
3. Dacryocystitis and dacryoadenitis.
4. Bacterial endophthalmitis. Amikacin is the aminoglycoside of choice for the treatment of Gram-negative bacterial endophthalmitis, because it is thought to be less toxic to intraocular structures than gentamicin and tobramycin.
5. Prophylaxis of post-operative infections. Tobramicin and neomycin are used for prophylaxis against infections following ocular surgery. Tobramycin is said to be less allergenic than neomycin. In addition, neomycin use is limited by the side-effect of contact dermatitis, which is said to occur in up to 4% of patients.

Adverse Effects and Interactions

The toxicities of aminoglycosides include nephrotoxicity, ototoxicity (vestibular and auditory) and, rarely, neuromuscular blockade and hypersensitivity reactions.

Ototoxicity is usually irreversible. Originally, ototoxicity was believed to result from transiently high peak serum concentrations, resulting in a high concentration of drug in the inner ear. Recent studies in animal models have indicated that aminoglycoside accumulation in the ear is dose-dependent but saturable. Once a threshold concentration of the antibiotic has been reached, increasing the drug concentration results in no further uptake.

Nephrotoxicity, which is usually reversible, is mostly associated with systemic treatment by aminoglycosides, though the case of acute renal failure after topical fortified gentamicin has also been repoted.[55] Nephrotoxicity results from renal cortical accumulation resulting in tubular cell degeneration and sloughing. Examination of urine sediment may reveal dark-brown, fine or granulated casts consistent with acute tubular necrosis but not specific for aminoglycoside renal toxicity. Monitoring of serum creatinine level may indicate renal toxicity, although it is more reflective of glomerular damage. Certain medications such as loop diuretics, ACE inhibitors, amphotericin and other nephrotoxic medications may increase the risk of renal toxicity with aminoglycoside use.

Contraindications

Aminoglycosides are contraindicated for use in patients with allergic reactions to aminoglycosides, myasthenia gravis, severe cardiovascular pathology, severe renal diseases and uremia, disorders of cerebral circulation, pregnancy and breastfeeding.

SULFONAMIDES

Sulfonamides were the first antibacterial agents used systemically for the treatment of bacterial infections. They are synthetic derivatives of para-aminobenzene sulfonamide (sulfanilamide). They are widely used antibacterial agents because they are relatively cheaper than other anti-bacterial agents. They are rarely used alone today. Often, they are combined with trimethoprim, which is not chemically related but is considered here because their modes of action are complementary. The sulfonamide that is most commonly used to treat ocular infection is sulfacetamide (Fig. 8.13).

Classification

Sulfonamides are classified on the basis of rapidity of their absorption and excretion (Table 8.9).

Mechanism of Action

Sulfonamides

Sulfonamides are derived from sulfanilamide, which is similar in structure to para-aminobenzoic

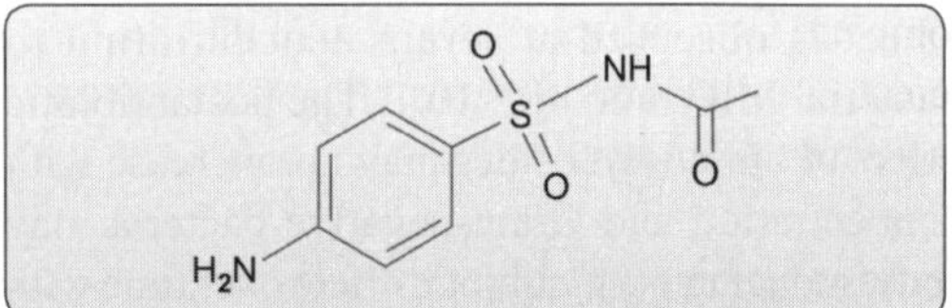

Figure 8.13 Structure of sulfacetamide

acid (PABA), a factor required by bacteria for folic acid synthesis (Fig. 8.14). Sulfonamides are competitive antagonists of PABA and inhibit the bacterial enzyme, dihydropteroate synthase that is responsible for incorporation of PABA into dihydrofolic acid, the precursor of folic acid. Thus sulfonamides inhibit the biosynthesis of folic acid, which is essential for the growth of susceptible organisms as folic acids is essential for the synthesis of purine nucleotides for DNA and RNA.

Only organisms that have to synthesize their own folic acid are inhibited by sulfonamides. Animal cells and bacteria that are capable of utilizing folic acid precursors or preformed folic acid are not affected by these drugs. The antibacterial activity of the sulfonamides decreases in the presence of blood or purulent exudates, which contain PABA.

Sulfonamides are bacteriostatic drugs and final eradication of infection depends also on cellular and humoral defense mechanisms of the host.

Trimethoprim (TMP)

Trimethoprim is a potent inhibitor of the bacterial enzyme dihydrofolate reductase and interferes

Table 8.9 Classification of sulfonamides

Class	Drugs
Absorbed and excreted rapidly	Sulfisoxazole Sulfamethoxazole Sulfadiazine
Well-absorbed and excreted slowly (long-acting)	Sulfadoxine
Poorly absorbed	Sulfasalazine
Topically used	Sulfacetamide Silver sulfadiazine

competitively with the conversion of dihydrofolic acid to tetrahydrofolic acid (Fig. 8.14). It is a bacteriostatic drug.

Cotrimoxazole

Cotrimoxazole is a combination of a sulfonamide (sulfamethoxazole) and trimethoprim. Combined administration of both trimethoprim and sulfonamides exerts synergistic antimicrobial activity leading to bactericidal effect. The synergistic effect is because of sequential blockade of two steps in the same metabolic pathway of folic acid synthesis. The regular strength cotrimoxazole tablets contain trimethoprim and sulfamethoxazole in the ratio of 1:5 (80 mg of trimethoprim and 400 mg of sulfamethoxazole). This proportion provides an ideal blood ratio of 1:20 and provides synergy.

Antibacterial Spectrum

Initially sulfonamides possessed a wide range of antimicrobial activity against both Gram-positive and Gram-negative bacteria such as *Staphylococcus aureus, Streptococcus pneumoniae, Streptococcus pyogenes, Neisseria meningitidis, Haemophilus influenzae, Escherichia coli, Shigella* species, *Klebsiella* species However, acquired bacterial resistance has now diminished the clinical usefulness of sulfonamides.

Pharmacokinetics

All orally administered sulfonamides are rapidly absorbed and are distributed throughout the body. They are metabolized in the liver by glucuronidation. The free drug and its metabolites are excreted in the urine. Sulfonamides compete for bilirubin-binding sites on albumin. Sulfacetamide sodium is suitable for ophthalmic use because it is freely soluble in water and less alkaline and, therefore, less irritating to the conjunctiva than other sulfonamides.

Trimethoprim is well absorbed and excreted by the kidneys.

Administration and Dosage

Sulfonamides generally are used in the oral form, though parenteral preparations are also available. Sulfacetamide sodium is a white, odorless, crystalline powder with a bitter taste and is freely soluble in water and sparingly soluble in alcohol. Commercially available 30% ophthalmic solutions of sulfacetamide sodium have a pH of 6.8–7.5, whereas, the solutions of other sulfonamides are highly alkaline.

Therapeutic Uses

Treatment of conjunctivitis, corneal ulcers, and other superficial infections of the eye caused by susceptible *Staphylococcus aureus, Streptococcus pneumoniae, Streptococcs viridans, Haemophilus influenzae, Enterobacter, Escherichia coli*, and *Klebsiella*.

Adverse Effects

Topical

The most frequently reported adverse effects following topical application of sulfacetamide sodium ophthalmic preparations are local

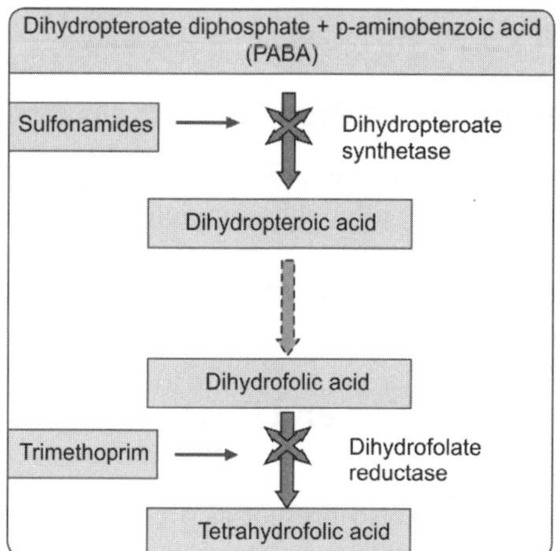

Figure 8.14 Biosynthetic pathway of tetrahydrofolic acid with PABA and sites of action of sulfonamides and trimethoprim

irritation, stinging, and burning. Conjunctivitis, conjunctival hyperemia, and secondary infections have been reported less frequently.

Topical application of sulfonamides may produce sensitization and subsequent systemic use should be avoided. Similarly for patients sensitized following systemic use, topical application should be avoided. Stevens-Johnson syndrome following use of sulfacetamide sodium ophthalmic ointment has been reported in a patient with history of bullous lesions with systemic sulfonamide therapy. Local hypersensitivity that progressed to a fatal syndrome resembling systemic lupus erythematosus has also been reported.

Systemic

Systemic adverse effects associated with sulfonamides include folate deficiency, hyperkalemia (trimethoprim can decrease renal tubular potassium excretion) and renal insufficiency. Nausea, vomiting, and rash are more common. Patients with AIDS have a high incidence of adverse effects, especially fever, rash and neutropenia.

Folate deficiency may result in macrocytic anemia. Use of folinic acid can prevent or treat macrocytic anemia, leukopenia and thrombocytopenia, which sometimes occur with prolonged cotrimoxazole use.

Rarely, severe hepatic necrosis occurs. The drug may also cause a syndrome resembling aseptic meningitis. Like other broad spectrum antibiotics, the use of sulfonamides may result in the overgrowth of non-susceptible organisms including fungi (superinfection).

Contraindications

The possibility of adverse reactions associated with systemic use of sulfonamides should be considered in patients receiving topical sulfonamides. Sulfonamides are contraindicated in patients who have previously exhibited hypersensitivity to sulfonamides or other ingredients in the formulations.

Interactions

Gentamicin sulfate antagonizes the action of sulfacetamide sodium, so concomitant administration should be avoided.

BACITRACIN

Bacitracin, an antibiotic substance derived from the cultures of *Bacillus subtilis*, has antibacterial action *in vitro* against a variety of Gram-positive and a few Gram-negative organisms. It is not used parenterally because it can cause renal necrosis with systemic use. It is mainly reserved for topical use.

Mechanism of Action

Bacitracin inhibits synthesis of cell wall by inhibiting the precursor peptidoglycan from migrating from the cytoplasm through the cell wall for incorporation into the peptidoglycan layer.

Antibacterial Spectrum

Bacitracin has a narrow antibacterial spectrum. Gram-positive bacteria such as *Staphylococcus* species and *Streptococcus* species are susceptible. Gram-negative bacteria are mostly resistant, except *Neisseria* species.

Pharmacokinetics

It is not absorbed after topical application or oral administration, although completely absorbed following intramuscular injection. It is slowly excreted by glomerular filtration and appears in urine within 24 hours.

Administration and Dosage

Bacitracin is available as a single-agent preparation and is also present as a component in a fixed-combination preparation. The topical, preparation of bacitracin is in the form of ointment as the drug is not stable in solution. However, more commonly a combination of neomycin, polymyxin and bacitracin ointment is used to treat superficial infections of conjunctiva, eyelids and cornea.

Therapeutic Uses

Bacitracin is never used as a systemic agent because it causes serious nephrotoxicity. It is usually used in combination with polymixin B and neomycin, both of which have antibacterial activity against Gram-negative bacteria, thereby, complementing the antibacterial activity of bacitracin, which has activity against Gram-positive bacteria. Hence, the antibacterial spectrum of the preparation is enhanced and the preparation is effective against common pathogens causing ocular surface infections.

Types of Ocular Infection Suitable for Treatment by Bacitracin

1. Acute and chronic conjunctivitis and blepharitis caused by *S. aureus* and other susceptible bacteria.
2. Keratitis and corneal ulcers caused by Gram-positive flora.

Adverse Effects

Topical

Hypersensitivity reactions, though rare, can manifest as contact dermatitis.

Systemic

The most serious systemic adverse effect is nephrotoxicity.

Contraindications

Bacitracin should be avoided in patients with known sensitivity toward it and those with impaired renal function.

Interactions

Like other cell wall inhibitors, bacteriostatic drugs could antagonize bacitracin. There is no known specific interaction with other drugs.

POLYMYXIN B

Polymyxins are a group of antibiotics derived from *Bacillus polymyxa*.

Mechanism of Action

Polymyxin B is a cell membrane inhibitor and is bactericidal. It interferes with the phospholipids in the cell membrane. This disrupts the membrane integrity and the bacterial cell loses its selective permeability leading to bacterial cell lysis and death.

Antibacterial Spectrum

Polymixin B is effective against Gram-negative bacteria including *E.coli*, *Klebsiella* species, *Salmonella* species, *Shigella* species, *Pasteurella*, *Acinetobacter* and *Pseudomonas aeruginosa*. *Proteus* and *Serratia* species are intrinsically resistant.

Pharmacokinetics

Polymixin B has no oral absorption and it is poorly absorbed from mucous membranes. It is excreted by kidney.

Therapeutic Uses

Polymixin B is not used systemically as it causes neurotoxicity and nephrotoxicity. Topically, it is used in combined preparations with other anti-infectives such as bacitracin (see section on bacitracin). A combination of polymixin B and trimethoprim is also complementary because although trimethoprim is active against many Gram-positive and Gram-negative bacteria but it is not active against *Pseudomonas aeruginosa,* which is susceptible to polymixin B. Trimethoprim/polymixin B ophthalmic preparation is available as ointment and solution. Polymixin B is also available for subconjunctival injections.

Types of Ocular Infection Suitable for Treatment by Polymyxin

1. Conjunctivitis, blepharitis and blepharoconjunctivitis due to Gram-negative infection.
2. Keratitis and corneal ulcers.

Adverse Effects and Drug Interaction

Topical use of polymyxin B does not produce systemic adverse effect due to poor systemic absorption.

GRAMICIDIN

Like polymyxin B, gramicidin changes the permeability of the cellular membrane and kills the bacteria. In contrast to bacitracin, gramicidin is effective against Gram-positive bacteria. It replaces bacitracin in some fixed-combination preparations used to treat ocular surface infections.

REFERENCES

1. Wainwright M, Swan HT. CG Paine and the earliest surviving clinical records of penicillin therapy. Med Hist. 1986;30(1):42–56.
2. James CW, Gurk-Turner C. Cross-reactivity of beta lactam antibiotics. Bayl Univ Med Cent Proc. 2001;14(1):106–7.
3. Demchick PH, Koch AL. The permeability of the wall fabric of *Escherichia coli* and *Bacillus subtilis.* J Bacteriol. 1996;178(3):768–73.
4. White D. The physiology and biochemistry of prokaryotes. 3rd ed. Oxford University Press Inc, 2006.
5. Bush K, Jacoby GA, Medeiros AA. A functional classification scheme for beta lactamases and its correlation with molecular structure. Antimicrob Agents Chemother. 1995;39(6):1211–33.
6. Barry G Hall, Miriam Barlow. Revised Ambler classification of β-lactamases. Antimicrob. Chemother. 2005;55(6):1050–1.
7. Saravanan M, Nanda A. Incidence of methicillin resistant *Staphylococcus aureus* (MRSA) from septicemia suspected children. Ind J Science Technol. 2009;2(12):36–9.
8. Haas W, Pillar CM, Torres M, Morris TW, Sahm DF. Monitoring antibiotic resistance in ocular microorganisms: Results from the Antibiotic Resistance Monitoring in Ocular Microorganism (ARMOR) 2009 surveillance study. Am J Ophthalmol. 2011;152(4):567–74.
9. Kaplan EL, Berrios X, Speth J, Siefferman T, Guzman B, Quesny F. Pharmacokinetics of benzathine penicillin G: serum levels during the 28 days after intramuscular injection of 1,200,000 units. J Pediatr. 1989;115(1):146–50.
10. Muller AE, De Jongh J, Bult Y, Goessens WH, Mouton JW, Danhof M, et al. Pharmacokinetics of penicillin G in infants with a gestational age of less than 32 weeks. Antimicrob Agents Chemother. 2007;51(10):3720–5.
11. Javiya VA, Ghatak SB, Patel KR, Patel JA. Antibiotic susceptibility patterns of Pseudomonas aeruginosa at a tertiary care hospital in Gujarat, India. Indian J Pharmacol. 2008;40(5):230–4.
12. Jones RN, Stilwell MG, Rhomberg PR, Sader HS. Antipseudomonal activity of piperacillin/tazobactam: more than a decade of experience from the Sentry Antimicrobial Surveillance Program (1997-2007). Diagn Microbiol Infect Dis. 2009;65(3): 331–4.
13. Workowski KA, Berman SM. Sexually transmitted diseases treatment guidelines, 2006. MMWR Recomm Rep 2006;55(RR11):1–94.
14. Browning DJ. Posterior segment manifestations of active ocular syphilis, their response to a neurosyphilis regimen of penicillin therapy, and the influence of human immunodeficiency virus status on response. Ophthalmol. 2000; 107(11):2015–23.
15. Williams JD. Classification of cephalosporins. Drugs 1987;34(2):15–22.
16. Haimovici R, Roussel TJ. Treatment of gonococcal conjunctivitis with single-dose

intramuscular ceftriaxone. Am J Ophthalmol. 1989;107(5):511–4.

17. Briscoe D, Rubowitz A, Assia EI. Changing bacterial isolates and antibiotic sensitivities of purulent dacryocystitis. Orbit. 2005;24(2):95–8

18. Raju B, Bali T, Thiagarajan G, Rao V, Das T, Sharma S. Physicochemical properties and antibacterial activity of the precipitate of vancomycin and ceftazidime: implications in the management of endophthalmitis. Retina. 2008;28(2):320–5.

19. Gualino V, San S, Guillot E, Korobelnik JF, Colin J, Trout H, et al. Intracameral cefuroxime injections in prophylaxis of postoperative endophthalmitis after cataract surgery: implementation and results. J Fr Ophtalmol. 2010;33(8):551–5.

20. Chau MT, Kaori T, Yuka Y, Takatsugu G, Hiroshige M, Kunitomo W. In Vitro antimicrobial activity of razupenem (SMP-601, PTZ601) against anaerobic bacteria. Antimicrob agents chemother. 2011;55(5):2398-402.

21. Schauersberger J, Amon M, Wedrich A, Nepp J, El Menyawi I, Derbolav A, et al. Penetration and decay of meropenem into the human aqueous humor and vitreous. Ocul Pharmacol Ther. 1999;15(5):439–45.

22. Miño de Kaspar H, Engelbert M, Thiel M, Grasbon T, Ta CN, Klauss V, et al. Intravenous imipenem prophylaxis in experimental endophthalmitis. Graefes Arch Clin Exp Ophthalmol. 2002;240(7):557–64.

23. Perez PA, Gomez MM, Minguez MA, Trampal GA, de Paz AS, Rodríguez MM. Aztreonam and ceftazidime: Evidence of in vivo cross allergenicity. Allergy, 1998;53(6):624–5.

24. Beasley H, Boltralik JJ, Baldwin HA. Chloramphenicol in aqueous humour after topical application. Arch Ophthalmol. 1975;93(3):184–5.

25. Seal DV, Barrett SP, McGill JI. Aetiology and treatment of acute bacterial infection of the external eye. Br J Ophthalmol 1982;66(6):357–60.

26. Doona M, Walsh JB. Use of chloramphenicol as topical eye medication: time to cry halt? BMJ. 1995;310(6989):1217–8.

27. Titcomb LC. Ophthalmic chloramphenicol and blood dyscrasias - a review. Pharm J. 1997;258:28–35.

28. Walker S, Diaper CJM, Bowman R, Sweeney G, Seal DV, Kirkness CM. Lack of evidence for sytemic toxicity following topical chloramphenicol use. Eye. 1998;12(Pt 5):875–9.

29. Lancaster T, Swart AM, Jick H. Risk of serious haematological toxicity with use of chloramphenicol eye-drops in a British general practice database. BMJ. 1998;316(7132):667.

30. Wilholm B, Kelly JP, Kaufman D, Issaragrisil S, Levy M, Anderson T, et al. Relation of aplastic anemia to use of chloramphenicol eye-drops in two international case-control studies. BMJ. 1998;316(7132):666.

31. Hooper DG. Quinolones. Mandell GL, Bennett JE, Dolin R (eds). Mandell, Douglas, and Bennett's Principles and Practice of Infectious Diseases, 6th (edn). Churchill Livingstone. 2005. pp. 451–67.

32. Güngör SG, Akova YA, Bozkurt A, Yasar Ü, Babaoğlu MÖ, Çetinkaya A, et al. Aqueous humour penetration of moxifloxocin and gatifloxacin eye drops in different dosing regimens before phacoemulsification surgery. Br J Ophthalmol. 2011;95(9):1272–5.

33. Solomon R, Donnenfeld ED, Perry HD, Snyder RW, Nedrud C, Stein J, et al. Penetration of topically applied gatifloxacin 0.3 %, moxifloxacin 0.5 % and ciprofloxacin 0.3 % into the aqueous humor. Opthalmology. 2005, 112(3):466–9.

34. Power WJ, Collum LMT, Easty DL, Bloom PA, Laidlaw DAII, Libert J, ct al. Evaluation of efficacy and safety of ciprofloxacin ophthalmic solution versus chloramphenicol. Eur J Ophthalmol. 1993;3(2):77–82.

35. Liebowitz HM. Antibacterial effectiveness of ciprofloxacin 0.3 per cent ophthalmic solution in the treatment of bacterial conjunctivitis. Am J Ophthalmol. 1991;112(4):29S–33S.

36. Keating GM. Levofloxacin 0.5% ophthalmic solution: a review of its use in the treatment of external ocular infections and in intraocular surgery. Drugs. 2009;69(9):1267–86.

37. De Kaspar HM, Chang RT, Shriver EM, Singh K, Egbert PR, Blumenkranz MS, et al. Three-day application of topical ofloxacin reduces the contamination rate of microsurgical knives in cataract surgery: a prospective randomized study. Ophthalmology. 2004;111(7):1352–5.

38. Parks DJ, Abrams DA, Sarfarazi FA, Katz HR. Comparison of topical ciprofloxacin to conventional antibiotic therapy in the treatment

of ulcerative keratitis. Am J Ophthalmol. 1993;115(4):471–7.

39. Herrin S. What's new in antibiotics: Ciloxan vs Ocuflox: The debate continues. Rev Ophthalmol. 1996;3:106–7.

40. Hoban DJ, Doern GV, Fluit AC, Roussel-Delvallez M, Jones RN. Worldwide prevalence of antimicrobial resistance in *Streptococcus pneumoniae, Haemophilus influenzae*, and *Moraxella catarrhalis* in the Sentry Antimicrobal Surveillance Program, 1997–1999. Clin Infect Dis. 2001;32(2):S81–S93.

41. David M, Rumelt S, Weintraub Z. Efficacy comparison between povidone iodine 2.5% and tetracycline 1% in prevention of ophthalmia neonatorum. Ophthalmology. 2011;118(7):1454–8.

42. Darling EK, McDonald H. A meta-analysis of the efficacy of ocular prophylactic agents used for the prevention of gonococcal and chlamydial ophthalmia neonatorum. J Midwifery Womens Health. 2010;55(4):319–27.

43. Bryskier AJ, Agouridans C, Gasc JC. Classification of macrolide antibiotics. In: Bryskier AJ, Butzler JP, Tulkens PM (eds). In: Macrolides. Chemistry, Pharmacology and Clinic Uses. Paris. 1993; pp. 5-66.

44. Barry A, Fusch P, Brown S. Relative potencies of azithromycin, clarithromycin and five other orally administered antibiotics. J Antimicrob Chemother. 1995;35(4):552–5.

45. Slaney L, Chubb H, Ronald R, Brunham R. In vitro activity of azithromycin, erythromycin, ciprofloxacin and norfloxacin. Neisseria gonorrhoeae, Haemophilus ducreui, Chlamydia trachomatis. J Antimicrob Chemother. 1990:25(A):1–5.

46. Johnston NJ, de Avazedo JC, Kelner JD,Low DE. Prevalence and characterization of the mechanisms of macrolide, lincosamide, and streptogramin resistance in isolates of Streptococcus pneumoniae. Antimicrob Agents Chemother. 1998;42(9):2424–6.

47. Bahal N, Nahata MC. The new macrolide antibiotics: azithromycin, clarithremycin, dirithromycin, and roxithromycin. Ann Pharmacother. 1992;26(1):46–55.

48. Wise R. The pharmacokinetics of azithromycin. Rev Contemp Pharmacother. 1994;4:329–40.

49. Girard AE, Cimochowski CR, Faiella JA. Correlation of increased azithromycin concentrations with phagocyte infiltration into sites of localized infection. J Antimicrob Chemother. 1996;37(C):9–19.

50. Evans JR, Solomon AW. Antibiotics for trachoma. Cochrane Database Syst. Rev. 2011;16(3):1860.

51. Rubinstein E. Comparative safety of the different macrolides. Int J Antimicrob Agents. 2001;18(l):71–6.

52. Rapp RP. Pharmacokinetics and pharmacodynamics of intravenous and oral azithromycin: Enhanced tissue activity and minimal drug interactions. Ann Pharmacother. 1998;32(7-8):785–93.

53. Ray WA, Murray KT, Meredith S, Narasimhulu SS, Hall K, Stein CM. Oral erythromycin and the risk of sudden death from cardiac causes. N Engl J Med. 2004; 351:1089–96.

54. Shazi S, Rosina K, Raffaele Z, Asad UK. Aminoglycosides versus bacteria – a description of the action, resistance mechanism, and nosocomial battleground. J Biomed Science. 2008; 15(1):5–14.

55. Tang RK, Tse RK. Acute renal failure after topical fortified gentamicin and vancomycin eyedrops. J Ocul Pharmacol Ther. 2011; 27(4):411–3.

CHAPTER 9

Antiviral Drugs

OVERVIEW

Ocular diseases due to viral infection are one of the most challenging in terms of diagnosis and treatment. Firstly, viruses are obligate intracellular parasites that are too small to be observed with light microscope. Secondly, virus particles have rugged molecular machinery that has evolved over time to ensure efficient transfer of genetic material between cells in stepwise manner (attachment, penetration, and initiation of a new replication cycle) and mechanisms to safeguard encoded information sufficient to ensure their own continued propagation and escape. Thirdly, the molecular organization of viruses is still incompletely understood as it is highly nascent and keeps modifying as per environmental conditions. Fourthly, the preponderance of variety in viral machinery like polymerases, envelope/ non-envelope, double-stranded (ds) DNA/RNA/ nucleic acids and regulatory proteins can lead to lysis or stimulation or even transformation of host cells, making these agents difficult to read and predict. Last but not the least, despite aggressive treatment the virus can survive as latent infection making the host its long-standing carrier and reactivate later in severe and fatal form.

Detection of cell-associated viral antigen for diagnosing infection using conventional staining techniques such as Papanicolaou and Giemsa stain is although, rapid and inexpensive, but self-limiting owing to non-specificity and low sensitivity. For example, these stains cannot differentiate the intra-nuclear inclusions of *Herpes Simplex Virus* (HSV) from that of *Varicella Zoster Virus* (VZV).

Direct and indirect immunofluorescence, indirect immunoperoxidase assays are rapid, specific and sensitive test systems that can be used in the diagnosis of HSV, VZV keratitis, and adenoviral keratoconjunctivitis. Indirect immunoperoxidase (IP) assay is preferred as it can be applied on paraffin embedded tissue, allows preparation of permanent records and needs ordinary light microscope for visualization. In contrast, the indirect immunofluorescence is usually conducted on frozen tissue sections, quenching leads to fading of records and requires sophisticated and expensive fluorescence microscope for visualization.[1,2]

Conventional practice of viral isolation using cell lines such as HeLa, Vero, HEp 2 and MRC-5 are very sensitive and useful in providing evidence for the presence of virus in ocular scrapings and samples. However, this can be time and technically demanding, as it requires special and expensive virology laboratory set up. In recent advancement, merely demonstration of presence of viral genetic material in clinical samples is taken as evidence of its presence and the need for isolation has been done away with.[1,2]

The current bouquet of antiviral agents is effective and has been in ophthalmic use for long, but is fraught with some limitations. Most antiviral agents that are available to treat dsDNA viruses inhibit the same target, the viral DNA polymerase. Hence, with increasing reports of the development of resistance to these drugs, new antiviral agents are urgently needed for management of HSV, *Cytomegalovirus* and Hepatitis B virus (HBV) infections. Further, there is paucity of drugs that are available for the treatment of DNA virus infections including *Adenovirus*, smallpox, *Molluscum contagiosum*, and *BK virus*.

Following is the detailed discussion of antiviral drugs that are currently in ophthalmic use (Table 9.1).

Table 9.1 Antiviral drugs

Drug	Mechanism of action	Antiviral activity	Therapeutic uses
Idoxuridine (IDU)	Replaces thymidine in viral DNA, inhibits viral DNA polymerase and interferes with other cellular enzymes	HSV-1- and -2	Superficial herpes simplex keratitis
Trifluridine	Same as IDU	HSV-1 and -2; *Vaccinia, Adenovirus* and *Cytomegalovirus*	Primary and recurrent herpes simplex keratoconjunctivitis, dendritic and geographic ulcers
Vidarabine	Inhibits viral DNA polymerase, competes with adenosine triphosphate for incorporation into viral DNA	HSV-1 and -2, *Vaccinia* and VZV	Herpes simplex keratoconjunctivitis and iritis, herpetic ulcers
Acyclovir (Valacyclovir is a prodrug of acyclovir)	Active form inactivates viral DNA polymerase. It replaces guanosine in viral DNA	HSV-1 and -2	Herpes simplex epithelial keratitis, stromal keratitis, dendritic herpetic ulcer, iritis and acute retinal necrosis; prophylaxis in patients undergoing keratroplasty for active herpes simplex keratitis and in immunosuppressed patients; herpes zoster and varicella infections
Famciclovir (A prodrug of penciclovir)	Inhibits DNA polymerase	HSV-1, HSV-2 and VZV	Herpes simplex infections, zoster ophthalmicus, acute retinal necrosis especially in cases of acyclovir resistance
Ganciclovir (Valganciclovir is an oral prodrug of ganciclovir)	Competes with deoxyguanosine triphosphate for incorporation into the viral DNA, inhibits viral DNA polymerase	*Cytomegalovirus*, HSV-1 and 2, *Epstein Barr Virus* and VZV	Cytomegalovirus retinitis, of severe cytomegalovirus infections such as respiratory, gastrointestinal and disseminated infections
Cidofovir	Inactivates viral DNA polymerase	*Cytomegalovirus* including strains resistant to ganciclovir, HSV-1 and -2, VZV, *Epstein Barr Virus*, Vaccinia and several adenoviruses	Cytomegalovirus retinitis
Foscarnet	Selective and noncompetitive inhibitor of viral DNA polymerases and reverse transcriptase	*Cytomegalovirus*, HSV-1 and -2, VZV and *Epstien Barr Virus*, HIV	Cytomegalovirus retinitis in HIV-infected patients, herpes simplex and zoster infections resistant to acyclovir in HIV patients

IDOXURIDINE (IDU)

IDU is the oldest antiviral drug that was used topically in ophthalmic practice. It was synthesized in 1959 as an anticancer drug but was later found to have antiviral properties.

Mechanism of Action

IDU is a thymidine analogue. The only difference in its structure from thymidine is that it consists of iodine at carbon 5 instead of methyl group and, therefore, its configuration resembles that of thymidine. Due to resemblance in structure, it replaces thymidine in viral DNA leading to production of faulty DNA. IDU is phosphorylated by viral and cellular kinases. IDU triphosphate inhibits viral DNA polymerase and, therefore, prevents viral replication. Additionally, IDU triphosphate terminates viral replication also by interfering with other cellular enzymes such as thymidine kinase, deoxycytidine monophosphate deaminase and cytidine diphosphate reductase. Similar effects in host cells lead to toxic effects of IDU.

Pharmacokinetics

Topically applied IDU penetrates the intact cornea poorly. It penetrates the cornea well only if the epithelium is damaged. Systemic absorption after ocular administration is unlikely. It is rapidly metabolized by deaminases or nucleotidases.

Antiviral Activity

IDU is effective against HSV-1- and -2. Modification of thymidine kinase gene results in emergence of resistance to IDU. IDU-resistant strains of HSV show cross-resistance to acyclovir and intermediate resistance to trifluridine but remain sensitive to vidarabine and ganciclovir.[3]

Therapeutic Uses

IDU is used topically for the treatment of herpes simplex keratitis. It is effective only for superficial epithelial infections and not for stromal keratitis or iritis as it does not penetrate the cornea well. Use of IDU has diminished now due to availability of newer antiviral agents.

Dosage and Administration

IDU for topical application is available as 0.1% drops and 0.5% ointment. In the treatment of herpetic keratitis, drops are instilled every 1–2 hour daily and ointment at bed time for 14 days.

Adverse Effects

Systemic use of IDU is minimally effective and highly toxic. It is teratogenic, mutagenic and potentially carcinogenic and, therefore, is not used systemically. Topical administration in eye may cause punctate epithelial keratitis, conjunctivitis, punctal stenosis, contact dermatitis and keratinization of lid margins. It interferes with stromal healing and may cause toxic epithelial changes.

TRIFLURIDINE

Trifluridine is a thymidine analogue. Its structure is similar to that of IDU except that it has 3 fluorine atoms attached to methyl radical replacing the iodine.

Mechanism of action

Although exact mechanism of antiviral effects of trifluridine is not known, it seems to act in the same way as IDU. It inhibits several steps in the synthesis of viral DNA. It is initially phosphorylated to trifluridine monophosphate, which is a potent inhibitor of thymidylate synthetase. It is further phosphorylated to its triphosphate compound, which competes with thymidine triphosphate for incorporation into the viral DNA.

Pharmacokinetics

In contrast to IDU, trifluridine penetrates the intact cornea well and in the presence of damaged cornea it achieves even higher aqueous humor levels. Systemic absorption after topical application is negligible.

Antiviral Activity

It is effective against HSV-1 and -2. It also has activity against *Vaccinia* and some adenoviruses.[4] Its activity against human *Cytomegalovirus* has also been reported.[5]

Resistance to trifluridine is rare and if it occurs, the mechanism is similar to that of IDU.

Therapeutic Uses

Trifluridine is effective in the treatment of primary and recurrent herpes simplex keratoconjunctivitis. In patients with dendritic ulcer, its efficacy is comparable to vidarabine and IDU. It may also be effective in patients with geographic ulcers. Average healing time is 6–7 days. Its efficacy is similar to topical acyclovir both in terms of healing rate and time for healing. It is especially useful for the treatment of ulcers not responding to IDU or vidarabine and in patients intolerant to IDU.[6]

Dosage and Administration

Trifluridine 1% solution is applied every 2 hours while awake to a maximum of 9 drops/day until cornea is re-epithelialized. Subsequently, dose is tapered to every 4 hours with a maximum of 5 drops/day for 7 days. Total duration of treatment should not be more than 21 days. In cases showing no response after 7 days of treatment or incomplete epithelialization after 14 days, change in therapy is indicated.

Adverse Effects

Topically applied trifluridine is well tolerated. Cross-toxicity with IDU or vidarabine is rare. Ocular adverse effects of topical application include transient burning and stinging, punctate epithelial keratitis, conjunctival hyperemia and chemosis, keratitis sicca, punctual stenosis, contact dermatitis, palpebral edema and poor stromal wound healing. Long-term use can cause conjunctival scarring.

It is too toxic for systemic use. Like IDU, it has teratogenic, mutagenic and carcinogenic properties.

VIDARABINE

Vidarabine is a guanosine analogue. It is obtained from fermentation cultures of *Streptomyces antibioticus*. It is also known as adenine arabinoside or Ara-A. Vidarabine was the first antiviral drug that became generally available for parenteral treatment of severe herpes infection in human. Besides its antiviral effects, it also possesses antineoplastic properties.

Mechanism of Action

Vidarabine has high affinity for viral encoded thymidine kinase, which converts it into vidarabine monophosphate. Further phosphorylation by viral and cellular kinases leads to formation of its triphosphate form. The triphosphate is both an inhibitor and substrate for viral DNA polymerase. Vidarabine triphosphate competes with adenosine triphosphate for incorporation into viral DNA leading to formation of faulty DNA and termination of viral replication.

Pharmacokinetics

Topically applied vidarabine penetrates the intact cornea poorly. Systemic absorption after topical administration is negligible.

Following intravenous administration, it undergoes rapid deamination by adenosine deaminase to form arabinosyl hypoxanthine, which has much less activity than vidarabine. To increase the antiviral activity of vidarabine it has been combined with inhibitors of deaminase. The combination, though increases the antiviral effects, the toxicity also increases.

Antiviral Activity

Vidarabine is effective against HSV-1 and -2, *Vaccinia* and VZV. It has poor activity against RNA viruses.

Resistance to vidarabine may emerge due to development of mutations in viral DNA polymerase gene.

Therapeutic Uses

Vidarabine ointment 3% has been shown to be effective in the treatment of herpes simplex keratoconjunctivitis and iritis. Its efficacy for promoting re-epithelialization is comparable to IDU, however, it is less toxic and even causes healing of IDU-resistant lesions. Topical vidarabine is also comparable to topical trifluridine and acyclovir in healing corneal herpetic lesions. Systemic vidarabine, although effective in the treatment of varicella and zoster ophthalmicus, is not a preferred choice.

Adverse Effects

The toxicity of both, the topical and systemic, vidarabine is negligible. Systemic administration of vidarabine requires large volume of fluid due to its relative insolubility and, therefore, may cause cardiovascular and renal homeostatic consequences. It also has teratogenic, mutagenic and carcinogenic potential. Therefore, systemic use of vidarabine is limited to life-threatening infections not responsive to other drugs.

VALACYCLOVIR AND ACYCLOVIR

Acyclovir is a synthetic guanosine analogue with selective anti-herpes activity. It was discovered in 1974 and was subjected to clinical trials in 1977. Topical preparation of acyclovir first became available for use in 1982. Valacyclovir, a prodrug, is L -valyl ester of acyclovir and was synthesized to enhance oral bioavailability of acyclovir.

Mechanism of Action

It is concentrated in viral infected cells and has high affinity for viral-induced thymidine kinase. Inside the infected cells, viral thymidine kinase converts acyclovir to acyclovir monophosphate, which undergoes further phosphorylation by host cellular enzymes to diphosphate and triphosphate. Acyclovir triphosphate is the active forms of the drug that inactivates viral DNA polymerase. It also gets incorporated in viral DNA causing its termination.

Pharmacokinetics

After oral administration, bioavailability of acyclovir is 20%. However, oral valacyclovir is rapidly metabolized in intestine and liver to acyclovir and bioavailability of acyclovir following oral dose of valacyclovir increases by 3–5 times. The plasma protein binding ranges from 9–33%. It is adequately distributed in tissues. The intracellular half-life of acyclovir is 0.7 and 1 hours in HSV-1 and -2 infected cells, respectively, and 0.8 hours in VZV infected cells as detected from *in vitro* experiments.[7] It undergoes minimal metabolism and is primarily excreted unchanged in urine after glomerular filtration and tubular secretion. The half-life of acyclovir is significantly affected by change in renal function and, therefore, dose adjustment is required in patients with impaired renal function. Elderly may require a lower dose due to age-related changes in renal function.[8] Regular intravenous administration of 5 mg/kg, 3 times a day provides the vitreous levels that are in excess of minimum inhibitory concentration for HSV-1- and -2, VZV and Epstein Barr virus.

Antiviral activity

Acyclovir is known as a selective anti-herpes agent as it is highly active against HSV-1 and -2, less effective against VZV and even less against *Epstein Barr Virus* and *Cytomegalovirus*. Uninfected and normal cells remain unaffected.

Chronic and intermittent administration of acyclovir, especially in AIDS patients, may result in development of resistance and failure of therapy. Development of resistance often results from quantitative or qualitative changes in virus-induced thymidine kinase or DNA polymerase.

Therapeutic Uses

Acyclovir is used in the treatment of epithelial keratitis, stromal keratitis, dendritic herpetic ulcer, iritis and acute retinal necrosis caused by herpes simplex. Oral administration of acyclovir causes significantly faster healing of dendritic herpetic corneal ulcer.[9] Herpetic eye disease study group examined the role of long-term acyclovir treatment in prevention of recurrent ocular herpes in immunocompetent patients.[10] It was observed that cumulative probability of recurrence of any type of ocular HSV disease during the 12 month treatment period was 19% in the acyclovir-treated group compared to 32% in the placebo group. Among patients with stromal keratitis, the most severe form of the disease, acyclovir reduced the recurrence rate to 14%. Recurrence of nonocular herpes was also reduced. Success rate for healing of corneal ulcers with acyclovir is comparable to IDU, trifluridine and adenine arabinoside.[11-13] Acyclovir is used for prophylaxis in patients undergoing keratroplasty for active herpes simplex keratitis and in immunosuppressed patients such as those with AIDS, blood dyscrasias or the organ transplant recipients. It is also used for the treatment of herpes zoster and varicella infections, however, the dose required are as high as 800 mg 5 times a day. It is recommended that for zoster infection, acyclovir should be initiated within first 72 hours for better outcome. Oral acyclovir also reduces the incidence and duration of zoster-associated postherpetic neuralgia. For the treatment of acute retinal necrosis, systemic acyclovir is the treatment of choice. However, it takes about 2 days before the disease progression can be prevented. Recent experiments in rabbit have shown that intravitreal acyclovir can be of use to provide coverage during initial few days of therapy and 1 mg dose was found to be safe and well tolerated.[14]

Valacyclovir is primarily used in the treatment of herpes zoster and herpes simplex infections in immunocompetent patients and its efficacy is comparable to oral acyclovir. It is more effective than acyclovir in reducing the severity of post-herpetic neuralgia. It has been shown to inhibit reactivation of ocular herpes simplex after excimer laser keratectomy or laser-assisted in-situ keratomileusis (LASIK).[15,16] Valacyclovir as a sole agent has been shown to provide complete resolution of retinitis.[17]

Dosage and Administration

Acyclovir is available as 3% ointment for topical application. For herpes simplex keratitis, it is used 5 times a day for 2 weeks and is then gradually tapered to twice a day. Acyclovir for oral administration is available as 200–800 mg tablets and is administered in a total daily dose of 1 gram. In immunosuppressed patients, it is administered at a dose of 5–10 mg/kg or 500 mg/m^2. Acyclovir is administered at a dose of 5 mg/kg body weight 8 hourly for 5–10 days intravenously. Acyclovir for injection is available in 20 and 40 mL vials containing 25 mg/mL of acyclovir. Intravitreal acyclovir 0.5 µg/100 µL has been used in the treatment of acute retinal necrosis. For the treatment of zoster, oral valacyclovir is administered 1 g thrice daily for 7 days.

Adverse Effects

Topically applied acyclovir ointment is well tolerated. The most common adverse effects include superficial punctate keratopathy and burning or stinging on application of the ointment. Other adverse effects are conjunctivitis and pain in the treated eye.[18] Systemic acyclovir can cause gastrointestinal disturbances, anorexia, dizziness, rash, edema and lymphadenopathy. Rapid intravenous injection can cause renal dysfunction. Other adverse effects include sweating, emesis, hypotension and neurological manifestations. Valacyclovir is not used in immunosuppressed as it can cause thrombotic thrombocytopenic purpura and hemolytic uremic syndrome in these patients.

FAMCICLOVIR AND PENCICLOVIR

Famciclovir is a potent and selective antiviral agent with activity against herpes viruses. It is a synthetic acyclic guanine derivative and is a prodrug of penciclovir.

Mechanism of Action

Famciclovir after oral administration undergoes rapid metabolism to penciclovir. Like acyclovir, penciclovir also undergoes phosphorylation to monophosphate by virus-induced thymidine kinase and subsequently to triphosphate by cellular kinases. Penciclovir triphosphate inhibits DNA polymerase and, thereby viral replication.

Pharmacokinetics

Famciclovir is well absorbed and is converted to penciclovir with bioavailability of 65–77% after oral administration. *In vitro*, intracellular half-life of penciclovir triphosphate is up to 10–12 hours in cells infected with HSV-1 and -2 and 9–14 hours in VZV infected cells. Oral famciclovir results in vitreal concentrations of penciclovir that are within the inhibitory range for HSV and VZV.[19] The prolonged intracellular half-life provides persistent antiviral activity. Less than 20% of penciclovir is plasma protein bound. Famciclovir is primarily excreted by kidneys. In patients with normal or mild renal impairment, dose adjustment is not required.[7]

Antiviral activity

Famciclovir is effective against herpesvirus family, including HSV-1, HSV-2 and VZV virus. Potency and spectrum of antiviral activity is similar to acyclovir.

Resistance may develop to famciclovir and the mechanism of resistance involves mutation of viral thymidine kinase and DNA polymerase genes. Acyclovir-resistant mutant strains that are negative for thymidine kinase show resistance to famciclovir.

Therapeutic Uses

Famciclovir is effective in the treatment of immunocompetent patients with herpes zoster or genital herpes infection. Its therapeutic efficacy in these infections is similar to oral acyclovir, however, famciclovir can be administered in more convenient dosage regimen. In the treatment of herpes zoster ophthalmicus also, its efficacy and safety profile is comparable to acyclovir. Oral famciclovir can also be an alternative to intravenous acyclovir in the treatment of acute retinal necrosis especially in cases of acyclovir resistance or for patients intolerant to prolonged intravenous treatment.[19]

Dosage and Administration

Famciclovir is available for oral administration as tablets containing 125, 250 and 500 mg of famciclovir. It is administered in the dose of 500 mg thrice a day in the treatment of herpes zoster ophthalmicus.

Adverse Effects

Most common adverse effects of famciclovir include gastrointestinal disturbance, headache and nausea. It can also cause rash, fatigue, paresthesia and dysmenorrhea.

GANCICLOVIR AND VALGANCICLOVIR

Ganciclovir is a synthetic acyclic guanosine analogue, which was the first drug to be approved for the treatment of cytomegalovirus infection. Valganciclovir is an oral prodrug of ganciclovir.

Mechanism of Action

After oral administration valganciclovir is converted to ganciclovir. Ganciclovir is concentrated in the virus-infected cells and undergoes phosphorylation by virus-encoded kinases. Further phosphorylation by cellular kinases leads to the formation of ganciclovir triphosphate, which competes with deoxyguanosine triphosphate for incorporation into the viral DNA and produces faulty DNA. It also inhibits viral DNA polymerase and hence inhibits viral replication.

Pharmacokinetics

The oral bioavailability of ganciclovir is poor amounting to about 5% under fasting condition. In the presence of fatty meal, bioavailability increases to 30%. Only 1–3% of the drug in circulation is plasma protein bound and up to 90% of the plasma ganciclovir is excreted unchanged by kidneys after glomerular filtration and tubular secretion. The half-life of intravenously administered ganciclovir is 2.5–3.6 hours and it is 3.1–5.5 hours after oral administration. In the presence of renal dysfunction, half-life increases significantly.

Antiviral Activity

It is active against *Cytomegalovirus*, HSV-1 and -2, *Epstein Barr Virus* and VZV. It has widely been used for the treatment of cytomegalovirus infections.

Resistance to ganciclovir may develop in patients with AIDS and cytomegalovirus retinitis receiving long-term treatment as well as those who have not received treatment previously. Mechanism of resistance is attributed to development of mutations of viral genes encoding kinases and DNA polymerase.

Therapeutic Uses

It is used both for induction and maintenance treatment of cytomegalovirus retinitis in patients with AIDS and other immunocompromized patients. It is also used for the treatment of severe cytomegalovirus infections such as respiratory, gastrointestinal and disseminated infections.

For induction, 5 mg/kg is administered over hours and is repeated every 12 hours for 2–3 weeks. Following induction, maintenance treatment can be given intravenously (5 mg/kg over 1 hour once daily, 7 days a week) or orally (1000 mg thrice a day with food). Ganciclovir is used for prevention of cytomegalovirus retinitis in high risk patients. Topical application of ganciclovir 0.15% gel is effective in herpes simplex keratitis and the efficacy is comparable to acyclovir ointment.[20]

Dosage and Administration

Ganciclovir is available as capsule containing 250 and 500 mg of the drug. For intravenous administration, ganciclovir sodium is available in vials containing 500 mg. Reconstitution in 10 mL of sterile water provides a concentration of 50 mg/mL. Ganciclovir is administered intravenously by slow injection and not as bolus or rapid injection to avoid toxicity caused by excessive plasma levels. Intramuscular or subcutaneous injections may cause severe tissue irritation due to alkaline pH of the solution. Weekly intravitreal injections of ganciclovir 2 mg in 0.05–0.1 mL are also used for the treatment of cytomegalovirus retinitis.

Ganciclovir is also available as a non-biodegradable intravitreal implant. This implant is made of ethylene-vinyl acetate copolymer (EVA) and polyvinyl alcohol (PVA). It contains ganciclovir 4.5 mg, which is released over 6–8 months by passive diffusion through a small opening in the EVA at the base of the device.[21] Besides the complications associated with the surgical procedure of implanting the device inside the eye, there are concerns of the risk of spread of infection to the unaffected eye and other parts of body. The biodegradable polylactide (PLA) containing ganciclovir implants are being developed. Such devices can be implanted into the vitreous from the sclerotomy site at the pars plana. The device does not disturb the transparency of the ocular medium and releases the active ingredient directly into the vitreous for up to one year.

Adverse Effects

Adverse effects of ganciclovir include pancyto-penia, gastrointestinal symptoms and acute renal failure.

CIDOFOVIR

Cidofovir is a newer antiviral drug that is classified as acyclic phosphonate cytosine analogue. It belongs to the family of phosphonyl methoxyalkyl derivative of purines and pyrimidines.

Mechanism of Action

Cidofovir is taken up by virus-infected and uninfected cells. It exists in monophosphate form and, therefore, does not require phosphorylation by viral thymidine kinase to get activated. Cellular kinases convert it into diphosphate, which inactivates viral DNA polymerase with 25–50 times higher specificity than human DNA polymerase.

Pharmacokinetics

After intravenous administration, the half-life of cidofovir is 2.4–3.2 hours. However, the intracellular half-life of cidofovir diphosphate is more than 48 hours resulting in long lasting antiviral effects. Its protein binding is less than 6% and it is eliminated in urine. It is administered with probenecid, which delays its renal clearance. Cidofovir in a crystalline lipid prodrug form, octadecyloxyethyl-cyclic-cidofovir, has shown prolonged vitreous half-life when injected intravitreally in rabbits.[22]

Antiviral Activity

Cidofovir is effective against *Cytomegalovirus* including strains resistant to ganciclovir. It is also effective against HSV-1 and -2, VZV, *Epstein Barr Virus*, *Vaccinia* and several adenoviruses.

Resistance for cidofovir is associated with prior treatment with oral ganciclovir or intravenous cidofovir. Resistant strains have mutation in UL97 and polymerase gene.

Therapeutic Uses

Cidofovir, due to its high efficacy and therapeutic margin, is currently the firstline drug for the treatment of cytomegalovirus retinitis. It can be given either intravenously or intravitreally. Cidofovir has also been found to be effective in the treatment of ocular infections caused by adenoviruses 1, 5 and 6 in rabbit.[23,24] Topical cidofovir 1% and 0.5% have also shown efficacy in treating HSV-1 in rabbits and effects were comparable to trifluridine and acyclovir.[23,25]

Dosage and Administration

For cytomegalovirus retinitis, cidofovir is given by intravenous infusion of 5 mg/kg once weekly for 2 weeks followed by either high dose (5 mg/kg) or low dose (3 mg/kg) weekly administration. It can also be given intravitreally 10–20 µg every 5–6 weeks and up to 10 injections may be given.

Adverse Effects

In the treatment of cytomegalovirus retinitis two most notable adverse effects, regardless of route of administration, are hypotony and nongranulomatous iritis. Topical administration may cause punctal stenosis.

Nephrotoxicity is the major dose-limiting toxicity and may occur in 50% of patients receiving maintenance dose of 5 mg/kg once in two weeks. Neutropenia may develop in 20% of the patients on maintenance doses.

FOSCARNET

Foscarnet is a non-nucleoside antiviral drug. It is a trisodium salt of phosphoformic acid.

Mechanism of Action

Foscarnet does not require phosphorylation for activation. It directly interacts with pyrophosphate binding site of viral DNA polymerases. It is a selective and noncompetitive inhibitor of viral DNA polymerases and reverse transcriptase at concentrations that do not affect the host DNA polymerase. Since it does not require phosphorylation by virus, the strains with mutant gene for thymidine kinase are sensitive to foscarnet.

Pharmacokinetics

The half-life of foscarnet is 4 hours. It is well distributed in tissues and achieves 43% of plasma levels in cerebrospinal fluid. It accumulates in bone marrow and in AIDS patients up to 20% of the administered dose can accumulate in bone marrow. It is metabolized and is excreted unchanged by kidneys.

Antiviral Activity

Foscarnet is active against all herpes viruses including *Cytomegalovirus*, HSV-1 and -2 and *Epstien Barr Virus*. It is also effective against HIV.

Foscarnet-resistant strains of herpes simplex have recently been reported. These strains were also resistant to acyclovir, though thymidine kinase gene mutations have not been observed in these strains.

Therapeutic Uses

The main therapeutic indication for foscarnet is cytomegalovirus retinitis in HIV-infected patients. It is also used for the treatment of herpes simplex and zoster infections resistant to acyclovir in HIV patients. The efficacy of foscarnet is comparable to ganciclovir, although foscarnet may prolong the survival due to its anti-HIV effects. Intravitreal foscarnet for cytomegalovirus retinitis is not approved by FDA, however, one study has reported that 4 out of 5 patients showed complete healing in 3 weeks when 2.4 µg/0.1 mL of foscarnet was injected intravitreally along with intravenous maintenance doses.[26]

Dosage and Administration

For intravenous administration foscarnet is available in 250 and 500 mL bottles containing 25 mg/mL of the drug. It is given as infusion either undiluted in the central vein or diluted with normal saline or 5% dextrose in peripheral vein. Initial dose is 60 mg/kg every 8 hours for 2–3 weeks. Maintenance dose is 90–120 mg/kg over 2 hours every day. During infusion good hydration must be maintained to avoid renal complications.

Adverse Effects

Nephrotoxicity is the major adverse effect that occurs in up to 45% of AIDS patients. Creatinine levels and electrolyte changes must be monitored during therapy. Intermittent dosing and good hydration during therapy helps to prevent nephrotoxicity. Other adverse effects include anemia in up to 50% of patients, elevated hepatic enzyme, headache, central nervous system dysfunction, gastrointestinal disturbances, mucosal erosions, nephrogenic diabetes insipidus and neutropenia.

REFERENCES

1. Sharma S, Sreedharan A. Diagnostic procedures in infectious keratitis. In: Nema HV, Nema N (eds).Diagnostic Procedures in Ophthalmology 2nd edn. Jaypee Brothers Medical Publishers (P) Ltd., New Delhi; 2009. pp. 316–32.
2. Johnson FB, Luker G, Chow C. Comparison of shell vial culture and the suspension-infection method for the rapid detection of HSVes. Diagn Microbiol Infect Dis. 1993;16:61–6.
3. Fardeau C, Langlois M, Nugier F, Asselot C, Aymard M, Denis J. Cross-resistances to antiviral drugs of IUdR-resistant HSV-1 in rabbit keratitis and in vitro. Cornea. 1993;12:19–24.
4. Schaeffer HJ, Beauchamp L, de Miranda P, Elion GB, Bauer DJ, Collins P. 9-(2-Hydroxyethoxymethyl) guanine activity against viruses of the herpes group. Nature. 1978;272:583–5.
5. Spector SA, Tyndall M, Kelley E. Inhibition of human cytomegalovirus by trifluorothymidine. Antimicrob Agents Chemother. 1983;23(1): 113–8.
6. Carmine AA, Brogden RN, Heel RC, Speight TM, Avery GS. Trifluridine: a review of its antiviral activity and therapeutic use in the topical treatment of viral eye infections. Drugs. 1982; 23(5):329–53.
7. Crumpacker C. The pharmacological profile of famciclovir. Semin Dermatol. 1996;15(2 Suppl 1):14–26.
8. de Miranda P, Blum MR. Pharmacokinetics of acyclovir after intravenous and oral administration. J Antimicrob Chemother. 1983;12 Suppl B:29–37.
9. Hung SO, Patterson A, Clark DI, Rees PJ. Oral acyclovir in the management of dendritic herpetic corneal ulceration. Br J Ophthalmol. 1984; 68(6):398–400.
10. The herpetic eye disease study group. Acyclovir for the prevention of recurrent HSV eye disease. N Engl J Med. 1998;339:300–6.

11. Coster DJ, Wilhelmus KR, Michaud R, Jones BR. A comparison of acyclovir and idoxuridine as treatment for ulcerative herpetic keratitis. Br J Ophthalmol. 1980;64:763–5.

12. la Lau C, Oosterhuis JA, Versteeg J, van Rij G, Renardel de Lavalette JG, Craandijk A, et al. Acyclovir and trifluorothymidine in herpetic keratitis: a multicentre trial. Br J Ophthalmol. 1982;66:506–8.

13. Collum LM, Logan P, McAuliffe-Curtin D, Hung SO, Patterson A, Rees PJ. Randomised double blind trial of acyclovir (zovirax) and adenine arabinoside in herpes simplex amoeboid corneal ulceration. Br J Ophthalmol 1985;69:847–50.

14. Damico FM, Scolari MR, Ioshimoto GL, Takahashi BS, Cunha Ada S Jr, Fialho SL, et al. Vitreous pharmacokinetics and electroretinographic findings after intravitreal injection of acyclovir in rabbits. Clinics (Sao Paulo). 2012;67(8):931–7.

15. Dhaliwal DK, Romanowski EG, Yates KA, Hu D, Mah FS, Fish DN, et al. Valaciclovir inhibition of recovery of ocular HSV Type 1 after experimental reactivation by laser in situ keratomileusis. J Cataract Refract Surg. 2001;27:1288–93.

16. Asbell P. Valaciclovir for prevention of recurrent HSV eye disease after Excimer laser photokeratectomy. Trans Am Ophthalmol Soc. 2000; 98:285–303.

17. Taylor SR, Hamilton R, Hooper CY, Joshi L, Morarji J, Gupta N, et al. Valacyclovir in the treatment of acute retinal necrosis. BMC Ophthalmol. 2012;12:48.

18. Grant DM. Acyclovir (zovirax) ophthalmic ointment: a review of clinical tolerance. Curr Eye Res. 1987;6(1):231–5.

19. Chong DY, Johnson MW, Huynh TH, Hall EF, Comer GM, Fish DN. Vitreous penetration of orally administered famciclovir. Am J Ophthalmol. 2009;148(1):38–42.

20. Kaufman HE, Haw WH. Ganciclovir ophthalmic gel 0.15%: safety and efficacy of a new treatment for herpes simplex keratitis. Curr Eye Res. 2012; 37(7):654–60.

21. Bausch & Lomb. Vitrasert_: sterile intravitreal implant with Cytovene_ (ganiciclovir, 4.5 mg) [online]. Available from URL: http://www.bausch.com/en_US/package_insert/surgical/vitrasert_pkg_insert.pdf.

22. Lingyun C, James BR, Ajay T, Karl HY, Carl H, William FR. Intraocular Pharmacokinetics of a crystalline lipid prodrug, octadecyloxyethyl-cyclic-cidofovir, for cytomegalovirus retinitis. J Ocul Pharmacol Ther. 2011; 27(2):157–62.

23. Romanowski EG, Gordon YJ, Araullo-Cruz T, Yates KA, Kinchington PR. The antiviral resistance and replication of cidofovir-resistant adenovirus variants in the New Zealand white rabbit ocular model. Invest Ophthalmol Vis Sci. 2001;42:1812–5.

24. Romanowski E, Gordon Y. Efficacy of topical cidofovir on multiple and adenoviral serotypes in the New Zealand ocular model. Invest Ophthalmol Vis Sci. 2000;41:460–3.

25. Romanowski E, Bartels S, Gordon Y: Comparative antiviral efficacies of cidofovir, trifluridine and acyclovir in the HSV-1 rabbit keratitis model. Invest Ophthalmol Vis Sci. 1999;40:378–84.

26. Studies of ocular complications of AIDS (SOCA) research group and the AIDS clinical trials group. Combination foscarnet and ganciclovir therapy versus monotherapy for the treatment of relapsed cytomegalovirus retinitis in patients with AIDS. Arch Ophthalmol. 1996;114:22–33.

CHAPTER 10

Antifungal Drugs

OVERVIEW

Although the fungi community is a large one, it is surprising but fortunate that only a few species are pathogenic to the eye. Some of the pathogenic fungi affecting the eye include *Candida, Aspergillus, Fusarium , Curvularia.* As with bacteria, fungal virulence includes factors that facilitate the infection and factors that affect the host. Ability of fungi to attach to host cells and presence of a polysaccharide capsule to prevent phagocytosis by macrophages facilitates fungal invasion into the host cells. Fungi cause host tissue damage by invoking an inflammatory reaction by the polysaccharide capsule and through cytokines production. They also cause direct tissue damage through mycotoxin production.

Fungi can affect almost every structure of the eye such as cornea, conjunctiva, lens, ciliary body and the uveal tract. Factors predisposing to fungal infection include prolonged use of oral or topical steroids, a suppressed immune system, contaminated contact lenses and injury or trauma to ocular structures. The source of infection can be through the blood from a systemic infection or through direct inoculation of the fungi to the ocular structures.

The approach to diagnose fungal infection of the eye is similar to diagnosing fungal infection of the skin or any other anatomical part of the body. Although often not diagnostic for a fungal ocular infection, history and clinical examination must be taken to decide if the ocular infection is part of a systemic one or if it is a localized ocular infection. Confirmation of a fungal infection is very important as treatment is often a prolonged one. Laboratory investigations to confirm fungal infection include microscopic examination of a smear or scrapping with or without the use of stains. Determining the susceptibility of the fungus to antifungal drugs and their MIC would aid in choosing appropriate treatment and dose.

There are some general limitations for the use of antifungals, which include their adverse effects, narrow antifungal spectrum, poor tissue penetration, drug interactions and drug resistance. There are four main classes of anti-fungals: polyenes, pyrimidines, azoles and echinocandins.

The clinical efficacy of an antifungal agent in ocular mycosis depends to a great extent on the concentration of the drug achieved in the target ocular tissue. Factors affecting the concentration achieved include the molecular mass, concentration of the drug, the route by which it has been administered, duration of contact with the target ocular tissue and the ability of the compound to penetrate the ocular tissue.

POLYENES

Polyenes were the first effective antifungal agents discovered. These compounds share a common molecular structure consisting of a conjugated double-bond linked to mycosamine, an amino acid sugar. Members of this group are classified according to the number of double-bonds present.

Polyene antifungal drugs include: Natamycin, nystatin and amphotericin B. Nystatin was the first polyene identified. Amphotericin B is derived from the bacteria, *Streptomyces nodosus*. Amphotericin B is a broad spectrum antifungal drug and was the first polyene used for systemic mycosis.

Mechanism of Action

Polyenes bind to the ergosterol present in the fungal cell membrane and disrupt the membrane permeability of the organism, which interferes with the osmotic regulation of the fungal cells.[1] Mammalian cells contain cholesterol instead of ergosterol and, therefore, they are much less susceptible to polyenes. The size of the polyene affects the molecular interaction between the drug and fungal cell membrane ergosterol. Larger drug molecules such as nystatin and amphotericin B bind to the cell membrane and create channels spanning across the cell membrane and allow electrolyte movement, whereas small polyenes like natamycin alter membrane permeability by creating localized disruptions in the membrane.[2] The activity of polyenes is concentration dependant; lower doses inhibit fungal growth (fungistatic) and higher doses are fungicidal.

Antifungal Activity

Polyenes have variable antifungal activity. The antifungal spectrum of polyenes is presented in the Table 10.1. Amphotericin B also has activity against some protozoa such as *Leishmania* species and *Naegleria fowleri*.

Fungal Resistance

Generally, fungi do not demonstrate significant level of resistance against polyenes, however, some isolates of *Candida* and *Aspergillus* are resistant to nystatin and amphotericin B. The most common mechanism of polyene resistance among mutant fungi is replacement of ergosterol with certain precursor steroids.

Pharmacokinetics

All polyenes are insoluble. They practically are not absorbed from gastrointestinal tract and mucous

Table 10.1 Antifungal activity of polyenes

Amphotericin B	Nystatin	Natamycin
Candida species, *Cryptococcus neoformans*, *Blastomyces dermatitidis*, *Histoplasma capsulatum*, *Aspergillus* species, *Coccidioides* species, *Sporothrix schenckii*, *Paracoccidioides braziliensis*	*Candida* species, *Cryptococcus*	*Candida* species, *Cryptococcus neoformans*, *Aspergillus* species, *Fusarium* species

membranes. The corneal epithelium appears to be a powerful barrier to corneal penetration of the polyenes. Amphotericin B was only available in the injectable form as oral administration produces low bioavailability. Recently special lipid formulations became available for both oral and intravenous use with good bioavailability, same spectrum of activity, better therapeutic indices and less risk of nephrotoxicity. Amphotericin B is currently available as conventional amphotericin B (C-AMB), liposomal amphotericin B (L-AMB), amphotericin B colloidal dispersion (ABCD) and amphotericin B lipid complex (ABLC).[3] Injectable form of amphotericin B reaches aqueous humor in two-thirds of plasma concentration and that covers the MICs of most fungi.[4] Nystatin is also available in liposomal formulation which is effective in the treatment of systemic mycosis.[5]

Natamycin, like other polyenes is insoluble in water. It is unstable to light and extreme temperatures. The ophthalmic preparation of natamycin 5% is available in 15 mL glass bottles from Alcon Laboratories. It can be stored at room temperature or refrigerated, but may not be placed in freezers. Natamycin is only for topical use and not systemic. It adheres to areas of corneal ulceration, thereby prolonging the duration of contact. Although natamycin is well absorbed by the cornea, only small amounts are bioactive. Despite that, natamycin is an effective ophthalmic antifungal agent because the relatively high total corneal drug concentration ensures that adequate amounts of bioactive drug are available.

Therapeutic Uses

Polyenes are drugs of choice in the treatment of fungal keratitis. Nystatin has limited use in the treatment of ocular infections because it has poor ocular penetration and causes corneal toxicity. Natamycin is the only polyene antifungal that is approved for topical application for ocular fungal infection. It is available as a 5% suspension. Natamycin is most effective against the filamentous fungi especially in most cases of keratitis caused by *Fusarium* and *Aspergillus*.[6] There are, however, reports of treatment failures with these and other filamentous fungi. Yeasts such as *Candida* species tend to be less sensitive to treatment with natamycin than filamentous fungi.

Amphotericin B is most efficacious in the treatment of keratitis caused by yeasts, particularly *Candida* and *Cryptococcus* species It is less effective in filamentous fungal infections.[6] The routes of administration of amphotericin B in the treatment of keratomycoses include topical, subconjunctival, intracameral and intravenous. Topical amphotericin B has been used to treat mycotic keratitis since 1959, although toxicity has been a troublesome complication. Low dilutions (0.15% and 0.05%) of amphotericin B have been shown to be efficacious and produce far less toxic effects than higher concentrations previously used. Subconjunctival administration of amphotericin B has been advocated for the treatment of fungal keratitis and in severe cases, especially ulcers with anterior chamber reaction.[7,8] However, the injections are quite painful and poorly tolerated. Ulceration and necrosis of the overlying conjunctival epithelium may occur. Intravenous administration carries a serious risk of systemic toxicity including renal toxicity, chills, fever, phlebitis and anemia. For this reason, intravenous amphotericin B is rarely used in the treatment of keratomycoses.

Regarding fungal endophthalmitis, to preserve visual function and eliminate the fungal pathogen, topical, systemic and intraocular amphotericin B therapy is used, though it achieves very poor concentrations in the posterior segment of the eye.[9]

Adverse Effects

Local

The toxic effects of topical amphotericin B appear to be related in part to the effects of the bile salt deoxycholate used as a solubilizer. They include chemosis, burning, epithelial clouding, and punctate epithelial erosions. In extreme cases, the cornea may assume a greenish hue. Intravenous administration causes phlebitis. Topical natamycin is usually well tolerated. Rarely, corneal toxicity manifested as a form of punctate keratitis may occur.

Systemic

Amphotericin B causes chills and rigors with infusion. Often, antipyretics and anti-histamines have to be administered to patients receiving infusion of amphotericin B. The serious adverse effect of this drug, which has limited its use, is nephrotoxicity. For patients on long-term treatment with amphotericin B, it is imperative to monitor patient's renal function.

Contraindications

Polyenes are contraindicated in patients with previous history of hypersensitivity towards it. Amphotericin B is to be used with caution in very young or elderly patients and patients with pre-existing renal disease to reduce the risk of nephrotoxicity.

PYRIMIDINES

Pyrimidines are antimetabolites which impair fungal DNA synthesis. Flucytosine (5-fluorocytosine) is a fluorinated pyrimidine and is the prototype drug for this drug class. First synthesized in 1957 as an antimetabolite for the treatment of leukemia, the antifungal properties of flucytosine were first described by Grunberg and colleagues in 1963.

Mechanism of Action

Flucytosine is a fungistatic drug. It is transported across the fungal cell membrane by a specific permease. Once inside the cell, it is metabolized by deamination to fluorouracil, a thymidine analogue that blocks further fungal thymidine synthesis, thereby impairing RNA and DNA synthesis. Flucytosine has selective toxicity toward fungal cells and not the mammalian cells as it is not metabolized due to lack of cytosine deaminase in mammalian cells.[3]

Antifungal Activity

Flucytosine is effective against *Candida spp.* and *Cryptococcus*. Monotherapy with flucytosine may result in fungal resistance. The mechanism of resistance is associated with the deficiency of specific permease required to transport the drug into the cell.

Pharmacokinetics

Flucytosine is moderately soluble in water. Given orally, the drug is well absorbed by the gastrointestinal tract. Therapeutic levels can be achieved in adults with the administration of a dose of 50–150 mg/kg/day in divided doses. Tissue penetration with 1% solution is good.

Flucytosine is widely distributed in the body. It is mostly excreted unchanged by the kidneys and can be cleared by hemodialysis. A topical preparation is made by dissolving the contents in a capsule of flucytosine in artificial tears. The solution is filtered before use to remove any undissolved flucytosine. Flucytosine has been used with success as a 1% solution topically in the treatment of keratitis.

Therapeutic Uses

Flucytosine is best used as an adjunct therapy in the treatment of fungal keratitis. With a narrow anti-fungal spectrum, the clinical uses of flucytosine are limited. It is effective against *Candida* with some moderate activity against *Aspergillus*. Because resistance to flucytosine is a major problem among fungi, it is often not effective as monotherapy and has to be used in combination with other anti-fungal drugs such as amphotericin B, natamycin and miconazole.[10]

Adverse Effects

Local

Topical flucytosine is well-tolerated.

Systemic

Flucytosine causes gastrointestinal adverse effects such as nausea, vomiting and diarrhea with oral administration. It is hepatotoxic and, therefore, monitoring of the liver function is essential for patients on this drug. As with other hepatotoxic drugs, withdrawal of the drug should be considered with increase in the levels of serum transaminases and alkaline phosphatase as these changes are reversed when the drug is discontinued. At concentrations higher than 100 µg/mL, flucytosine can cause bone marrow suppression.[10]

Contraindications

Flucytosine is contraindicated in patients who have a previous history of hypersensitivity towards it. It is also contraindicated in patients with bone marrow suppression and should be used cautiously in patients with liver dysfunction and renal impairment.

AZOLES

Thiabendazole, an antiprotozoal drug was found to have antifungal properties. This led to the discovery of a potent and effective antifungal class of azoles. Azoles are divided into two groups, imidazoles and triazoles (Table 10.2), both have the same mechanism of action.

The most commonly used azoles in ophthalmology are clotrimazole, ketoconazole,

Table 10.2 Classification of azole antifungal agents

Imidazoles		Triazoles	
Systemic	Topical	Systemic	Topical
Ketoconazole	Miconazole	Fluconazole	Terconazole
	Clotrimazole	Itraconazole	
	Econazole	Ravuconazole	
	Butoconazole	Posaconazole	
	Bifonazole	Voriconazole	
	Tioconazole		
	Oxiconazole		
	Fenticonazole		
	Sertaconazole		
	Sulconazole		

miconazole, itraconazole, fluconazole and voriconazole.

Mechanism of Action

All azoles inhibit 14-α-sterol demethylase enzyme, which is involved in fungal ergosterol synthesis. Therefore, they impair ergosterol biosynthesis for the cytoplasmic membrane and cause accumulation of ergosterol precursor 14-α-methylsterol. Methylsterol disrupts the structure of cytoplasmic membrane and membrane associated enzymes responsible for the fungal growth.[3]

The imidazoles, except for ketoconazole, are fungistatic *in vitro* at low concentrations and fungicidal at high concentrations. The high concentrations required for fungicidal effect is not easily attainable in the ocular tissue. Therefore, in the treatment of ocular infections, the viewpoint accepted is that the azoles have a fungistatic effect.

Antifungal Activity

Azoles are generally active against *Candida* species, *Aspergillus* species, *Histoplasma capsulatum*, *Cryptococcus neoformans*, *Blastomyces dermatitidis*, *Coccidioides* species, *Sporothrix schenckii*, and *Paracoccidioides braziliensis*.

Secondary azole resistance emerges due to prolonged use and is associated with several mechanisms such as the alteration of 14-α-sterol demethylase, increased production of 14-α-sterol demethylase and azole efflux.

Pharmacokinetics

Systemic Azoles

The systemic azoles such as ketoconazole, itraconazole, fluconazole and voriconazole are well absorbed from gastrointestinal tract and are widely distributed in tissues. They achieve adequate concentrations in the cornea when administered topically, or orally. With oral administration, it also achieves high concentrations in the aqueous humor. They are used in the treatment of systemic mycoses because of their pharmacokinetic properties and good safety.

Topical Azoles

Topical azoles are usually poorly absorbed from mucous membranes and are used for the treatment of superficial mycoses. Azoles like clotrimazole are used topically. Although they are well absorbed orally, their use is limited to topical because of their significant systemic toxicity. Ketoconazole primarily was introduced in clinical practice as systemic antifungal drug but it has been replaced by intraconazole and other triazoles because of their better safety profile. Currently, ketoconazole is available for topical use. Miconazole preparations for topical administration are available in the form of 1% drop in arachis oil or as cream (2%). It is also available in an injectable form for subconjunctival injection, which can also be used as topical application. Miconazole can achieve high concentrations in the cornea and the aqueous humor with topical and subconjunctival administration. It can be given intravenously to treat corneal fungal infections.

Therapeutic Uses

Fungal keratitis is very commonly caused by three fungal species: *Aspergillus spp., Candida spp.* and *Fusarium spp.* Ketoconazole is effective in the treatment of keratitis and corneal ulcers caused by all three causative agents. It can be administered orally to treat corneal ulcers or as a topical agent at a concentration of 1–5%. Combined therapy of oral ketoconazole and topical and subconjunctival miconazole can be used effectively to treat corneal ulcers. An alternative treatment to ketoconazole specially in yeast infections is fluconazole 0.5% and miconazole 1%.[11] Voriconazole is rapidly becoming the drug of choice for all fungal keratitis because of its wide spectrum of antifungal activity and ability to achieve high concentration in the cornea.[12] Combination therapy of topical amphotericin B eye drops with subconjunctival injection of fluconazole is more effective than the use of topical amphotericin B eye drops alone and may be recommended in complicated cases with corneal perforation.[13]

Candida and *Aspergillus* are most common causative agents for fungal endophthalmitis. The major problem in the treatment of fungal endophthalmitis is a highly variable penetration of systemically administered antifungal agents into the posterior segment of the eye. Fluconazole and voriconazole are the drugs of choice because they achieve therapeutic concentration in the vitreous for both, *Candida* and *Aspergillus.*[9] The combination of intravitreal amphotericin B with fluconazole or itraconazole is also a very common mode of treatment in patients with fungal endophthalmitis.[14,15]

Adverse Effects

Local

Generally azoles are well tolerated. However, patients can develop punctate keratopathy and ocular irritation on prolonged use.

Systemic

Nausea, vomiting, diarrhea, abdominal cramps are most common adverse drug reactions associated with azoles. Systemic azoles especially ketoconazole and itraconazole can cause serious hepatotoxicity. The liver dysfunction is reversible on cessation of therapy. Monitoring of liver function is indicated in patients on long-term oral ketoconazole and itraconazole treatment. Voriconazole and some other azoles cause QT interval prolongation and may provoke arrhythmias specially if co-administered with drugs that also prolong QT interval (amiodarone, sotalol, quinidine, procainimide, etc.). Most of systemic azoles are teratogenic (category C and D of risk in pregnancy) and they are contraindicated during gestation.[16] Allergic reactions such as rash, anaphylaxis, Stevens-Johnson syndrome may occur during azole treatment.

Drug Interactions

Azoles are potent inhibitors of cytochrome P450. Thus, co-administration of azoles with drugs undergoing cytochrome metabolism may lead to elevation of their plasma levels and appearance of toxic effects. Drugs manifesting elevated plasma levels due to co-administration with azoles include carbamazepine, digoxin, glipizide, haloperidol, losartan, lovastatin, methylprednisolone, omeprazole, phenytoin, quinidine, sirolimus, tacrolimus, warfarin, zidovudine and zolpidem.

ECHINOCANDINS

The echinocandins are systemic antifungal agents that were discovered in 1970s as the products of fungal fermentation. Three echinocandins are approved for clinical use currently: caspofungin, anidulafungin, and micafungin. [17]

Mechanism of Action

All echinocandins noncompetitively inhibit 1, 3-β- and 1,6-β-D-glucan synthase, an enzyme involved in the synthesis of 1,3-β-D-glucan, an essential polysaccharide compound for the fungal cell walls. Changes in the cell wall structure due to abnormality of glucan synthesis leads to osmotic instability and lysis of fungal cells.[17]

Antifungal Activity

The echinocandins show high fungicidal activity against *Candida spp.* including the strains that are fluconazole-resistant. Echinocandins also have also fungistatic activity against *Aspergillus spp.*

Pharmacokinetics

All echinocandins have very low oral bioavailability and, therefore, they are administered only intravenously.[17] They have high protein binding and are widely distributed in the body. However, cerebrospinal fluid and intravitreous penetrations are minimal.[18] The clinical significance of low brain and ocular barrier penetration is questionable. There are some reports of clinical failure as well as successful use of caspofungin monotherapy in the treatment of *Candida albicans* endophthalmitis.[19]

Following initial distribution, echinocandins are metabolized in liver (caspofungin and micafungin) and red blood cells (micafungin). Metabolites are mostly excreted in the bile. They are not dialyzable and do not require dose adjustment in patients with renal failure.

Therapeutic Uses

The echinocandins are the drugs of choice in the treatment of systemic yeast infection, especially for empirical treatment of systemic candidiasis. Unfortunately echinocandins are of limited use in ophthalmology due to their poor intravitreous penetration. Nevertheless, echinocandins may be used in the treatment of fungal endophthalmitis usually in combination with other antifungal agents.

Adverse Effects

Generally echinocandins are relatively safe and well-tolerated drugs. Micafungin and anidulafungin show lower frequency of adverse drug reactions as compared to caspofungin. However, it might be explained by the longer history of caspofungin's clinical use compared to two other echinocandins.[19]

There is insufficient data regarding the safety of caspofungin and other echinocandins in pregnancy. Echinocandins belong to pregnancy category C and should be avoided during gestation and breast feeding.[16]

Drug Interactions

Generally echinocandins neither serve as a substrates nor are potent inducers/inhibitors of cytochrome P450 and, therefore, have minimal risk of involvement in drug-drug interactions even in combinations with other antifungal agents.[18] Caspofungin slightly increases tacrolimus plasma level, while no such effects of micafungin and anidulafungin have been reported [3].

GRISEOFULVIN

Griseofulvin is one of the oldest antifungal drug. It was isolated in 1939 from some strains of *Penicillium griseofulvum.*

Mechanism of Action

Griseofulvin binds to tubulin and inhibits microtubule formation during mitosis, thereby affects fungal cell division. Thus, the mechanism of action of griseofulvin is similar to that of vinca alkaloids but the sites of binding are different. Similarities of the mechanisms of action make griseofulvin potentially interesting as anticancer drug.[20]

Antifungal Activity

Griseofulvin is fungistatic and is most effective against dermatophytes including various species of *Microsporum (Microsporum audouinii, Microsporum canis, Microsporum gypseum), Epidermophyton (Epidermophyton floccosum)*, and *Trichophyton (Trichophyton rubrum, Trichophyton tonsurans, Trichophyton mentagrophytes, Trichophyton interdigitalis, Trichophyton verrucosum, Trichophyton megnini, Trichophyton gallinae, Trichophyton crateriform, Trichophyton sulphureum, Trichophyton schoenleini).*

Pharmacokinetics

Griseofulvin is used orally. It is highly lipophilic and is well absorbed from gastrointestinal tract. Fatty meal increases the systemic bioavailability of griseofulvin. Bioavailability of microcrystalline (Grifulvin V) and ultra-microcrystalline (Gris-PEG) preparations of griseofulvin is reported to be higher and this allows use of two-third of the normal dose of griseofulvin. However, there is currently no evidence that this lower dose confers any significant clinical differences with regard to safety and/or efficacy.

Griseofulvin is distributed and mainly deposited in keratin precursor cells. Long-term persistence of griseofulvin in keratin prevents fungal invasion into the disease free tissues until they are replaced by non-griseofulvin containing cells.[3]

Therapeutic Uses

Griseofulvin is indicated for the treatment of the ringworm infections (*Tinea corporis, Tinea pedis, Tinea cruris, Tinea barbae, Tinea capitis, and Tinea unguium*).[21] In ophthalmology practice, griseofulvin may be used for the treatment dermatomycoses affecting eyebrows and periorbital skin.

Adverse Effects

Griseofulvin is a relatively safe drug. The most common adverse drug reactions due to griseofulvin are headache, fatigue, vertigo and peripheral neuritis. Other adverse effects include hepatotoxicity, neutropenia and severe skin reactions (Stevens-Johnson syndrome, toxic epidermal necrolysis). Estrogen-like effects have been observed in children.

Drug Interactions

Griseofulvin induces hepatic cytochrome enzymes and, therefore, may reduce the efficacy of the drugs like warfarin and oral contraceptives.[22]

Contraindications

Griseofulvin is contraindicated in patients with severe liver failure and hypersensitivity to griseofulvin. Chronic use of griseofulvin causes increased level of protoporphyrins, thus, it is also contraindicated in patients with porphyria.[3]

ALLYLAMINES

Allylamines are synthetic antifungal agents including systemic terbinafine and topical naftifine, amorolfine, and butenafine.

Mechanism of Action

Allylamines inhibit the synthesis of ergosterol by inhibiting squalene epoxidase, an enzyme involved in ergosterol synthesis. Ergosterol is essential for the structure of fungal cytoplasmic membranes and interruption of its synthesis leads to disruption of cytoplasmic membranes.

Antifungal Activity

The antifungal spectrum of all allylamines is similar to that of griseofulvin and includes species of *Microsporum, Epidermophyton*, and *Trichophyton.*

Pharmacokinetics

Terbinafine is well absorbed, but its bioavailability is significantly decreased due to first-pass metabolism in the liver. Terbinafine is lipophilic and is well distributed in the tissues. It accumulates in the skin, nails and fat. It is metabolized in liver by the cytochrome P450.[3]

Therapeutic Uses

Naftifine, amorolfine, and butenafine are administered topically in the form of a cream and nail lacquer. Terbinafine is used topically as well as systemically. Terbinafine is mostly used in the treatment of tinea infections and onychomycosis.[21] Topical applications of terbinafine, naftifine, and butenafine are sometimes used for the treatment of cutaneous candidiasis. In ophthalmology terbinafine may be used in the treatment of dermatomycosis of the periorbital skin.

Adverse Effects

Terbinafine is well tolerated and may be safely used even in children. Rarely, it may cause hepatotoxicity and severe neutropenia. Stevens-Johnson syndrome may also occur.

Drug Interations

Terbinafine has a low potential for drug interactions.[22] However, terbinafine is metabolized by cytochrome so it may interacts with drugs significantly affecting cytochrome P450 activity, such us phenobarbital, rifampin and cimetidine.

REFERENCES

1. Baginski M, Czub J. Amphotericin B and its new derivatives - mode of action. Curr Drug Metab. 2009;10(5): 459–69.
2. Te Welscher YM, Ten Napel HH, Balagué MM, Souza CM, Riezman H, de Kruijff B, et al. Natamycin blocks fungal growth by binding specifically to ergosterol without permeabilizing the membrane. J Biol Chem. 2008; 283(10):6393–401.
3. Bennet JE. Antifungal agents. In: Brunton LL, Chabner BA, Knollmann BC (eds). Goodman and Gilman's The Pharmacological Basis of Therapeutics, 12th edn. Mc Graw Hill Medical. 2011;1571–92.
4. Qu L, Li L, Xie H. Corneal and aqueous humor concentrations of amphotericin B using three different routes of administration in a rabbit model. Ophthalmic Res. 2010;43(3):153–8.
5. Offner F, Krcmery V, Boogaerts M, Doyen C, Engelhard D, et al. Liposomal nystatin in patients with invasive aspergillosis refractory to or intolerant of amphotericin B. Antimicrob Agents Chemother. 2004;48(12):4808–12.
6. Tuli S S. Fungal keratitis. Clin Ophthalmol. 2011;5:275–9.
7. Carrasco MA, Genesoni G. Treatment of severe fungal keratitis with subconjunctival amphotericin B. Cornea. 2011;30(5):608–11.
8. Yilmaz S, Ture M, Maden A. Efficacy of intracameral amphotericin B injection in the management of refractory keratomycosis and endophthalmitis. Cornea. 2007;26(4):398–402.
9. Riddell J 4th, Comer GM, Kauffman CA. Treatment of endogenous fungal endophthalmitis: focus on new antifungal agents. Clin Infect Dis. 2011;52(5):648–53.
10. Vermes A, Guchelaar HJ, Dankert J. Flucytosine: a review of its pharmacology, clinical indications, pharmacokinetics, toxicity and drug interactions. J. Antimicrob Chemother. 2000;46(2):171–9.
11. Manzouri B, Vafidis GC, Wyse RK. Pharmacotherapy of fungal eye infections. Expert Opin Pharmacother. 2001;2(11):1849–57.
12. Hariprasad SM, Mieler WF, Lin TK, Sponsel WE, Graybil JRl. Voriconazole in the treatment of fungal eye infections: a review of current literature. Br J Ophthalmol. 2008;92(7):871–8.
13. Mahdy RA, Nada WM, Wageh MM. Topical amphotericin B and subconjunctival injection of fluconazole (combination therapy) versus topical amphotericin B (monotherapy) in treatment of keratomycosis. J Ocul Pharmacol Ther. 2010;26(3):281–5.
14. Chakrabarti A, Shivaprakash MR, Singh R, Tarai B, George VK, Fomda BA, et al. Fungal endophthalmitis: fourteen years' experience from a center in India. Retina. 2008;28(10):1400–7.
15. Khan FA, Slain D, Khakoo RA. Candida endophthalmitis: focus on current and future

antifungal treatment options. Pharmacotherapy. 2007; 27(12):1711–21.

16. Moudgal VV, Sobel JD. Antifungal drugs in pregnancy: a review. Expert Opin Drug Saf. 2003; 2(5):475–83.

17. Sucher AJ, Chahine EB, Balcer HE. Echinocandins: the newest class of antifungals. Ann Pharmacother. 2009; 43(10):1647–57.

18. Denning DW. Echinocandin antifungal drugs. Lancet. 2003; 4;362(9390):1142–51.

19. Eschenauer G, DePestel DD, Carver1 PL. Comparison of echinocandin antifungals. Ther Clin Risk Manag. 2007; 3(1):71–97.

20. Panda D, Rathinasamy K, Santra MK, Wilson L. Kinetic suppression of microtubule dynamic instability by griseofulvin: implications for its possible use in the treatment of cancer. Proc Natl Acad Sci USA. 2005;102(28): 9878–83.

21. Huang DB, Ostrosky-Zeichner L, Wu JJ, Pang KR, Tyring SK. Therapy of common superficial fungal infections. Dermatol Ther. 2004;17(6):517–22.

22. Albengres E, Le Louët H, Tillement JP. Systemic antifungal agents. Drug interactions of clinical significance. Drug Saf. 1998;18(2):83–97.

CHAPTER 11

Drugs Used in Ocular Pain and Inflammation

OVERVIEW

As with several other clinical conditions, pain is also a frequent accompaniment of many ophthalmic disorders. Pain localized to the eye and surrounding structures shares causes, which are similar to the ones responsible for pain in other parts of the body such as trauma (including surgical), inflammation, and neoplasia. Raised intraocular pressure and refractive errors also lead to pain. While correction of the underlying cause is important for effective pain relief in the latter, pain control itself is an important priority in the former.

The two major classes of drugs that have long been used for analgesic purpose are the "opiates" and the "non-steroidal anti-inflammatory drugs" (NSAIDs) or non-opioid analgesics. Both morphine (the prototype opiate) and aspirin (the earliest NSAID) are still in use but several new members of each class have been developed over the years. Under certain circumstances some non-analgesic drugs may be used to relieve pain (e.g. anticonvulsants, tricyclic antidepressants or serotonin/norepinephrine reuptake inhibitors for neurogenic pain, ergot alkaloids for migraine and nitroglycerine for pain of angina pectoris) but these are not classified among the analgesic drugs.

In this chapter, we discuss the pharmacology of the 'classical' analgesics viz. the opiates and NSAIDs. The use of opiates in ophthalmic practice does not differ greatly from its use in other fields, hence these are only dealt with in brief. NSAIDs find a greater use, particularly those for which suitable topical formulations are available, since topical use is associated with fewer adverse events as compared to systemic administration. Available topical preparations are listed in Table 11.8.

Following better understanding of the mechanisms involved in pain generation and transmission, recent strategies have targeted newer approaches for analgesia. Some of these are described in the later part.

MECHANISMS OF PAIN

Pain is a subjective phenomenon generally regarded as being associated with tissue damage, injury or inflammation. However, not only is pain often experienced in the apparent absence of any overt signs of such processes (e.g. neuralgias), the intensity of the pain experienced in the presence of tissue damage or inflammation can also exhibit wide variations. Thus, pain cannot be considered simply to be a response to tissue damage but rather a complex interplay of processes comprising of physiological, neural, psychological and emotional components.

Despite the complexities involved, we now have a fairly clear understanding of many of the processes involved in the initiation, the pathways of transmission and the central mechanisms pertaining to the perception of pain. Several chemical mediators that either stimulate or enhance the sensitivity (thereby lowering their excitation threshold) of nociceptors and thus, play a role in the initiation and amplification of the pain stimulus are well recognized. Similarly, the processes involved in the transmission of the pain stimulus from the site of generation to the central nervous system and the mechanisms, chemical signaling molecules and receptors involved therein, leading to the perception of pain, have been worked out in substantial detail. The role of prostaglandins, in the generation of the pain stimulus and that of the endogenous peptides and their receptors in the central processing of pain have been the subject of great attention and also the major targets for pain control strategies. Despite so many advances, the two major groups of analgesics that have dominated for more than a century, and still continue to dominate, are the NSAIDs, which inhibit prostaglandin synthesis, and opiate derivatives (including synthetic) which act on specific receptors (mu, kappa and delta) that are the targets of endogenous opioid peptides viz. endorphin and encephalin. Other targets, which have of late received attention for possible approaches towards analgesic drug development, include ion channels involved in nociceptive nerves, neuropeptides like somatostatin, glutamate receptors and cannabinoid receptors. Most of these are still under experimental or early clinical evaluation.

OPIOID (NARCOTIC) ANALGESICS

For many centuries crude opium, derived from the opium poppy, has been in use (and abuse) for its analgesic, sedative and euphoric effects. Serturner isolated the pure alkaloid in 1803 and named it morphine (after *Morpheus* the Greek god of dreams). It is surprising that even after more than two centuries, during which tremendous advances have been made in the field of synthetic drugs, not only is morphine still in clinical use but is also the standard against which all other analgesics of this class are compared. Several derivatives obtained from natural sources, by chemical modifications of the opium alkaloids or through *de novo* synthesis, sharing similar properties and mechanisms of action are grouped together as opioids (*the term 'opiate' is reserved for drugs obtained from the opium plant*).

Mechanism of Action

Opioid analgesics produce analgesia by binding to specific G-protein coupled receptors. These receptors are classified into three types and denoted by the Greek characters μ (mu), K (kappa) and δ (delta). Each of these receptors also has subtypes. The μ and δ have two subtypes viz. μ_1, μ_2 and δ_1, δ_2 while K has three subtypes K_1, K_2 and K_3. These receptors are located in regions of the brain and spinal cord, which are involved in the transmission and processing of pain. Opioid receptors are also present at nerve terminals in the periphery and may be involved in the modulation of release of neurotransmitters from the sensory nerve terminals. The inhibition of the release of substance P in the dorsal horn of the spinal cord by morphine is one of the mechanisms involved in its analgesic effect. Although all the opioid receptors are involved with pain regulation, the principal receptor for analgesic action of opioids appears to be the μ receptor.

Physiologically the opioid receptors are targets for a group of peptides, which are richly present in regions of the CNS concerned with pain modulation and themselves possess analgesic, sedative and other pharmacological properties that are similar to the opioids. These peptides, therefore, have been termed as the endogenous opioid peptides.

Three families of peptides (Table 11.1) derived from pre-proopiomelanocortin (POMC) have been characterized and studied in extensive detail viz. the endorphins, encephalins (leu-enkephalin and met-enkephalin) and the dynorphins. These peptides display varying affinities for the opioid receptor subtypes but all of them are involved in endogenous pain control mechanisms and are released in response to painful and other stressful stimuli. Besides, they are also involved in other physiological functions.

In addition, another receptor-ligand system has also been identified. The endogenous ligand for this system is nociceptin, which differs from dynorphin only marginally with the N-terminal tyrosine being absent. This receptor ligand system

Table 11.1 Opioid receptor subtypes and the opioid peptides

Endogenous opioid peptide	Receptor affinity	Function
Endorphin	$\mu > \kappa$ or δ	Analgesia (spinal and supraspinal), respiratory depression, decrease in GI motility, neuroendocrine modulation
Enkephalin	$\delta > \mu$ or κ	Analgesia (spinal and supraspinal), neuroendocrine modulation
Dynorphins	$\kappa > \mu$ or δ	Analgesia[#], decrease in GI motility, psychotomimetic effects

[#]Dynorphin has also been reported to produce a hyperalgesic action at the spinal dorsal horn level through κ receptors

is widely represented in the central nervous system and also in the periphery. However, in contrast to endorphins, it opposes μ receptor mediated pain suppression besides involvement in other behavioral functions.

Interaction of opioids with the G protein coupled receptors affects gating of ion channels to modulate ion fluxes across neuronal membranes. Receptor actions of opioids bring about a closure of voltage dependent Ca^{++} channels on presynaptic nerve terminals causing a decrease in the neurotransmitter release. An inhibitory action on presynaptic release of neurotransmitters by opioids has been demonstrated for several neurotransmitters including norepinephrine, serotonin, acetylcholine, substance P and glutamate. Post-synaptically, an increase in K^+ efflux (by opening K^+ channels) by opioids hyperpolarizes the membrane to reduce neuronal activity. Sites that are concerned with the regulation of pain exhibit a rich distribution of opioid receptors as shown in Table 11.2.

Morphine: The Prototype Opioid Drug

Morphine is the major analgesic drug present in crude opium derived from the poppy plant. It acts on all three subtypes (μ, K and δ) of opioid receptors, possesses powerful analgesic actions and also displays the full range of effects of opioid drugs on other tissues and systems. It is, therefore, taken as a prototype for this class against which all other drugs are compared. Codeine, is also present in the extract of the opium plant but has substantially lower analgesic activity. Other opioids may differ from morphine in their analgesic as well as other actions because of one or more of the following reasons:

i. Preferential affinity for only particular (and not all) receptor subtypes
ii. Partial agonist action at the opioid receptors on which they act
iii. Mixed actions, i.e. agonist at one or more receptor subtype and antagonist at other/s

Table 11.2 Distribution of opioid receptors and their role in analgesia

Site	Suggested role
Spinal cord (substantia gelatinosa)	Suppression of upward transmission of afferent sensory information from the periphery
Medial hypothalamus	Modulate perception of deep (poorly localized) pain
Limbic system	Not involved directly with analgesia but may be important for emotional reaction to painful stimuli
Peripheral sensory nerve terminals	Inhibit release of pro-inflammatory substances

Classification

Due to differences in receptor actions and pharmacokinetics, opioids display differences in their efficacies for pain relief, with some like morphine and fentanyl possessing powerful analgesic actions, even against high intensity pain, while others, like codeine and pentazocine, display only limited effects. Further, differences are also observed in their propensity for inducing adverse effects. Opioids can thus be classified either on the basis of their pain relieving potential (Table 11.3) or on the basis of their receptor actions (Table 11.4). The former is more relevant with regard to the choice for clinical use while the latter is important for an understanding of their actions and some of their adverse effects. For example, the drugs like buprenorphine, which have partial agonist action at μ receptors, have less potential for severe respiratory depression as compared to full agonists. Alternatively, opioids can also be classified according to their chemical structure.

Table 11.3 Classification of opioids based on their efficacy

High efficacy	Morphine, meperidine, fentanyl, methadone, nalbuphine, buprenorphine
Moderate efficacy	Hydrocodone, oxycodone, pentazocine
Low efficacy	Codeine

Pharmacokinetics

Absorption: Opioids are most frequently administered through the parenteral route. Most opioids are well absorbed after intramuscular or subcutaneous administration. Morphine is absorbed from the gut after oral administration although the absorption is slow, often erratic and subject to considerable first-pass metabolism. Consequently the oral dose of morphine is usually several folds higher than its equivalent parenteral dose. Extended release forms of morphine are often used orally to achieve more consistent plasma levels. Codeine does not undergo extensive first pass metabolism and is used orally.

Distribution: Following absorption opioids rapidly enter most tissues with greater localization in the highly perfused tissues such as the brain, lungs , liver, kidney and spleen. Morphine is less lipophilic than many other commonly used opioids and only a small fraction crosses the blood brain barrier. In contrast, other agents like methadone, fentanyl and heroin are more lipophilic and readily enter the brain. Morphine, however, crosses the placental barrier and can affect the fetus and is, therefore, not recommended during labor. Highly lipophilic agents like fentanyl tend to accumulate in fatty tissue, especially following high doses or continuous perfusion.

Metabolism: Conjugation with glucuronic acid in the liver converts morphine to more

Table 11.4 Classification of opioids based on their receptor actions

Agonists	Partial agonists	Mixed agonist-antagonists	Antagonists
Morphine (μ,κ,δ)	Buprenorphine (μ)	Pentazocine (P-Ag κ; Ant μ, δ)	Naloxone (μ, κ, δ)
Meperidine (μ,κ)		Nalbuphine	Naltrexone
Fentanyl		Butorphanol	Nalmefine
Alfentanil			Naloxonazine
Sufentanil			
Ramifentanil			
Methadone			
Oxycodone			
Codeine			
Propoxyphene			
Heroin			

P-Ag: partial agonist; Ant: antagonist

polar forms, which are rapidly excreted by the kidneys and to a lesser extent in bile. Morphine-3-glucuronide, the major metabolite, exhibits some neuroexcitatory properties, which are not entirely mediated through opioid receptors. Up to 10% of morphine gets converted to morphine-6-glucuronide, which shows considerably more potent analgesic potency as compared to the parent compound. These metabolites are not considered to be of significance for effects following acute administration since being polar they are not able to readily cross the blood brain barrier. Administration of large doses or in patients with compromised renal functions the accumulation of these metabolites may result in adverse effects. Morphine administration is not recommended in neonates because the conjugating enzymes are not fully developed. Pethidine (meperidine) and fentanyl and other phenylpiperidine derivatives are primarily degraded by hepatic oxidative metabolizing enzymes to inactive products. Normeperidine, the metabolite of pethidine has potential for inducing seizures and its accumulation after high doses or in patients with compromised renal functions may be dangerous. The pharmacokinetic properties of some commonly used opioids are given below (Table 11.5).

Pharmacological Actions

The most notable effects of opioid agonists are on the central nervous system. Members that have affinity for μ receptors display a range of effects related to the central nervous system.

Analgesia: Opioids are effective in relieving both the sensory as well as emotional components of pain. Through a combination of effects at the spinal and supraspinal levels they cause not only an increase in the threshold for pain perception by the brain but also alter the emotional reaction to pain whereby the awareness of pain sensation is no longer unpleasant and, thereby, more tolerable.

Euphoria: Morphine produces a strong sense of well-being, a floating sensation and a decrease in anxiety especially after intravenous administration – the major reason for its abuse by intravenous drug users. As opposed to euphoria, dysphoria – an unpleasant state of restlessness – may result in some individuals.

Sedation: Mental clouding, drowsiness and induction of sleep are commonly associated with administration of morphine. These effects are potentiated by concomitant use of other CNS depressants like sedative-hypnotics.

Respiratory depression: Morphine and other opioid drugs can produce respiratory depression by decreasing the sensitivity of neurons in the respiratory center in the brain stem to carbon dioxide. This occurs with usual doses of morphine and becomes more pronounced with increasing doses. Very high doses can result in a complete suppression of respiratory function. Failure of respiration is the most common cause of death from opioid overdose. Thus, respiratory depression constitutes the most important limitation to

Table 11.5 Pharmacokinetic properties of some commonly used opioids

Drug	Approximate equivalent doses (parenteral)	Route/s of administration	Duration of analgesic action
Morphine	10 mg	IV, IM, SC, PO	4–5 h
Meperidine	100 mg	IM, IV, SC	3–4 h
Fentanyl	0.1 mg	IV	0.75–1.0 h
Pentazocine	30 mg	IV, IM, PO	Up to 4 h
Buprenorphine	0.3 mg	IV, IM	Up to 8 h
Codeine	30–60 mg	Oral	3–4 h

effective use of opioids for pain control. The presence of increased intracranial tension or chronic obstructive pulmonary disease (COPD) increases the susceptibility for this untoward outcome. Some opioids like buprenorphine exhibit a 'ceiling effect' in this regard. Thus with increasing doses the respiratory depressant effects seems to level off, providing some margin of safety.

Suppression of cough reflex: Suppression of cough reflex is a well known effect of opioids and codeine in particular is used as an antitussive. The mechanism of cough suppression appears to be somewhat different from the analgesic effects of opioids and does not correlate with analgesic potency.

Emesis: Morphine stimulates the chemoreceptor trigger zone in the area postrema and produces nausea and vomiting.

Miosis: Miosis is produced by most opioids. An increase in parasympathetic influence on the eye due to stimulation of μ and K receptors in the Edinger-Westphal nucleus of the oculomotor nerve is responsible for this effect. Pin-point pupils are a diagnostic sign for opioid poisoning even in chronic drug users since little tolerance develops to this effect.

Other CNS-mediated effects of opioids include alterations of homeostatic regulation of body temperature, supraspinally mediated exaggeration of the tone of trunk muscles, a central depression of vasomotor tone and neuroendocrine effects. Opioids also produce several peripheral effects, which include effects on:

Smooth muscles: Intestinal motility is diminished due to an increase in the tone of the circular smooth muscle through an action on the enteric nervous system leading to constipation. Some opioid congeners with restricted peripheral smooth muscle actions like loperamide and diphenoxylate are indeed used as antidiarrheals. Constriction of the biliary smooth muscle as well as the sphincter of Oddi may result in biliary colic.

Uterus: Labor is prolonged by opioid analgesics.

Renal effects: A decrease in renal plasma flow caused by opioids results in a decrease in renal function.

Histamine release: Morphine releases histamine from the mast cells. This often results in urticaria, vasodilatation and sweating following intravenous administration.

Tolerance and Dependence

On continued use of morphine and other opioids, tolerance often develops for some of the effects. Effects which display a high level of tolerance development include analgesia—the major therapeutic purpose for which opioids are generally used—necessitating an increase in dosage to achieve an acceptable therapeutic effect, euphoria, sedation, nausea and vomiting and respiratory depression. Cross tolerance among different members is commonly seen. Tolerance is minimal or absent for constipation and miosis.

Emergence of tolerance following frequent and repeated use of opioids is also accompanied by the development of physical dependence. Stopping the drug in such individuals, results in the appearance of a 'withdrawal syndrome' characterized by restlessness, excitatory symptoms and drug craving. The mechanisms for development of tolerance and physical dependence are complex and involve an interplay of adaptive changes occurring at the level of receptors, neurotransmitters and other molecular targets.

Therapeutic Uses

Analgesia: Morphine and other high efficacy opioids (Table 11.3) occupy an important place in the management of moderate to severe pain. Constant and sustained pain responds better while sharp, intermittent pain appears to be less effectively controlled with opioids. The pain associated with cancer almost always requires the use of opioid analgesics on a long-term basis and some degree of tolerance and dependence are often encountered during such use. However, the possibility of inducing tolerance and dependence should not constrain the use of opioid analgesics in such conditions since the benefits in terms of relief of pain and the consequent enhancement of quality of life far outweigh the risks associated with dependence in these patients. Severe visceral pains arising from conditions such as biliary and renal colics and the pain of myocardial infarction often require opioids. Opioids are also used during obstetric labor but caution is required since opioids can cross the placenta and cause fetal respiratory depression. Meperidine (pethidine) is less likely to produce fetal respiratory depression and is preferred over morphine for obstetric use.

Acute pulmonary edema: Dramatic relief of dyspnea can be achieved in pulmonary edema associated with acute left ventricular failure with administration of intravenous morphine. A decrease in anxiety and reduced cardiac preload and afterload (due to reduced venous and arteriolar tones) contribute to these effects.

Diarrhea: Morphine has a constipating effect due to effects on intestinal motility and circular smooth muscle tone thus providing effective control of diarrhea. Synthetic derivatives such as diphenoxylate and loperamide, which have relatively selective gastrointestinal action with minimal effects on the central nervous system, are used as antidiarrheals.

Cough suppression: Opioids suppress cough by a central action at doses lower than those required for analgesia. Codeine has greater antitussive action as compared to morphine. Synthetic derivatives such as dextromethorphan and levopropoxyphene are more selective as cough suppressant and are devoid of other opioid effects.

Anesthesia: Opioids have important applications in anesthesia both as premedication and as a component of the anesthetic regimen. In addition, epidural and subarachnoid application of opioids is often used for producing regional analgesia for operative purposes or for pain control.

Adverse Effects

The adverse effects of opioids are generally an extension of their pharmacological actions. Thus sedation, respiratory depression, nausea, vomiting and constipation are the adverse effects commonly encountered during opioid use. With high doses severe respiratory depression can be a serious and life threatening problem. Patients with respiratory insufficiency are especially prone to respiratory depressant effects and require careful monitoring if opioids have to be used at all in this group. Other adverse effects include dysphoria occurring occasionally, postural hypotension which is exacerbated by hypovolemia, itching and urticaria, an elevation of intracranial pressure and acute urinary retention in patients with benign prostatic hyperplasia. Development of tolerance and physical dependence (see above) require consideration during chronic opioid use.

Contraindications

The use of opioids in certain conditions might constitute an increased risk for adverse effects and toxicity. Under such situations their use is either contraindicated or, in case there is no alternative to their use, extreme caution and monitoring is required.

Head injury: In head injury, the intracranial pressure is usually raised. Opioids can further worsen this by producing dilatation of cerebral vessels due to their depressant effects on respiration and consequent carbon dioxide retention. Additionally, the CNS effects of opioids can complicate the signs of altered consciousness making identification and interpretation of the clinical signs of the head injury difficult.

Reduced pulmonary function: Respiratory depressant effects of opioids can lead to acute respiratory failure in patients with compromised respiratory function and reduced respiratory reserve such as those with emphysema and COPD. Bronchoconstriction might further aggravate respiratory insufficiency in COPD and asthma patients.

Impaired hepatic or renal functions: The half-life of morphine and other opioids is prolonged in the presence of reduced hepatic and renal functions. Consequently, accumulation of the parent drug and/or active metabolites is likely to occur if this is not compensated by an adequate downward adjustment of the dose.

Combination of more than one opioids: Since the mechanism of action of all opioids is similar, a simultaneous use of more than one opioids is not justified and may not yield additional therapeutic benefit while increasing the risk of additive toxicity. Further, if a partial agonist or mixed agonist-antagonist (e.g. pentazocine) is administered together with a full agonist (e.g. morphine) the combined analgesic effect might actually be reduced. Opioids can, however, be combined with other non-opioid analgesics (NSAIDs) for additive effects.

Drug Interactions

Concurrent administration of opioids with other sedative hypnotic drugs tends to potentiate the CNS and respiratory depressant effects. Increased sedation is also encountered with combined use of opioids and tricyclic antidepressant drugs. Monoamine oxidase (MAO) inhibitors used either during therapy with opioids (particularly meperidine), or within the last 14 days may result in hyperpyrexia and hypertension.

Tramadol

Tramadol is a synthetic drug, which produces centrally mediated analgesia like the opioids but has only a weak agonist activity at μ-receptors. Its analgesic action is thought to be related more to its serotonin re-uptake blocking activity. It is orally effective for mild to moderate pain with less risk for respiratory depression. It is, however, associated with an increased risk of seizures and is not recommended for patients with history of seizures.

Opioid Antagonists

Structural modifications of morphine and other opioid drugs have yielded pure opioid receptor antagonists like naloxone, naltrexone and nalmefine. These agents have high affinity for μ opioid receptors and lower activity on δ and K receptors. Several other non-peptide antagonists have been developed such as β-flunaltrexamine, which is relatively specific for μ receptors and naltrindole a δ receptor antagonist. The major utility of opioid receptor antagonists is in the management of opioid overdose.

Topical Ocular Use of Opioids

Systemic use of opioids in ophthalmic practice is generally limited to pain control following surgery. However, there is some clinical and experimental data to support potential topical use of opioids for ophthalmic pain control.[1] Topical opioids have been shown to alleviate pain following corneal abrasions without significantly delaying corneal healing.[2] Moreover, topical opioid use may also have application in lowering intraocular pressure and in reversal of mydriasis following an ophthalmic examination. Opioid antagonist naltrexone might have a potential use in enhancing corneal wound healing.[3] Further development of opioid formulations for ophthalmic use might provide safe alternatives for treatment of ophthalmic pain, glaucoma and corneal wound healing, without the concomitant adverse effects associated with systemic opioid use.

NON-STEROIDAL ANTI-INFLAMMATORY DRUGS (NSAIDs; NON-NARCOTIC ANALGESICS)

Non-steroidal anti-inflammatory drugs (NSAIDs) have an important place in ophthalmic practice for the treatment of intraocular inflammation. The use of aspirin and other salicylic compounds for the treatment of ophthalmic inflammation has been described almost a century ago.[4] The time since then has seen the development of many other drugs with anti-inflammatory, analgesic and antipyretic properties. While traditionally these drugs have been employed via the systemic route of administration, the availability of topical preparations for some of them has promoted renewed interest in their use for ophthalmic purposes.

Pharmacokinetics

NSAIDs are rapidly absorbed following oral administration and are readily distributed to most tissues. Following entry into circulation most NSAIDs are extensively bound to plasma proteins. Peak concentrations are achieved between 1–3 hours for different drugs. In general, food delays absorption but peak concentrations are usually unaffected. Plasma half-life for most is between 2–4 hours but may be longer for some like naproxen (14 hours) and meloxicam (upto 20 hours). The half-life of aspirin can be prolonged to more than 15 hours with toxic doses as compared to around 1 hour with the therapeutic doses. NSAIDs are mostly biotransformed by the hepatic microsomal enzymes. Unchanged drug and the metabolites are eliminated by the kidneys. In patients with compromised liver function or renal failure the elimination may be greatly delayed leading to an increased risk for adverse effects. Sulindac, a prodrug, is transformed to the active form through metabolism.

Mechanism of Action

Aspirin and other NSAIDs produce anti-inflammatory action primarily by inhibiting cyclooxygenase (COX), which is involved in the synthesis of prostaglandins (PGs). PGs are autacoids that are synthesized by almost all tissues for a variety of physiological purposes. Arachidonic acid, the precursor for PGs, is a component of the cell membrane phospholipids, and is released by the action of phospholipase A_2 and other hydrolases on cell membranes. Free arachidonic acid is metabolized along two separate metabolic pathways, viz. COX pathway – to produce PGs, prostacyclin and thromboxane (TXA) – and the lipoxygenase (LOX) pathway, to yield leukotrienes (LTs; Fig. 11.1). While PGs have a diverse range of physiological functions, they are also intimately involved, together with

the leukotrienes, in the process of inflammation which occurs in response to tissue insult. PGs lower the threshold of the nociceptors of the C fibers and inhibition of PG synthesis by NSAIDs reverses this sensitization of pain receptors to mechanical and chemical stimulation.

Two isoforms of cyclooxygenase enzyme (termed COX-1 and COX-2) are known to occur. COX-1 has been identified as the constitutive or 'house-keeping' isoform involved with physiological and homeostatic functions while COX-2 is induced during the inflammatory process and has pro-inflammatory actions. Although a third isoform, COX-3, of cyclooxygenase, has also been described[5] with an attempt to explain the analgesic and antipyretic action of acetaminophen – a weak inhibitor of COX-1 and COX-2 in the periphery – its exact significance still remains controversial.

Aspirin, the prototype NSAID, irreversibly inhibits both COX-1 and COX-2. Other older NSAIDs are also COX inhibitors with little selectivity for either COX-1 or COX-2. In contrast to aspirin, the inhibition of COX by other NSAIDs is reversible. Some NSAIDs possess additional mechanisms, which possibly contribute to their anti-inflammatory effects. Recognition of separate identities and functions of the two isoforms triggered the development of selective COX-2 inhibitors with the inherent hope that such agents would provide anti-inflammatory

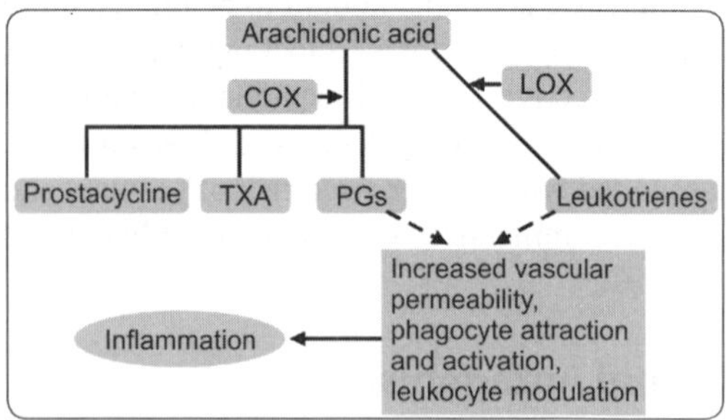

Figure 11.1 Arachidonic acid metabolism and generation of inflammatory mediators

The generation of prostaglandins and leukotrienes from arachidonic acid through the actions of COX and LOX, respectively, and some of the mechanisms by which PGs and LTs produce inflammation is shown.

action with a reduced liability for adverse effects as compared to non-selective COX inhibitors. Selective COX-2 inhibitors are comparable with non-selective members with regard to their anti-inflammatory activity with greater safety in terms of gastrointestinal adverse effects. Selective COX-2 inhibitors do not possess anti-platelet-aggregatory activity. NSAIDs are usually classified on the basis of their chemical structure and COX selectivity (Table 11.6).

Inhibition of COX is the common mechanism shared by all NSAIDs but additional mechanisms may also be involved with the actions of some of them. Inhibition of interleukin-1 actions on the hypothalamic thermoregulatory centers is considered to be mechanism responsible for antipyretic action of aspirin.

Pharmacological Actions

The major pharmacological effects of NSAIDs can be summarized as anti-inflammatory, analgesic, antipyretic and antiplatelet. Aspirin, which irreversibly inhibits COX, displays all

Table 11.6 Classification of NSAIDs

Class	Comments
Salicylates Aspirin Diflunisal	 Salicylate is the anti-inflammatory metabolite Not metabolized to salicylic acid
Indole acetic acid derivatives Indomethacin Sulindac (prodrug) Ketorolac Etodolac	Very potent; high toxicity; *ocular preparation available* Prodrug Potent analgesic; *ocular preparation available*
Propionic acid derivatives Ibuprofen Fenoprofen Ketoprofen Naproxen Flurbiprofen	Better tolerated as a class Anti-inflammatory and analgesic *Ocular preparation available*
Phenylacetic acid derivatives Diclofenac	 *Ocular preparation available*
Fenamates Mefenamic acid Meclofenamate Nepafenac	Efficacy, GI side-effects similar to aspirin *Ocular preparation available*
Oxicam derivatives Piroxicam Meloxicam	Long half-life; single daily dose is effective Relatively more selective for COX-2
Para-aminophenol derivative* Acetaminophen	Weak inhibitor of COX ; only analgesic and antipyretic
Selective COX-2 inhibitors# Celecoxib Valdecoxib	Inhibits CYP2D6 Inhibits CYP2C9; increased risk of stroke, MI

Ocular preparations for topical ophthalmic use are available only for some NSAIDs.
* Does not have anti-inflammatory activity. Central actions may be involved in its analgesic and antipyretic actions.
# Use of some COX-2 inhibitors has been linked with increased risk for vascular accidents and rofecoxib was withdrawn from clinical use.

these actions and is considered as the prototype against which all other drugs are compared. The relative degree of these actions may vary in different members. For example, while ibuprofen produces analgesic, antipyretic and anti-inflammatory effects, relatively higher doses are usually necessary for anti-inflammatory effects. Although all non-selective COX inhibitors inhibit platelet function, only aspirin can do so in a sustained manner and in low doses due to irreversible inhibition of the enzyme in platelets, thus making it therapeutically relevant. NSAIDs have also been shown to reduce generation of free radicals, adhesion molecules and cytokines. But these effects are seen at higher concentrations and their relevance to the pharmacological effects is a subject of debate.

Analgesic Action: Several chemical mediators released during tissue injury or inflammation are responsible for eliciting the pain response. These include bradykinin, serotonin, leukotrienes, neuropeptides, prostaglandins and other mediators. PGE_2 and PGI_2 formed as a result of induction of COX-2, sensitize the peripheral nociceptors and increase their excitability. The reversal of nociceptor sensitization by inhibition of COX-2-induced PG synthesis is thought to be the major determinant for the peripheral analgesic action of NSAIDs. A central component in the analgesic action of NSAIDs has also been suggested and involves similar effects at spinal and supraspinal levels to reduce PG mediated central sensitization, which might contribute to hyperalgesia and allodynia.

Anti-inflammatory action: Increased PGE_2 and PGI_2 synthesis during inflammation, mainly through induction of COX-2 contributes, together with other mediators, to local vasodilatation, increase in vascular permeability and infiltration of leucocytes, thereby sustaining the inflammatory process. By inhibiting PG synthesis, NSAIDs tend to reverse the inflammation.

Antipyretic Action: Increased formation of cytokines such as interleukins, tumor necrosis factor and interferons destabilizes the thermoregulatory mechanisms at the preoptic hypothalamic area. PGE_2 formed in the region of the preoptic hypothalamus in response to these cytokines cause an elevation of the thermoregulatory 'set point' resulting in an elevation of body temperature. Inhibition of PGE_2 synthesis by NSAIDs reverses this response to produce an antipyretic action.

Antiplatelet Action: Aspirin irreversibly acetylates platelet COX-1 causing suppression of thromboxane A_2 (TXA_2) formation and consequent loss of platelet function. Adult platelets lack the enzymatic machinery for fresh synthesis of COX, therefore, once it is inhibited by aspirin the platelet is unable to synthesize TXA_2 and suffers an irreversible loss of its capacity to aggregate with consequent prolongation of bleeding time. The bleeding time remains prolonged till a sufficient number of fresh platelets with functional COX are formed and released. The duration of effect is thus dependent upon the turnover rate of platelets and may last for 4–7 days after cessation of administration. The dose of aspirin required for antiplatelet action is much lower (less than 100 mg/day) as compared to the anti-inflammatory or antipyretic doses. Other NSAIDs, which are reversible inhibitors of COX do not have such long lasting antiplatelet effects while selective COX-2 inhibitors as well as acetaminophen are devoid of this property.

Therapeutic Uses

Analgesic: NSAIDs are used for analgesic, antipyretic and anti-inflammatory purposes in a wide variety of conditions. They are effective against mild to moderate pain of somatic origin especially where the pain is associated with inflammation. The response to moderate or severe visceral pain is often not satisfactory and NSAIDs can be combined with opioid analgesics, whereby, they synergistically enhance the analgesia providing improved pain control and a consequent reduction of opioid dose requirement. Such combinations are often employed for the treatment of cancer pain. Acetaminophen, is devoid of any appreciable anti-inflammatory activity and is used mainly for its analgesic and antipyretic actions. It is well tolerated and is almost free from GIT irritation, which together with its over-the-counter availability, makes it the most widely used analgesic. Although safe in usual doses, in very high (toxic) doses or in presence of pre-existing hepatic damage, it can lead to severe hepatic cellular necrosis due to a toxic metabolite N-acetyl-p-benzoquinone. Ketorolac is another NSAID that is recommended mainly as an analgesic, although it has significant anti-inflammatory activity. It has strong analgesic action and can substitute for opioids for relief of post-surgical pain in some cases.

Antipyretic: Aspirin, acetaminophen and some other NSAIDs have an important place in the control of pyrexia of varied origins. Central mechanisms are thought to be involved in this effect and not all NSAIDs are equally effective as antipyretics.

Anti-inflammatory: NSAIDs have a major role in the treatment of somatic inflammatory disorders most notably rheumatoid arthritis. Therapeutic benefits in this situation result from reduced inflammation as well as pain relief. However, when used for this purpose, NSAIDs have to be employed for relatively longer periods and are thus more likely to give rise to adverse effects. All NSAIDs are more or less equally effective as anti-inflammatory agents but may differ in their adverse effects and tolerability. Selective COX-2 inhibitors have lower potential for adverse gastrointestinal effects but concerns remain about the increased incidence of stroke and MI with their use and have led to the withdrawal of some members (rofecoxib) for this reason.

Antiplatelet Action: Among the NSAIDs, only aspirin is used for antiplatelet and cardioprotective action. The low dose of aspirin required to achieve antiplatelet action is more easily tolerated with negligible side effects in most cases. Since the life of platelets is approximately 10 days, a subject on antiplatelet therapy requires a period of 7–10 days to regain normal platelet function (by the time new platelets with functional TXA_2 replace the old platelets) after aspirin is stopped, a fact that has to be borne in mind, if a surgical procedure is planned.

Besides their above mentioned uses, NSAIDs have also been found to be of some value in other conditions, which include systemic mastocytosis[6] and prevention of colorectal cancer.[7]

Adverse Effects

Major adverse effects of aspirin and other non-selective COX inhibitors are related to gastric irritation and intolerance. Microscopic blood loss in the feces is common with aspirin therapy but frank ulceration of the gastric and duodenal mucosa also occurs. Locally present PGs in the gastric mucosa normally serve a protective function against mucosal damage and the loss of this protection due to inhibition of PG synthesis, besides the direct irritant effects of NSAIDs, contributes to the mucosal damage. As mentioned earlier, selective COX-2 inhibitors and acetaminophen have a better safety profile in this respect. Bleeding time is increased by NSAIDs due to their inhibitory effects on platelet TXA_2 synthesis. This can manifest as easy bruising or enhanced bleeding following trauma or surgical procedures as also the enhanced risk of intracranial bleeds.

NSAIDs are generally regarded as nephrotoxic especially in individuals with pre-existing renal or hepatic disease, congestive heart failure, cirrhosis or other conditions associated with decreased renal perfusion. In such situations PGs serve a critical role in maintaining renal perfusion and by inhibiting PG synthesis, NSAIDs can severely compromise renal function. High doses of aspirin can cause nausea, vomiting, tinnitus and impaired hearing, which are together referred to as *salicylism.* Hyperventilation also occurs with high doses of aspirin. Since all NSAIDs share the same mechanism of action, many of their adverse effects are also shared. The shared adverse effects of NSAIDs are listed in Table 11.7.

Topical Ocular Use of NSAIDs

Until recently the topical use of glucocorticoids has been the mainstay of treatment for ophthalmic inflammatory conditions as well as for pre- and postoperative control of inflammation. Corticosteroid therapy provides powerful anti-inflammatory response but is also associated with some inherent risks such as increase in intraocular pressure, delayed healing and cataract formation. Availability of topical preparations of some NSAIDs has provided an alternative for ocular anti-inflammatory therapy without these disadvantages. NSAIDs now find important uses in ophthalmic practice for prevention of intraoperative miosis, reduction of post-surgical inflammation and in the treatment of ocular inflammatory conditions.[8] Use of topical NSAIDs prior to cataract surgery has been reported to facilitate a safer and more efficient surgical procedure (due to a mydriatic effect), reduce postoperative pain and inflammation and also decrease the risk of post-operative cystoids macular edema. Beneficial effects on pain and inflammation have also been reported in refractive surgery.[9] Topical use of NSAIDs is generally safer as compared to their systemic use because of the smaller doses and limited absorption into systemic circulation. Topical application of NSAIDs, may sometimes cause local irritation and discomfort, which can affect patient compliance. Further,

these agents should not normally be used in patients who are sensitive or intolerant to aspirin or other NSAIDs. Exacerbation of bronchospasm in asthmatic patients has been reported with topical use of NSAIDs.[10] Topical NSAIDs have been reported to cause corneal complications such as keratitis, epithelial breakdown, erosion, ulceration, perforation and rarely, corneal melting.[11-13] The exact mechanism for these complications is not clear but a careful monitoring for epithelial damage is necessary and any evidence of same warrants discontinuation of topical NSAIDs.

Five topical preparations are currently available for ophthalmic use. The preparations and their recommended uses are given in Table 11.8.

Several clinical trials to compare the relative efficacy and safety of different topical preparations did not reveal any marked superiority of any one agent over another when used during cataract or corneal surgery.[15-18] Nepafenac, however, has been reported to be less effective than ketorolac in preventing miosis during cataract surgery[19] and not effective for relieving pain and inflammation following keratectomy.[20]

In addition to their use during ophthalmic surgery, NSAIDs also find use in the treatment of ocular inflammatory disorders such as scleritis, episcleritis and iridocyclitis. Topical or systemic NSAIDs may be used as an adjunct

Table 11.7 Adverse effect common to most NSAIDs

Gastrointestinal tract[1]	Intolerance, irritation, ulceration, hemorrhage, perforation, diarrhea.
Platelets[1]	Increased bleeding and clotting time, risk of hemorrhage, bruising
Uterus	Prolongation of labor
Electrolytes	Salt and water retention
Vascular[2]	Closure of ductus arteriosus
Kidney	Decreased renal function (specially in pre-existing renal or cardiac disease)
CNS	Headache, dizziness, vertigo, confusion
Hypersensitivity	Asthma, urticaria, angioneurotic edema, asthma[3]

[1]Less with COX-2 selective agents
[2]Indomethacin has been used for closure of patent ductus arteriosus
[3]Pre-existing asthma may be worsened due to diversion of arachidonic acid via the LOX pathway for increased leukotriene production.

Table 11.8 Topical ophthalmic NSAIDs and their uses

Drug	Indications	Comments
Diclofenac* 0.1%	Cataract surgery: Reduction of pain, inflammation and photophobia; Refractive surgery	Start 24 hours postoperative then continue for 2 weeks
		Start preoperative and then continue postoperative for 3 days
Nepafenac 0.1%	Cataract surgery: Reduction of pain and inflammation	Begin preoperative and then continue for upto 2 weeks
Bromfenac 0.09%	Cataract surgery: Reduction of postoperative inflammation	Begin 24 hours postoperative then continue for 2 weeks
Ketorolac* 0.4%; 0.5%	Seasonal allergic conjunctivitis	
	Cataract surgery: Reduction of pain and inflammation	Begin 24 hours postoperative and then continue for 2 weeks
Flurbiprofen 0.03%	Refractive surgery: Reduction of pain	Postoperative upto 4 days
	Cataract surgery: To minimize miosis	Begin 2 hours preoperative

*Topical ketorolac and diclofenac have also been used for cystoid macular edema following cataract surgery[14]

in their management. Their use in inflammation associated with infective disorders of the eye has been suggested especially since corticosteroid use under such conditions is associated with a risk of exacerbating the infection.

REFERENCES

1. Abelson MB, Dewey-Mattia D, Shapiro A. Finding new uses for ancient drugs. Review of Ophthalmology. [updated 2009 NOV 06]. *Available from:* http:// www.revophth.com/ content/d/ therapeutic_topics/c/22882.
2. Peyman GA, Rahimy MH, Fernandes ML. Effects of morphine on corneal sensitivity and epithelial wound healing: Implications for topical ophthalmic analgesia. Br J Ophthalmol. 1994;78(2):138–41.
3. Klocek MS, Sassani JW, McLaughlin PJ, Zagon IS. Topically applied naltrexone restores corneal reepithelialization in diabetic rats. J Ocul Pharmacol Ther. 2007;23(2):89–102.
4. Gifford H. On the treatment of sympathetic ophthalmia by large doses of salicylate of sodium aspirin or other salicylic compounds. Ophthalmoscope. 1910;8:257–9.
5. Chandrasekharan NV, Dai H, Roos LT, Evanson NK, Tomsik J, Elton TS, et al. COX-3, a cyclooxygenase-1 variant inhibited by acetaminophen and other analgesic/antipyretic drugs: cloning, structure, and expression. Proc Natl Acad Sci USA. 2002;99(21):13926–31.
6. Butterfield JH. Survey of aspirin administration in systemic mastocytosis. Prostaglandins Other Lipid Mediat. 2009;88(3-4):122–4.
7. Kune GA, Kune S, Watson LF. Colorectal cancer risk, chronic illnesses, operations and medications: case control results from the Melbourne Colorectal Cancer Study. Cancer Res. 1998;48(15):4399–404.
8. Schalnus R. Topical nonsteroidal anti-inflammatory therapy in ophthalmology. Ophthalmologica. 2003;217(2):89–98.
9. Trattler W. Topical NSAIDs for pain and inflammation. Review of ophthalmology [Internet]. 2006 [updated 2010 Dec 06]. Available from: http://www.revophth.com/content/d/ features/i/1306/c/25129.
10. Sitenga GL, Ing EB, Van Dellen RG, Younge BR, Leavitt JA. Asthma caused by topical application of ketorolac.Ophthalmology. 1996;103(6): 890–2.

11. Gaynes BI, Fiscella R. Topical nonsteroidal anti-inflammatory drugs in ophthalmic use: a safety review. Drug Saf. 2002;25(4):233–50.

12. Flach AJ. Corneal melts associated with topically applied nonsteroidal anti-inflammatory drugs. Trans Am Ophthalmol Soc. 2001;99:205–12.

13. Lin JC, Rapuano CJ, Laibson PR, Eagle RC, Cohen EJ. Corneal melting associated with use of topical nonsteroidal anti-inflammatory drugs after ocular surgery. Arch Ophthalmol. 2000, 118(8):1129–32.

14. Weisz JM, Bressler NM, Bressler SB, Schachat AP. Ketorolac treatment of pseudophakic cystoids macular edema identified more than 24 months after cataract extraction. Ophthalmology. 1999;106:1656–9.

15. Koçak I, Yalvaç IS, Koçak A, Nurözler A, Unlü N, Kasim R, et al. Comparison of the anti-inflammatory effects of diclofenac and flurbiprofen eye drops after cataract extraction. Acta Ophthalmol Scand. 1998;76(3):343–5.

16. Flach AJ, Dolan BJ, Donahue ME, Faktorovich EG, Gonzalez GA. Comparative effects of ketorolac 0.5% or diclofenac 0.1% ophthalmic solutions on inflammation after cataract surgery. Ophthalmology. 1998;105(9):1775–9.

17. Flach AJ, Dolan BJ. Incidence of postoperative posterior opacification following treatment with diclofenac 0.1% and ketorolac 0.5% ophthalmic solutions: 3-year randomized, double masked, prospective clinical investigation. Trans Am Ophthalmol Soc. 2000;98:101–5.

18. Narvaez J, Krall P, Tooma TS. Prospective, randomized trial of diclofenac and ketorolac after refractive surgery. J Refract Surg. 2004;20(1):76–8.

19. Bucci Jr F, Waterbury L, Amico L. Prostaglandin E2 inhibition and aqueous concentration of ketorolac 0.4% (Acular LS) and nepafenac 0.1% (nevanac) in patients undergoing phacoemulsification. Am J Ophthalmol. 2007; 144(1):146–7.

20. Colin J, Paquette B. Comparison of the analgesic efficacy and safety of nepafenac ophthalmic suspension compared with diclofenac ophthalmic solution for ocular pain and photophobia after excimer laser surgery: a phase II, randomized, double-masked trial. Clin Ther. 2006;28(4): 527–36.

CHAPTER 12

Corticosteroids

OVERVIEW

Corticosteroids have been used for the treatment of ocular inflammatory diseases for more than 60 years. They are the most prescribed pharmacological group in ophthalmology because large number of acute ocular diseases are inflammatory in nature such as non-infectious conjunctivitis, uveitides, episcleritis, inflamed pingueculae, chemotoxic keratoconjunctivitis, phlyctenular keratoconjunctivitis, contact lens associated red eye, allergic conjunctivitis, blepharitis, corneal infiltrates, ocular trauma, recurrent corneal erosions, etc. Though many aspects of their adverse effects still remain open, anti-inflammatory and immunosuppressive actions are valuable therapeutic effects in ophthalmic diseases. This chapter describes the pharmacological aspects of corticosteroids in ophthalmology.

HISTORY

Tadeusz Reichstein, Edward Calvin Kendall and Philip Showalter Hench were awarded the Nobel Prize for physiology and medicine in 1950 for their work on hormones of the adrenal cortex, which culminated in the isolation of cortisone. The history of corticosteroids in ophthalmic therapy starts with Elkinton and co-authors (1949), who first applied ACTH therapy in patients with inflammatory hemorrhagic retinopathy associated with "generalized collagen diseases".[1] Later, ACTH was reported to be effective in various inflammatory conditions of eyes. One of the earliest works on usage of corticosteroids in ophthalmology was the study of Wood (1950) demonstrating efficacy of ACTH and cortisone in 14 patients with inflammatory ocular diseases.[2] Mann and Markson (1950) showed positive result of ACTH application in patients with uveitis and episcleritis.[3]

The next important step for progression of anti-inflammatory therapy in ophthalmology was introduction of topical formulations of cortisone. Their clinical use was accompanied by rapidly growing number of indications in 1950's, including vernal conjunctivitis, episcleritis, scleritis as well as inflammatory conditions of the uvea. After introduction of prednisone and prednisolone by Schering in mid-1960s under the brand names Meticorten and Meticortelone, ophthalmologists received a therapeutic instrument that was 10 time stronger in its anti-inflammatory action in comparison with cortisone. However, within a few years, a number of ophthalmic adverse effects, such as cataract and elevated intraocular pressure, were reported.[4] Additionally, it was established, that there is a close correlation between anti-inflammatory potency of applied corticosteroids and risk of ocular hypertension.

PHARMACOLOGY OF CORTICOSTEROIDS

Classification

The chemical structure of all corticosteroids is ketone based except for loteprednol, which is ester based. The most commonly prescribed steroids, prednisolone and dexamethasone, are ketone-based. Other classification is based on the strength of action and classifies corticosteroids in two groups of maximum and moderate strength steroids (Table 12.1).

Pharmacokinetics

Topical application of ophthalmic formulations (drops, ointments) is the most common route of administration of corticosteroid to the eye. Although, the clinical benefits and adverse events associated with systemic corticosteroid use are well documented, their basic pharmacokinetics after topical application is yet to be fully elucidated.

Most of the pharmacokinetic studies of topical corticosteroids have been done in rabbits and the data obtained from these experiments may not be suitable to extrapolate in human because of the anatomical and physiological differences between the rabbit and human eye. Despite these differences, there are similarities between the two eyes allowing extrapolation of data from rabbit to human.

Most topically applied corticosteroids penetrate the eye via cornea. Following a single drop topical application, steroids have been detected in measurable quantity in human aqueous humor within 15–30 minutes.[6] Some pharmacokinetic parameters of topical corticosteroids indicating rate and extent of corneal permeation are summarized in Table 12.2.[7]

Corneal penetration studies conducted in unanesthetized rabbits have described transfer through the epithelium as the rate-limiting step for absorption of hydrophilic compounds, whereas transfer through the stroma is rate-limiting for hydrophobic compounds. However,

Table 12.1 Classification of corticosteroids based on the strength of their action[5]

Generic name	Brand name	Manufacturer	Preparation	Contents
Maximum strength (steroids)				
Difluprednate 0.05%	Durezol	Sirion Therapeutics	Emulsion	5 mL
Loteprednol etabonate 0.5%	Lotemax	Bausch and Lomb	Suspension	2.5 mL, 5 mL, 10 mL, 15 mL
Prednisolone acetate 1%,	Pred Forte, generic	Allergan and generic	Suspension	1 mL, 5 mL, 10 mL, 15 mL
Prednisolone sodium phosphate 1%	Generic	Generic	Solution	5 mL, 10 mL, 15 mL
Rimexolone 1%	Vexol	Alcon	Suspension	5 mL, 10 mL
Moderate strength (steroids)				
Fluorometholone acetate 0.1%	Flarex and generic	Alcon	Suspension	5 mL, 10 mL
Fluorometholone alcohol 0.1%	FML and generic	Allergan	Suspension	5 mL, 10 mL, 15 mL
Fluorometholone alcohol 0.1%	FML SOP	Allergan	Ointment	3.5g
Prednisolone acetate 0.12%	Pred mild and generic	Allergan	Suspension	5 mL, 10 mL
Medrysone 1%	HMS (Medrysone ophthalmic suspension)	Allergan	Suspension	5 mL, 10 mL

Table 12.2 Human aqueous humor concentration of corticosteroids following topical and subconjunctival application (according to Awan[7] with modification)

Drug	Route	Dose (Number of drops, frequency of instillation)	Mean peak aqueous concentration (ng/mL)	Time to peak concentration (minutes)	Aqueous concentration at 12 hours (ng/mL)	Aqueous concentration at 24 hours (ng/mL)
Dexamethasone alcohol	Topical (drops)	0.1% (1)	31	90–120	3.1	NA
Dexamethasone – cyclodextrin-polymer co-complex	Topical (drops)	0.32% (1)	140	150	NA	NA
Dexamethasone disodium phosphate	Topical (drops)	0.1% (10)	30.5	55	NA	NA
Prednisolone acetate	Topical (drops)	1% (1)	669.9	120	99.5	28.4
Prednisolone acetate	Topical (drops)	1% (1)	1130	30–45	NA	NA
Prednisolone sodium phosphate	Topical (drops)	0.5% (1)	25.6	90–240	0	NA
Betamethasone phosphate	Topical (drops)	0.5% (1)	7.7	90–120	2.5	0.4
Fluorometholone alcohol	Topical (drops)	0.1% (1)	5.1	31–60	NA	NA
Clobetasone butyrate	Topical (ointment)	0.1% (1)	0.1	810	0.1	NA
Betamethasone phosphate	Topical (ointment)	0.1% (1)	20.3	810	20.3	NA
Hydrocortisone acetate 2.5%	Subconjunctival	0.5 mL (1)	214×10^3	10	NA	103×10^3
Dexamethasone sodium phosphate 0.4%	Subconjunctival	0.5 mL (1)	268×10^3	10	NA	123×10^3

very low molecular weight compounds penetrate well through the corneal epithelium and appear rapidly in aqueous humor. These observations are in accordance with the proposed "pore" model for the penetration of drugs through the cornea. According to this proposed model, corneal permeability of drugs depends on both the partition coefficient and molecular-weight.[7] It has also been demonstrated in a rabbit study that cornea becomes significantly less permeable with age, particularly for large hydrophilic compounds.

Different topical formulations may show marked differences in pharmacokinetic behavior despite identical concentrations of the same steroid. Therefore, it cannot be assumed that equivalent steroid contents in a formulation assure equivalent efficacy. Based on the duration of action, ophthalmic corticosteroid formulations can be placed in the following ascending order: *drops → cream → ointment*. The rate and extent of corneal permeation is affected by not only the drug's concentration and its physiological properties but also by several excipients used in the formulation. Therefore, even small modifications in the composition of formulation can significantly affect intraocular drug concentration.

The role of peribulbar injection is limited to the operating room and to a few other selected situations where frequent topical medication is not suitable. Subconjunctivally injected steroids enter the eye via sclera. Topical and local administration of steroids appears preferable to systemic administration wherever possible. However, the limitations of, and alternatives to, subconjunctival injection should be carefully considered, should the possibility of adrenal suppression following intensive topical corticosteroid therapy arise in children and small adults. The local administration of ocular corticosteroids enables the use of smaller doses for equivalent or greater local corticosteroid concentration, more target-specific drug application and reduced risk of systemic adverse events.

Mechanism of Action

The pharmacological effects of corticosteroids are mediated through the glucocorticoid receptor, which is located in the cytoplasm. Due to the ubiquitous nature of the glucocorticoid receptor, corticosteroids act on a wide variety of cell types. Glucocorticoid receptor is expressed in almost all tissues and cells, and the effects, both beneficial and unwanted, of corticosteroids are mediated through reversible binding to this receptor. After binding to the receptor, the drug-receptor complex translocates into the nucleus, binds to DNA, and hence activates or represses gene transcription through different mechanisms. The complexes may induce the transcription of mRNA leading to synthesis of new proteins (transactivation). Such proteins include lipocortin, a protein known to inhibit phospholipase A_2 and, thereby block the synthesis of prostaglandins and leukotrienes. Glucocorticoids also inhibit the production of other mediators including arachidonic acid metabolites such as cytokines, the interleukins, adhesion molecules, and enzymes such as collagenase. Transactivation was also found to be associated with several side-effects of corticosteroids. The transrepression, repression of transcription factors such as nuclear factor-kB and activator protein-1, seems to be responsible for the anti-inflammatory effect.[8-10]

Pharmacological Effects

Anti-Inflammatory

Corticosteroids are potent anti-inflammatory agents and inhibit inflammatory processes above the site of action of NSAIDs (Fig. 12.1). Corticosteroids inhibit the generation of prostaglandins by producing proteins called lipocortins. Lipocortins exert their effect on the prostaglandin cascade by inhibiting phospholipase A_2. The major effect is inhibition of migration of inflammatory cells (including neutrophils and monocyte-macrophages) into the site of inflammation. They also inhibit lysosomal enzyme release. Inhibition of prostaglandin E_2 may be the dominant mechanism for their anti-inflammatory effects. There is also evidence for anti-interleukin-1 and anti-TNFα effects.

Immunosuppression

Corticosteroids suppress the cell-mediated immunity. They act by inhibiting genes that code for the cytokines such as interleukin-2 and interferon-γ, the most important of which is IL-2. Reduced cytokine production prevents the T cell proliferation.

Corticosteroids also suppress the humoral immunity, causing B cells to express smaller amounts of IL-2 and of IL-2 receptors. This diminishes both B cell clone expansion and antibody synthesis. The diminished amounts of IL-2 also cause fewer T lymphocyte cells to be activated.

Therapeutic Uses

Corticosteroids remain the first line treatment in non-infectious ocular inflammation and can be administered topically, periocularly, intravitreally and systemically. Corticosteroids do not appear to have specific effects but exert a broad spectrum of anti-inflammatory activity. They are more effective in acute than in chronic inflammatory conditions. Some aspects of corticosteroid-induced effects are of particular importance for the treatment of ocular diseases. For example, the

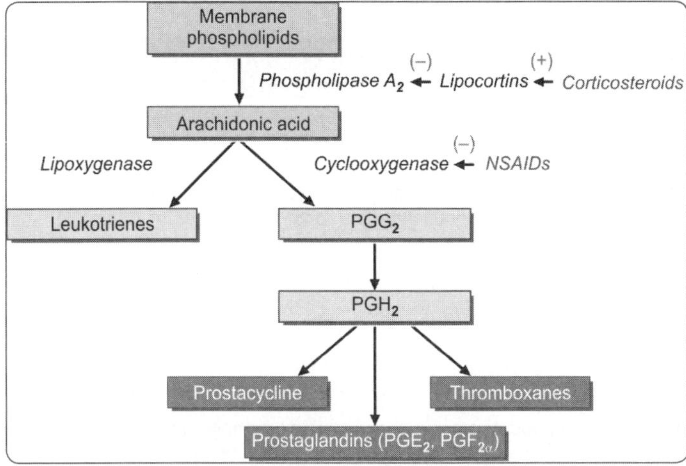

Figure 12.1 Prostaglandin synthesis inhibition. NSAIDs–Non-steroidal anti-inflammatory drugs, PGG$_2$–prostaglandin G2, PGH$_2$–prostaglandin H$_2$, PGE$_2$–prostaglandin E$_2$, PGFα$_2$–prostaglandin Fα$_2$; (+) stimulating effect; (−) inhibiting effect

reduction of fibrinoid exudation and inhibition of corneal scar formation are important to prevent secondary complications of ocular inflammation and to maintain corneal transparency. If a long-term anti-inflammatory effect is needed, less potent corticosteroids should be slowly replaced because of the potential side-effects of long-term use, such as cataract, glaucoma and local immunosuppression.

Ocular Indications for Topical Corticosteroid Use

Topical corticosteroids are indicated in the treatment of corticosteroid-responsive allergic and inflammatory conditions of the palpebral and bulbar conjunctiva, cornea and anterior segment diseases (Table 12.3). Topical corticosteroids suppress all aspects of the inflammatory process such as edema, fibrin deposition, capillary dilation, leukocyte migration, capillary proliferation, deposition of collagen, scar formation, and fibroblastic proliferation. Topical corticosteroids are effective in acute inflammatory conditions of the conjunctiva, sclera, cornea, lids, iris, and anterior segment of the globe as well as in ocular allergic conditions (Table 12.3). Fluorometholone (0.1%), medrysone, or prednisolone (0.125%) may be preferred for long-term treatment because they are least likely to increase intraocular pressure.

The ocular surface may exhibit a wide variety of immunologic responses that may result in conjunctival and corneal inflammation and may in certain instances be the specific and only target affected by certain autoimmune diseases. Topical steroids are very effective in treating signs and symptoms of allergic and autoimmune ocular diseases.

Ocular Indications for Periocular Corticosteroid Use

Periocular administration is used when more posterior effects are needed or if the patient is non-compliant.[11] Several techniques have been advocated for the periocular application of corticosteroids, including subconjunctival, sub-Tenon's, transeptal, orbital floor, and retrobulbar injections.[11]

Table 12.3 Ocular indications for topical corticosteroid use

Pathology localization	Clinical Use
Eyelids	Blepharitis, chalazia, dermatitis, burns
Conjunctiva	Conjunctivitis (various types), mucocutaneous lesions, burns
Cornea	Edema, graft rejection, rosacea keratitis, dry eye syndrome, interstitial keratitis, herpes simplex (stromal) keratitis, herpes zoster keratitis, post-Herpes zoster neuralgia, infiltrates, marginal ulcers, burns
Uvea	Iridocyclitis, uveitis, traumatic hyphema, sympathetic ophthalmia
Sclera	Episcleritis, scleritis
Retina	Vasculitis, chorioretinitis
Optic nerve	Neuritis, temporal arteritis
Orbit	Endophthalmitis, pseudotumor cerebri, Grave's ophthalmopathy

Ocular Indications for Intraocular (Intravitreal) Corticosteroid Use

Intraocular injections of corticosteroid can also be used to deliver a high concentration of corticosteroids, to treat inflammation involving both anterior and posterior segments.[11] Often the intraocular concentrations of topically applied steroids fail to achieve therapeutic levels and, therefore, intraocular injections may be of benefit in certain ocular disorders including diabetic macular edema, cystoid macular edema, age-related macular degeneration, retinal vascular occlusion and uveitis.[12] Intravitreal triamcinolone acetonide provides an effective short-term treatment for persistent macular edema and may be a useful adjunctive treatment for choroidal neovascularization. The side-effect profile of intravitreal corticosteroids is significant and includes increase in corticosteroid-induced intraocular pressure. With long-term studies, the rate of posterior subcapsular cataract formation is higher, and there is a small but potential risk of endophthalmitis.[13] Recently, sustained-release intraocular corticosteroid implants are emerging as potential treatments for macular edema due to uveitis, diabetic macular edema or retinal vascular occlusion.[12, 14-16]

Ocular Indications for Systemically Administered Corticosteroid

Systemic steroids can be used to treat ocular inflammation recalcitrant to topical and periocular-injections or when the uveitis is associated with systemic disease. A concerning ocular side-effect of corticosteroids is ocular hypertension especially with long-term use (more than three months). Systemically administered steroids are used less often in ocular diseases. Ocular indications for oral or injectable steroids include the following:

- Uveitis not responding to topical therapy
- Posterior uveitis and/or chorioretinitis
- Orbital pseudotumor
- Acute ocular allergic response not responding to topical therapy
- Scleritis—subconjunctival injections are contraindicated
- Temporal arteritis/arteritic anterior ischemic optic neuropathy
- Optic neuritis
- Severe burns
- Underlying autoimmune diseases (collagen-vascular disorders).

Adverse Effects

Corticosteroids are one of the most potent and effective drug classes available in the treatment of ocular inflammation. However, they can produce variety of adverse ocular and systemic effects. Corticosteroid-induced ocular hypertension and glaucoma are significant risks of local and systemic administration. Posterior subcapsular cataract, observed after about 4 months of topical corticosteroids use, is supposed to be due to covalent binding of corticosteroid to lens proteins with subsequent oxidation. Inappropriate use of topical corticosteroids in the presence of corneal infections also continues to be a cause of ocular morbidity. Corticosteroids may cause retardation of corneal epithelialization, i.e. the time required for epithelial regeneration is increased in eyes treated with steroids. Effects on collagen synthesis and fibroblast activity have been proposed as a possible mechanism. Paradoxically, the topical use of dexamethasone or prednisolone can lead to acute inflammation of the anterior segment of the eye (corticosteroid uveitis). The incidence is higher in the black population (5.4%) than in the white population (0.5%). Corticosteroids increase susceptibility to microbial infections. Prolonged use may aid in the establishment of secondary ocular infections from fungi and viruses.

Other risks of locally administered ophthalmic corticosteroids include: epithelial toxicity, crystalline keratopathy, decreased wound strength, orbital fat atrophy, ptosis, limitation of ocular movement, inadvertent intraocular injection, and reduction in endogenous cortisol.

Almost all the side-effects—most notably cataracts and increased intraocular pressure – are minimal or absent with the ester-based formulation, and only occasionally are problematic even with the ketone formulation. The key to these differences is that the human body possesses abundant esterases, but has no ketones. Ketone-based steroids such as prednisolone and dexamethasone linger in tissues, which renders good therapeutic effect but concurrently places patients at risk for undesirable side-effects such as posterior subcapsular cataracts and increased IOP. In contrast, ester-based steroids provide a potent anti-inflammatory effect and as they undergo enzymatic degradation, the potential for development of adverse side-effects minimizes.

Contraindications

Corticosteroids are contraindicated in patients with viral infections, fulminant bacterial infections, fungal infections, injuries and glaucoma.

Corticosteroids used in Ophthalmic Diseases

Prednisolone Acetate 1% as Pred Forte (*Allergan*) is a highly prescribed topical steroid. Prednisolone acetate is a suspension and is, therefore, optimally suited for penetrating the cornea and the anterior chamber. This makes it effective for treating anterior chamber inflammation and it remains the drug of choice in treating anterior uveitis. Prednisolone acetate 1% is used for moderate to severe forms of ocular inflammation such as episcleritis, iritis, inflammatory keratitis, chemical or thermal burns of the cornea. Prednisolone acetate is available in 1% and 0.125% concentrations.

Prednisolone sodium phosphate 1% solution as Inflamase Forte (*Novartis*) is a commonly prescribed steroid solution. It penetrates less readily into the aqueous and is not as effective as suspensions in treating uveal inflammation. It is, however, an excellent choice for treating moderate to severe inflammatory disorders of the ocular surface. It is used for the treatment of episcleritis, acute allergic inflammation, superior limbic keratoconjunctivitis, traumatic inflammation and other advanced ocular surface diseases.

Dexamethasone (as **dexamethasone alcohol 0.1%** and **dexamethasone disodium phosphate 0.1%**) is more potent and longer acting, but its corneal penetration is less than that of prednisolone acetate. Dexamethasone achieves its peak concentration in aqueous humour between 91 and 120 minutes following instillation (mean concentration, 31 ng/mL) and is still detectable in the aqueous 12 hours after instillation.[17] The dexamethasone has the highest propensity for increasing intraocular pressure, particularly in the long term. Thus, there is little reason to use dexamethasone monotherapy. However, for short-term use in combination products, it is effective in treating moderate inflammation. Dexamethasone (Maxidex® and Ak-Dex, Dexasol) is approved by FDA for the treatment of inflammatory conditions of the palpebral and bulbar conjunctiva, cornea, and anterior segment of the globe and corneal injury. Dexamethasone (Ozurdex™) is FDA-approved for treatment of macular edema following branch retinal vein occlusion or central retinal vein occlusion.

Rimexolone 1% suspension as Vexol (Alcon) has similar anti-inflammatory activity as corticosteroids such as 1% prednisolone acetate. It is used for the treatment of uveitis and post-surgical inflammation. A double-blind, randomized, crossover study of corticosteroid responders compared the effects of 1% rimexolone on intraocular pressure with those of 1% prednisolone and 0.1% fluorometholone. The results suggested that the intraocular pressure elevating potential was comparable to that of fluorometholone.[18, 19] Its safety profile is similar to the fluorometholones, which gives it an enhanced margin of safety. Rimexolone is used for the treatment of anterior uveitis and also is the first FDA-approved ophthalmic product for post-operative care of cataract surgery patients.

Betamethasone is potent and long-acting, but does not penetrate well. Betamethasone concentration is highest during 91–120 minutes following topical administration (mean peak concentration 7.7 ng/mL). At 12 hours post-instillation, the mean concentration of betamethasone is 2.5 ng/mL, and detectable levels are still measurable in the aqueous humor 24 hours after application.[20] Steroid-induced cataracts and glaucoma have been reported, most often in patients receiving betamethasone eyedrops. It is available as eyedrop solution.

Fluorometholone alcohol is moderate-strength ophthalmic suspension. It is used to treat mild to moderate ocular surface inflammatory conditions. It is also a useful drug in treating chronic inflammations requiring long-term (beyond 3 to 4 weeks) therapy. Fluorometholone alcohol is available in both 0.1% and 0.25% suspensions and 0.1% ointment. The 0.25% suspension offers little, if any, clinical advantage over the 0.1%, and is rarely used. Fluorometholone alcohol's value in chronic care lies in its reduced tendency to cause secondary IOP increase.

Fluorometholone acetate is a more potent form of fluorometholone, and is used for moderate to moderately severe conditions. It has relatively low IOP-sparing effect. The peak aqueous humor level of fluorometholone is 5.1 ng/mL between 31 and 60 minutes, and significant concentrations of fluorometholone (mean level 4.3 ng/mL) were detected between 181 and 240 minutes.[21] This drug does not have quite the clinical efficacy of 1% prednisolone acetate, yet can be useful in a wide array of ocular inflammatory conditions. As acetate ophthalmic suspension, fluorometholone (Flarex®) is FDA-approved for use in the treatment of inflammatory conditions of the palpebral and bulbar conjunctiva, cornea, and anterior segment of the eye.

Loteprednol etabonate is ester-based class of steroids. It is an entirely new generation of corticosteroids using an ester base.[22] Loteprednol is structurally similar to other corticosteroids. However, the ketone group at position number 20 is absent. It is highly lipid soluble, which enhances its penetration into cells. Loteprednol is synthesized through structural modifications of prednisolone-related compounds so that it undergoes a predictable transformation to an inactive metabolite. Based upon in vivo and in vitro preclinical metabolism studies, loteprednol undergoes extensive metabolism to inactive carboxylic acid metabolites. Primary site of deactivation of the topically applied drug is the corneal tissue. A substantial amount of metabolites were also detected in the iris, although these were lower than in the cornea. The amount of drug and metabolites in the aqueous humor was low.[23] Loteprednol is indicated for the treatment of inflammation of the eye due to allergies, as well as chronic forms of keratitis (adenoviral and Thygeson's keratitis), vernal keratoconjunctivitis, pingueculitis, and episcleritis. The drug renders a potent anti-inflammatory effect and is subsequently broken down into inert components by resident tissue esterases. It is available in both a 0.5% suspension (Lotemax™) and a 0.2% suspension (Alrex). Lotemax™ is food and drug administration (FDA) approved for treatment of inflammatory conditions of the palpebral and bulbar conjunctiva, cornea, and anterior segment of the globe, treatment of post-operative inflammation following ocular surgery. Lotemax™ and Alrex are approved for treatment of ocular allergy, including dry eye.

Clobetasone butyrate (0.1%) is a topical corticosteroid ophthalmic preparation for the treatment of ocular inflammation. Clobetasone butyrate had significantly less effect on raising intraocular pressure than dexamethasone.

Difluprednate 0.05% ophthalmic emulsion (Sirion Therapeutics) is the first "emulsion" formulation of corticosteroid to come to the market. Unlike a suspension, an emulsion does not require shaking because emulsions maintain homogenous molecular distribution within the vehicle. It is a difluorinated derivative of prednisolone and, therefore, another ketone-based corticosteroid, similar to dexamethasone. The emulsion vehicle allows for enhanced ocular surface contact time, thereby allowing less frequent instillation, as compared to non-emulsion delivery systems. Durezol (Durezol™) is FDA-approved specifically for the "management of inflammation and pain after intraocular surgery".[24]

Medrysone is indicated for the treatment of allergic conjunctivitis, vernal conjunctivitis, episcleritis, and epinephrine sensitivity. Adverse reactions include occasional transient stinging and burning on instillation. Increased intraocular pressure and posterior subcapsular cataract formation have been reported rarely with the use of medrysone. Systemic absorption and side-effects may result with the use of topical corticosteroids. It is available as ophthalmic suspension. Medrysone was historically marketed to treat ocular allergies, but newer, better choices have made it obsolete.

Triamcinolone acetonide (Intravitreal) is used to deliver a high concentration of corticosteroids to the anterior and posterior segments of eye for the treatment of inflammatory conditions. Recent studies have reported increasing use of intravitreal triamcinolone acetonide in the treatment of other intraocular proliferative, edematous and neovascular diseases.[12,14-16] The complications of intravitreal triamcinolone therapy include: secondary ocular hypertension, medically uncontrollable high intraocular pressure, posterior subcapsular and nuclear cataract and post-operative infectious endophthalmitis. Intravitreal triamcinolone injection can be combined with other intraocular surgeries, including cataract surgery, particularly in eyes with iris neovascularization.[25] In non-vitrectomized eyes, the duration of the effect and side-effects of a single intravitreal injection of triamcinolone is about 6–9 months for a dosage of about 20 mg, and about 2–4 months for a dosage of 4 mg.[25] Triamcinolone acetonide (Triesence™) is approved by FDA for the treatment of sympathetic ophthalmia, temporal arteritis, uveitis, and ocular inflammatory conditions unresponsive to topical corticosteroids.

CONCLUSION

Corticosteroids are some of the most potent and effective drugs for the treatment of ocular inflammation. However, despite the continuing development of techniques and vehicles for local administration of corticosteroids, both systemic and ocular adverse events continue to be reported with ocular corticosteroid preparations. Although non-steroidal anti-inflammatory drugs have been shown to challenge the therapeutic efficacy of corticosteroids in a number of ophthalmic conditions without the associated risk of elevated intraocular pressure, decreased wound strength or predisposition to infection, topical corticosteroids remain a fundamental component of the ophthalmic therapeutic strategy.

REFERENCES

1. Elkinton JR, Hunt AD Jr, Godfrey L, McCory WW, Rogerson AG, Stokes J Jr. Effects of pituitary adrenocorticotropic hormone (ACTH) therapy. JAMA. 1949;141:1273–9.
2. Woods AC. Clinical and experimental observations on the use of ACTH and cortisone in ocular inflammatory disease. Am J Ophthalmol. 1950;33:1325–49.
3. Mann WA, Markson DE. A case of recurrent iritis and episcleritis on a rheumatic basis treated with ACTH. Am J Ophthalmol. 1950;33:459–61.
4. Sherif Z, Pleyer U. Corticosteroids in ophthalmology: Past – Present – Future. Ophthalmologica. 2002;216(6):305–15.
5. Clinical guide to ophthalmic drugs. In: Melton, Randall T (Ed). Review of Optometry. 2009; 15A–9A.
6. McGhee CN. Pharmacokinetics of ophthalmic corticosteroids. Br J Ophthalmol. 1992;76: 681–4.
7. Awan MA, Agarwal PK, Watson DG, McGhee CN, Dutton GN. Penetration of topical and subconjunctival corticosteroids into human aqueous humour and its therapeutic significance. Br J Ophthalmol. 2009;93(6):708–13.
8. Oakley RH, Cidlowski JA. The glucocorticoid receptor: expression, function, and regulation of glucocorticoid responsiveness. In: Goulding NJ, Flower RJ. ed. Glucocorticoids. Basel, Switzerland: Birkhaeuser Verlag; 2001;pp. 55–80.
9. Goulding NJ, Flower RJ. Glucocorticoid biology: a molecular maze and clinical challenge. In: Goulding NJ, Flower RJ, editors. Glucocorticoids. Basel, Switzerland: Birkhaeuser Verlag; 2001; pp. 3–15.
10. Schacke H, Schottelius A, Docke WD, Strehlke P, Jaroch S, Schmees N, et al. Dissociation of transactivation from transrepression by a selective glucocorticoid receptor agonist leads to separation of therapeutic effects from side effects. Proc Natl Acad Sci. 2004;101(1):227–32.
11. Bodh SA, Kumar V, Raina UK, Ghosh B, Thakar M. Inflammatory glaucoma. Oman J Ophthalmol. 2011;4(1):3–9.
12. Kiernan DF, Mieler WF. The use of intraocular corticosteroids. Expert Opin Pharmacother. 2009;10(15):2511–25.
13. Conti SM, Kertes PJ. The use of intravitreal corticosteroids, evidence-based and otherwise. Curr Opin Ophthalmol. 2006;17(3):235–44.
14. Yilmaz T, Cordero-Coma M, Lavaque AJ, Gallagher MJ, Padula WV. Triamcinolone and intraocular sustained-release delivery systems in diabetic retinopathy. Curr Pharm Biotechnol. 2011;12(3):337–46.
15. Hunter RS, Lobo AM. Dexamethasone intravitreal implant for the treatment of noninfectious uveitis. Clin Ophthalmol. 2011;5:1613–21.
16. Schwartz SG, Flynn HW Jr. Fluocinolone acetonide implantable device for diabetic retinopathy. Curr Pharm Biotechnol. 2011; 12(3):347–51.
17. Watson D, Noble MJ, Dutton GN, Midgley JM, Healey TM. Penetration of topically applied dexamethasone alcohol into human aqueous humor. Arch Ophthalmol. 1988;106(5): 686–7.
18. Hirnei C, Neubauer AS, Kampik A, Schönfeld C L. Comparison of prednisolone 1%, rimexolone 1% and ketorolac tromethamine 0.5% after cataract extraction. A prospective, randomized, double-masked study. Graefe's Arch Clin Exp Ophthalmol. 2005;243(8):768-773.
19. Solomon KD, Vroman DT, Barker D, Gehlken J. Comparison of ketorolac tromethamine 0.5% and rimexolone 1% to control inflammation after cataract extraction: prospective randomized double-masked study. J Cataract Refract Surg. 2001;27(8):1232–7
20. Watson DG, McGhee CN, Midgley JM, Dutton GN, Noble MJ. Penetration of topically applied betamethasone sodium phosphate into human aqueous humour. Eye. 1990;4(4):603–6.
21. McGhee CN, Watson DG, Midgley JM, Dutton GN, Fern AI. Penetration of synthetic corticosteroids into human aqueous humour. Eye. 1990;4(3):526–30.
22. Pavesio CE, Decory HH. Treatment of ocular inflammatory conditions with loteprednol

etabonate. Br J Ophthalmol. 2008;92(4): 455–9.

23. Druzgala P, Wu WM, Bodor N. Ocular absorption and distribution of loteprednol etabonate, a soft steroid, in rabbit eyes. Curr Eye Res. 1991;10(10):933–7

24. Yamaguchi M, Yasueda S, Isowaki A, Yamamoto M, Kimura M, Inada K, et al. Formulation of an ophthalmic lipid emulsion containing an anti-inflammatory steroidal drug, difluprednate. Int J Pharm. 2005;301(1-2):121–8

25. Jonas JB. Intravitreal triamcinolone acetonide for treatment of intraocular oedematous and neovascular diseases. Acta Ophthalmol Scand. 2005;83(6):645–63.

Website Links

1. Clinical Guide to Ophthalmic Drugs (http://www.eyeupdate.com/pages/corticosteroids/corticosteroids.html)
2. FDA MedWatch (www.fda.gov/medwatch/index.html) the National Registry of Drug Induced Ocular Side-Effects (www.eyedrugregistry.com or http://piodr.sterling.net)

CHAPTER 13

Drugs Used in Ocular Allergy

OVERVIEW

Allergies frequently affect ocular structures, most commonly the conjunctivae. Allergic manifestations in the form of conjunctival congestion, burning, itching, increased secretions and swelling of eyelids may be triggered by localized contact of environmental antigens with the eye surface or may form a part of a systemic response to some exogenous or intrinsic allergens. Sympathomimetic drugs with vasoconstrictor actions are effective in reducing conjunctival congestion and reducing secretions. Since histamine has a well established role in acute allergic disorders, drugs which interfere with either the release of histamine from the mast cells by inhibiting degranulation, or those which block the H_1 histamine receptors are useful in the management of allergic disorders. Although both, sympathomimetic decongestants as well as antihistaminic drugs may be used by the systemic route, for ophthalmic purposes local instillation is the commonly employed method. Several ocular preparations containing antihistaminic agents, decongestants or their combinations are available.

Some fraction of the drugs administered topically to the eye is likely to get absorbed into the systemic circulation via nasolacrimal drainage and subsequent swallowing. However, systemic adverse effects following topical use are much smaller in magnitude as compared to systemic administration.

This chapter includes a brief discussion on the role of mast cells and histamine in allergic disorders. Antagonists of histamine H_2 receptors are discussed here mainly for comparison with H_1 receptor blockers. They do not have any uses specific to the eye. Mast cell stabilizers which inhibit release of histamine and other inflammatory mediators during allergic response are discussed as are drugs with combined antihistamine and mast cell stabilizing effects. Ocular decongestants that are clinically useful belong to the group of sympathomimetics, which reduce hyperemia by virtue of their vasoconstrictor effects. Only the role of sympathomimetic drugs as vasoconstrictors and decongestants is discussed in this chapter and their other ocular uses have not been included.

HISTAMINE

Histamine is a biologically active endogenous amine, which serves complex physiological as well as pathological functions through multiple receptors. It occurs both, as a neurotransmitter in neurons originating mainly from the posterior hypothalamus[1,2] and as an autacoid released locally by tissues. The central role of histamine in initiating the allergic response has been well established following its isolation from mammalian tissues over a hundred years back. Sir Henry Dale demonstrated that histamine application could mimic a type 1 (immediate hypersensitivity) anaphylactic response in sensitized tissue both *in vivo* and *in vitro*. Locally applied histamine has been shown to produce swelling, redness and edema while its administration intravenously produces symptoms identical to systemic anaphylaxis.

The discovery of histamine in mast cells led to further elucidation of its biological activity and role in antigen-antibody mediated allergic reactions. Histamine is synthesized from histidine by enzymatic action of histidine decarboxylase. It is found in mast cells and basophils in almost all tissues with particularly high concentrations in lungs, skin and the gastrointestinal tract. In addition, it is also present in 'histaminocytes' in the stomach and in histaminergic neurons in the brain. Formed histamine in mast cells and basophils is stored in intracellular granules complexed with a protein and heparin and is released by exocytosis during antigen-antibody reactions triggering inflammatory responses. The complement system activated during the antigen-antibody reaction acts on specific cell surface receptors to trigger an increase in cytosolic calcium, which then causes release of histamine in a fashion similar to other secretory processes. Histamine can also be released from the mast cells directly by certain chemicals and drugs such as morphine and d-tubocurarine as also by mechanical injury to mast cells. Contrary to this, agents such as β-adrenoceptor agonists, which increase intracellular cAMP formation inhibit the release of histamine. Two enzymes, histaminase and N-methyltransferase are responsible for the breakdown of released histamine.

Organ System Effects of Histamine

Among the important physiologic functions of histamine in humans is its role in secretion of gastric acid and as a neurotransmitter/neuromodulator. A role of histamine in chemotaxis has also been suggested. Histamine exerts its physiologic and pharmacologic effects through specific cell surface G-protein coupled receptors belonging to the seven membrane-spanning receptor superfamily. Four distinct histamine receptors, designated H_1-H_4 have been cloned. While H_1 receptor has been widely accepted to play a major role in allergic diseases, all four receptor types have been implicated in the inflammatory response.[3] Important characteristics of histamine receptors are summarized in Table 13.1 and the pharmacological effects of histamine on tissue and organ system are given in Table 13.2.

"Triple response": Experimental intradermal injection of histamine produces a characteristic response manifesting as a red spot, a raised wheal (edema) and surrounding reddish flare. Itching is also seen in and around the site of injection. These responses result from the effects of histamine on the vascular smooth muscle (redness), the vascular endothelium (edema due to increased permeability) and the sensory nerve endings (itching due to direct effects and reddish flare surrounding the wheal due to an axon reflex). This response is almost identical to that seen after insect bites or on local contact with allergens.

Table 13.1 Subtypes of histamine receptors[4-8]

Receptor	Major presence	Agonist	Classical effect	Antagonist
H_1	Smooth muscles, endothelium, brain	Histamine, Methylhistaprodifen	Smooth muscle contraction (except blood vessels)	Mepyramine
H_2	Gastric mucosa, myocardium, mast cells, brain	Histamine Dimaprit Amthamine	Stimulation of gastric secretion; cardiac stimulation	Cimetidine Ranitidine
H_3	Brain, myenteric plexus	Histamine R-alpha methylhistamine	Presynaptic inhibition of the release of neurotransmitters	Thioperamide
H_4	Eosinophils, neutrophils, T-cells	Histamine Clobenpropit, Clozapine	Chemotaxis; may play a role in inflammation and allergy	JNJ7777120 Thioperamide

Table 13.2 Tissue and organ system effects of histamine

Tissue/organ system	Major action	Receptor type	Manifestations
Nervous system			
Sensory nerves	Stimulation	H_1	Urticaria, reaction to insect bites and stings
Presynaptic action	Inhibition of the release of neurotransmitter	H_3	↓ Release of Ach[1], peptide and amine transmitters
Cardiovascular system			
Vascular smooth muscle	Relaxation	H_1 and H_2[2]	↓ Systolic and diastolic BP
Vascular endothelium	Increased permeability	H_1	Edema, urticaria
Heart	Stimulation	H_2	↑ HR (direct) and reflex[3]
Respiratory system			
Bronchial smooth muscle	Contraction	H_1	Asthmatic attacks
Gastrointestinal system			
Smooth muscle	Contraction	H_1	Diarrhea
Gastric secretions	Increased	H_2	↑ gastric acid, pepsin

[1]Acetylcholine;
[2]H_2 receptors also mediate dilatation at higher doses;
[3]Due to vasodilatation and fall in BP.

ANTIALLERGIC DRUGS

Since allergic disorders of the eye, especially those affecting the conjunctiva, are most often due to environmental antigens, a modification of the patients environment or limiting his exposure to the antigens may, at least theoretically, be attempted to mitigate the symptoms. However, this may not be practically feasible or effective in many cases, thus requiring the use of antiallergic medication. Systemic administration of antiallergic drugs may be required for some cases, such as those arising as a consequence of constitutional disorders or affecting deeper structures, but in most cases of allergic conjunctivitis local application is sufficient to control the symptoms with minimum liability for systemic adverse effects.

Antiallergic drugs that are in clinical use can be categorized in three groups viz:

i. *Antihistamines:* Competitive blockers of histamine receptors;
ii. *Mast cell stabilizers:* Which prevent mast cell degranulation and
iii. *Dual action drugs:* Which possess combined properties of the above two groups. Additio-nally, corticosteroids may also sometimes be employed for their antiallergic and anti-inflammatory actions.

Antihistamines

These are compounds, which competitively block histamine receptors. H_1 receptor blockers have been used for a long time as antiallergic agents. There are many members in this class and are generally classified into two generations: 1st generation (older) agents, which block H_1 receptors and also manifest moderate to marked sedation as a side effect as well as other CNS actions; 2nd generation agents, which do not readily cross into the CNS and hence have minimal sedating effects. The histamine H_2 receptor blockers are used primarily for reducing gastric acid secretion but some use for these has also been suggested in allergic disorders.

H_1 Receptor Blockers

All the H_1 receptor antagonists have an amine structure with attached chemical groups that differentiate them into various subgroups (Table 13.3). All of these competitively block histamine H_1 receptors on the effector sites thus preventing histamine from initiating an action. They have little effect on H_2 or H_3 receptors. The binding of H_1 receptor antagonists is reversible thus their efficacy is dependent on their concentration relative to that of the local histamine levels at the site. In addition, the 1st generation agents are also likely to block other autonomic receptors. This might explain some of their other effects such as antiemetic, anticholinergic and antiparkinsonian.

Pharmacokinetics: H_1 receptor antagonists are rapidly absorbed after oral administration and are widely distributed throughout the body. Peak concentrations following oral administration are achieved within 1–2 hours. Symptomatic relief may begin to appear within half an hour and lasts up to 4–6 hours with most agents. Duration of action is longer with many 2nd generation agents and may be up to 12 hours or more. The 1st generation agents cross the blood-brain barrier to enter the brain while 2nd generation agents do not readily do so, which explains the lack of sedating effects with the latter. 2nd generation agents are less lipid soluble as well as they are substrates for P-glycoprotein reverse transporter in the blood-brain barrier, both of which limit their entry into the brain. These agents are mostly metabolized in the liver by the hepatic microsomal cytochrome P450 enzymes and metabolites are excreted in the urine within 24 hours. Metabolites of some agents also retain activity and active metabolites of some like hydroxyzine, terfenadine and loratidine (cetirizine, fexofenadine and desloratidine, respectively) are themselves used as antihistaminc drugs.

H_1 receptor antagonists that are available for topical ophthalmic use are formulated in a suitable water-soluble form (such as maleate or phosphate). Following topical application, they distribute in the preocular tear film and also penetrate into the conjunctival layer and corneal stroma. Systemic absorption of such topically applied drugs occurs primarily through nasopaharyngeal and oropharyngeal mucosa following drainage via the nasolacrimal duct.

Other Pharmacological Effects: Apart from their antiallergic effects, H_1 receptor antagonists also produce several other pharmacological effects many of which are not related to blockade of H_1 receptors.

Sedation: This is seen mostly with the 1st generation H_1 receptor antagonists, although, the extent varies among different classes (Table 13.3). Toxic doses may result in marked CNS excitation leading to convulsions. Children may occasionally display excitement even with normal doses. 2nd generation members are relatively free of sedative effects and are thus preferred for daytime use.

Anticholinergic effects: As shown in Table 13.3 below, many 1st generation agents also possess antimuscarinic actions. This may result in drying of mucosal secretions (beneficial for rhinorrhea), dry mouth, urinary retention and blurring of vision.

Antiemetic effects: Some 1st generation H_1 receptor antagonists, mainly belonging to phenothiazine group are useful as antiemetics, while the piperazines have been found to be effective for prophylaxis of motion sickness.

Antiparkinsonian effects: Diphenhydramine shows significant inhibition of extrapyramidal effects. This may be related to its marked anticholinergic activity. It is useful for controlling antipsychotic induced extrapyramidal effects as well as for adjuvant therapy for some cases of Parkinson's disease.

Other miscellaneous effects: Phenothiazine H_1 receptor blockers also possess some á-adrenergic receptor blocking action and may result in orthostatic hypotension in some individuals. Local anesthetic activity is present in many 1st generation H_1 blockers due to a blocking action on sodium channels in a fashion similar to that of lidocaine. However, they are seldom used for local anesthetic purpose. Cyproheptadine also exhibits strong serotonin receptor blocking action and some of its pharmacological effects such as on

Table 13.3 Subclasses of H_1 antihistaminic drugs

Class	Members	Antimuscarinic activity	Comment
		First generation	
Ethylenediamines	Antazoline[1] Tripelennamine Pyrilamine[1]	Mild	Moderate sedative and GIT side-effects
Ethanolamines	Diphenhydramine Clemastine Dimenhydrinate Carbinoxamine Doxylamine	Marked	Significant antimuscarinic and sedative side-effects
Alkylamines	Pheniramine[1] Chlorpheniramine Brompheniramine Triprolidine	Mild	Mild sedation; rarely CNS stimulation
Phenothiazines	Promethazine Trimeprazine Methdilazine	Marked	Marked sedative and antimuscarinic effects; used as antiemetics
Piperazines	Hydroxyzine Meclizine Cyclizine Buclizine	–	Moderate to marked sedation; cyclizine and meclizine useful for motion sickness; hydroxyzine used for sedation and as antiemetic
Piperidines	Azatadine Cyproheptadine[2]	Mild	Moderate sedation
		Second generation	
Piperidines	Fexofenadine Loratidine Desloratidine	–	Relatively non-sedating
Piperazines	Cetirizine	–	Relatively non-sedating

[1] Ophthalmic preparations;
[2] Also possesses antiserotonergic activity; useful for controlling serotonin syndrome; is sometimes also used as appetite stimulant

appetite may be related to this action. Cetirizine also inhibits mast cell release of histamine and other mediators and this may be an additional mechanism for its antiallergic actions.

Adverse Effects: The most commonly encountered adverse effects with H_1 receptor antagonists are sedation and antimuscarinic effects, which are described above. Sedation is specially a problem with some of the 1st generation agents and these are best avoided for daytime use and in persons working with machinery or driving. As mentioned above, paradoxical excitation and convulsions may occur in children. Antimuscarinic adverse effects are usually mild in normal individuals but might be troublesome in the elderly or patients with benign prostatic hyperplasia in whom they can cause acute urinary retention. Marked antimuscarinic effects, typically resembling atropine overdose, are usually seen with high or toxic doses of drugs, which have significant muscarinic receptor blocking activity (Table 13.3). Postural hypotension can occasionally result following use of drugs, which have alpha adrenergic receptor blocking activity. The 2nd generation antihistaminic agents are relatively well-tolerated and are devoid of troublesome side-effects. However, earlier members of this group viz. astemizole and terfenadine were found to induce cardiac arrhythmias and have now gone out of use.

Interactions: Since most H_1 receptor antagonists utilize CYP enzymes, inhibition of these enzymes by other concomitant medications is likely to increase the circulating levels of the antihistaminic agent. This was typically illustrated by the interaction between, the now withdrawn 2nd generation H_1 blocker, terfenadine and the antifungal drug ketoconazole. The latter inhibits metabolism by CYP3A4 and increases the circulating concentrations of the former resulting in an increased incidence of cardiac arrhythmias. Other antimicrobial agents like the macrolide antibiotics (e.g. erythromycin) also inhibit CYP3A4 and thus can cause an increase in circulating levels of antihistaminic drugs. 1st generation agents, which have marked sedative effects can potentiate the effects of other CNS depressants.

Use of H_1 Antihistaminic Drugs for Ophthalmic Allergy: There appears to be no strong justification for systemic use of antihistaminic drugs for ocular allergies since i) ocular allergy is mostly a local condition ii) topical administration of antiallergic drugs achieves higher concentrations at the target site more quickly thus resulting in faster onset of relief and iii) the total dose of the drug required to be administered for achieving the desired concentration at the target site is much lower as compared to that which would be required by systemic route. Thus, even allowing for significant absorption into the systemic circulation, the incidence and intensity of adverse effects like sedation is likely to be lower with topical administration of H_1 receptor blockers. The second generation H_1 receptor antagonists have a lower risk for sedation and anticholinergic adverse effects and may be used by systemic route for alleviating itching, swelling and hyperemia without major systemic side-effects. However, topical application of olopatadine (H_1 antagonist and mast cell stabilizer) was found to be more efficacious than one of the most effective systemic antihistaminic agents, loratidine, in experimental allergen induced conjunctivitis.[9]

H_1 Receptor Blockers for Topical Ocular Use: Of the older H_1 receptor antagonists only three – antazoline phosphate (0.5%), pheniramine maleate (0.3 %) and pyrilamine maleate (0.1%) –are available for ocular use and these are available in over-the-counter preparations mostly in combination with sympathomimetic, ocular decongestants. Some newer H_1 receptor antagonists have also been developed for topical ocular use. These include levocabastine hydrochloride (0.05%) olopatadine (0.1%), and emedastine (0.05%). These have been found to be effective in controlling itching and hyperemia in allergic conjunctivitis. In addition, there are dual action agents with combined antihistaminic and mast cell stabilizing activities. These are discussed below.

H_2 Receptor Blockers

The main motivation for development of H_2 receptor selective antagonists was to target the stimulatory action of histamine on gastric acid secretion. The first two compounds, burimamide and metiamide that displayed selective H_2 receptor antagonism, however, were later found to be toxic and did not come into clinical use. The first drug of this class that was put to widespread clinical use in peptic ulcer disease was cimetidine. Several congeners have since been developed and include ranitidine and famotidine, which are one of the most widely prescribed drugs world over. There use largely remains confined to the inhibition of gastric acid secretion in peptic ulcer disease, gastro-oesophageal-reflux disease (GORD) and in hospitalized patients for control of stress-induced ulceration of the gastric mucosa.

H_2 receptor antagonists are not used in ophthalmic disorders. However, histamine induced vasodilatation involves both H_1 and H_2 receptors (Table 13.2), hence there appears to be a theoretical basis for the use of H_2 receptor blockers in combination with H_1 antihistaminic agents for additional benefits in relation to control of hyperemia that is associated with allergic conjunctivitis. Combined use of cimetidine (for which an ophthalmic formulation is available) with H_1 receptor blocker pyrilamine, has been shown to reduce the conjunctival hyperemia produced by local histamine challenge.[10] Although, currently there is no ophthalmic use of H_2 receptor antagonists, it is likely that they may find a place in the treatment of ophthalmic allergies.

Mast Cell Stabilizers

IgE antibodies develop on first exposure to an environmental antigen, which then becomes attached to the surface of the mast cells and basophils (known as sensitization). On subsequent contact with the same allergen IgE antibodies on the surface of the sensitized mast cells interact with the antigen to trigger an influx of calcium into the mast cells with consequent degranulation and release of histamine and some other mediators of inflammatory response. Histamine receptor blockers can prevent histamine from acting on the receptors on target sites, but for this they would have to be present in sufficient local concentration at the site when the antigen-antibody reaction occurs. This is usually not feasible since exposure to allergens is unpredictable. The role of H_1 receptor blockers is thus primarily to reverse the effects and reduce the symptoms after the allergic response has set in. Mast cell stabilizers are compounds which, as the name suggests, stabilize the mast cell membrane and prevent release of histamine and other mediators by degranulation following the antigen-antibody interaction.

The first mast cell stabilizing compound that came into clinical use was disodium chromoglycate (cromolyn). It was derived, like many other drugs, from a plant through chemical structure modifications of the parent benzopyrine molecule. It was shown to provide protection against attacks of experimentally induced bronchial asthma.[11]

Pharmacokinetics: Disodium chromoglycate is moderately soluble in water and almost insoluble in alcohol. It is poorly absorbed by the gastrointestinal route (oral capsules are used for local action within the gut for gastrointestinal allergies) and is not subject to metabolic transformation. For both asthma and ocular allergies, it has to be administered topically, i.e. by inhalation and as eyedrops respectively. Less than 10% is absorbed into the systemic circulation when chromoglycate is given by inhalation and is almost completely eliminated within 24 hours mostly in unchanged form.

For ocular use a water soluble form of sodium chromoglycate is available as eyedrops (4% solution). Pharmacokinetic details following topical ophthalmic use in humans are not available. However, it is well distributed in the surface tear film and also penetrates the conjunctival epithelium and substantia propria. Systemic absorption following repeated instillation is negligible (less than 0.1% in rabbits) and this occurs via drainage into the oropharynx and nasopharynx through the nasolacrimal duct.

Mechanism of Action: Cromolyn prevents the release of histamine and slow reacting substance of anaphylaxis (SRS-A) from mast cells. Cromolyn binds to a specific cromolyn-binding protein on the mast cell surface in the presence of calcium. The binding protein for cromolyn on the mast cell surface has been suggested to be a calcium transporter. This transporter once occupied by the drug is unable to transport calcium which is essential for degranulation and release of histamine and other mediators following antigen-antibody interaction. Chromoglycate also chelates calcium and several other divalent cations but calcium chelating action is not considered to be responsible for preventing degranulation. Phospholipase A-induced degranulation of non-sensitized mast cells and release of chemical mediators, in vitro, is inhibited by Cromolyn and this does not appear to be due to inhibition of enzymatic activity of phospholipase A. Another suggested mechanism thus for cromolyn induced suppression of degranulation of mast cells is the phosphorylation of a 78000 Da membrane bound protein in the mast cells, which is integral to the process of histamine release. The time course of phosphorylation by cromolyn of the membrane bound protein and its inhibitory action on histamine release are similar thus lending weight to the possibility of such a mechanism being responsible for the observed effects.

Cromolyn does not appear to possess any intrinsic antihistaminic, vasoconstrictor, bronchodilator, anticholinergic or anti-inflammatory activity. Other mast cell stabilizers, viz. nedocromil sodium (2%), lodoxamide (0.1%) and pemirolast (0.1%), that are available for ophthalmic use are similar in action to chromoglycate.

Use of Mast Cell Stabilizers in Ocular Allergic Disorders: The actions of mast cell stabilizer are due to inhibition of the release of mediators from the sensitized mast cells when they come in contact with the antigen. Hence their therapeutic role is mainly prophylactic whereby in the presence of the drug, even when sensitized mast cells are challenged by antigenic exposure the release of histamine and other mediators and the subsequent allergic manifestations do not follow.

Cromolyn sodium (ophthalmic solution 4%) is employed as eyedrops for vernal conjunctivitis or keratoconjunctivitis. The drops are to be administered 4 to 6 hourly. The ocular preparations of mast cell stabilizers that are available for ophthalmic use are given in Table 13.4.

Adverse effects: Sodium chromoglycate is well tolerated at therapeutic doses. Since topical administration does not result in significant absorption, the incidence of systemic adverse effects is low. Local effects such as irritation, redness and ocular and periocular itching might be seen with topical administration but these are usually mild and transient. Incidence of systemic adverse effects with other mast cell stabilizers is also low primarily because of low absorption into circulation. Headache, however, is a common adverse effect observed especially with pemirolast and local irritant effects may also be seen. Mast cell stabilizers are contraindicated in patients sensitive to the drug or other constituents in the ophthalmic solution.

Dual Action Agents

H_1 receptor blockers provide symptomatic relief by preventing action of histamine that is released by degranulation of mast cells during the allergic episode. Mast cell stabilizers on the other hand are effective in preventing the release of histamine and other inflammatory mediators and hence are effective for preventing the attack but are of little value once the mediators have been released. Dual action agents combine receptor blocking and mast cell stabilizing actions and are thus useful for both symptomatic relief as well as for prevention of further attacks. Agents with both H_1 receptor blocking and mast cell stabilizing activities are given below in Table 13.5. Some of them also possess additional activity against other inflammatory mediators.

Adverse effects of dual action agents: Like the mast cell stabilizers, headache, burning and irritation are common side-effects of dual action drugs. Other effects include a feeling of foreign body in the conjunctiva, dry eyes and itching in and around the eyes. Systemic adverse effects are not marked mainly due to small amounts absorbed from the ocular site. With azelastine a bitter taste may be felt as the drug drains into the oropharynx.

Table 13.4 Ophthalmic preparations of mast cell stabilizers

Drug	Concentration in eye drops	Administration
Disodium Chromoglycate (cromolyn sodium)	4%	1 to 2 drops 4–6 times daily
Nedocromil sodium	2%	1 to 2 drops twice a day
Lodoxamide tromethamine	0.1%	1 drop 4 times a day[1]
Pemirolast potassium	0.1%	1 to 2 drops 4 times daily

[1] Two times may be sufficient in some cases

Table 13.5 Antiallergic drugs with combined H_1 receptor blocking and mast cell stabilizing activities

Drug	Concentration in eyedrops	Comment
Azelastine	0.05%	Also blocks effects of other pro-inflammatory mediators like leukotrienes; inhibits eosinophil chemotaxis and activation
Epinastine	0.05%	Also inhibits eosinophil chemotaxis; additionally blocks H_2 and α receptors; rapid onset of relief after local instillation
Ketotifen	0.025%	Also blocks H_2 and H_3 receptors; decreases chemotaxis and eosinophil activation
Olopatadine	0.1%	Also inhibits production of inflammatory cytokines

Other Drugs for Ocular Allergies

Non-steroidal anti-inflammatory drugs have been considered for use in ocular allergies. However, only ketorolac (0.5% ophthalmic solution) has been found to provide beneficial effects in seasonal allergic conjunctivitis and is approved for such use. Ketorolac belongs to the group of non-selective cyclooxygenase inhibitors, the pharmacology of which has been discussed in chapter 11. A 0.4 or 0.5% solution of ketorolac tromethamine is effective for seasonal allergic conjunctivitis.

Glucocorticoids are also beneficial in ocular allergies. Besides their powerful anti-inflammatory actions these drugs also display other mechanisms of action which make them useful in allergic disorders. These mechanisms include inhibition of the release of histamine and other mediators from the mast cells, basophils and neutrophils and decreased synthesis of inflammatory mediators. The detailed pharmacology of corticosteroids is discussed in Chapter 12. Loteprednol etabonate (0.2%) is a steroid specifically designed for ophthalmic allergic conditions.

A comparative evaluation of different ocular antiallergic drugs shows that topical antihistamines, especially those with dual actions (e.g. olopatadine), are superior to mast cell stabilizers or topical NSAIDs.[12] Oral antihistamines are not recommended as first line option for allergic conjunctivitis due to their adverse systemic effects, including chances of causing dry eyes. However, for seasonal allergic rhinoconjunctivitis, second generation oral antihistamines may provide an advantage in terms of combined effects on nasal and ocular symptoms. Ketotifen, which is a mast cell stabilizer with additional effects on release of inflammatory mediators, has good efficacy in allergic conjunctivitis and is available as a preparation without preservatives. This makes it especially suitable for use in patients who wear contact lenses. Topical corticosteroids are effective but carry the risk of ocular side-effects, which include glaucoma, corneal ulcers and cataract. However, other more severe forms of ocular allergies such as vernal keratoconjunctivitis and atopic conjunctivitis, which are chronic allergic disorders with complex pathophysiological mechanisms, may respond better to topical corticosteroids than to antihistamines.

OCULAR DECONGESTANTS

Decongestant drugs achieve their effect primarily by causing vasoconstriction. Most such agents are sympathomimetic drugs, which act directly or indirectly (by releasing noradrenaline) on α adrenergic receptors on blood vessels to cause vasoconstriction and consequently a decrease in hyperemia and a reduction in edema and mucous secretion. Sympathomimetic drugs like ephedrine and pseudoephedrine act indirectly by increasing noradrenaline release while phenylephrine and naphazoline are α receptor agonists. When administered by systemic route their effects are widespread and may lead to generalized increase in vascular tone resulting in hypertension. Other systemic effects like excitation, sleeplessness, anxiety, nervousness and dizziness can also result. Because of these limitations, topical use of these agents is preferable. Ocular decongestants for topical use include phenylephrine, naphazoline, oxymetazoline and tetrahydrozoline. They are often combined with antihistaminic drugs for ocular use and such combinations are also available in several ophthalmic preparations. Table 13.6 summarizes the properties of the commonly used ocular decongestant preparations and Table 13.7 shows some decongestant-antihistamine combinations that are available in commercial formulations.

Topical administration of ophthalmic solutions of these agents into the eye produces a reduction in conjunctival injection and reduces watering and irritation. Other effects on the eye include dilatation of pupil and changes in intraocular pressure (Table 13.6). While dilatation of pupil may produce some blurring of vision in otherwise normal individuals, it may be especially dangerous in those with closed angle glaucoma in whom drainage from the anterior chamber might become further compromised resulting in dangerous increase in intraocular pressure.

Adverse effects: Systemic effects following topical use are usually unremarkable in normal individuals, because of the relatively small amounts entering the general circulation. However, caution is required while prescribing these drugs in the presence of conditions like hypertension or cardiovascular disorders, hyperthyroidism and diabetes where even mild sympathomimetic effects might prove dangerous.

Local adverse effects in the eye following topical use of decongestants are usually a sharp irritation and a stinging sensation, which is transient. Blurring of vision might occur due to dilatation of pupil. The frequency of administration should be as low as possible but in any case should not exceed four times daily. Tachyphylaxis can develop as also the incidence of rebound congestion and epithelial erosion can increase following repeated and frequent use of these agents. Decongestants are contraindicated in subjects with closed angle glaucoma due to the reasons described above.

Table 13.6 Ophthalmic decongestants

Drug[1]	Concentration	Pupil dilatation	Effect on IOP[2]
Phenylephrine	0.12%	±	±
Naphazoline	0.012–0.1%	↓	↑
Oxymetazoline	0.025%	±	-
Tetrahydrozoline	0.05%	±	may ↓

[1]All are formulated as hydrochloride salts for ophthalmic solution.
[2]IOP: Intraocular pressure

Table 13.7 Decongestant-antihistamine combinations

Decongestant	Antihistaminic		
	Pyrilamine	Pheniramine	Antazoline
Phenylephrine 0.12% 0.125%	0.1% -	- 0.5%	- -
Naphazoline 0.025% 0.05%	- -	0.3% -	- 0.5%

FUTURE DIRECTIONS

In the past, development of drugs for relief of episodic allergies has remained focused mainly on histamine and mast cells as the targets. Over the last two decades several other aspects have attracted the attention of researchers. Thus, although histamine is the primary chemical mediator which triggers allergic response and the accompanying symptoms, other mediators are also involved in allergic response. Some of these may be released during mast cell degranulation and are involved in the inflammatory response and contribute to the overall manifestations. Prostaglandins have been recognized as powerful itch producing substances in the conjunctiva, thus inhibition of local prostaglandin synthesis has been targeted in trials with ocular preparations of NSAIDs. Ketorolac tromethamine, as mentioned above, is already approved for use in conjunctival allergies. Trials with other NSAIDs like flurbiprofen and diclofenac have also yielded promising results. Steroids have multiple mechanisms by which they inhibit allergic response. Site specific steroids such as loteprednol etabonate and rimexolone are topically effective in treating allergic conjunctivitis with reduced potential for adverse effects such as cataract formation or increase in intraocular pressure that are seen with classical steroids. Other mediators such as leukotrienes and platelet activating factor, which are co-released from mast cells could also be targeted in future to develop agents, that will inhibit their actions. Peptide derivatives from the human IgE have been found to competitively inhibit binding of IgE to the target cells and block the type I hypersensitivity response on subsequent exposure to the antigen.[13] Pentigetide, a synthetic pentapeptide has been found to inhibit allergic response in sensitized individuals[14] and clinical trials with this agent showed promising results in allergic conjunctivitis.[15] The emerging role of the H_4 histamine receptors in the pathophysiology of allergic disorders and the fact that these are co-localized with H_1 receptors with a higher sensitivity to histamine, has led to the suggestion that these may be playing a significant role in conditions like allergic conjunctivitis.[16] Some H_4 receptor antagonists are currently in the stage of early clinical trials.[17-19] These and other similar agents may be added in future to the drugs that are available for the treatment of ocular allergies.

REFERENCES

1. Sakata T, Yoshimatsu H, Kurokawa M. Hypothalamic neuronal histamine: implication of its homeostatic control of energy metabolism. Nutrition. 1997;13(5):403–11.
2. Schwartz JC, Arrang JM, Garbarg M, Pollard H, Ruat M. Histaminergic transmission in the mammalian brain. Physiol Rev. 1991;71(1):1–51.
3. Gutzmer R, Diestel C, Mommert S, Köther B, Stark H,Wittmann M, et al. Histamine H_4 receptor stimulation suppresses IL-12p70 production and mediates chemotaxis in human monocyte-derived dendritic cells. J Immunol. 2005;174(9): 5224–32.
4. Malinowska B, Piszcz J, Schlicker E, Kramer K, Elz S, Schunack W. Histaprodifen, methylhistaprodifen, and dimethylhistaprodifen are potent H_1-receptor agonists in the pithed and in the anaesthetized rat. Naunyn-Schmiedeberg's Arch Pharmacol. 1999;359(1): 11–16.
5. Seeley N, Sturman G. Effect of amthamine, a histamine H2-agonist, in two mouse chemical-induced seizure models. Inflamm Res. 2001; 50(2):S82–S3.
6. Krause M, Stark H, Schunack W. Azomethine prodrugs of (r)-alpha-methylhistamine, a highly potent and selective histamine H_3-receptor agonist Curr Med Chem. 2001;8(11):1329–40.
7. Sugata Y, Okano M, Fujiwara T, Matsumoto R, Hattori H, Yamamoto M, et al. Histamine H_4 receptor agonists have more activities than H_4 agonism in antigen-specific human T-cell responses. Immunology. 2007;121(2): 266–75.
8. Thurmond RL, Desai PJ, Dunford PJ, Fung-Leung W, Hofstra CL, Jiang W, et al. A potent and selective histamine H_4 receptor antagonist with anti-inflammatory properties. JPET. 2004; 309:404–13.
9. Abelson MB, Welch DL. An evaluation of onset and duration of action of Patanol (olopatadine hydrochloride ophthalmic solution 0.1%) compared to Claritin (loratidine 10 mg) tablets

in acute allergic conjunctivitis in the conjunctival allergen challenge model. Acta. Ophthalmol Scand. 2000;78(230):60–3.

10. Leon J, Charap A, Duzman E, Shen C. Efficacy of cimetidine/pyrilamine eyedrops, a dose response study with histamine challenge. Ophthalmology. 1986;93(1):120–3.

11. Altounyan REC. Inhibition of experimental asthma by a new compound, disodium cromoglycate, 'INTAL'. Acta Allergol. 1967;22:487.

12. del Cuvillo A, Sastre J, Montoro J, Jauregui I, Davila I, Ferrer M, et al. Allergic conjunctivitis and H_1 antihistamines. J Investig Allergol Clin Immunol. 2009;19(1):11–8.

13. Geha RS, Helm B, Gould H. Inhibition of the Prausnitz-Kustner reaction by an immunoglobulin E-chain fragment synthesized in *E. coli*. Nature. 1985;315(6020):577–8

14. Hamburger RN. Peptide inhibition of the Prausnitz-Kustner reaction. Science. 1975;189 (4200):389–90.

15. Kalpaxis JG, Thayer TO. Double-blind trial of pentigetide ophthalmic solution, 0.5%, compared with cromolyn sodium, 4%, ophthalmic solution for allergic conjunctivitis. Ann Allergy. 1991; 66(5):393–98.

16. Abelson MB, McLaughlin J. Ocular antihistamines revisited: Beyond H_1. Rev Ophthalmol. 2011;18(4):66–70.

17. Torkildsen G, Shedden A. The safety and efficacy of alcaftadine 0.25% ophthalmic solution for the prevention of itching associated with allergic conjunctivitis. Curr Med Res Opin. 2011;27(3):623–31.

18. Engelhardt H, Smits RA, Leurs R, Haaksma E, de Esch IJ. A new generation of anti-histamines: Histamine H4 receptor antagonists on their way to the clinic. Curr Opin Drug Discov Devel. 2009;12(5):628–43.

19. Strakhova MI, Cuff CA, Manelli AM, et al. In vitro and in vivo characterization of A-940894: A potent histamine H4 receptor antagonist with anti-inflammatory properties. Br J Pharmacol. 2009;157(1):44–54.

CHAPTER 14

Local Anesthetics in Ophthalmology Practice

OVERVIEW

Anesthesia for ophthalmic surgery has undergone tremendous changes over the past few decades. The earliest authentic description on this subject was probably provided by the ancient Indian surgeon Sus'ruta in 600 BC. Since those days, ophthalmic surgery has reshaped by evolution of anesthesia, both in terms of the introduction of new local anesthetic agents as well as development of new techniques of administration.

Currently, there are two major approaches for ophthalmic anesthesia—general anesthesia and local anesthesia. The decision to choose between these two approaches involves the surgeon in terms of suitability for the type of surgery; the anesthesiologist in terms of appropriateness of the patient's general physical condition to that specific anesthetic approach and lastly and equally important, is the patient's acceptability.[1] Nowadays, majority of the ophthalmic surgeries can be performed under local anesthesia, while, general anesthesia is kept as an alternative option for special situations like uncooperative patients (e.g. children), bilateral surgery, and extensive or lengthy procedures. This preference for local anesthesia despite insignificant difference in morbidity and mortality profiles is due to several advantages that local anesthesia offers over general anesthesia such as less post-operative risk of nausea and vomiting, superior post-operative pain control, shorter post-operative recovery time and ability of the patient to maintain mental alertness during surgical procedure. Furthermore, local anesthesia in an expert hand carries a very low risk of serious complications.[2] Even though, in one of the studies, patients reported seeing light flashes during the surgery that were considered terrifying experience for significant number of them,[2] regional or topical anesthesia is still the most popular type of anesthesia for ophthalmic surgery.[3] The relevant anatomical considerations for the techniques of administration of local anesthesia are described in Chapter 1.

PHARMACOLOGY OF LOCAL ANESTHETIC AGENTS

Local anesthetic agents are used to produce transient loss of sensation and motor paralysis in a specific area or part of the body. These agents are capable of producing reversible block of action potential propagation, which is responsible for nerve conduction in any part of nervous system and in all types of nerves including sensory and motor nerves.

Cocaine was the first local anesthetic agent isolated by Niemann in 1860 and was used at first for ophthalmic anesthesia. Although, it was soon discovered that cocaine is highly addicting, it remained in use for about 30 years until procaine was synthesized by Einhorn in 1905.[4] An ideal local anesthetic is expected to provide rapid onset and long duration of action without local and systemic toxicity. None of the currently available agent possesses all desirable properties and synthesis of newer agents continues.

Local anesthetic agents consist of a lipophilic group linked to an ionizable group by an intermediate chain. This intermediate chain is either an ester or an amide link (Fig. 14.1).

Besides the chemistry and general physical properties, specific stereochemical configurations of local anesthetic agents also determine their potency. Based on their chemical structure, local anesthetic agents are divided into two classes:

1. Amino esters: Possess an ester linkage between the benzene ring and the amine side chain.
2. Amino amides: Possess an amide linkage between the benzene ring and the amine side chain.

At present, all commonly used topical anesthetics are of the ester type except lidocaine gel, while all injectable local anesthetics are of amide type (except procaine). The reason behind replacement of injectable esters by amides apart from cocaine's addiction risk is that they are metabolized to para-aminobenzoic acid (PABA) which is known for its potential to cause allergy.[4] For topical use, the case is different as there is less systemic absorption and much lower risk of allergic reaction due to PABA. At the same time, amino-esters provide rapid onset of action, which lasts for brief duration.

Topical and injectable anesthetics used in ophthalmic practice are listed in Table 14.1 and 14.2.

Pharmacokinetics

Local anesthetics are injected or instilled locally close to nerve fibers that need to be blocked. Uniquely, local anesthetics reach their site of action before they reach the vascular compartment, in contrast to other drugs that are distributed from the vascular compartment to their sites of action. In other words, the appearance of local anesthetic in the vascular compartment represents the termination of their action. Therefore, the duration of their action is affected by the rate at which they are removed from their local site of injection or instillation into the systemic circulation. The extent of their systemic absorption also determines the likelihood of their systemic adverse effects.[6]

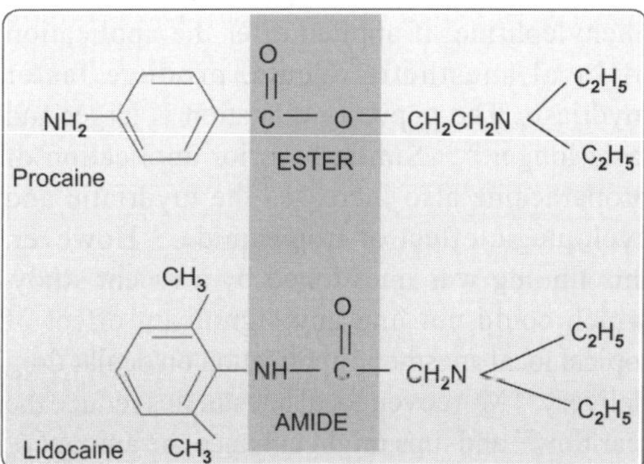

Figure 14.1 Chemical structure of local anesthetics

Table 14.1 Topical anesthetics

Preparation	Class	Formulation	Onset	Duration	Commonly used preservative
Tetracaine hydrochloride	Ester	0.5% solution	1 minute	15–20 minutes	Chlorobutanol (0.4%)
Proparacaine hydrochloride	Ester	0.5% solution	6–20 seconds	10–15 minutes	Benzalkonium chloride (0.01%), Chlorobutanol (0.2%)
Proparacaine hydrochloride with fluorescein	Ester	0.5% solution with 0.25% sodium fluorescein	6–20 seconds	10–15 minutes	Thimerosal (0.01%)
Benoxinate hydrochloride with fluorescein	Ester	0.4% solution with 0.25% sodium fluorescein	1–2 minutes	10–15 minutes	Chlorobutanol (1.0%)
Lidocaine gel	Amide	1.5, 2, 3.5 and 4% gel	1–5 minutes	15–40 minutes	Preservative free

Table 14.2 Injectable anesthetics

Preparation	Class	Formulation (% solution)	Onset (min)	Duration (min)
Procaine	Ester	1, 2, 10	7–8	30–45
Lipocaine	Amide	0.5, 1, 1.5, 2, 4	4–6	40–60
Mepivacaine	Amide	1, 1.5, 2	3–5	120–180
Bupivacaine	Amide	0.25, 0.5, 0.75	5–10	240–720
Etidocaine	Amide	1, 1.5	3–5	180–600
Prilocaine	Amide	4%	2–3	150–108

Local Absorption and Distribution

The availability of a local anesthetic agent to nerves depends upon its ability to diffuse through the tissue and the outer lipid membrane of nerve fibers to reach its site of action. The movement through the nerve fiber membranes depends upon the lipid solubility of the local anesthetic agent. The small and highly lipid soluble molecules interact faster with the sodium channel receptors. While lipid solubility helps in penetration through the neuronal membrane, water solubility helps the local anesthetic to be in the cationic form, which binds to anionic fragments of the specific receptor sites in voltage gated sodium channels.[7]

Therefore, the potency of local anesthetic agents is positively correlated with their lipid solubility, as long as the water solubility is retained.

The pH of the tissue in which the drug is injected also affects its diffusion. Local anesthetic agents are weak bases but for clinical use they are available as salts to increase their solubility and stability. The pK_a of the local anesthetic solutions ranges from 8.00 – 9.00. Therefore, when injected in the body, at physiological pH their larger fraction exists as charged cationic form[8,9] as is shown by Henderson-Hesselbalch's equation:

$$\text{Log (cationic form/unionized form)} = pK_a - pH$$

The unionized form, being highly lipid soluble helps in the penetration of drug through the outer lipid membranes of nerve fibers whereas ionized form is most active at the receptor site as it cannot easily leave the closed channels. Therefore, when injected in infected and inflamed tissue, local anesthetics have poor efficacy as they exist largely in ionized form due to highly acidic local pH and penetrate the lipid membranes poorly.[9,10]

It has been reported that topical application of local anesthetics increases corneal permeability of subsequently applied drugs and mydriatics, like phenylephrine, if applied after the application of local anesthetic agents, produce faster mydriasis. The pupillary dilatation is larger and lasts longer.[10-12] Similarly, prior application of proparacaine also increases the mydriatic and cycloplegic effect of tropicamide.[13] However, this finding was questioned by a recent study, which could not find any significant effect of topical local anesthetic application on ocular drug delivery.[14] Moreover, local anesthetics reduce the tear flow[15] and thus might enhance the amount of drug absorption through cornea by reducing the washout effect of tear flow.[16] Increased corneal absorption reduces the amount of systemic absorption, thus reducing the systemic toxicity.

Systemic Absorption and Distribution

Systemic absorption of local anesthetics is the means for their local elimination and termination of action. The extent and rate of systemic absorption of local anesthetics is determined by the dose, site of injection, extent of tissue protein binding, physicochemical properties and presence of vasoconstrictor substance. Injection of a local anesthetic agent in a highly vascular area (e.g. muscles) will lead to higher amount of systemic absorption as compared to that after its injection in a poorly vascularized area (e.g. subcutaneous tissue). The duration of action of local anesthetics is proportional to the time for which they remain in contact with nerve or local tissue. All local anesthetic agents have intrinsic vasodilating activity except cocaine, which has vasoconstrictor activity. Thus, local anesthetic agents promote their own removal from the site of injection, which affects their duration of action. For example, lidocaine has shorter duration of action as compared to mepivaciane due to its enhanced vasodilating property.[17] Drugs like bupivacaine and etidocaine have high protein binding, which reduces the amount of free drug available to interact with the receptor. But this high protein binding acts as a drug reservoir and prolongs the duration of action of these drugs.[7] Addition of a vasoconstrictor such as epinephrine causes local vasoconstriction, thereby reducing the rate and extent of systemic absorption. This causes increased local availability of the local anesthetic and enhanced neuronal uptake. Co-administration of epinephrine, therefore, improves the onset, provides better quality and increases duration of anesthesia. Epinephrine also reduces local bleeding and the risk of systemic toxicity to local anesthetic agent by reducing its systemic absorption. Epinephrine can delay the wound healing and can occasionally cause tissue necrosis due to intense vasoconstriction.[7] Epinephrine can also cause anxiety, restlessness, tremors, palpitations, pallor, hypertension, headache and precordial discomfort. The usual concentration of epinephrine used in ophthalmic preparations ranges from 1:50,000 to 1:200,000. The effect of adding epinephrine is especially prominent with short- and medium acting local anesthetics. Relatively less efficacy of epinephrine to prolong action of long-acting agents is due to their high lipid solubility and high tissue protein binding.[18] Addition of a vasoconstrictor has no effect on the duration of topical anesthesia but increases the risk of systemic adverse effects, and therefore, is not recommended. Use of epinephrine is relatively contraindicated in patients with hypertension and ischemic heart disease. In patients with glaucoma, epinephrine can cause severe local vasospasm and permanent loss of vision. Nevertheless, a balance should be always sought between the cardiac risk and the benefits of epinephrine with regards to the quality and duration of anesthesia and level of pain control.[19]

The enzyme hyaluronidase is often added to local anesthetic solution for retrobulbar and peribulbar injections to facilitate its local distribution. Hyaluronidase depolymerizes the hyaluronic acid, which is a component of connective tissue and acts as tissue cement. The breakdown of hyaluronic acid allows easy spread of the solution in the tissue.[18] A usual dose of 75 units (0.5 mL) per 10 mL of anesthetic solution produces enhanced akinesia and anesthesia.[20]

Once into the systemic circulation, amide local anesthetics are widely distributed. At first into the highly vascular tissues like CNS, liver, kidney and brain, followed by less vascular tissues like gastrointestinal tract and muscles. Ester type of agents have a very short half-life as they undergo rapid metabolism before they are distributed to various tissues.

Metabolism and Excretion

Metabolism of local anesthetics in plasma or liver converts them into highly water soluble forms for easy excretion in urine. Ester type of local anesthetics such as procaine is quickly metabolized by pseudocholinesterase (butyrylcholinesterase) and, therefore, has a short half-life. Amide types are metabolized by hepatic microsomal cytochrome P450. Individual amide agents are metabolized at different rates by microsomal enzymes. Concomitant use of other drugs that inhibit the same cytochrome enzyme may potentiate the action of amide type of local anesthetic agents. Toxicity of amide types is also more likely in patients with impaired liver functions or reduced hepatic blood flow due to their reduced hepatic metabolism.[7]

Mechanism of Action

Local anesthetics act by blocking the voltage-gated sodium channels in nerve fibers. The action of sodium pump is crucial in maintaining the transmembrane ionic gradients required for impulse conduction in excitable membranes such as neuronal fibers and cardiac muscles. During excitation the resting membrane potential of –90 to –60 mV changes to +40 mV due to rapid influx of sodium ions through the open sodium channels. During this membrane depolarization, sodium channels pass into an active stage and potassium channels open. Outward flow of potassium ions causes membrane repolarization, return of membrane potential to –95 mV and return of sodium channels to resting stage. Sodium channels in resting stage can again pass into active stage at the arrival of new impulse.

During the entire process of membrane depolarization and repolarization, the sodium channels pass through three conformational changes or stages, the resting stage in which the entry of sodium is blocked at its activation gate near extracellular site, activated stage in which both the inactivation and activation gates are open to allow rapid entry of sodium ions and finally inactive stage when the inactivation gates near intracellular site are closed and sodium entry is blocked. The inactive channels are in a refractory stage and must return to resting stage before they become available for activation once again. The return of inactive channels to resting stage is time dependent.[8]

Local anesthetics bind to the receptors near the intracellular end of sodium channel and block them in the inactive and active stages, while resting stage is relatively resistant to the blocking effect of local anesthetics. Rapidly firing nerves are more susceptible to the action of local anesthetic agents as their membrane voltage is more positive than normal, which facilitates the interaction of local anesthetic molecule with the receptor.[9] Additionally, rapidly firing neurons pass through the open and inactive stages of sodium channels more often than the resting fibers and, therefore, are more sensitive to the action of local anesthetics. Recovery of sodium channels from inactive to resting stage after being blocked by local anesthetics is much slower as compared to that from normal inactivation. Local anesthetics, therefore, increase the refractory period and reduce the frequency of nerve conduction (Fig. 14.2).

As mentioned before, sodium channels in resting stage are less sensitive to local anesthetic action as compared to open and inactive channels and thus, increased extracellular calcium concentration partially antagonizes the action of local anesthetics by favoring the resting stage, whereas increased extracellular potassium enhances the effect of local anesthetics by favoring the inactive stage of sodium channels.[7]

The susceptibility of nerve fibers to blockade of impulse conduction by local anesthetics is also influenced by: size of the nerve fibers, myelination and position of nerve fiber in the nerve bundle. The fibers with smaller diameter are blocked faster than those with larger diameter. Myelinated nerves are blocked faster than the unmyelinated

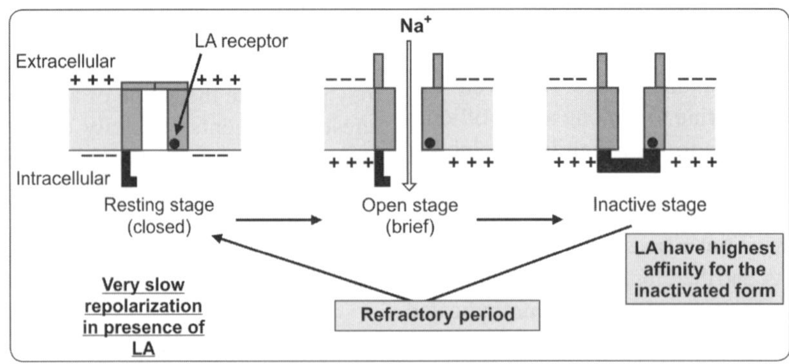

Figure 14.2 Representation of voltage-gated sodium channels showing the site and mechanism of action of local anesthetics

nerves of the same diameter. In large peripheral nerves, motor fibers are located peripherally and are, therefore, exposed first to locally administered anesthetic agent. As a consequence, motor nerve block may appear faster than the sensory block. In the extremities, sensory fibers for proximal parts are located outside the sensory fibers for distal parts. Therefore, sensory loss appears first for proximal areas followed by distal areas.[10]

The local anesthetics act on all excitable membranes, such as CNS neurons and cardiac cells, in the same way as on peripheral neuronal membranes. Therefore, at very low concentration they can be useful as antiarrhythmic agents but at high concentration are likely to cause arrhythmias and CNS adverse effects.

Adverse Effects

Local

Topically applied local anesthetics, like tetracaine, cause mild local stinging and burning sensation. Such symptoms are short lasting and do not require specific treatment. In some patients corneal epithelial damage occurs due to tear film instability caused by decreased reflex tearing, increased tear evaporation and infrequent blinking.[21] Superficial punctate keratopathy is infrequent and usually mild. Local allergic reactions are uncommon. They may present as conjunctival hyperemia, chemosis, swelling of eyelids, lacrimation and itching. The allergic reactions are more likely with ester types as compared to amides.

Repeated long-term administration of topical anesthetics causes delayed wound healing and is associated with infiltrative keratitis. Local anesthetics may be used to relieve initial ocular pain and should not be prescribed for self-administration as virtually all local anesthetics can cause corneal damage on prolonged use.[22] Frequent instillation of local anesthetics even for a few days causes increased corneal permeability and loss of corneal epithelium and tear film instability. Reduced corneal sensations cause reduced blinking, which further enhances corneal

drying. Clinically, the changes manifest as eyelid edema, conjunctival hyperemia, papillary hypertrophy, mucopurulent discharge, corneal epithelial defects which can progress to stromal infiltration, keratic precipitates, anterior uveitis, hypopyon and hyphema. Appearance of a dense yellowish white stromal ring is characteristic of corneal damage due to anesthetic misuse and abuse.[23]

Systemic

Systemic toxicity to topically applied anesthetics is relatively uncommon and is usually seen with drug overdose. Drug overdose can cause high blood levels leading to toxicity.

Injectable local anesthetics can cause systemic adverse effects after extravascular administration. Inadvertent intravenous injection can cause serious toxicity. The degree of systemic toxicity correlates with the potency of the anesthetic agent. Accordingly, bupivacaine and tetracaine are more likely to cause toxicity as compared to prilocaine and lidocaine. Among the agents with similar potency, the likelihood to cause toxicity varies according to the extent of absorption and metabolism. For example: after subcutaneous administration, prilocaine is less readily absorbed and is more readily metabolized as compared to lidocaine and, therefore, toxicity of prilocaine is 60 percent lower than that of lidocaine. The systemic adverse effects of local anesthetic agents mainly involve CNS and cardiovascular system.[9]

The *central nervous system* excitation represents the earliest sign of toxicity. Initial symptoms consist of a feeling of light headedness, dizziness followed by visual disturbances, tinnitus, drowsiness, disorientation, slurred speech, muscle twitching and temporary loss of consciousness. Tremors of face and extremities may be followed by convulsions. The CNS excitation may be followed by respiratory arrest and generalized CNS depression.[7]

Cardiovascular adverse effects of local anesthetics are attributed to their direct action on heart, peripheral actions on blood vessels and blockade of conduction in autonomic fibers. Myocardial suppression and vasodilation due to direct relaxant effect on blood vessels causes decrease in cardiac output. All local anesthetic agents show similar cardiovascular toxicity.[7]

Methemoglobinemia leading to cyanosis is an adverse effect of the high doses of prilocaine. Prilocaine metabolizes to orthotoluidine, which upon accumulation, oxidizes hemoglobin to methemoglobin. Reducing agents like methylene blue or ascorbic acid are used to reduce methemoglobin to hemoglobin.[7]

Allergic reactions to amino-esters are seen in small percentage of population. Esters metabolize to PABA, which is responsible for allergic reactions such as dermatitis and rashes. Amino-amides do not metabolize to PABA and, therefore, allergic reactions with amides are rare.[7]

Contraindications

Patients with previous history of hypersensitivity should not be given the same anesthetic agent. However, an agent from different chemical group may be tried. Amide type of local anesthetic agents are metabolized in liver and, therefore, should be used with caution in patients with impaired liver function. Ester type of local anesthetics are metabolized by plasma pseudocholinesterase and, therefore, are contraindicated in patients with genetic deficiency of the enzyme. Topically applied anesthetics cause tear film instability and reduced reflex tearing and thus can complicate the clinical picture in dry eye patients. In such cases anesthetic agents should be used after complete evaluation for dry eye condition.[23] In conditions requiring collection of specimen from ocular surface for culture, instillation of anesthetic agent should be done after specimen collection as many of these agents have antimicrobial activity, though, it is suggested that proxymetacaine 0.5% can be used as it has minimal antibacterial effects *in vitro*.[24] In patients with perforating

injury, topical application of anesthetic agents can cause endothelial damage.

TYPES OF LOCAL ANESTHESIA

Types of local anesthesia that are used for ophthalmic procedures include:
1. Retrobulbar block
2. Peribulbar block
3. Sub-Tenon's block
4. Local infiltration
5. Topical

Retrobulbar Block

Retrobulbar block is a suitable anesthetic technique for majority of ophthalmic surgical procedures (such as cataract extraction, glaucoma filtering procedures, iris surgery, trans-pars-plana vitrectomy, or orbital exploration) with or without addition of a second injection in the superior nasal quadrant.[25]

It is performed by injecting the local anesthetic solution inside the muscle cone behind the globe (Fig 14.3). The injection is made just above the inferior orbital margin in the inferotemporal quadrant. The needle is inserted parallel to the orbital floor and then is directed upwards and medially and local anesthetic is injected after ruling out intravascular location of the needle. Retrobulbar block provides global and conjunctival anesthesia due to the conduction block in the intraorbital sensory division of the ophthalmic branch of trigeminal nerve. For global akinesia, conduction block of oculomotor, trochlear and abducent nerve is required. Since the injection is made inside the cone and trochlear nerve runs an extraconal course, activity of superior oblique muscle is retained.

This block requires merely, 2 to 4 mL, of local anesthetic to produce adequate retrobulbar anesthesia. Almost any of the local anesthetic agents can be used but many ophthalmologists favor a combination of bupivacaine and lidocaine.[26]

Conversely, for peribulbar approach, needle does not advance into the muscle cone and, therefore, slightly larger volume, 4-6 mL is needed.

Peribulbar Block

Peribulbar block is achieved by injecting local anesthetic outside the muscle cone (Fig 14.3). This helps to avoid proximity of the needle to optic nerve. The method requires larger quantities of local anesthetic solution. The injection is made just above the lateral one third of inferior orbital rim. If a second injection is required it is made in more medial position to achieve complete akinesia.[27] A pressure lowering device is used to spread the anesthetic agent and soften the eye.

Sub-Tenon's Block

Sub-Tenon's block requires administration of anesthetic agent under the Tenon's fascia. Tenon's fascia is incised 5–10 mm lateral to limbus. A cannula is inserted under the Tenon's fascia for injection of local anesthetic agent.[27,28]

Local Infiltration

Injection of local anesthetic agent by local infiltration is commonly used for eyelid surgery. To achieve anesthetic effect in anterior lamella

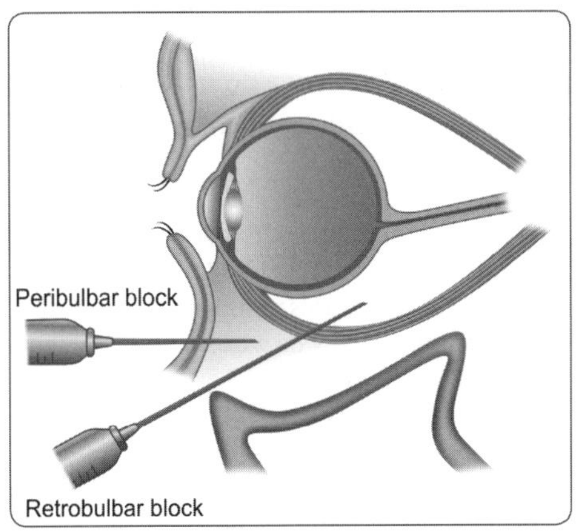

Figure 14.3 Schematic diagram showing sites of injection for retrobulbar and peribulbar block

including skin, orbicularis muscle, orbital septum and anterior tarsal surface, a pretarsal block is given. For surgery involving palpebral conjunctiva and posterior tarsal surface, a retrotarsal block is given. The procedure requires subcutaneous administration of 0.5 to 1.0 mL of solution along the proximal tarsal border. A gentle massage over the injected area facilitates spread of solution and reduces the chance of hematoma formation.[27,28]

Topical

Topical application is the most commonly used method of administering local anesthesia. Majority of topically applied local anesthetic agents provide similar onset, depth and duration of anesthesia. Topical anesthesia is used for common diagnostic procedures such as applanation tonometry and gonioscopy. Procedures like removal of small superficial foreign body, suture removal can be done under topical anesthesia. Intraocular procedures such as phacoemulsification are now done under topical anesthesia. Some specialized procedure like forced duction test, electroretinography, corneal epithelial debridement are also performed under topical anesthesia.[27,28]

FUTURE OF LOCAL ANESTHETICS IN OPHTHALMIC SURGERY

Future advances in local anesthetic use in ophthalmic surgery might involve the topical application of a new local anesthetic like neosaxitoxin, which is a phycotoxin. It has the capability of reversibly blocking neuronal voltage-gated sodium channels.[29] It has been shown in a recent study that neosaxitoxin has a promising long acting profile of local anesthetic effect when compared to bupivacaine for post-operative pain control.[30] Furthermore, future prospects might not be limited to merely prolongation of local anesthetic effect, but could extend to the control of the duration of action of the local anesthetics. For example use of a reversibly acting vasodilator phentolamine mesylate,has been shown to have a safe profile and a promising success in decreasing the duration of local anesthesia in dental practice.[31,32] In a recent clinical study, it was found that phentolamine mesylate has a high rate of acceptance from both the patients and the dentists.[33] Its utility in ophthalmic practice remains to be determined.

REFERENCES

1. Vann MA, Ogunnaike B, Joshi G. Sedation and anesthesia care for ophthalmologic surgery during local/regional anesthesia. Anesthesiology. 2007;107(3):502–8.
2. Grzybowski A. The history of cocaine in medicine and its importance to the discovery of the different forms of anaesthesia. Klin Oczna. 2007; 109 (1-3):101-5.
3. Ang CL, Eong KGA, Tan CSH, Lee SSG, Chan SP. Patients' expectation and experience of visual sensations during phacoemulsification under topical anesthesia. Eye. 2007;21(9):1162–7.
4. Kumar C, Dowd T. Ophthalmic regional anesthesia. Curr Opin Anesthesiol. 2008; 21(5): 632–7.
5. Horton C. Better living through chemistry: Anesthetic pharmacology. In: Anesthesia Crash Course, 1st edn. New York: Oxford University Press. 2009. pp.27–45.
6. Howe JP, Fee JPH. Local anesthetics. In: Pharmacology for anesthesiologists, 1st edn New York: Taylor & Francis; 2005. pp. 79–92.
7. Barash PG, Cullen BF, Stoelting RK, Cahalan MK, Stock MC. Local anesthetics. In: Clinical anesthesia, 6th edn. Philadelphia: Lippincott Williams & Wilkins; 2009. pp. 531–49.
8. Brunton L, Parker K. Local anesthetics. In: Goodman and Gilman's manual of pharmacology and therapeutics, 1st edn. New York: McGraw-Hill. 2007; pp. 241–52.
9. Stoelting RK, Hillier SC. Local anesthetics. In: Handbook of pharmacology and physiology in anesthetic practice, 2nd edn. Philadelphia: Lippincott Williams & Wilkins; 2005. pp. 179–210.
10. Lyle WM, Bobier WR. Effects of topical anesthetics on phenylephrine induced mydriasis. Am J Optom Physiol Opt. 1977;54(5):276–81.
11. Jauregui MJ, Polse KA. Mydriatic effect using phenylephrine and proparacaine. Am J Optom Physiol Opt. 1974;51(8):545–9.
12. Kubo DJ, Wing TW, Polse KA, Jauregui MJ. Mydriatic effect using low concentration of phenylephrine hydrochloride. J Am Optom Assoc. 1975;46(8):817–22.
13. Mordi JA, Lyle WM, Mousa GY. Does prior instillation of topical anesthetic enhances the effect of tropicamide? Am J Optom Physiol Opt. 1986;63(4):290–3.
14. Haddad DE, Rosenfield M, Portello JK, Krumholz DM. Does prior instillation of a topical anesthetic alter the pupillary mydriasis produced by tropicamide (0.5%)? Ophthalmic Physiol Opt. 2007;27(3):311–4.
15. Nwaji ECS, Barrah GHO. The effect of local anesthetics on tear production. J Nigerian Optometric Assoc. 2005;12:27–9.
16. Florence AT, Attwood D. Parenteral routes of drug administration. In: Physicochemical Principles of Pharmacy, 5th edn. London: Pharmaceutical Press. 2011; pp. 389–97.
17. Calvey N, Williams N. Local Anesthetics. In: Principles and Practice of Pharmacology for Anesthetists, 5th edn. Oxford: Blackwell Publishing. 2008; pp. 149–70.
18. Nicoll JMV, Treren B, Acharya PA, Ahlen K, James M. Retrobulbar anesthesia: the role of hyaluronidase. Anaesth Analg. 1986; 65(12):1324–8.
19. Malamed SF. Questions. In: Handbook of Local Anesthesia, 6th edition. Mosby, an imprint of Elsevier Inc. 2013; pp. 383.
20. Simonson D. Retrobular block: a review for the clinicians. AANA J. 1990;58(6):456–61.
21. McGee HT, Fraunfelder FW. Toxicities of topical ophthalmic anesthetics. Expert Opin Drug Saf. 2007;6(6):637–40.
22. Patel M, Fraunfelder FW. Toxicity of topical ophthalmic anesthetics. Expert Opin Drug Metab Toxicol. 2013; 9(8):983-988.
23. Gunaydin B. Hazards of topical ophthalmic drug administration: why do we care? J Br Ophthalmic Anesth Soc. 2008;15:8–13.
24. Pelosini L, Treffene S, Hollick EJ. Antibacterial activity of preservative-free topical anesthetic drops in current use in ophthalmology departments. Cornea. 2009;28(1):58–61.
25. Chelly JE. Single-Injection Peripheral Blocks: Retrobulbar block. In: Peripheral Nerve Blocks:

A Color Atlas, 3rd edn. Lippincott Williams & Wilkins. 2008; pp.173–7.

26. Brown DL. Head and Neck Blocks: Retrobulbar (Peribulbar) Block. In: Atlas of Regional. Anesthesia, 4th edition. Saunders, Elsevier. 2010; pp.171-76.

27. Hadzic A. Chapter 18 Local & Regional Anesthesia for Eye Surgery. In: Textbook of Regional Anesthesia and Acute Pain Management, 1st edn. The McGraw-Hill Companies. 2007.

28. Basta SJ. Chapter 65 Anesthesia for Ophthalmic Surgery. In: Longnecker et al. Anesthesiology. The McGraw-Hill Companies. 2008; pp. 1565-71.

29. Rodríguez-Navarro AJ, Lagos N, Lagos M, Braghetto I, Csendes A, Hamilton J, et al. Neosaxitoxin as a Local Anesthetic: Preliminary Observations from a First Human Trial. Anesthesiology. 2007;106(2):339–45.

30. Rodríguez-Navarro AJ, Berde CB, Wiedmaier G, Mercado A, Garcia C, Iglesias V, et al. Comparison of Neosaxitoxin versus bupivacaine via port infiltration for postoperative analgesia following laparoscopic cholecystectomy: A randomized, double-blind trial. Reg Anesth & Pain Med. 2011; 36(2):103-9.

31. Tavares M, Goodson JM, Studen-Pavlovich D, Yagiela JA, Navalta LA, Rogy S, et al. Soft Tissue anesthesia reversal group. Reversal of soft-tissue local anesthesia with phentolamine mesylate in pediatric patients. J Am Dent Assoc. 2008;139(8):1095–104.

32. Laviola M, McGavin SK, Freer GA, Plancich G, Woodbury SC, Marinkovich S, et al. Randomized Study of phentolamine mesylate for reversal of local anesthesia. J Dent Res. 2008; 87(7):635–9.

33. Saunders TR, Psaltis G, Weston JF, Yanase RR, Rogy SS, Ghalie RG. In-Practice Evaluation of OraVerse® for the reversal of soft-tissue anesthesia after dental procedures. Compend Contin Educ Dent. 2011;32(5):58–62.

CHAPTER 15

Immunomodulators

OVERVIEW

Classically, immunity is defined as the defense mechanism of body that is responsible for prevention of entry and elimination of pathogens and other exogenous agents (dust, pollens, foods, drugs, microbiologic agents, chemicals, and many blood products). In the absence of systematic immune response, contact with antigen can lead to acute or chronic inflammation and tissue damage. In the condition of blood transfusion reactions and organ/tissue graft rejection, immune reactions have been established to be evoked by endogenous homologous tissue antigens. Another category of immune reactions is initiated by self or autologous antigens, and is categorized as autoimmune diseases.

Hypersensitivity reactions are immune responses caused by humoral or cell-mediated immune mechanisms in response to exogenous antigen and usually vary from itching of skin, to bronchial asthma. On the basis of the immunologic mechanism that mediates the disease, hypersensitivity reactions can be further classified as—*Type I* or immediate, *Type II* or antibody-mediated, *Type III* or immune complex-mediated and *Type IV* or cell-mediated.

The cell-mediated hypersensitivity is initiated by antigen-activated T lymphocytes (CD 4^+ and $CD8^+$ T cells) and may manifest as delayed type hypersensitivity reaction or direct cell cytotoxicity. This type of hypersensitivity reaction is commonly seen in rheumatoid arthritis, transplant rejection, tumor immunity, etc. In order to manage Type IV hypersensitivity reactions, immunosuppressive therapy is routinely adopted; the mainstay of which is the drug, cyclosporine (CsA). In addition, drugs such as azathioprine, steroids, rapamycin and mycophenolate mofetil are also used to widen the umbrella of immunomodulation.

OCULAR ALLERGIES

Industrialized countries are witnessing a spate of allergic conditions as about 30% of people are reported to have one or the other form of allergic disease and more importantly, 40–80% of these have allergic symptoms in the eyes.[1] Ocular inflammation is usually a localized allergic condition that manifests as red and itchy eyes, lacrimation that may sometimes be associated with rhinitis. Clinically, conjunctivitis, blepharitis, blepharoconjunctivitis, or keratoconjunctivitis are identified as conditions of ocular inflammation.

In the cascade of events leading to ocular inflammation, two phases have been identified-early and late. In the early phase, the mast cells are activated, and in late phase the inflammatory cells are recruited to the site of inflammation. As part of the first response to allergen insult, the mast cells degranulate to release histamine from intracellular storage sites and at the same time initiate the *de novo* synthesis of other mediators like leukotrienes and prostaglandins. These events can be observed within first fifteen minutes of the antigen attack. Mast cell degranulation also activates vascular endothelial cells and fibroblasts that help to amplify inflammation. Further, in response to the chemotactic factors that are released by mast cells, an accumulation of eosinophils and neutrophils at the site of inflammation can be observed.

Lymphocytes (T and B cells) are also important mediators of allergic reactions and are divided into CD4$^+$ helper T cells (Th) and CD8$^+$ killer T cells (Tk). The antigen-presenting cells (APCs) in the conjunctiva present the antigen to CD4$^+$ T cells, which then initiate the inflammatory reaction.

In most cases of ocular inflammation, normal visual acuity is maintained. But some severe forms of ocular inflammation such as allergic conjunctivitis and vernal keratoconjunctivitis (VKC), may culminate in visual impairment, due to corneal damage or corneal curvature change.

Therefore, the main goal in the management of allergic eye diseases is to reduce inflammation followed by prevention of the associated complications such as vision impairment, dry eye, etc.

Current Immunomodulatory Option for Ocular Allergies

Current drug treatment for ocular allergy focuses on control of inflammation. Conventionally, besides antihistaminics, corticosteroids have been used as the mainstay in the management of ocular allergies. Severe morbidities associated with the use of corticosteroids and their failure to treat the cause of allergy and prevent its recurrence, has become the major limitation and this has lead to development of alternative management modalities. Detailed pharmacology of corticosteroids, antihistaminics and mast cell stabilizers is discussed in Chapters 12 and 13.

The complete bouquet of immunomodulating drugs available for treatment of ocular allergy are subdivided into the following categories based on their specific mechanism of action:
1. Calcineurin inhibitors: CsA, tacrolimus and sirolimus

2. Alkylating agents: Cyclophosphamide and chlorambucil
3. Antimetabolites: Methotrexate, mycophenolate mofetil and azathioprine
4. Viral replication Inhibitors: Human Recombinant Interferon (INFα2a, INFα2b)

These immunomodulating agents provide alternative to corticosteroid-based immunosuppressive therapy. Currently, these agents are also indicated as first-line therapy for the treatment of systemic inflammatory diseases with destructive ocular sequela, e.g. Behçet's disease and granulomatosis with polyangiitis (Wegener's). However, use of systemic immunosuppressive agents has to be carefully monitored in order to derive maximum therapeutic benefit, and minimize the potential side-effects, to afford favorable long-term outcome. In fact, it is now advocated that in cases of therapy-resistant, severe ocular allergies (like conjunctivitis or rhinoconjunctivitis), the immunotherapy should be initiated early so that the quality of life and patient compliance is improved.

CYCLOSPORINE

CsA, a cyclic polypeptide of 11 amino acids, is produced by the fungus *Beauveria nivea*. CsA ophthalmic emulsion (Restasis®, 0.05%) is the only formulation currently approved by the Food and Drug Administration as topical immunomodulator with anti-inflammatory effects for the treatment of dysfunctional tear syndrome and in patients whose tear production is presumed to be suppressed due to ocular inflammation, associated with keratoconjunctivitis sicca. Another topical ophthalmic preparation of CsA (0.1%) is under investigation in Phase II trials for immunomodulator and immunosuppressive action.

Mechanism of Action

CsA has been shown to be effective in suppression of T-cell dependent immune reactions and humoral immunity-mediated ocular allergic inflammation. It mainly acts by suppression of Th2-lymphocyte proliferation, interleukin (IL)-2 and IL-5 production and chemotaxis of eosinophils.

At the outset of inflammatory reaction, when antigen binds to the receptor located on T-cell membrane it leads to increase in intracellular calcium levels (Fig. 15.1). Intracellular calcium stimulates dephosphorylation of Nuclear Factor of Activated T-cells (NFAT), and simultaneously translocates to nucleus. Consequently, transcription of immunoproliferating genes is activated with release of cytokines such as IL-2, IL-5.

On the other hand, CsA exerts immuno-suppressive action by selective inhibition of IL-2 release during T-cell activation. CsA forms a complex with cyclophilin, a cytoplasmic-receptor protein present in target cells (Fig. 15.1). CsA-cyclophilin complex further binds to calcineurin and this complex inhibits Ca^{2+} stimulated dephosphorylation of the cytosolic component of NFAT. As translocation of cytoplasmic dephosphorylated NFAT to the nucleus is required for activation of immunoproliferating gene transcription, the cascade is truncated at this stage leading to failure of T-cell activation in response to specific antigenic stimulation.

Cyclosporine Formulations

CsA is a lipophilic drug and ensuring its absorption into ocular tissues following topical administration is a challenge. Consequently, CsA is formulated for clinical administration using castor oil. In order to increase the therapeutic efficacy of CsA and decrease its adverse effects, various drug development approaches such as preparation of solid formulations, liposomes, micelles, emulsions and microemulsions, microspheres, nanoparticles, and physical or chemical enhancers have been adopted. Another strategy to enhance the penetration of the lipophilic CsA through ocular tissues is the synthesis of a chemically modified pro-drug, which is hydrophilic. This form of CsA is inactive and is transformed into the active form within the tissues and provides efficient delivery of the drug.

Other developments regarding delivery of CsA to ocular tissue include preparation of punctal plug that is composed of Hydroxyl Ethyl Methacrylate (HEMA) and Ethylene Glycol Dimethacrylate (EGDMA).[2]

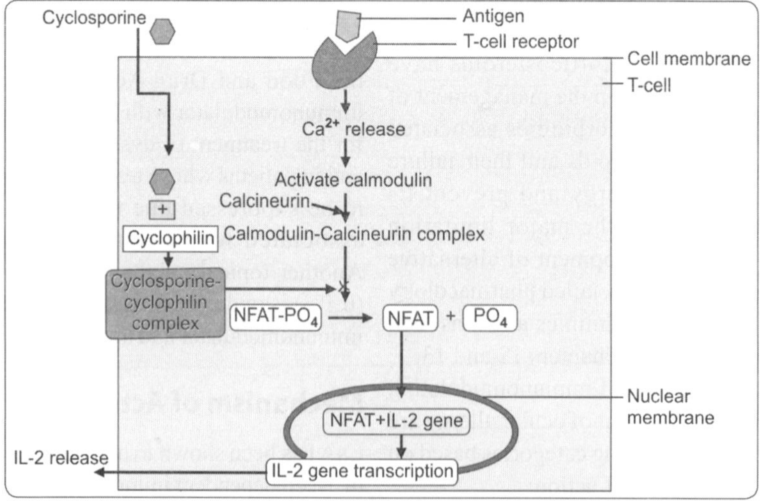

Figure 15.1 CsA—cyclophilin A complex binds to calcineurin to inhibit intracellular signaling process involved in inflammation

Therapeutic Uses

Dry Eye Syndrome

Healthy tears are essential for protecting and nourishing the ocular surface and serve as a protective sheath. However, the condition of dysfunctional tears clinically manifest as Dry Eye Syndrome (DES) that has become a growing problem in urban cities owing to various factors such as pollution, stress, etc. Central to the etiology of DES lies ocular surface inflammation and conventional management includes application of topical anti-inflammatory drugs, on one hand and promoting the secretion of healthy tears on the other. Wide variety of artificial tear formulations containing electrolytes and solutes and having compatible osmolarity, viscosity, preservatives etc., are available. The pharmacology of these therapeutic options is discussed in Chapter 18. Autologous serum eye drops and topical steroids are also used for management of DES but at best provide short-term relief and their chronic use is associated with high risk of complications.

Increasingly, preparations of CsA (0.05%) are finding use as effective treatment of inflammation of ocular surface and moderate-to-severe dry eye. Topical, subconjunctival, and systemic routes have been studied for CsA delivery in the treatment of DES. It acts by inhibiting inflammation of subconjunctival and lacrimal gland, that leads to increase in tear production and conjunctival goblet cell density.[3,4]

Atopic Keratoconjunctivitis (AKC)

Although topical CsA is being used to provide clinical and symptomatic relief in AKC, the basis of this therapy is still under investigation. Limited preliminary data from controlled clinical trials indicates that topical CsA treatment may be efficacious and safe and may help to reduce use of topical steroids in cases with steroid-dependent or resistant AKC.

Adverse Effects and Drug Interactions

The principal adverse reactions to CsA therapy are renal dysfunction, hypertension, tremor, hirsutism, hyperlipidemia and gum hyperplasia.

Sirolimus aggravates CsA-induced renal dysfunction, while CsA increases Sirolimus-induced hyperlipidemia and myelosuppression. This has led to the recommendation that the administration of the two drugs should not be done at the same time.

Tacrolimus

Two calcineurin phosphate inhibitors namely, Tacrolimus (Protopic®, 0.03% and 0.1% ointments) and Pimecrolimus (1% cream) are also available for ophthalmic use. Tacrolimus (FK506) is an 822 kd lipophilic immunosuppressant belonging to the class of macrolides and isolated from a strain of *Streptomyces*. Both these drugs act on T lymphocytes, and bind to macrophilin-12, an intracellular protein. This complex inhibits the phosphorylase enzyme, calcineurin, which prevents translocation of the NFAT. The signaling pathway for NFAT targets specific genes in T cells, including IL-2, 3, 4 and 10, IFN-γ, and granulocyte-macrophage colony-stimulating factor. Topical tacrolimus effectively reduces inflammatory cells like eosinophils in the conjunctiva to control inflammation. In addition, it inhibits the release of histamine from mast cells and reduces prostaglandin synthesis.

Tacrolimus, first used for the treatment of atopic dermatitis, now also finds use in the treatment of atopic blepharoconjunctivitis and other severe ocular inflammatory conditions such as Behcet's disease and uveitis in the dose range of 1–2 mg/day. Tacrolimus ointment provides therapeutic relief in atopic lid eczema without any serious side-effects. It offers the advantage of being more effective than CsA or corticosteroids with less likelihood of side-effects.

Pimecrolimus (Elidel®, 1%), sirolimus, voclosporin are some of the other calcineurin inhibitors that are fast replacing corticosteroids for the management of inflammatory conditions of the eye (Table 15.1).

INTERFERONS

IFNs are natural multifunctional proteins that belong to the cytokine family and are responsible for the innate immunity in humans.

Table 15.1 Immunodulators for ophthalmic use

S No.	Drug	Trade name	Formulation/dosage	Indication
1.	Cyclosporine	Restasias®	Ophthalmic emulsion 0.05%	Keratoconjunctivitis sicca
2.	Tacrolimus	Protopic®	Ointment 0.03% Ointment 0.1%	Vernal keratoconjunctivitis Uveitis Atopic keratoconjunctivitis Postoperative management of trabeculectomy Management of graft rejection Atopic eyelid disease
3.	Pimecrolimus	Elidel®	Suspension 0.3% Suspension 1.0%	Severe keratoconjunctivitis sicca
4.	Voclosporin	LX214	Nanomicelle 0.02% Nanomicelle 0.2%	Dry eye syndrome Uveitis (phase II/III)
5.	Sirolimus	DE109	Liquid formulation— Subconjunctival injection Intravitreal injection	Uveitis (phase I) Diabetic macular edema (phase II)
6.	Azathioprine	Imunran®	Oral	Behçet's disease Multifocal choroiditis
7.	Methotrexate	Rheumatrex® Folex® Mexate® Trexall® Abitrexate®	Oral	Mild to moderate scleritis, Vasculitis
8.	Mycophenolate Mofetil	Cellcept®	Capsule 250 mg, tablet 500 mg, suspension, injection	To prevent organ transplant rejection
9.	Infliximab, Chimeric human-murine antibody to TNF	Remicade®	Intravenous	Under investigation for serious sight-threatening uveitis[7]
10.	Daclizumab, humanized monoclonal antibody to IL-2 receptor	Zenapax®	Intravenous	Under investigation for ophthalmic inflammatory disorders[8]
11.	Anakinra, IL-1 receptor antagonist	Kineret®	100 mg/day, subcutaneous	Under investigation (phase I/II) for Behcet's disease, uveitis[9]
12.	Interferon IFNα2a	Human Recombinant IFNα2a	6 million units, subcutaneous	Viral keratitis Vernal keratoconjunctivitis Behçet's disease[10]

Type I IFNs are produced by almost every cell in the body and impart resistance to host cells against viral infection. On the basis of their amino acid sequence they may be classified as alpha, beta, gamma IFN. Type II IFNs are specifically produced by Natural Killer cells and T-lymphocytes and are responsible for their cytotoxic and anti-proliferative properties.

Mechanism of Action

Interferons are characteristic products of the host cells but function non-specifically against various viruses by inhibiting their replication. IFN bind to cell surface proteins to initiate intracellular signalling pathways resulting in induction of protein kinases and phosphorylation of protein synthesis factors. In addition, enzyme-2′, 5′ oligoadenylate synthetase is also activated, which in turn activates IFN-specific RNAase. This enzyme can cleave viral RNA and inhibit viral replication. Based on this mechanism, IFNs have been implicated with anti-proliferative, immunomodulatory and anti-angiogenic properties and are employed for anti-neoplastic, anti-infective, anti-inflammatory and anti-fibrotic uses in ophthalmology practice.

Adverse Effects

The most common adverse effects associated with systemic IFN therapy are flu-like symptoms, depression, suicidal tendencies and increase in liver enzymes.[5] On topical ocular administration, vision loss, retinopathy and retinal hemorrhage, ischemic optic neuropathy have been reported.[6]

Various immunomodulators including calcineurin inhibitors, corticosteroids, antime-tabolites, biologics and IFN that are marketed or currently under investigation are summarized in Table 15.1 and also find detailed discussion in other chapters in this book.

REFERENCES

1. Kari O, Saari MK. Updates in the treatment of ocular allergies. J Asthma Allergy. 2010;3: 149–58.
2. Sall K, Stevenson OD, Mundorf TK, Reis BL. Two multicenter randomized studies of the efficacy and safety of cyclosporine ophthalmic. emulsion in moderate to severe dry eye disease. Ophthalmology. 2000;107(4):631–9.
3. Wilson SE and Perry HD. Long-term resolution of chronic dry eye symptoms and signs after topical cyclosporine treatment. Ophthalmology. 2007; 114(1):76–9.
4. Yavuz B, Pehlivan SB, Unlu N. An overview on dry eye treatment: approaches for cyclosporin a delivery. The Scientific Journal 2012; Article ID 194848. doi: 10.1100/2012/19848.
5. Stubiger N, Winterhalter S, Pleyer U, et al. Effects and side-effects of interferon therapy in ophthalmology. Ophthalmology. 2011;108(3): 204–12.
6. Hayasaka S, Nagaki Y, Matsumoto M, et al. Interferon associated retinopathy. Br J Ophthalmol. 1998;82: 323–5.
7. Lindstedt EW, Baarsma GS, Kuijpers RWAM, van Hagen PM. Anti-TNF-a therapy for sight threatening uveitis. Br J Ophthalmol 2005; 89:533–6.
8. Papaliodis GN, Chu D, Foster CS. Treatment of ocular inflammatory disorders with daclizumab. Ophthalmology. 2003;110(4):786–9.
9. http://clinicaltrials.gov/show/NCT01441076
10. Gantyala SP, Shekhar H, Vanathi M, Sinha R, Titiyal JS. Interferons in ophthalmology current status and advancing trend. Delhi Journal of Ophthalmology. 2013;23(4):295–7.

CHAPTER 16

Antiglaucoma Drugs

Glaucoma is an optic neuropathy characterized by structural and functional changes in the optic disc. The pathophysiology of glaucoma is multifactorial and involvement of several risk factors has been described. However, currently the management of glaucoma primarily aims to lower intraocular pressure (IOP), which is then expected to arrest the retinal ganglion cell apoptosis. IOP lowering can be achieved by reducing the rate of aqueous humor production, improving its outflow or both. The groups of pharmacological agents used as IOP lowering agents include the following:

1. Cholinomimetic drugs
2. Sympathomimetics and sympathetic blockers
3. Carbonic anhydrase inhibitors
4. Prostaglandin analogs
5. Systemic hyperosmotic agents

CHOLINOMIMETIC DRUGS

Cholinomimetic drugs were the first ones used in the treatment of glaucoma. These drugs mimic the action of acetylcholine (ACh) either because they bind directly with ACh receptors and activate them or they inhibit the enzyme acetylcholinesterase (AChE), which is responsible for degradation of ACh to inactive metabolites.

Neurotransmission in Eye

Both the sympathetic and parasympathetic components of autonomic nervous system innervate the ocular structures. The details of sympathetic and parasympathetic pathways are presented in Chapter 1. ACh is the neurotransmitter at both the sympathetic and parasympathetic preganglionic sites. Most postganglionic parasympathetic fibers are also cholinergic (secrete ACh) except some that utilize nitric oxide or peptides for neurotransmission. Most postganglionic sympathetic fibers are noradrenergic (secrete norepinephrine) but those supplying sweat glands are cholinergic and the ones supplying renal vascular smooth muscles are dopaminergic (secrete dopamine).

Acetylcholine

ACh is synthesized in the cytoplasm of the cholinergic nerves from acetyl-CoA and choline and requires presence of the enzyme, choline acetyltransferase (ChAT). Acetyl-CoA comes from mitochondria in the cell and choline is transported from outside the cell by a sodium-dependent carrier. ACh once synthesized is transported into the vesicles using a transporter. Action potential triggers the influx of Ca^{2+} into the nerve terminal. Increased intracellular Ca^{2+} destabilizes the ACh containing vesicles, which move towards the surface and fuse with the nerve membrane to release their contents into the synapse. The process of release of ACh is blocked by botulinum toxin. Released ACh acts on the cholinergic receptors and is eventually inactivated by AChE, which splits it into choline and acetate (Fig. 16.1). Most

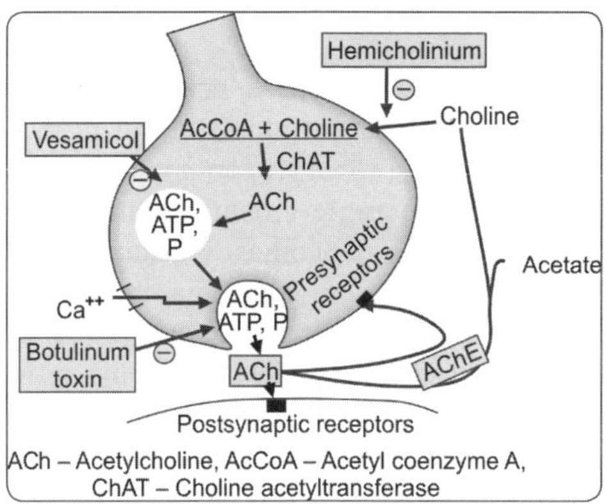

Figure 16.1 Synthesis, storage, release, degradation and action of ACh on presynaptic and postsynaptic neurons

of the cholinergic synapses are richly supplied with AChE. AChE is also present in other tissues like red blood cells. Another cholinesterase, butryl or pseudocholinesterase, which has a low specificity for ACh is present in plasma, liver and many other tissues.

Cholinergic Receptors

Cholinergic receptors are of two types—nicotinic and muscarinic. The subtypes of these cholinergic receptors and their distribution are shown in Table 16.1.

The circular muscle of iris, ciliary muscle and lacrimal glands consist of M_3 muscarinic receptors. Stimulation of muscarinic receptors in the circular muscle of iris results in pupillary constriction. Ciliary muscle contraction causes relaxation of suspensory ligaments of lens, which makes the lens more convex and eye gets accommodated for near vision, an effect known as spasm of accommodation. Ciliary muscle contraction and pupillary constriction widen the angle of eye and pull the scleral spur so as to open the canal of Schlemm more widely. This action facilitates outflow of aqueous humor. Better aqueous humor drainage helps to lower the IOP.

Cholinomimetic Drugs: Classification

The cholinergic drugs used in the treatment of glaucoma are classified in two categories based on their mechanism of action:

1. Direct-acting cholinergic drugs: Pilocarpine, carbachol
2. Indirect-acting cholinergic drugs: Ecothiophate

Table 16.1 Cholinergic receptors—types, subtypes, distribution and intracellular signaling

Receptor types	Nicotinic		Muscarinic		
Receptor sub-types	N_M	N_N	M_1	M_2	M_3
Distribution	Neuromuscular junctions	Autonomic ganglia brain	Sympathetic ganglia Gastric parietal cells Cerebral cortex	Myocardial and smooth muscle cells Presynaptically in peripheral and central neurons	Glands Visceral and vascular smooth muscles, Endothelium
Intracellular signaling	Depolarization of postsynaptic membrane subsequent to opening of Na+, K+ channels	Depolarization of postsynaptic membrane subsequent to opening of Na+, K+ channels	G-protein activation → Formation of IP_3+DAG → Increased intracellular calcium	Opening of K+ channel → Inhibition of adenylyl cyclase	G-protein activation → Formation of IP_3+DAG → Increased intracellular calcium

Pilocarpine

Pilocarpine is an alkaloid derived from the leaves of tropical American shrubs of the genus *Pilocarpus*. It is a direct-acting cholinomimetic drug, i.e. it directly interacts with muscarinic receptors and produces actions similar to ACh. Both the central and peripheral muscarinic receptors are stimulated. The ocular responses to pilocarpine like ACh include miosis, spasm of accommodation and reduction in IOP.[1] Pilocarpine reduces IOP in both the normal and glaucomatous eyes by about 15%.[2] It can be used in combination with other IOP lowering drugs. Pilocarpine hydrochloride 0.25–10% and pilocarpine nitrate 1–4% are available in solution. Use of higher concentration generally does not yield additional advantage; however, patients with pigmented iris may respond poorly and require higher concentrations. Pilocarpine is also available in 4% concentration in gel form. Other preparations of pilocarpine include ocusert Pilo-20 and 40. These are sustained release membrane bound dosage forms, which release pilocarpine at the rate of 20 and 40 µg/hour, respectively.

The frequency of instillation with pilocarpine solutions is usually 4 times a day but if the nasolacrimal occlusion is performed, good IOP control can be maintained with twice a day instillations.[3] Pilocarpine gel 4% is used by applying ½ inch ribbon in the lower conjunctival sac once a day at bedtime. Ocuserts offer the advantage of reduced dosing frequency. The peak IOP lowering appears 2 hours after insertion and lasts for about 7 days. The hypotensive effect of ocusert Pilo-20 equals that of pilocarpine solution 1–2%, four times a day and the effect of ocusert Pilo-40 is equivalent to pilocarpine solution 2–4%, four times a day. Despite the benefit of reduced frequency of dosing, ocusert is rarely used in practice because of its several disadvantages. The main problems of using ocusert are difficulties of insertion and removal, possibility of membrane rupture causing sudden release of excessive quantity of drug, foreign body sensation, unnoticed loss of the device and high cost.

Therapeutic Uses

Among the cholinomimetic drugs, pilocarpine is the most useful antiglaucoma drug in the management of primary open-angle glaucoma (POAG), acute angle-closure glaucoma and many secondary glaucomas. During the acute attack of angle-closure glaucoma, the sphincter muscle of iris is often ischemic due to high IOP. Pilocarpine instillation under such conditions may be ineffective and use of systemic IOP lowering drugs is indicated. Use of pilocarpine has also been described during laser iridotomy to facilitate stretching of iris.[4]

Adverse Effects

Ocular adverse effects

The ocular adverse effects of pilocarpine are significant especially on long-term use and require discontinuation of therapy in large number of patients. The troublesome adverse effects are primarily attributed to ciliary spasm and miosis. Ciliary spasm lasts for 2–3 hours after instillation and is especially troublesome for patients younger than 40 years of age. Older patients generally tolerate it better as the ciliary muscle contractility reduces with age.[5] Miosis interferes with vision especially in patients with nuclear or subcapsular cataract and under dim illumination. Long-term use of pilocarpine causes loss of tone of radial muscle of iris and fibrosis of sphincter muscle resulting in permanent miosis.[6] The actions of pilocarpine also cause forward displacement of iris-lens diaphragm and, therefore, long-term instillation of pilocarpine can cause pupillary block and subsequent angle closure.[7] Forward displacement of iris-lens diaphragm also predisposes to retinal detachment.[8] Long-term use of pilocarpine is also associated with cataract development.[9] Periodic examination of retina and optic disc with pupillary dilatation after discontinuation of pilocarpine helps not only in early detection of drug-related adverse effects but also helps to avoid some of the adverse effects due to sustained pilocarpine action such as permanent miosis.

Other adverse effects of pilocarpine include ciliary and conjunctival congestion, frontal headache and ocular and periorbital pain. These effects are short-lasting and disappear with continued therapy.

Systemic adverse effects

The systemic adverse effects of pilocarpine are rare but with the use of high concentration, systemic symptoms such as salivation, lacrimation, diarrhea and bronchospasm may appear.

Contraindications

Use of pilocarpine is contraindicated in patients younger than 40 years of age and in those with acute angle-closure glaucoma, cataract or history of retinal detachment. Patients with myopia are at high risk of retinal detachment. Pilocarpine should also be avoided in patients with neovascular and uveitic glaucoma and those with history of bronchial asthma.

Carbachol

Carbachol, like pilocarpine, is a direct acting cholinergic drug with same mechanism of action. However, its duration of action is longer than pilocarpine as it is completely resistant to hydrolysis by AChE. It requires 8 hourly instillations but with nasolacrimal occlusion good IOP control can be achieved with twice a day instillation. Carbachol chloride solution is available for topical use in the concentration range of 0.75–3%. Preservative-free carbachol solution is available for intracameral use in 0.1% concentration, of which 0.5 mL is applied by gentle irrigation postoperatively.

Therapeutic Uses

The most common use of carbachol is by intracameral injection in patients undergoing phacoemulsification and posterior chamber lens implantation to induce miosis and achieve better IOP control postoperatively. It can also be used in primary and secondary glaucomas but due to its more severe ocular adverse effects, pilocarpine is a preferred choice among cholinergic drugs.

Adverse Effects and Contraindications

Ocular adverse effects of carbachol are similar to pilocarpine but are more severe. Systemic adverse effects and contraindications are also the same as those of pilocarpine.

Ecothiophate

Ecothiophate is an indirect-acting cholinomimetic drug. It acts by inhibiting the enzyme AChE, thereby increasing the concentration of endogenous ACh. The inhibitors of AChE belong to two categories—reversible inhibitors and irreversible inhibitors. Reversible inhibitors of AChE, like physostigmine, form a complex with AChE, which dissociates quickly to make the enzyme free for its action on ACh. Thus the action of reversible AChE inhibitors is short-lasting. Irreversible AChE inhibitors like ecothiophate make a stable complex with AChE, which dissociates very slowly and, therefore, such drugs have long duration of action. The effects of ecothiophate on iris, ciliary body and IOP are same as that of pilocarpine. After topical application, miosis begins in 10–30 minutes and lasts for 1–4 weeks. Maximum IOP reduction is achieved at 24 hours and lasts for days or weeks. Ecothiophate iodide is available for topical instillation in concentration range of 0.03–0.25%. It is supplied in powder form, which requires reconstitution and storage in refrigerator for stability. Despite its potent action, it is not used in glaucoma due to its severe adverse effects and narrow therapeutic index.

Adverse Effects and Contraindications

Development of cataract is the major ocular complication of ecothiophate. Other ocular adverse effects of ecothiophate are similar to pilocarpine but are more severe. Significant systemic absorption of ecothiophate can cause serious toxicity such as intestinal cramps, hypotension, cardiac arrest, respiratory failure and CNS symptoms. In patients already receiving anticholinesterases, such as in myasthenia gravis, are likely to have serious systemic toxicity. Ecothiophate can prolong the duration of action of succinylcholine by lowering the concentration of plasma pseudocholinesterase, which is required for the breakdown of succinylcholine. Therefore, patients receiving general anesthesia with succinylcholine as muscle relaxant can develop respiratory paralysis. The patients exposed to insecticides may show additive effects causing systemic toxicity.

The contraindications for the use of ecothiophate are same as those of pilocarpine. Drug requires discontinuation several weeks before the general anesthesia with succinylcholine is planned. Similar discontinuation is also required before intraocular surgery to allow time for conjunctival and ciliary congestion to subside before surgery.

SYMPATHOMIMETICS AND SYMPATHETIC BLOCKERS

Adrenergic agonists are the drugs that act by stimulating sympathetic receptor actions or they mimic the action of catecholamines (sympathetic neurotransmitters). Sympathetic blockers are antagonists at sympathetic receptors and act by blocking sympathetic transmission. Three endogenous catecholamines include norepinephrine, epinephrine and dopamine. Norepinephrine is the major neurotransmitter at postganglionic sympathetic sites. Epinephrine is secreted by adrenal medulla. Dopamine is the sympathetic neurotransmitter at various sites in brain and renal blood vessels (Fig. 16.2).

Intraocular sympathetic innervation is primarily restricted to radial muscles of iris. Circular muscles of iris do not receive sympathetic supply. The smooth muscles of eyelids are also supplied by sympathetic nerves. Details of sympathetic innervations of eye are described in Chapter 1.

Catecholamines

Biosynthesis of catecholamines utilizes dietary amino acid L-phenylalanine, which gets oxidized to L-tyrosine in liver. Circulating L-tyrosine is actively taken up by adrenergic neurons. In the neuronal cytoplasm L-tyrosine is hydroxylated to L-dopa by the enzyme tyrosine hydroxylase. This is a rate-limiting step in the synthesis of catecholamines and is inhibited by negative feedback in the presence of sufficient quantities of catecholamine in the nerve terminal. L-dopa is then carboxylated to dopamine in the presence of the enzyme L-amino acid decarboxylase. Dopamine is transported inside the storage vesicles where it undergoes further conversion to norepinephrine by dopamine $-\beta$-hydroxylase. In the adrenal medulla, norepinephrine is converted to epinephrine in the presence of the enzyme phenylethanolamine-N-methyltransferase. Catecholamines are stored in storage vesicles complexed with ATP. An action potential triggers the inflow of Ca^{++} and causes vesicle disruption and release of catecholamines. The action of adrenergic neurotransmitters is terminated primarily by neuronal re-uptake and remaining is metabolized by the enzymes monoamine oxidase (MAO) or catechol-O-methyl transferase (COMT) (Fig 16.2).

Sympathetic Receptors

Released norepinephrine and epinephrine act on sympathetic receptors, which belong to two main categories: alpha (α) receptors and beta (β) receptors. Alpha receptors are of two subtypes i.e. α_1 and α_2 whereas β receptors are of three subtypes i.e. β_1, β_2 and β_3. The distribution of α and β receptors is shown in Table 16.2. All sympathetic receptors are G-protein linked.

α_1 receptors are predominantly located postsynaptically in vascular smooth muscles. The catecholamine actions through postsynaptic

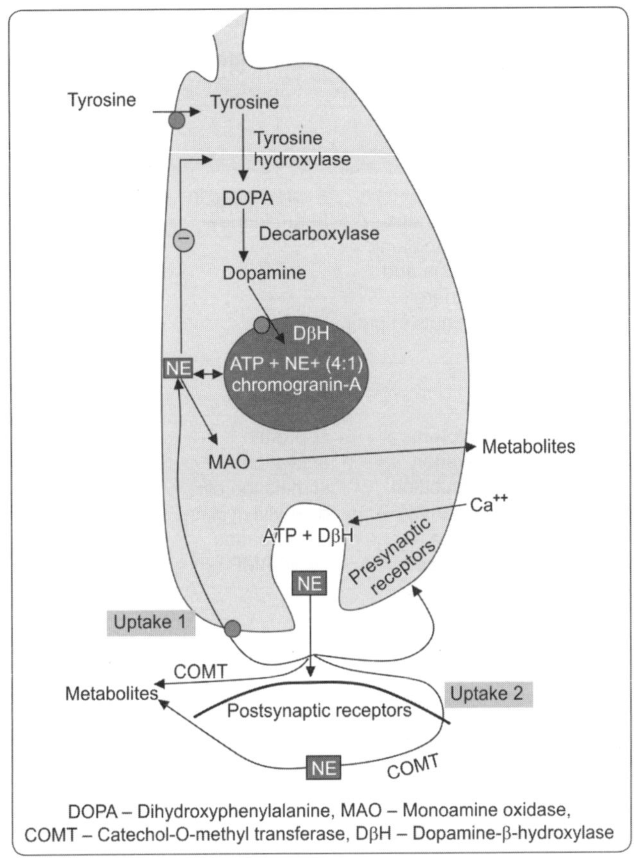

Figure 16.2 Synthesis, storage, release, degradation and action of norepinephrine on presynaptic and postsynaptic neurons

α_1 receptors are mediated through formation of IP_3 and DAG leading to increased intracellular calcium and muscle contraction. α_2 receptors are predominantly presynaptic and mediate their action through inhibition of adenylyl cyclase causing reduced cellular cAMP. This action leads to decreased catecholamine release from presynaptic nerves. The postsynaptic β receptors stimulate adenylyl cyclase and increase cellular cAMP levels.

In eye, α_2 receptors have been identified on the presynaptic sympathetic nerve terminals and postsynaptically in the ciliary body. β_2 receptors are present postsynaptically in ciliary body and upon activation increase the aqueous humor production. β_1 receptors are also said to be present in ciliary body and affect aqueous humor production. Therefore, reduced β receptor activity such as in the presence of β-blockers reduces aqueous humor production and IOP. Presynaptic α_2 receptor activation reduces catecholamine release and henceforth reduces its availability and stimulation of postsynaptic α_2 and β_2 receptors. Besides aqueous humor production, outflow facility and arterial and venous pressure are also modulated by α_2 receptor activity.

Antiglaucoma drugs acting through sympathetic receptors are classified in two categories:

1. Sympathetic agonists

    a. α_2 Agonists: Apraclonidine, brimonidine, dipivefrin

Table 16.2 Sympathetic receptor subtypes, distribution and intracellular signaling mechanisms

Receptor types	Adrenergic receptors				
Receptor sub-types	α_1	α_2	β_1	β_2	β_3
Distribution	Vascular smooth muscles, salivary glands, bronchi, uterus, radial muscle of iris, liver cells	Presynaptic on sympathetic postganglionic neurons and cholinergic terminals in gut Brain	Postsynaptic in heart, kidney	Postsynaptic in bronchi, blood vessels in skeletal muscles, coronaries, uterus, GIT Cardiac muscle	Adipocytes
Intracellular signaling	G-protein activation → Formation of IP_3+DAG → increased intracellular calcium	G-protein activation → inhibition of adenylyl cyclase → decreased cyclic AMP	G-protein activation → stimulation of adenylyl cyclase → increased cyclic AMP	G-protein activation → stimulation of adenylyl cyclase → increased cyclic AMP Activation of cardiac Gi under some conditions	G-protein activation → stimulation of adenylyl cyclase → increased cyclic AMP

2. Sympathetic blockers
   a. Non-selective β-blockers: Timolol, levobunolol, metipranolol, carteolol
   b. β_1-selective blocker: Betaxolol

Apraclonidine

Apraclonidine is a relatively selective α_2 agonist and reduces IOP in both the normal and glaucomatous eyes. Following instillation, the effect appears within 1 hour, reaches peak in about 3–5 hours and lasts for 12 hours. An average of 20% reduction is achieved with both 0.5% and 1.0% solutions.[10] This initial effect on IOP is primarily due to reduced aqueous production.[11] After continued treatment for more than 8 days the IOP reduction is primarily due to improved uveoscleral outflow of aqueous humor.[12] With long-term treatment, the ocular hypotensive effect of apraclonidine reduces due to development of tachyphylaxis. The age, race and color of iris do not affect the IOP lowering by apraclonidine.

Therapeutic Uses

Apraclonidine hydrochloride is available in 0.5 and 1% concentrations. Its 0.5% concentration is used three times a day as short-term add on therapy in patients inadequately controlled with other maximally tolerated medications. Long-term use is not satisfactory due to development of tachyphylaxis. Primary as well as secondary glaucomas respond equally but congenital glaucoma responds poorly. Apraclonidine 1% is used to control postoperative IOP elevation in patients undergoing anterior segment laser surgery and for short-term IOP control in open-angle glaucoma before filtration procedure.

Adverse Effects and Contraindications

Conjunctival blanching, eyelid retraction and mydriasis are the most common side-effects due to α_1 receptor activation. Instillation may be associated with discomfort, burning, itching and dryness. Ocular hypersensitivity reaction can appear specially on long-term use. Systemic absorption is poor because of the poor lipophilicity of the drug and systemic adverse effects, therefore, are dose-dependent. Common systemic adverse effects include dry mouth, dry nose, headache, lethargy, chest heaviness, shortness of breath and taste abnormalities.

Use of apraclonidine is contraindicated in patient on monoamine oxidase inhibitors and those with allergy to clonidine. A cautious use is indicated in patients with hypertension or severe cardiovascular disease.

Brimonidine

Brimonidine is a highly selective α_2 agonist and like apraclonidine reduces IOP in both the normal and glaucomatous eyes. Reduction of IOP by brimonidine occurs by the similar mechanism as apraclonidine, i.e. reduced aqueous production on initial use and improved uveoscleral outflow on prolonged use. Additionally, brimonidine has been shown to provide neuroprotective effect and protects the retinal ganglion cells from apoptosis.[13,14] Brimonidine binds with ocular melanin, which prolongs its half-life. The peak IOP lowering by brimonidine appears 2 hours post-instillation and lasts for 12 hours. A mean IOP reduction by 6.5 mm Hg from baseline has been reported with 0.2% concentration.[15] The IOP lowering effect of 0.2% brimonidine is comparable to 0.5% timolol and is higher than 0.5% betaxolol.[16,17]

Therapeutic Uses

Brimonidine tartrate 1%, two or three times a day is used topically for the treatment of open-angle glaucoma and ocular hypertension. It is also effective in attenuating the IOP spiking after laser trabeculoplasty. Like apraclonidine, it can be used as add on or replacement therapy in patients showing inadequate control with maximally tolerated medical therapy.

Adverse Effects and Contraindications

The most common ocular adverse effects include hyperemia, burning, stinging and foreign body sensation. Ocular allergy may manifest as lid edema, conjunctivitis and conjunctival follicles. Incidence of ocular allergy with brimonidine is much lower as compared to that with apraclonidine. Systemic adverse effects and contraindications are similar to apraclonidine.

Dipivefrin

Dipivefrin is a prodrug, which metabolizes to epinephrine and provides enhanced corneal permeability compared to epinephrine. It acts by stimulating α- and/or β_2-adrenergic receptors resulting in improved uveoscleral outflow. Trabecular outflow is affected to a lesser extent. After topical application, the IOP lowering effect appears in 30 minutes, reaches peak in 1 hour and persists for 12 hours or more.

Therapeutic Uses

Dipivefrin hydrochloride is indicated as initial therapy for controlling IOP in chronic open-angle glaucoma. It is administered twice daily and reduces IOP by 20–24% in 3–5 months.

Therapeutic response to dipivefrin ophthalmic solution twice daily is somewhat less than 2% epinephrine twice daily. Controlled studies showed statistically significant differences in IOP lowering in response to dipivefrin 0.1% and 2% epinephrine. In controlled studies involving patients with a history of epinephrine intolerance, only 3% patients treated with dipivefrin ophthalmic solution exhibited intolerance, while 55% of those treated with epinephrine again developed intolerance.

Therapeutic response to dipivefrin twice daily therapy is comparable to 2% pilocarpine four times daily. Controlled clinical studies comparing dipivefrin ophthalmic solution and 2% pilocarpine, showed no statistically significant differences in the maintenance of IOP levels. Dipivefrin does not produce miosis or accommodative spasm. Night blindness often associated with miotic agents is not associated with dipivefrin therapy. Patients with cataract avoid the inability to see around lenticular opacities caused by constricted pupil.

Adverse Effects and Contraindications

Photosensitivity, conjunctival hyperemia and blephroconjunctivitis are the common ocular adverse effects. Systemic adverse effects such as tachycardia, arrhythmias and hypertension are rare. Use of dipivefrin is contraindicated in patients with angle-closure glaucoma or in patients predisposed to angle closure. Use of dipivefrin requires caution in patients with cardiac diseases.

Timolol

Timolol is a non-selective β-blocker without intrinsic sympathomimetic activity. It acts by reducing aqueous humor production and has no effect on aqueous outflow. The peak IOP lowering appears in about 1 hour post-instillation and lasts for 12 hours. A twice daily instillation is often recommended, however, once daily use has also shown similar efficacy. An IOP reduction of more than 30% has been reported.[18] The maximal efficacy of timolol in concentrations ranging from 0.1–0.5% is similar. But patients with dark iris may require higher concentration to achieve the same effect because of the melanin binding of the drug. The other eye effect due to systemic absorption is significant. The IOP lowering effect of timolol is additive with other IOP lowering drugs. On long-term use 5–10% of the patients per year have been reported to develop tolerance and require additional medications.[19] On discontinuation of therapy, the IOP lowering effect of timolol lasts for up to 2 weeks or longer in patients with dark iris.[20]

Therapeutic Uses

Timolol maleate and timolol hemihydrate are available for topical use in concentration of 0.25 and 0.5%. It is used in the treatment of POAG, ocular hypertension and secondary glaucomas. It is also effective in the prophylactic treatment of IOP elevation due to laser iridotomy or posterior capsulotomy and cataract surgery.

Adverse Effects and Contraindications

Ocular irritation on instillation is not seen frequently, however, local allergic reaction can occur. Allergy manifests as lid edema and conjunctivitis and may require replacement by another beta blocker or a drug from other pharmacological group. Due to the membrane stabilizing properties, beta-blockers produce corneal anesthesia. However, the anesthetic effect of timolol is least among all beta blockers and is not significant clinically. Other ocular adverse effects of timolol include dry eye symptoms and sometimes superficial punctate keratitis.

Significant systemic absorption of timolol can give rise to bradycardia, systemic hypotension, heart block, bronchospasm, diarrhea, lethargy, amnesia, emotional instability and sexual dysfunction. Topical timolol can adversely affect the carbohydrate and lipid metabolism but has not been associated with increased risk of coronary artery disease. The systemic effects are more likely in elderly due to coexisting systemic illnesses and non-compliance.

Timolol is contraindicated in patients with bronchial asthma, chronic obstructive pulmonary disease, bradycardia, congestive cardiac failure, heart block and sensitivity to drug. Topical timolol can mask the symptoms of thyrotoxicosis and hypoglycemia and, therefore, should be used with caution in patients with diseases like diabetes mellitus. In patients already on systemic beta-blocker therapy, drugs from other classes are preferred. Combination of two beta blockers needs to be avoided as it does not increase the effectiveness of the therapy but risk of systemic adverse effects increases.

Levobunolol

Levobunolol, like timolol is a non-selective β blocker without intrinsic sympathomimetic activity but unlike timolol it has no local anesthetic activity. The mechanism of IOP lowering by levobunolol is the same as that of timolol. Levobunolol metabolizes to an equipotent metabolite and has efficacy similar to timolol. The IOP reduction following topical application of levobunolol is similar to timolol in terms of peak effect as well as the duration of action. Both the 0.25 and 0.5% concentrations are equally effective and once daily instillations are as effective as twice daily. Development of tolerance on chronic use is also the same as with timolol.

Therapeutic Uses

Levobunolol hydrochloride is available in 0.25 and 0.5% concentrations. It is used in the treatment of POAG and ocular hypertension. Like timolol it is also effective in the prophylactic treatment of IOP elevation due to laser iridotomy or posterior capsulotomy and cataract surgery.

Adverse Effects and Contraindications

The ocular adverse effects of levobunolol are similar to timolol but it does not produce corneal anesthesia and dry eye symptoms. It can produce allergic blephroconjunctivitis but in patients showing allergy to timolol it can be used as replacement.

The adverse effects due to its systemic absorption and contraindications are same as those with timolol.

Betaxolol

Betaxolol is a β-blocker with relative specificity for β_1 receptors. It reduces IOP by reducing the aqueous humor formation, however, its efficacy in reducing IOP is lower than that of timolol and levobunolol.[21] Additionally, betaxolol has calcium channel blocking action in ocular vasculature as well as retinal ganglion cells. Blockade of calcium channels causes vasorelaxation and improves retinal blood flow.[22] In the retinal ganglion cells betaxolol prevents glutamate-mediated calcium influx and cell death.[23] Thus, betaxolol may possess additional neuroprotective properties.

Therapeutic Uses

Racemic betaxolol hydrochloride (0.25%) suspension is used twice a day topically in the treatment of ocular hypertension and open-angle glaucoma. Due to its relatively specific β_1 effects it is safer in patients with coexisting pulmonary disease, however, its efficacy is less than the non-selective β-blockers. The levo isomer of betaxolol is used as 0.5% suspension and has efficacy similar to timolol maleate 0.5%. It is also less effective in preventing IOP elevations after cataract surgery and is, therefore, not the agent of choice.

Adverse Effects and Contraindications

Ocular irritation and stinging due to instillation is much less with 0.25% concentration but is significant with 0.5% concentration. The effects of systemic β-blockade are significantly less than non-selective β-blockers, however, the IOP control is poorer. The use of betaxolol is contraindicated in patients with sinus bradycardia, heart block, congestive cardiac failure and cardiogenic shock. Although the drug has relatively less effects on pulmonary functions it should be used with caution in patients with bronchial asthma and chronic obstructive pulmonary disease. The drug is also contraindicated for use in patients with hypersensitivity to any of its components.

Metipranolol

Metipranolol is a non-selective β-blocker with no local anesthetic and intrinsic sympathomimetic activity. Like timolol it acts by reducing the aqueous humor formation and its efficacy in reducing IOP is comparable to other non-selective β-blockers.

Therapeutic Uses

Racemic metipranolol hydrochloride 0.1–0.6% is used twice daily in the treatment of ocular hypertension and glaucoma.

Adverse Effects and Contraindications

Topical instillation is associated with allergic blepharoconjunctivitis, uveitis and periorbital dermatitis. The ocular side-effects occur more often with the use of higher concentrations.

The adverse effects due to its systemic absorption and contraindications are same as those with timolol.

Carteolol

Carteolol is a non-selective β-blocker but possesses local anesthetic and intrinsic sympathomimetic activity. It reduces IOP by reducing aqueous humor formation. The IOP lowering efficacy of carteolol 1% is comparable to timolol 0.5%.[24]

Therapeutic Uses

Racemic carteolol hydrochloride 1% is used twice daily in the treatment of ocular hypertension and glaucoma.

Adverse Effects and Contraindications

The ocular irritation due to 1% carteolol is less than 0.5% timolol. Although the systemic adverse effects are same as timolol, due to its intrinsic sympathomimetic activity, effects on pulmonary functions and heart are less pronounced. Contraindications for the use of carteolol are same as those of timolol.

CARBONIC ANHYDRASE INHIBITORS

Carbonic anhydrase inhibitors (CAIs) reduce the IOP by inhibiting the enzyme carbonic anhydrase and reducing aqueous humor production. Carbonic anydrase is one of the key enzymes in aqueous humor production in non-pigmented ciliary epithelium.

In ciliary epithelial cells bicarbonate ions (HCO_3^-), which are the main anions, are generated in the presence of carbonic anhydrase. Carbonic anhydrase catalyzes the reaction of CO_2 with water resulting into the formation of carbonic acid (H_2CO_3), which dissociates quickly into H^+ and HCO_3^-. The sodium ions (Na^+), which are the main cations, are transported into the cells either by diffusion or by Na^+-H^+ exchanger.

Na^+-K^+- ATPase transports Na^+ accompanied with HCO_3^- into the lateral intercellular space. Some chloride ions (Cl^-) are also transported into the lateral intercellular space, however, mechanism of their transport is not known. This movement of ions in the lateral intercellular space creates hypertonicity and attracts water by osmosis. As there are tight junctions between the ciliary epithelial cells on stromal side, the newly formed fluid moves into the posterior chamber.

CAIs reduce the formation of HCO_3^- by inhibiting the activity of CA. Moreover, CAIs alter the intracellular pH, which affects the activity of Na^+-K^+-ATPase and transport of Na^+ is also inhibited. Thus inhibition of CA by CAIs reduces aqueous humor production by reducing transport of Na^+, HCO_3^- and water into the intercellular spaces and subsequently to posterior chamber. The amount of CA present in tissues is much higher than the physiological requirement and, therefore, to inhibit aqueous humor production at least 99% of the enzyme in ciliary processes must be inhibited. This is easily achieved with systemic CAIs and newly developed topical CAIs. CAIs are classified in two categories:

1. Systemic CAIs: Acetazolamide, Methazolamide, Dichlophenamide.
2. Topical: Dorzolamide, Brinzolamide

Acetazolamide

Acetazolamide is administered orally as 125 or 250 mg tablets or 500 mg sustained release capsules. The recommended dose is 250 mg 6 hourly or 500 mg capsule twice a day. The ocular hypotensive effect after oral 250 mg tablet appears in 2 hours and lasts for 6 hours. The effect of sustained release capsule appears in 2 hours and lasts for 6–18 hours. Although the duration of IOP reduction is higher with sustained release preparation, the magnitude of IOP reduction is less as compared to 6-hourly tablets. Acetazolamide is also available for intravenous use in 500 mL vial. After intravenous administration the IOP lowering effect persists for 4 hours.

Acetazolamide is readily absorbed after oral administration and attains peak plasma levels in 2–4 hours. Peak level with 250 mg tablet is maintained for 4-6 hours but up to 10 hours with sustained release preparation. The peak levels achieved with sustained release are lower than that with tablets. Acetazolamide is extensively bound to plasma proteins (90–95%) and the free form is in unionized form, which can easily penetrate through cell membranes. It is not metabolized and is excreted unchanged in urine by tubular secretion. Because of its renal action, acetazolamide promotes HCO_3^- excretion in urine and makes it alkaline. Alkaline pH keeps acetazolamide in ionized form and favors its excretion.

Therapeutic Uses

Acetazolamide is used as an add on therapy in the treatment of POAG when topical drugs provide insufficient control of IOP. In combination with timolol, the IOP lowering effect is additive as both the drugs act by reducing aqueous humor production. Timolol does not reduce nocturnal aqueous humor production but acetazolamide can reduce it by 24%. Therefore, the bed-time instillation of timolol is not required and it is added to as day time instillation. Topically used CAIs are now preferred over acetazolamide due to low risk of adverse effects. In the treatment of acute angle-closure glaucoma acetazolamide is used preoperatively along with timolol. In such condition, acetazolamide can be administered intravenously especially if the patient is not able to take orally due to vomiting.

Adverse Effects

Although, the incidence of adverse effects varies with dose and formulation, intolerable adverse effects are experienced by up to 80% of the patients and tolerability is often poor. The most common but tolerable adverse effects

are tingling and numbness in fingers, toes and perioral region and metallic taste. On prolonged use a symptom complex characterized by malaise, fatigue, weight loss, depression, anorexia and loss of libido may appear.[25] Oral acetazolamide can also cause cramps, nausea and diarrhea due to gastrointestinal irritation. In kidney, acetazolamide prevents HCO_3^- excretion and, therefore, causes alkaline urine and metabolic acidosis. Besides, excretion of citrate is also inhibited. Low citrate and alkaline pH of urine favor calcium phosphate precipitation in urine. Acetazolamide can also cause blood dyscrasias such as thrombocytopenia, agranulocytosis and aplastic anemia. Myopic shift in refractive error may also occur.

Contraindications

Acetazolamide is unsubstituted aromatic sulfonamide. Although, its structure significantly differs from the antibacterial sulfonamides, hypersensitivity reactions have been reported. Therefore, in patients with history of hypersensitivity to sulfonamides, acetazolamide should be avoided. It should also be used with caution in patients with impaired renal and hepatic functions. In presence of renal failure the drug may accumulate in plasma as it is excreted unchanged in urine. Alkaline pH of urine caused by acetazolamide prevents excretion on NH_4^+ and thus can significantly increase ammonia levels in patients with impaired hepatic function. Patients with diabetic nephropathy can develop serious acidosis. Acetazolamide should also be avoided in patients with chronic obstructive pulmonary disease as the acid-base imbalance can precipitate acute respiratory failure. In patients with significant outflow obstruction, CAIs are not as useful because they act by decreasing the aqueous humor production without any effect on outflow. Moreover, the production reduces only by 45–55%, which may not be enough to reduce IOP. Acetazolamide should also be avoided in pregnant.

Acetazolamide induced hypokalemia is exaggerated if the patient is also taking a thiazide diuretic. Digitalis toxicity may be precipitated in presence of hypokalemia. The alkalinization of urine by acetazolamide increases tubular reabsorption of some drugs like tricyclic antidepressants, quinidine and amphetamine. Consequently, the action of these drugs is prolonged. Concurrent use of aspirin and acetazolamide increases serum levels of unionized salicylic acid.

Methazolamide

Methazolamide structurally resembles acetazolamide. However, its efficacy in reducing IOP is achieved at 100 mg dose compared to 250 mg of acetazolamide. The peak levels of methazolamide are maintained for 8 hours as compared to 4–6 hours with acetazolamide. The half-life of methazolamide is 14 hours as compared to 5 hours of acetazolamide.

Dichlophenamide

Dichlophenamide is also an orally administered carbonic anhydrase inhibitor. Its pharmacological actions are similar to acetazolamide, however, the diuresis persists even after long-term use and hypokalemia is more likely. The drug has clinical use limited to patients not able to tolerate acetazolamide and methazolamide.

Dorzolamide

Dorzolamide is a topically administered carbonic anhydrase inhibitor. It reduces the rate of aqueous humor secretion by inhibiting the isoenzyme II in the ciliary processes. It also inhibits membrane-bound isoenzyme IV. The effect of dorzolamide on aqueous humor secretion is less as compared to acetazolamide, due to incomplete inhibition of the enzyme isoforms. The peak IOP reduction occurs 2 hours post-instillation. When instilled 3 times a day, 2% concentration produces an IOP reduction of 22–26%.[26] The night time aqueous humor secretion is inhibited more effectively with topical carbonic anhydrase inhibitors as compared to timolol. Dorzolamide has additive effect with timolol.[27]

Therapeutic Uses

Dorzolamide 2% is used three times a day for IOP reduction in patients with ocular hypertension and open angle glaucoma. It can be used as monotherapy or in combination with other IOP lowering drugs. Topical carbonic anhydrase inhibitors do not reduce IOP as effectively as systemic drugs, therefore, their use is limited to management of chronic glaucoma. It is also effective in the prophylactic treatment of IOP spiking after YAG laser capsulotomy, argon laser trabeculoplasty or laser iridotomy.

Adverse Effects and Contraindications

The most common ocular adverse effects following topical instillation include stinging, burning, foreign body sensation and blurred vision. Dorzolamide 2% solution has a pH of 5.6 and, therefore, the local irritation is possibly related to the acidic pH. Topical dorzolamide can also cause local allergic reactions involving lids and conjunctiva. Dorzolamide also inhibits carbonic anhydrase II in corneal endothelium and, therefore, can cause corneal edema and decompensation specially in patients who have undergone intraocular surgery.[28] Although topical dorzolamide does not cause significant systemic adverse effects, its concomitant administration with systemic carbonic anhydrase inhibitors is not recommended. Safety of dorzolamide in children and pregnant is not established. It should also be avoided in patients with history of allergy to sulfonamides.

Brinzolamide

Brinzolamide, like dorzolamide, is a topically administered carbonic anhydrase inhibitor. Its action on carbonic anhydrase and effect on aqueous humor secretions are same as those of dorzolamide. The extent of IOP reduction is comparable to dorzolamide. It causes less ocular irritation as compared to dorzolamide. Therapeutic uses, adverse effects and contraindications for brinzolamide are same as those of dorzolamide.

PROSTAGLANDIN ANALOGS

Prostaglandins used topically in the treatment of glaucoma are $PGF_{2\alpha}$ analogs. Prosatglandin analogs lower the IOP by increasing the aqueous outflow exclusively through uveoscleral pathway.[29] The action of $PGF_{2\alpha}$ analogs is mediated through activation of prostanoid FP receptors, which are located in the ciliary muscle, circular muscle of iris and aqueous outflow pathways. FP receptor stimulation is associated with substantial extracellular matrix remodeling and reduced collagen in the ciliary muscle and adjacent sclera secondary to activation of matrix degrading metalloproteinases. This action leads to reduced resistance to the outflow of aqueous humor.[30,31]

Latanoprost

Latanoprost was the first prostagladin used in the treatment of glaucoma. The peak IOP lowering effect of latanoprost appears 8 hours post-instillation and persists for 12–24 hours. Therefore, only once a day instillation is required. When instilled at bedtime, it provides effective IOP control throughout the day with minimal diurnal variations. Once a day latanoprost reduces IOP by about 27%, which is higher than the IOP lowering by timolol 0.5% twice a day.[32,33] Thus the patients showing inadequate IOP control with timolol monotherapy can be switched to latanoprost monotherapy to achieve higher IOP reduction. Moreover, due to its unique mechanism of action, it has additive effect when used in conjunction with other IOP lowering drugs such as timolol, pilocarpine, acetazolamide. Latanoprost, by virtue of its higher efficacy, once daily dosing, absence of systemic toxicity and excellent tolerability, is now considered as the first line drug in the treatment of glaucoma.

Therapeutic Uses

Latanoprost 0.005% is used once a day in the evening or bedtime in the treatment of ocular hypertension and POAG. The IOP lowering by latanoprost in pigmentary glaucoma is higher than that caused by timolol. It is also effective for IOP reduction in patients with normal tension glaucoma.

Adverse Effects and Contraindications

Latanoprost on continued use causes increased melanin accumulation in the iridial melanocytes, which is evidenced by darkening or iris color. This change is observed in 5–20% of patients and those with mixed color irides. The change is permanent and takes 4 weeks to several months to appear. Skin of eyelids can also show increased pigmentation. Prolonged latanoprost treatment also stimulates cell division and growth leading to hypertrichosis. The eyelashes become thick, long and dark. Eyelashes can also grow in areas adjoining the normal eyelash distribution. The change is especially noticeable in patients using latanoprost unilaterally. Conjunctival hyperemia has been reported in approximately one-third of the treated patients. Allergy to latanoprost may require discontinuation of treatment. Punctate epithelial corneal erosions and pseudodendritic corneal lesions resembling herpes simplex virus (HSV) infection have been reported in patients using latanoprost. Such changes can be attributed to the preservative used in the formulation rather than the latanoprost itself. Being a prostaglandin, latanoprost has been suggested to increase blood aqueous and blood-retinal barrier permeability leading to uveitis and cystoid macular edema (CME) respectively. However, such associations have not been confirmed in patients on long-term latanoprost treatment. Latanoprost has no significant systemic adverse effects.

Use of latanoprost is contraindicated in patients with history of HSV keratitis, uveitis, CME, pervious intraocular surgery especially with vitreous loss and diabetes mellitus. The risk of iris pigmentation and hypertrichosis must be explained especially to patients intending unilateral use.

Unoprostone

Unoprostone is a derivative of $PGF_{2\alpha}$ metabolite. The extent of IOP reduction and its duration is less than latanoprost. Unoprostone has been shown to improve blood flow in the optic nerve head, retina and choroid by antagonizing the endothelin-1 induced vasospasm. It is, therefore, especially useful in improving optic nerve circulation in patients with vasospasm.

Therapeutic Uses

Unoprostone isopropyl l0.12% is used twice a day in the treatment of ocular hypertension and POAG and is as efficacious as timolol 0.5% twice a day. Unoprostone also reduces IOP significantly in patients with normal tension glaucoma.

Adverse Effects and Contraindications

Prolonged use of unoprostone has not been shown to cause iris pigmentation as is the case with latanoprost. However, corneal surface abnormalities have been reported. Like latanoprost, it has no systemic adverse effects. Contraindications for its use are also the same as for latanoprost. Additionally, it should be used carefully in patients with dry eyes and in combination of other topical drugs that are likely to cause corneal epithelial damage.

Travoprost

Travoprost is a newer $PGF_{2\alpha}$ analog that produces significant IOP lowering with once daily instillation. It is most effective at 0.004% concentration. It is used in ocular hypertension, POAG and normal tension glaucoma.

Its adverse effects are generally mild and contraindications are same as those for latanoprost.

Bimatoprost

Bimatoprost 0.03% reduces IOP in patients with open-angle glaucoma. It should not be administered more than once daily as the IOP lowering effect may reduce when administered more frequently. Pressure starts reducing at about 4 hours post-instillation and a maximum effect is seen within 8 to 12 hours.

Its adverse effects and contraindications are the same as latanoprost.

Ocular Hypotensive Lipids

Ocular hypotensive lipids are also $PGF_{2\alpha}$ derivatives obtained by substituting carboxylic acid moiety with neutral substitutes. They do not act on prostanoid receptors but at a concentration of 0.01%, reduce the IOP as effectively as latanoprost 0.001%. This novel groups of compounds has shown promising results.

SYSTEMIC HYPEROSMOTIC AGENTS

Systemically administered hyperosmotic agents are especially useful in the management of acute angle closure glaucoma and for IOP control before intraocular surgery. One of the examples is glycerin. Oral form of glycerin creates osmotic gradient between plasma and ocular fluids and reduces IOP.

Ophthalmic use of 1 to 2 drops of glycerol reduces edema and removes the corneal haze by attracting water through semipermeable corneal epithelium so that the ophthalmoscopic and goniosopic examination becomes easy in patients with acute glaucoma. The detailed pharmacology of hyperosmotic agents is described in Chapter 19 (A).

RECENT ADVANCES IN PHARMACOTHERAPY OF GLAUCOMA

Recent advances in glaucoma are directed towards the better understanding of the pathways involved in retinal ganglion cell apoptosis, identification of therapeutic targets and, accordingly, development of therapeutic agents. Elevated IOP is only one of the risk factors for glaucoma and the hallmark of the disease, loss of retinal ganglion cells, is also observed in patients with normal IOP. Despite this fact, current pharmacotherapeutic approaches primarily focus on lowering the IOP. Studies are now being focused to explore the agents, which along with reducing the IOP can provide neuroprotection.

Use of neuroprotective drugs for the treatment of certain neurodegenerative disorders of the CNS such as Alzheimer's and Parkinson's disease led to the hypothesis of using neurotrophic (neuron survival) agents for the maintenance of normal vision in glaucoma.[34,35] Loss of neurotrophin function in retinal ganglion cells may be a contributing factor in the development of glaucomatous optic neuropathy. Acute IOP elevation has previously been shown to obstruct retrograde axonal transport in experimental glaucoma.[36] Receptors (TrkB) for brain derived neurotrophic factor (BDNF) have also been detected on retinal ganglion cells. In animal models of glaucoma with acute elevation of IOP, retrograde transport of target-derived BDNF to the retina was found to be decreased. After BDNF administration increased survival of ganglion cell axons was observed.[35,37-38] Studies have shown that Lentiviral transduced BDNF-producing mesenchymal stem cells can survive in eyes with chronic hypertension and can provide retina and optic nerve functional and structural protection. Therefore, transplantation of BDNF producing stem cells may be a viable treatment strategy for glaucoma.[39] Ciliary neurotrophic factor (CNTF) injected into the eyes of rats with increased IOP has also been shown to reduce apoptosis. Clinical trials are being undertaken using CNTF after observing its efficacy and safety in preclinical studies.[35] Efficacy of neurotrophic agents has also been observed in photoreceptor degenerations and similar neuropathies. Their safety and efficacy needs evaluation in preclinical glaucoma models. Clinical trials using BDNF in glaucoma may provide useful results. Drug delivery system like encapsulated cell technology is available and effective and should be considered for use in glaucoma.[35]

Another possible therapeutic agent in glaucoma is pigment epithelium-derived factor (PEDF).[40] Transfected PEDF is protective for ganglion cells in mouse glaucoma model as it showed anti-inflammatory effects in preserving ganglion cells.[41] It could possibly be useful in neovascular glaucoma and may protect from gliosis.

Brimonidine, an IOP-lowering agent has been reported to be a ganglion cell neuroprotectant.[42] Muscarinic receptors may also be good therapeutic targets for neuroprotection in glaucoma, as has been demonstrated using galantamine that activates M_1 and M_4 muscarinic receptors.[43] Alpha 2-macroglobulin has also been investigated as a target in ganglion cell neuroprotection.[44]

Role of glutamate-mediated excitotoxicity in retinal ganglion cell apoptosis has been investigated widely. Glutamate, a major excitatory neurotransmitter in the CNS and retina, is released by the presynaptic cells and acts on N-methyl-D-aspartate (NMDA), α-amino-3-hydroxy-5-methyl-4-isoxazolepropionic acid (AMPA), and kainite (KA) receptors.[45] Excessive amounts of glutamate results in excitotoxic neuronal death mainly mediated through NMDA receptors in retinal ganglion cells. Vitreal glutamate levels are increased in primary glaucoma. Fang et al. showed that bis(7)-tacrine had neuroprotective effects against glutamate-induced RGCs damage both *in vitro* and *in vivo*, possibly through the drug's anti-NMDA receptor effects. Therefore, it may potentially be useful for treating ischemic/traumatic retinopathies inclusive of glaucoma.[45]

High glutamate levels result in increased inflow of Ca^{2+} in ganglion cells. Ca^{2+}-dependent intracellular mechanisms that finally activate caspases underlie the pathological progression of neurodegeneration in glaucoma. Calcium channel blockers have been investigated for preventing apoptotic neuronal loss in glaucoma and caspase inhibitor nipradilol has shown antiapototic effects on retinal ganglion cells.[46-47]

Free radicals such as nitric oxide (NO) have also been shown to play a significant role in retinal ganglion cell loss by disrupting mitochondrial function, degrading DNA and causing apoptosis. Neufeld, et al. supported the theory that NO can cause neurotoxicity in the optic nerve head of patients with POAG.[48] Experiments using NO-inhibitors showed neuroprotection in animal models.[49] Levels of NO and endothelin-1 are increased in the aqueous humor of POAG patients and in patients with chronic closed-angle glaucoma.[50] A new compound comprising latanoprost and NO-donating moiety (NCX 125, BOL-303259-X) was synthesized and it was found to successfully lower IOP in rabbit, dog, and primate models of glaucoma. This compound is reportedly entering clinical trial.[51] Age-Related Eye Disease Study (AREDS) with a selected subset of antioxidative agents showed that antioxidants have neuroprotective effects by slowing down the disease progression. Several other antioxidant trials have been completed or are in progress. It is probable that antioxidants would be effective in slowing down the ganglion cell death.

Activation and proliferation of glial cells possibly significantly contributes to glaucomatous ganglion cell death.[52] Minocycline treatment has been shown to reduce retinal microglia activation and improvement in optic nerve integrity in mouse model.[53]

Several studies using herbal drugs have also shown promising results in lowering the elevated IOP in animal models. These plants were chosen on the basis of their antioxidant, anti-inflammatory, antihypertensive, antiangiogenic activities. These herbal formulations have not shown any side-effects in animal models of glaucoma and may have potential as antiglaucoma agents.[54-55] The clinical trials on herbal formulations are warranted.

REFERENCES

1. Taylor P. Cholinergic agonists. In Gillman AG, Rall TW, Nies AS, Taylor P. (eds). Goodman and Gillman's The pharmacological basis of therapeutics. New York: Pergamon Press, 1990; pp. 122–30.

2. Krill AE, Newell FN. Effects of pilocarpine on ocular tension dynamics. Am J Ophthalmol. 1964;57:34-41.

3. Zimmerman TJ, Sharir M, Nardin GF, Fuqua M. Therapeutic index of pilocarpine, carbachol and timolol with nasolacrimal occlusion. Am J Ophthalmol. 1992;114:1–7.

4. Fernandez-Bahamonde JL, Alcaraz-Michelli V. The combined use of apraclonidine and pilocarpine during laser iridotomy in a Hispanic population. Ann Ophthalmol. 1990;22(12):446–9.

5. Croft MA, Oyen MJ, Gange SJ, et al. Aging effects on accommodation and outflow facility responses to pilocarpine in humans. Arch Ophthalmol. 1996;114(5):586–92.

6. Chen HS, Steinmann WC, Spaeth GL. The effects of chronic miotic therapy on the result of posterior chamber intraocular lens implantation and trabeculectomy in patients with glaucoma. Ophthalmic Surg. 1989;20(11):784–8.

7. Van Buskirk EM. Hazards of medical glaucoma therapy in the cataract patient. Ophthalmology. 1982;89(3):238–41.

8. Weseley P, Leibmann J, Ritch R. Rhegmatogenous retinal detachment after initiation of ocusert therapy. Am J Ophthalmol. 1991;112(4):458–9.

9. Zimmerman TJ. Pilocarpine. Ophthalmology. 1981;88(1):85–8.

10. Araujo SV, Bond JB, Wilson RP, M R Moster, C M Schmidt, Jr, and G L Spaeth. Long-term effects of apraclonidine. Br J Ophthalmol. 1995;79(12):1098–101.

11. Koskela T, Bribaker RF. Apraclonidine and timolol combined effects in previously untreated normal subjects. Arch Ophthalmol. 1991;109(6):604–8.

12. Toris CB, Tafoya ME, Camras CB, Yablonski ME. Effect of apraclonidine on aqueous humor dynamics in human eyes. Ophthalmology. 1995;102(3):456–61.

13. Yoles E, Muler S, Schwartz M. Injury-induced secondary degeneration of rat optic nerve can be attenuated by alpha-2 adrenoreceptor agonist AGN 191103 and brimonidine. Invest Ophthalmol Vis Sci. 1996;3(Suppl.):S114.

14. Wheeler LA, Lai R, Woldemusie E. From the lab to the clinic: activation of an alpha-2 agonist pathway is neuroprotective in models of retinal and optic nerve injury. Eur J Ophthalmol. 1999;9(1):S17–S21.

15. Schuman JS, Horowitz B, Choplin NT, David R, Albracht D, Chen K. A 1-year study of brimonidine twice daily in glaucoma and ocular hypertension. Arch Ophthalmol. 1997;115(7):847–52.

16. Katz LJ. Brimonidine tartrate 0.2% twice daily versus timolol 0.5%twice daily: 1-year results in glaucoma patients. Brimonidine Study Group. Am J Ophthalmol. 1999;127(1):20–6.

17. Serle JB, The Brimonidine Study Group III. A comparison of the safety and efficacy of twice daily brimonidine 0.2%versus betaxolol 0.25% in subjects with elevated intraocular pressure. Surv Ophthalmol. 1996;41(Sppl. 1):S39–S47.

18. Zimmerman TJ, Kaufman HE. Timolol: dose response and duration of action. Arch Ophthalmol. 1977;95(4):605–7.

19. Levobunolol Study Group. Levobunolol: a four-year study of efficacy and safety in glaucoma treatment. Ophthalmology. 1989;96(5):642–5.

20. Silverstone DE, Arkfeld D, Cowan G, Lue JC, Novack GD. Long-term diurnal control of intraocular pressure with levobunolol and with timolol. Glaucoma. 1985;7:138–40.

21. Coulangeon LM, Sole M, Menerath JM, Sole P. Aqueous humor flow measured by fluorophotometry. A comparative study of the effect of various beta-blocker eyedrops in patients with ocular hypertension. Ophthalmology. 1990;4(2):156–61.

22. Yu DY, Su EN, Cringle SJ, Alder VA, Yu PK, DeSantis L. Systemic and ocular vascular roles of the antiglaucoma agents beta-adrenergic agonists and Ca2+ entry blockers. Surv Ophthalmol. 1999;43(Suppl 1):S214–S22.

23. Hirooka K, Kelly ME. Baldridge WH, Barnes S. Suppressive actions of betaxololon ionic currents in retinal ganglion cells may explain its neuroprotective effects. Exp Eye Res. 2000;70(5):611–21.

24. Stewart WC, Cohen JS, Netland PA, Weiss H, Nussbaum LL. Efficacy of carteolol hydrochloride 1% vs timolol 0.5% in patients with increased intraocular pressure. Am J Ophthalmol. 1997;124(4):498–505.

25. Epstein DL, Grant WM. Carbonic anhydrase inhibitor side effects. Serum chemical analysis. Arch Ophthamol. 1977;95(8):1378–82.

26. Lippa EA, Carlson LE, Ehinger B, et al. Dose response and duration of action of dorzolamide, a topical carbonic anhydrase inhibitor. Arch Ophthalmol. 1992;110(4):495–9.

27. Adamsons I, Clineschmidt C, Polis A, Taylor J, Shedden A, Laibovitz R. The efficacy and safety of dorzolamide as adjunctive therapy to timolol maleate gellan solution in patients with elevated intraocular pressure. J Glaucoma. 1998;7(4):253–60.

28. Konowal A, Morrison JC, Brown SV, Cooke DL, Maguire LJ, Verdier DV, et al. Irreversible corneal decompensation in patients treated with topical dorzolamide. Am J Ophthalmol. 1999;127(4):403–6.

29. Lindsey JD, Kashiwagi K, Kashiwagi F, Weinreb RN. Prostaglandins alter extracellular matrix adjacent to human ciliary muscle cells in vitro. Invest Ophthalmol Vis Sci. 1997;38(11):2214–23.

30. Sagara T, Gaton DD, Lindsey JD, Gabelt BT, Kaufman PL, Weinreb RN. Topical prostaglandin F2 treatment reduces collagen I, III and IV in the monkey uveoscleral outflow pathway. Arch Ophthalmol. 1999;117(6):794–801.

31. Weinreb RN, Kashiwagi K, Kashiwagi F, Tsukahara S, Lindsey JD. Prostaglandins increase matrix metalloproteinase release from human ciliary smooth muscle cells. Invest Ophthalmol Vis Sci. 1997;38:2772–80.

32. Mishima HK, Masuda K, Kitazawa Y, Azuma I, Araie M. A comparison of latanoprost and timolol in primary open angle glaucoma and ocular hypertension. A 12 week study. Arch Ophthalmol. 1996;114(8):929–32.

33. Camras CB and the United States Latanoprost Study Group. Comparison of latanoprost and timol in patients with ocular hypertension and glaucoma. A six-month, masked, multicenter trial in the United States. Ophthalmology. 1996;103(1):138–47.

34. Nilforushan N. Neuroprotection in glaucoma. J Ophthalmic Vis Res. 2012;7(1):91–3.

35. Chader GJ. Advances in glaucoma treatment and management: Neurotrophic agents. Invest Ophthalmol Vis Sci. 2012;53(5):2501–5.

36. Howell G, Macalinao D, Sousa G, et al. Molecular clustering identifies complement and endothelin induction as early events in a mouse model of glaucoma. J Clin Invest. 2011;121:1429–44.

37. Martin KR, Quigley HA, Zack DJ, et al. Gene therapy with brain derived neurotrophic factor as a protection: retinal ganglion cells in a rat glaucoma model. Invest Ophthalmol Vis Sci. 2003;44: 4357–65.

38. LaVail MM, Unoki K, Yasumura D, Matthes MT, Yancopoulos GD, Steinberg RH. Multiple growth factors, cytokines, and neurotrophins rescue photoreceptors from the damaging effects of constant light. Proc Natl Acad Sci. USA. 1992;89:11249–53.

39. Harper M, Grozdanic S, Blits B, et al. Transplantation of BDNF secreting mesenchymal stem cells provides neuroprotection in chronically hypertensive rat eyes. Invest Ophthalmol Vis Sci. 2011;52:4506–15.

40. Miyazaki M, Ikeda Y, Yonemitsu Y, et al. Pigment epithelium derived factor gene therapy targeting retinal ganglion cell injuries: neuroprotection against loss of function in two animal models. Hum Gene Ther. 2011;22:559–65.

41. Zhou X, Kong L, Chodosh J, Cao W. Anti-inflammatory effect of PEDF in DBA/2J mice. Mol Vis. 2009;15:438–50.

42. Lambert W, Ruiz L, Wheeler L, Calkins D. Brimonidine prevents axonal and somatic degeneration of retinal ganglion cell neuron. Mol Neurodegener. 2011;13:6.

43 Almasieh M, Kelly M, Casanova C, Di Polo A. Structural and functional neuroprotection in glaucoma: role of galantamine-mediated activation of muscarinic ACh receptors. Cell Death Dis. 2010;1:e27

44. Bai Y, Sivori D, Woo SB, Neet KE, Lerner SF, et al. During glaucoma, alpha-2-macroglobulin accumulates in aqueous humor and binds to nerve growth factor neutralizing neuroprotection. Invest Ophthalmol Vis Sci. 2011;52:5260–5.

45. Fang JH, Wang XH, Xu ZR, Jiang FG. Neuroprotective effects of bis(7)-tacrine against glutamate-induced retinal ganglion cell damage. BMC Neurosci. 2010;11:31–40.

46. Crish SD, Calkins DJ. Neurodegeneration in glaucoma: progression and calcium-dependent intracellular mechanisms. Neuroscience. 2011; 176:1–11.

47. Mavlyutov TA, Nickells R, Guo L. Accelerated retinal ganglion cell death in mice deficient in the Sigma-1 receptor. Mol Vis. 2011;17:1034–43.

48. Neufeld AH. Nitric oxide: a potential mediator of retinal ganglion cell damage in glaucoma. Surv Ophthalmol. 1999;43(Suppl 1):S129–S35.

49. Neufeld AH, Das S, Vora S, Gachie E, Kawai S, Manning PT, Connor JR. A Prodrug of a selective inhibitor of inducible nitric oxide synthase is neuroprotective in the rat model of glaucoma. J Glaucoma. 2002;11(3):221–5.

50. Ghanem AA, Elewa AM, Arafa LF. Endothelin-1 and nitric oxide levels in patients with glaucoma. Ophthalmic Res. 2011;46:98–102.

51. Borghi V, Bastia E, Guzzetta M, et al. A novel nitric oxide releasing prostaglandin analog, NCX 125, reduces intraocular pressure in rabbit, dog and primate models of glaucoma. J Ocul Pharmacol Ther. 2010;26:125–32.

52. Ganesh BS, Chintala SK. Inhibition of reactive gliosis attenuates excitotoxicity-mediated death of retinal ganglion cells. PLoS One. 2011;6:e18305.

53 Bosco A, Inman D, Steele M, et al. Reduced retina microglial activation and improved optic nerve integrity with minocycline treatment in DBA/2J mouse model of glaucoma. Invest Ophthalmol Vis Sci. 2008;49:1437–46.

54. Agarwal R, Gupta SK, Srivastava S, Agarwal P, Agrawal SS. Therapeutic potential of Curcuma longa, the golden spice of India, in drug discovery for ophthalmic diseases. Expert Opin Drug Discov. 2009;4:(2):147–58. (doi:10.1517/13543770802668117)

55. Agarwal R, Gupta SK, Srivastava S, Saxena R, Agrawal SS. IOP lowering effects of topical application of Aegle marmelos fruit extract in experimental models of glaucoma. Ophthalmic Res. 2009; 42:112–6.

CHAPTER 17

Drugs Used in Retinal Diseases

OVERVIEW

Retinal diseases such as age-related macular degeneration (AMD), retinal vein occlusion (RVO), retinal artery occlusion and diabetic retinopathy (DR), as a cause of visual impairment and blindness are of major concern because the treatment of these conditions faces serious challenges. AMD affects older individuals and can be nonexudative (dry) or exudative (wet). The condition involves macula leading to loss of central visual fields. Central retinal artery and vein occlusion lead to severe retinal damage due to ischemia. Among all, DR is the most prevalent affecting vision of millions of people around the world.

DIABETIC RETINOPATHY

Diabetic Retinopathy (DR) is a disorder of microvasculature of retina that occurs as a consequence of prolonged and uncontrolled hyperglycemic state. It has been reported that more than 4% of world population is diabetic and half of them are suffering from DR at some stage of disease progression. DR affects all patients with Type-1 diabetes and more than 70% of Type 2 diabetic patients develop DR after 15 years of diabetes. There are large number of studies conducted in western world to set up database for the epidemiology of DR.[1-8] However, there is a paucity of data on DR in India and other Asian countries despite the fact that DR has become the leading cause of vision loss in all Asian countries.

Based on the severity of the disorder, DR is classified into two types: Non-proliferative (NPDR) and proliferative (PDR).[9] NPDR, commonly known as background retinopathy, is an early stage of diabetic retinopathy. In this stage, blood or fluid leaks from tiny blood vessels within the retina. Leaking fluid causes the retina to swell or to form deposits called exudates. NPDR may be mild, moderate or severe.

i. Mild NPDR: It is the initial phase of NPDR and is characterized by the presence of at least one microaneurysm, and also dot, blot or flame-shaped hemorrhages. Hard exudates and cotton wool spots are usually not a feature of mild NPDR.

ii. Moderate NPDR: It is the next and more severe stage of NPDR. During this stage, some of the small blood vessels in the retina may become blocked. The blockade of these tiny blood vessels causes a decrease in the supply of nutrients and oxygen to certain areas of the retina (Figs 17.1A and B).

iii. Severe NPDR: In severe NPDR significant number of small blood vessels in the retina become blocked. As a result more areas of retina are deprived of nourishment and oxygen. Lack of sufficient oxygen supply to the retina results in retinal ischemia. To overcome ischemic insult a variety of compensatory growth factor cascade are activated eventually causing raised retinal Vascular Endothelial Growth Factor (VEGF) and Protein Kinase-C-β (PKC-β) levels. These angiogenic growth factors are responsible for

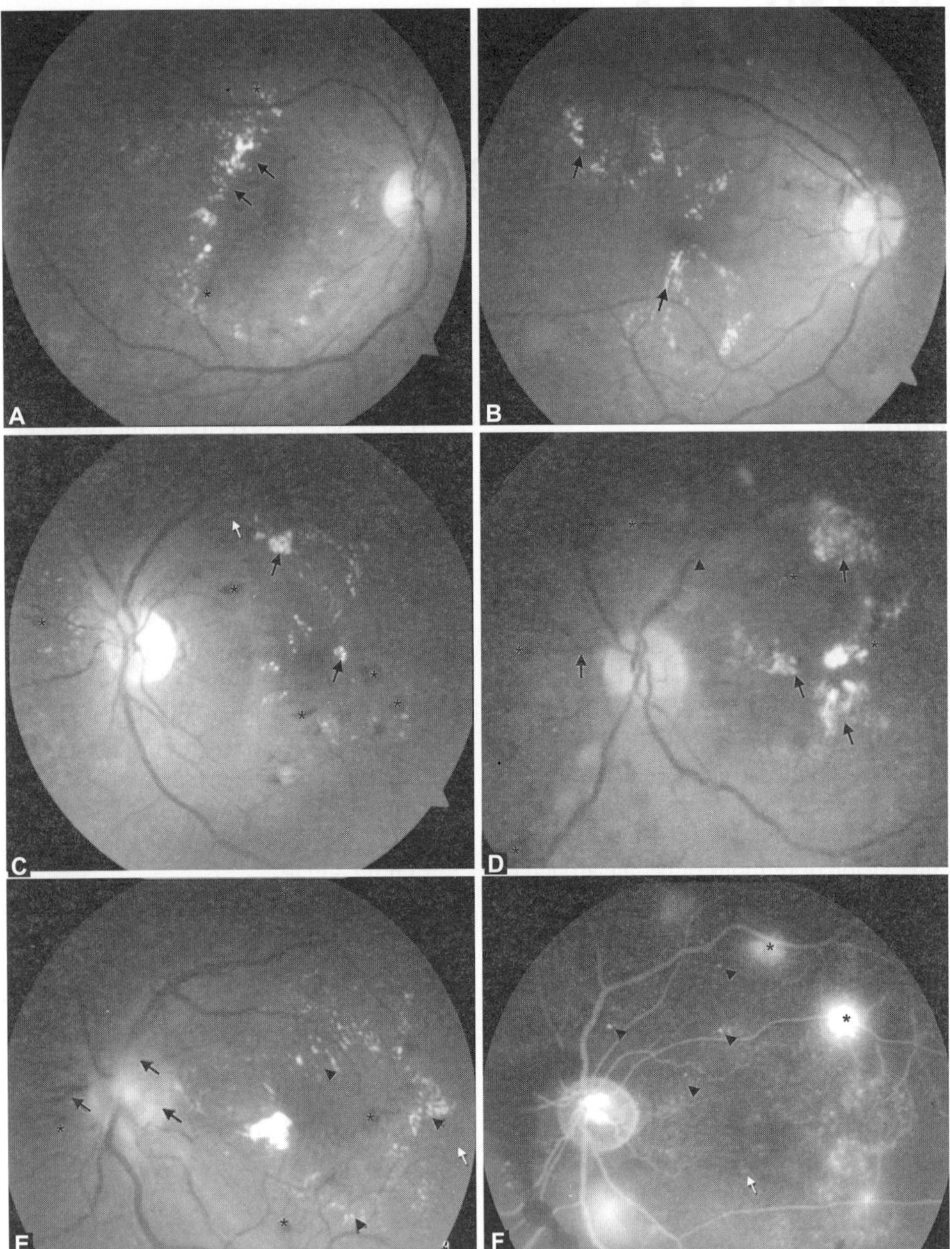

Figures 17.1A to F (A and B) Representative fundus photographs from patient with moderate NPDR showing significant accumulation of hard exudates (arrow), microaneurysms and leakages at some areas (asterisk); (C) Fundus photograph from patient with severe NPDR showing significantly high leakage at multiple areas (star) and appearance of hard exudates; (D) Fundus photograph from patient with severe NPDR showing tortuous blood vessels (arrow head), large deposits of hard exudates (arrow) and leakages in the fundus (star); (E) A representative image from patient with PDR as evident from neovascularization of the optic disc (arrow), tortuous vessel, appearance of hard exudates (arrow head) and retinal hemorrhage (star); (F) A fluorescein fundus angiogram from a patient with PDR showing significant leakage of sodium fluorescein (star) and appearance of microaneurysms in the form of hyperfluorescent dots (arrow heads)

the increased retinal vascular permeability and neovascularization (Figs17.1C and D).

PDR is a more advanced form of DR and a major cause of vision loss in diabetic patients. It is characterized by neovascularization on optic disc and in other areas of retina. Sometimes vessels grow out of inner limiting membrane and bleed in the vitreous leading to significant vision loss (Figs 17.1E and F).

Drugs Used in the Treatment of DR

Since the last two decades, there have been significant developments in the field of pharmaco-therapy of DR. For DR, the advent of laser photocoagulation three decades back, was really useful in limiting vision loss in most of the cases and is still considered the gold standard. However, corticosteroids and anti-VEGF agents have shown promising results with regards to the prevention of neovascularization, but remained limited in use due to their short-lasting effects. More importantly none of these agents have shown ability to substitute the remarkable durability and effectiveness of panretinal photocoagulation in preventing vision loss in the late stages of DR. Therefore, pharmacotherapy of DR is still an adjunct to panretinal photocoagulation (Table 17.1).

Anti-VEGF Drugs

VEGF is a secreted protein that stimulates the growth of vascular endothelial cells. It is known to play a significant role in ocular pathologies associated with neovascularization and is, therefore, a target for several pharmacological agents used to treat such conditions.

VEGF exists in at least 4 isoforms consisting of 121, 165, 189, and 206 amino acids. $VEGF_{165}$ has the greatest mitogenic activity and is the primary mediator of pathologic neovascularization. The mitogenic, angiogenic and permeability effects of VEGF are mediated through two tyrosine kinase receptors VEGFR1 and VEGFR2. Binding of VEGF with its receptor stimulates angiogenesis, induces inflammation and increases vascular permeability. Several anti-VEGF drugs have emerged as effective treatment modalities in pathological choroidal and retinal neovascularization.[10]

Pegaptanib (Macugen®): Pegaptanib is an aptamer, a pegylated modified oligonucleotide, which binds with extracellular $VEGF_{165}$ and prevents it from binding with the VEGF receptors.[11] Following intravitreal administration, it gets distributed into the retina, vitreous and aqueous and is slowly absorbed in the systemic circulation. It is metabolized by nucleases and is generally not affected by the cytochrome P450 enzymes. Pegaptanib requires repeated administration at 6 weeks intervals. At 0.3 mg dose, no dose reduction is required in patients with renal impairment.

It is available as preservative-free, sterile, aqueous solution in single dose pre-filled syringes. The active ingredient is 0.3 mg of the free acid form of the oligonucleotide without polyethylene glycol, in a volume of 90 µL. This dose is equivalent to 1.6 mg of pegaptanib sodium (pegylated oligonucleotide) or 0.32 mg as the sodium salt form of the oligonucleotide moiety.

The most frequently reported adverse events in patients treated with Macugen® 0.3 mg for up to two years were anterior chamber inflammation, blurred vision, cataract, conjunctival hemorrhage, corneal edema, eye discharge, eye irritation, eye pain, hypertension, increased intraocular pressure (IOP), ocular discomfort, punctate keratitis, reduced visual acuity, visual disturbance, vitreous floaters, and vitreous opacities.

Macugen® is contraindicated in patients with ocular or periocular infections. It is also contraindicated in patients with known hypersensitivity to pegaptanib sodium or any other excipient in this product.

Ranibizumab (Lucentis®): It is also available for intravitreal injection. It is a humanized monoclonal antibody fragment against VEGF derived from parent murine antibody bevacizumab (Avastin®). It is much smaller than parent molecule and binds more strongly with VEGF.[12] It differs from Macugen® in that it binds with all four isoforms of VEGF.

Table 17.1 Summary of currently available drugs for diabetic retinopathy and associated retinal pathology

Drug/formulation	Company	Category/ Mechanism	Clinical phase	Regulatory approval
Triesence (40 mg/mL),IVTA* Preservative-free Injection	Alcon Laboratories Inc.	Anti-inflammatory	-	FDA-approved
Trivaris (80 mg/mL), IVTA* Preservative-free Injection	Allergan Inc.	Anti-inflammatory	-	FDA-approved
I-vation, Intravitreal TA** Implant	Surmodics Inc.	Anti-inflammatory	Phase I completed	-
Iluvien, fluocinolone acetonide	Alimera Sciences	Anti-inflammatory	Phase III completed	Not FDA-approved
Ozurdex, Dexamethasone IV*** implant	Allergan Inc.	Anti-inflammatory	Under Phase III	FDA-approved for DME
Avastin, Bevacizumab	Genentech Inc.	Anti-VEGF	Under Phase III	Not FDA-approved
Lucentis, Ranibizumab	Genentech Inc.	Anti-VEGF	Under Phase III	FDA-approved for AMD
Macugen, Pegaptanib	EyeTech Pharmaceuticals and Pfizer	Anti-VEGF	-	FDA-approved
VEGF Trap- Eye	Regeneron and Bayer Healthcare Collaboration	Anti-VEGF	Phase II (DME)# Phase III (AMD and CRVO)	Not FDA-approved
Vitrase, hyaluronidase	ISTA Pharmaceuticals	Vitreous clearing agent	Undergoing Phase III	Not FDA-approved

*IVTA: Intravitreal triamcinolone acetonide;
**TA: Triamcinolone acetonide;
***IV: Intravitreal;
#Diabetic macular edema.
Source: Kumar B, Gupta SK, Saxena R, Srivastava S. Current trends in the pharmacotherapy of diabetic retinopathy. J Postgrad Med. 2012;58:132-9.

The drug has proven efficacy in wet AMD and macular edema caused by RVO. It is administered intravitreally once a month. The frequency of administration may be reduced to once in 3 months after 4 months of treatment but the efficacy reduces as compared to monthly injections. Ranibizumab has also been used along with verteporfin photodynamic therapy in the treatment of wet AMD.[13] Verteporfin is a liposomal preparation containing photosensitizer verteporfin. After intravenous administration, liposomes containing verteporfin accumulate in endothelial cells by endocytosis through LDL receptors.[14]

Ranibizumab is available for intravitreal injection as preservative-free sterile, colorless to pale yellow solution in single use vials containing 0.5 mL of 10 mg/mL of lucentis.

Besides the complications associated with injection procedure other adverse effects include conjunctival hemorrhage, eye pain, vitreous floaters, increased IOP, and intraocular inflammation. Use of intravitreal anti-VEGF agents is also associated with arterial thromboembolic events but the incidence is very low. Like other proteins, anti-VEGF agents can also produce immunoreactivity.

Lucentis® is contraindicated in patients with ocular or periocular infections. It is also contraindicated in patients with known hypersensitivity to lucentis or any other excipient in the product.

Bevacizumab (Avastin®): It is also a humanized monoclonal antibody, and was the first commercially available VEGF antibody. Like ranibizumab, it also targets all isoforms of VEGF. It is approved for use in many metastatic cancers such as colorectal, lung and breast. It prevents the tumor growth by inhibiting proliferation of new capillaries. It is a low-cost alternative to lucentis. Moreover, it has longer intravitreal half-life thus reducing the frequency of administration.[15,16] It has also been used in the treatment of PDR, neovascular glaucoma, diabetic macular edema, retinopathy of prematurity and macular edema secondary to RVO. Avastin® has no significant effect when used with laser photocoagulation in patients of DR with significant macular edema. However, it is effective in patients without significant macular edema.

Corticosteroids

Steroids are potent anti-inflammatory agents. They inhibit the production of VEGF and breakdown of blood-retinal barrier. Owing to these properties steroids have been the mainstay of treatment in several ocular diseases. For the treatment of ophthalmic diseases steroids can be administered by topical, systemic, retrobular or intraocular route. Steroids that are used for intravitreal injection include triamcenolone acetonide, dexamethasone and fluocinolone acetonide. Dexamethasone and fluocinolone acetonide are also available as intravitreal implant.

Triamcinolone acetonide modulates the epithelial cell resistance, reduces permeability of outer blood-retinal barrier, promotes exudate reabsorption and down-regulates inflammatory stimuli. Triamcinolone acetonide has been increasingly used in the treatment of diabetic macular edema, RVO and non-infectious uveitis. Usefulness of triamcinolone is limited in uveitis related macular edema due to recurrence of symptoms and adverse effects like elevated IOP and cataract. Another limitation for the use of this steroid is that repeated injections (every 4 month) are often required with standard 4 mg dose.

For intravitreal administration, triamcinolone acetonide is available as preservative-free sterile suspension at 40 and 80 mg/mL concentration. Particle dispersion from suspension can initiate macrophage reaction causing sterile endophthalmitis. Use of preparations with hydrogel base limits the particle dispersion and avoids sterile endophthalmitis.

Dexamethasone is one of the most potent corticosteroid. It is used in the treatment of persistent macular edema associated with diabetic retinopathy, RVO and non-infectious uveitis. Intravitreal dexamethasone causes significant improvement in visual acuity, fluorescein leakage and central retinal thickness in these patients.

The half-life of dexamethasone after intravitreal injection is short. A biodegradable dexamethasone intravitreal implant (Ozurdex/Posurdex) is now available, which provides extended release of a total dose of 0.35 or 0.7 mg dexamethasone. It is a rod shaped implant consisting of dexamethasone dispersed in poly (lactic-co-glycolic) acid (PLGA) matrix. The implant is placed through pars plana incision into the vitreous chamber outside the visual axis. It releases the active drug initially in high pulses for a few weeks and then maintains sustained release for about 6 months.[17-19] It is indicated for the treatment of macular edema following DR, branch retinal vein occlusion or central retinal vein occlusion.[20] The adverse effects include increased IOP, conjunctival hemorrhage, eye pain, conjunctival congestion, cataract, vitreous detachment and headache.

Use of intravitreal dexamethasone is contraindicated in patients with active or suspected ocular or periocular infections including most viral diseases of the cornea and conjunctiva (epithelial herpes simplex keratitis, vaccinia, varicella), mycobacterial infections and fungal diseases. It is also contraindicated in patients with advanced glaucoma and patients with known hypersensitivity to any of its components or to other corticosteroids.

Fluocinolone acetonide, a non-biodegradable sustained release intravitreal implant consisting of 0.59 mg of fluocinolone acetonide (Retisert®), is available for extended drug delivery.[21-23] The implant consists of fluocinolone acetonide 1.5 mm diameter pellet encased in a silicone elastomer cup with a release orifice.[24,25] The device is implanted in vitreous through a pars plana incision and after implantation, it releases active drug at a rate of 0.3–0.4 µg/day for a period of 30 months. It is used in the treatment of macular edema associated with DR, RVO and non-infectious uveitis. The implant is expensive and associated complications include cataract and elevated IOP.

Vitreolytic Agent

Vitrase (hyaluronidase ovine, ISTA Pharmaceuticals, Inc.) is the first and only pure, preservative-free, thimerosal-free, ovine hyaluronidase, which is FDA-approved as a spreading agent. Intravitreal vitrase has shown efficacy and safety in a Phase III clinical trial that investigated its ability to promote the clearance of vitreous hemorrhage in cases of PDR, although, the agent is not FDA-approved for this purpose.[26,27]

AGE-RELATED MACULAR DEGENERATION

Age-related macular degeneration (AMD) is a major cause of global visual morbidity after DR and is the leading cause of blindness among people over 50 years of age.[28] The prevalence of AMD varies widely among different ethnic groups and genetic make-up is a predisposing factor in the pathogenesis of AMD.[29] It is estimated that by the year 2020, at least 80 million people will be affected by AMD globally.[30]

AMD is classified into Dry or Wet (neovascular) AMD. Dry or nonexudative AMD affects 90% of the patients and is characterized by drusen and retinal pigment epithelium (RPE) mottling, hyperplasia, and atrophy. On the other hand, wet or exudative AMD affects only 10% of the patients but causes blindness among 90% of them. It is characterized by the growth of choroidal neovascular membranes.[31] Neovascular AMD results from repeated cycles of shedding, degradation, and resynthesis of photoreceptor outer segments, which induce metabolic stress within the outer retina and RPE. The resultant chronic ischemia and inflammation upregulates several inflammatory cytokines and growth factors such as VEGF, which promote the growth of choroidal neovascular membranes from the choriocapillaris into the sub-RPE space or subretinal space.[32]

Current Pharmacotherapy of AMD

Laser Photocoagulation

Thermal laser photocoagulation is a technique for treating a number of eye conditions including wet AMD. A thermal laser is directed into the eye at abnormal blood vessels growing beneath the retina. The heat from the laser closes off the unwanted blood vessels, preventing further leakage and vision loss. Apart from this, thermal laser can also destroy surrounding retinal tissue resulting in scotomas. The use of photocoagulation is effective for patients with lesions that are outside the center of the macula.[33]

Photodynamic Therapy

For photodynamic therapy, a light-sensitive dye, verteporfin (Visudyne), is injected intravenously. The dye accumulates in the neovascular tissue and is activated upon exposure to non-thermal light at 689 nm. Free radicals generated due to activation cause cell death and subsequent occlusion of abnormal new vessels with little or no damage to normal vessels. Although, photodynamic therapy is a FDA-approved method for the treatment of AMD, it has not succeeded in preventing vision loss in AMD patients.[34,35]

Nutritional Agents

Lutein and zeaxanthin are the two major carotenoids found in the human macula.[36-37] These are structurally similar to β-carotene and are found in various colored fruits and green leafy vegetables. Lutein and zeaxanthin have been reported to accumulate in the macular region of the retina where their contents are up to 5 fold higher than the peripheral retina.[36] Zeaxanthin preferentially accumulates in the foveal region, whereas lutein is abundant in the perifoveal region.[37,38] These pigments are collectively known as the macular pigment. Definitive role of these pigments in AMD is not known, however, a recent systematic review and meta analysis involving 6 longitudinal cohort studies has shown that dietary lutein and zeaxanthin is not significantly associated with a reduced risk of early AMD, but an increase in their intake may be protective against late AMD.[39]

Anti-angiogenic Agents

Antiangiogenic agents are of value in the treatment of AMD as they inhibit VEGF-mediated pathological changes in the retina. Ranibizumab and bevacizumab have been discussed in the previous section. Clinical trials with ranibizumab and bevacizumab have shown that patients receiving protocol-driven treatment have a 30–40% chance of achieving a 15-letter (halving of the visual angle) improvement in visual acuity.[40-42]

Aflibercept (EYLEA®) is a newer addition in this class of drugs. It was approved by FDA in November 2011 for use in neovascular AMD. It is a VEGF inhibitor administered as an intravitreal injection. It is a fully human recombinant fusion protein that binds all isoforms of VEGF and prevents their binding to VEGFR-1 and VEGFR-2. Aflibercept also binds to placental growth factor inhibiting its binding to VEGFR-1. Inhibition of the binding of VEGF to its receptors decreases inflammation and vascular permeability, prevents the progression of neovascular AMD, and prevents further loss of vision.

Aflibercept is indicated for the treatment of patients with wet AMD and macular edema following CRVO. The recommended dose is 2 mg (0.05 mL) administered by intravitreal injection every 4 weeks for the first 3 months, followed by 2 mg (0.05 mL) via intravitreal injection once every 8 weeks. It is available as 40 mg/mL solution in a single-use vial. Use of aflibercept is contraindicated in patients with ocular or periocular infection and active intraocular inflammation.

The most common adverse reactions ($\geq$ 5%) reported in patients receiving aflibercept are conjunctival hemorrhage, eye pain, cataract, vitreous detachment, vitreous floaters and increased intraocular pressure. Recent clinical studies comparing the efficacy and safety of aflibercept with ranibizumab over 2 years have shown no appreciable difference in the vision gain and retinal thickness between patients treated with aflibercept 2 mg every 4 weeks and ranibizumab. Both drugs were well tolerated and incidence of serious ocular events or systemic adverse effects was comparable between treatment groups.[43,44]

RETINAL VEIN OCCLUSION

RVO is the second largest cause of visual morbidity after DR. The prevalence of RVO has been shown to vary from 0.7 to 1.6%.[45,46] In a population-based study, an overall incidence of symptomatic RVO was found in 0.21% of patients aged 40 years or older.[47] Hayreh et al. (1990) investigated the demographic characteristics of various types of RVO in 1108 patients (1229 eyes).[48] In this study, a male: female ratio of 1.2:1 was noted. RVO is of two main types: Central Retinal Vein Occlusion (CRVO) and Branch Retinal Vein Occlusion (BRVO).

BRVO may result from one or more of the following primary mechanisms:

a. *Compression of the vein at the arteriovenous (A/V) crossing*: In majority of A/V crossings, the thin walled vein lies between the more rigid thick-walled artery and the highly cellular retina. The sharing of the common adventitial sheath by artery and vein and narrowing of the venous lumen that normally occurs at the A/V crossing results in the pathogenesis of BRVO.[49-52]

b. *Degenerative changes in the vessel wall*: It has been suggested that trophic changes in the venous endothelium and intima media , due to compression by overlaying artery, may underlie the pathogenesis of BRVO.[52,53-56]

c. *Abnormal hematological factors*: Several studies have shown a relation between BRVO and hyperviscosity due to high hematocrit. Higher blood viscosity causes poor blood flow and favors erythrocyte aggregation. Dysregulation of the thrombosis-fibrinolysis balance may also be a contributory mechanism.[52,57,58]

The pathogenesis of CRVO is not completely understood. The central retinal artery and vein share a common exit through optic nerve head and pass through a narrow opening in the lamina cribrosa. Therefore, the vessels are in a tight compartment with limited space for displacement. Apart from anatomical susceptibility, a combination of several other factors including slowing of the blood flow, vessel wall changes and rheological changes in the blood predispose to thrombus formation in the central retinal vein in the region of the lamina cribrosa.

Although, there is no specific risk factor identified for CRVO, some of the suggested ones include increasing age, hypertension, diabetes, arteriosclerotic vascular risk factors and glaucoma. Reduced incidence is seen with increased physical activity, alcohol consumption and use of estrogen therapy in postmenopausal women.[52]

Currently, pharmacotherapy has a very limited role in the treatment of RVO and laser therapy is commonly employed for the treatment of neovascular ischemic complications. Currently available therapeutic options are broadly classified into, (A) Drugs for the treatment of obstructed venous blood flow, and (B) Drugs for the treatment of complications of RVO such as macular edema and retinal ischemic neovascularization.

A. Drugs for the Treatment of Obstructed Venous Blood Flow

i. *Antiplatelet and thrombolytic agents*: Platelet aggregation has extensively been studied as a causal factor for the pathogenesis of RVO. Therefore, anti-platelet therapy improves retinal microcirculation and is considered effective. Ticlopidine has shown better results as compared to aspirin. Thrombolytic agents are used to lyse thrombus causing obstruction to venous blood flow.[59,60]

ii. *Hemodiluants*: Isovolemic hemodilution using hydroxyethyl starch or dextran has been investigated in several clinical trials but due to large variation in study protocols the evidence supporting their use remains incomplete.[61,62]

iii. *Troxerutin*: Troxerutin inhibits erythrocyte aggregation, thus reduces blood viscosity and increases the retinal microcirculation.[63-79]

B. Drugs for the Treatment of Complications

Drugs used for the treatment of complications associated with RVO include corticosteroids and anti-VEGF drugs. A detailed account of these drugs is presented under previous section on DR.

REFERENCES

1. Klein R, Klein BE, Moss SE. The Wisconsin epidemiologic study of diabetic retinopathy: an update. Aust N Z J Ophthalmol. 1990;18(1):19-22.

2. Diabetes Control and complications trial research group. Clustering long-term complications in families with diabetes in diabetes control and complications trial. Diabetes. 1997;40:1829–39

3. Klein R, Klein BE, Moss SE, Cruickshanks KJ. The Wisconsin Epidemiologic Study of Diabetic Retinopathy: XVII. The 14-year incidence and progression of diabetic retinopathy and associated risk factors in type 1 diabetes. Ophthalmology. 1998; 105(10):1801–15.

4. Kobrin Klein BE. Overview of epidemiologic studies of diabetic retinopathy. Ophthalmic Epidemiol. 2007;14(4):179–83.

5. Klein R, Knudtson MD, Lee KE, Gangnon R, Klein BE. The Wisconsin Epidemiologic Study of Diabetic Retinopathy XXIII: the twenty-five-year incidence of macular edema in persons with type 1 diabetes. Ophthalmology. 2009; 116(3):497–503.

6. Rema M, Deepa R. Diabetic retinopathy: an Indian perspective. Ind J Med Res. 2007; 125(3):297-310.

7. Rema M, Premkumar S, Anitha B, Deepa R, Pradeepa R, Mohan V. Prevalence of diabetic retinopathy in urban India: the Chennai Urban Rural Epidemiology Study (CURES) eye study, I. Invest Ophthal Vis Sci. 2005;46(7):2328-33.

8. Raman R, Rani PK, Reddi RS, Gnanamoorthy P, Uthra S, Kumaramanickavel G, et. al. Prevalence of diabetic retinopathy in India: Sankara Nethralaya diabetic retinopathy epidemiology and molecular genetics study report 2. Ophthalmology. 2009;116(2):311–8.

9. Frank RN. Diabetic retinopathy. N Engl J Med. 2004;1:350(1):48–58.

10. Andreoli CM, Miller JW. Anti-vascular endothelial growth factor therapy for ocular neovascular disease. Curr Opin Ophthalmol. 2007;18:502–8.

11. Ng EWM, Shima DT, Calias P, Cunningham ET Jr, Guyer DR, Adamis AP: Pegaptanib, a targeted anti-VEGF aptamer for ocular vascular disease. Nat Rev Drug Discov. 2006;5:123–32.

12. Ferrara N, Mass RD, Campa C, Kim R Targeting VEGF-A to treat cancer and age-related macular degeneration. Annu Rev Med. 2007;58: 491–504.

13. Lucentis Utilizing Visudyne (LUV Trial) combination therapy in the treatment of age-related macular degeneration (ClinicalTrials.gov identifier NCT00423189). US National Institutes of Health, Clinical Trials.gov (online). Available from URL: http://www.clinicaltrials.gov (Accessed 2012 Dec 16).

14. Amin K, Wasan KM, Albrecht RM, et al. Cell association of liposomes with high fluid anionic phospholipid content is mediated specifically by LDL and its receptor, LDLr. J Pharm Sci. 2002; 91(5):1233–44.

15. Bakri SJ, Snyder MR, Reid JM, Pulido JS, Ezzat MK, Singh RJ. Pharmacokinetics of intravitreal ranibizumab (Lucentis). Ophthalmology. 2007; 114:2179–82.

16. Bakri SJ, Snyder MR, Reid JM, Pulido JS, Singh RJ: Pharmacokinetics of intravitreal bevacizumab (Avastin). Ophthalmology. 2007; 114: 855–9.

17. Kuppermann BD, Blumenkranz MS, Haller JA, et al. An intravitreous dexamethasone bioerodible drug delivery system for the treatment of persistent diabetic macular edema (abstract no. 4289). Association for Research in Vision and Ophthalmology Annual Meeting; 2003 May 4-9; Fort Lauderdale (FL).

18. Haller JA, Blumenkranz MS, Williams GA, et al. Treatment of persistent macular edema associated with central and branch retinal vein occlusion with extended delivery of intravitreal dexamethasone (abstract no. 4311). Association for Research in Vision and Ophthalmology Annual Meeting; 2003 May 4-9; Fort Lauderdale (FL).

19. Williams GA, Blumenkranz MS, Haller JA, et al. Treatment of persistent macular edema (PME) associated with uveitis or Irvine-Gass syndrome (IGS) with an intravitreal bioerodible sustained dexamethasone release implant; a prospective controlled multi-center clinical trial (abstract no. 4309). Association for Research in Vision and Ophthalmology Annual Meeting. 2003 May 4-9; Fort Lauderdale (FL).

20. Allergan. Allergan receives FDA approval for OZURDEX_biodegradable, injectable steroid implant with extended drug release for retinal disease (online). Available from URL: http://agn.client.shareholder.com/releasedetail.cfm? Release ID = 390519 (Accessed Jan 2012).

21. Jaffe GJ, Ben-Nun J, Guo H, et al. Fluocinolone acetonide sustained drug delivery device to treat severe uveitis. Ophthalmology. 2000;107(11): 2024–33.

22. Jaffe GJ, Yang CH, Guo H, et al. Safety and pharmacokinetics of an intraocular fluocinolone acetonide sustained delivery device. Invest Ophthalmol Vis Sci. 2000;41(11):3569–75.

23. Jaffe GJ, McCallum RM, Branchaud B, et al. Long-term follow-up results of a pilot trial of a fluocinolone acetonide implant to treat posterior uveitis. Ophthalmology. 2005;112(7):1192–8.

24. Retisert_ (fluocinolone acetonide intravitreal implant) 0.59 mg: prescribing information. Rochester (NY):Bausch & Lomb Inc., 2009 Mar (online). Available from URL: http://www.bausch.com/en_US/downloads/ecp/pharma/general/retisert_prescinfopdf.pdf (Accessed 2012 Dec 20).

25. Retisert_ (fluocinolone acetonide intravitreal implant) 0.59mg – sterile: prescribing

information. Rochester (NY): Bausch & Lomb Inc., 2007 Apr [online]. Available from URL: http://www.bauschsurgical.com/vitreoretinal/pdf/prescribing_information_new.pdf (Accessed Dec 2012).

26. Kupperman BD, Thomas EL, de Smet MD, Grillone LR; Vitrase for Vitreous Hemorrhage Study Groups. Safety results of two phase III trials of an intravitreous injection of highly purified ovine hyaluronidase (Vitrase) for the management of vitreous hemorrhage. Am J Ophthalmol. 2005;140:585–97.

27. Lopez-Lopez F, Rodriguez-Blanco M, Gomez-Ulla F, Marticorena J. Enzymatic vitreolysis. Curr Diabetes Rev. 2009;5:57–62.

28. Klein R, Wang Q, Klein BE, Moss SE, Meuer SM. The relationship of age-related maculopathy, cataract, and glaucoma to visual acuity. Invest Ophthalmol Vis Sci. 1995;36:182–91.

29. Katta S, Kaur I, Chakrabarti S. The molecular genetic basis of age-related macular degeneration: an overview. J Genet. 2009:88,425–49.

30. Clemons TE, Milton RC, Klein R, Seddon JM, Ferris FL III and Age-Related Eye Disease Study Research Group. Risk factors for the incidence of advanced age-related macular degeneration in the age-related eye disease study (AREDS) AREDS report no. 19. Ophthalmology. 2005;112:533–9.

31. Ferris FL III, Fine SL, Hyman L. Age-related macular degeneration and blindness due to neovascular maculopathy. Arch Ophthalmol. 1984;102(11):1640–2.

32. Stewart MW. Clinical and differential utility of VEGF inhibitors in wet age-related macular degeneration: focus on aflibercept. Clinical Ophthalmol. 2012;6:1175–86.

33. Virgili G, Bini A. Laser photocoagulation for neovascular age-related macular degeneration. Cochrane Database of Systematic Reviews. 2007, Issue 3. Art. No.: CD004763. DOI: 10.1002/14651858.CD004763.pub2.

34. Treatment of Age-related Macular Degeneration with Photodynamic Therapy (TAP) Study Group. Verteporfin Therapy of Subfoveal Choroidal Neovascularization in Patients with Age-Related Macular Degeneration. Arch Ophthalmol. 2002;120:1443–54.

35. Bressler NM, Bressler SB. Photodynamic Therapy with Verteporfin (Visudyne): Impact on Ophthalmology and Visual Sciences. Invest Ophthalmol Vis Sci. 2000;41(39):10.

36. Handelman GJ, Dratz EA, Reay CC, van Kuijk JG: Carotenoids in the human macula and whole retina. Invest Ophthalmol Vis Sci. 1988; 29:850–5.

37. Bone RA, Landrum JT, Fernandez L, Tarsis SL: Analysis of the macular pigment by HPLC: retinal distribution and age study. Invest Ophthalmol Vis Sci. 1988;29:843–9.

38. Snodderly DM, Handelman GJ, Adler AJ: Distribution of individual macular pigment carotenoids in the central retina of macaque and squirrel monkeys. Invest Ophthalmol Vis Sci. 1991;32:268–79.

39. Ma L, Dou HL, Wu YQ, Huang YM, Huang YB, Xu XR, et al. Lutein and zeaxanthin intake and the risk of age-related macular degeneration: a systematic review and meta-analysis. Br J Nutr. 2012;107(3):350–9.

40. Rosenfeld PJ, Brown DM, Heier JS, et al. Ranibizumab for age-related macular degeneration. N Engl J Med. 2006;355:1419–31.

41. Brown DM, Kaiser PK, Michels M, et al. Ranibizumab versus verteporfin for neovascular age-related macular degeneration. N Engl J Med. 2006;334:1432–44.

42. Martin DF, Maguire MG, Ying G-S. Ranibizumab and bevacizumab for neovascular age-related macular degeneration. N Engl J Med. 2011;364(20):1897–908.

43. Vascular Endothelial Growth Factor (VEGF) Trap-Eye: Investigation of Efficacy and Safety in Wet Age-Related Macular Degeneration (AMD) (VIEW1). Available from: http://www.clinicaltrials.gov/ct2/show/NCT00509795?term=Aflibercept+VIEW+1andrank=1 (Last accessed on 2011 Nov 21).

44. Vascular Endothelial Growth Factor (VEGF) Trap-Eye: Investigation of Efficacy and safety in wet age-related macular degeneration (AMD) (VIEW 2) Available from: http://www.clinicaltrials.gov/ct2/show/NCT00637377?term=Aflibercept+VIEW+1andrank=2 (Accessed Nov 2011).

45. Klein R, Klein BE, Moss SE, Meuer SM. The epidemiology of retinal vein occlusion: The Beaver Dam Eye Study. Trans Am Ophthalmol Soc. 2000;98:133–41.

46. Mitchell P, SmithW, Chang A. Prevalence and associations of retinal vein occlusion in Australia. The Blue Mountains Eye Study. Arch Ophthalmol. 1996;114:1243–7.

47. David R, Zangwill L, Badarna M, Yassur Y. Epidemiology of retinal vein occlusion and its association with glaucoma and increased intraocular pressure. Ophthalmologica. 1988; 197:69–74.

48. Hayreh SS, Zimmerman B, Podhajsky P. Incidence of various types of retinal vein occlusion and their recurrence and demographic characteristics. Am J Ophthalmol. 1990;117:429–41.

49. Koyanagi Y. The role of arteriovenous crossing for occurring of retinal branch vein occlusion. Klin Monatsbl Augenheilkd. 1928;81:219–31.

50. Zhao J, Sastry SM, Sperduto RD, Chew EY, Remaley NA. Arteriovenous crossing patterns in branch retinal vein occlusion. Ophthalmology. 1993;100:423–8.

51. Duker JS, Brown GC. Anterior location of the crossing artery in branch retinal vein obstruction. Arch Ophthalmol. 1989;107:998–1000.

52. Rehak, J and Rehak, M. Branch Retinal Vein Occlusion: Pathogenesis, Visual Prognosis, and Treatment Modalities. Curr Eye Res. 2008, 33:111–31.

53. Jefferies P, Clemett R, Day T. An anatomical study of retinal arteriovenous crossings and their role in the pathogenesis of retinal branch vein occlusions. Aust N Z J Ophthalmol. 1993;21:213–7.

54. Seitz R. The Retinal Vessels: Comparative Ophthalmoscopic and Histologic Studies on Healthy and Diseased Eyes. St. Louis, MO: CV Mosby; 1964:28.

55. Frangieh GT, Green WR, Barraquer-Somers E, Finkelstein D. Histopathologic study of branch retinal vein occlusion. Arch Ophthalmol. 1982;100:1132–40.

56. Christoffersen NL, Larsen M. Pathophysiology and hemodynamic of branch retinal vein occlusion. Ophthalmology. 1999;106:2054–62.

57. Trope GE, Lowe GD, McArdle BM, Douglas JT, Forbes CD, Prentice CM, et al. Abnormal blood viscosity and haemostasis in longstanding retinal vein occlusion. Br J Ophthalmol. 1983;67:137–42.

58. McGrath MA, Wechsler F, Hunyor AB, Penny R. Systemic factors contributory to retinal vein occlusion. Arch Intern Med. 1978;138:216–20.

59. Chen HC, Wiek J, Gupta A, Luckie A, Kohner EM. Effect of isovolaemic haemodilution on visual outcome in branch retinal vein occlusion. Br J Ophthalmol. 1998;82:162–7.

60. Squizzato A, Manfredi E, Bozzato S, Dentali F, Ageno W. Antithrombotic and fibrinolytic drugs for retinal vein occlusion: a systematic review and a call for action. Thromb Haemost. 2010; 103:271–6.

61. McIntosh RL, Mohamed Q, Saw SM, Wong TY. Interventions for branch retinal vein occlusion: an evidence-based systematic review. Ophthalmology. 2007;114:835–54.

62. Mohamed Q, McIntosh RL, Saw SM, Wong TY. Interventions for central retinal vein occlusion: an evidence-based systematic review. Ophthalmology. 2007;114:507–24.

63. Houtsmuller AJ, Vermeulen JA, Klompe M, Zahn KJ, Henkes HE, Baarsma GS, et al. The influence of ticlopidine on the natural course of retinal vein occlusion. Agents Actions Suppl. 1984;15:219–29.

64. Glacet-Bernard A, Coscas G, Chabanel A, Zourdani A, Lelong F, Samama MM. A randomized, double-masked study on the treatment of retinal vein occlusion with troxerutin. Am J Ophthalmol. 1994;118:421–9.

CHAPTER 18

Drugs Used in the Treatment of Dry Eyes

OVERVIEW

Dry eye or keratoconjunctivitis sicca is defined as "a disorder of the tear film due to tear deficiency or excessive tear evaporation that causes damage to the interpalpebral ocular surface and is associated with symptoms of discomfort" (National Eye Institute, December 5–6, 1994). The discomfort may be intermittent or continuous with mild symptoms such as burning, itching or tearing and blurring of vision. At times condition may be severe leading to keratitis, conjunctivitis, corneal ulceration, scarring and permanent vision loss. Depending upon the predominant cause of dry eye condition, it can be divided in two categories: aqueous deficiency and evaporative. Aqueous deficient dry eye is the largest category and occurs due to reduced tear volume. Reduction in tear volume may be due to dysfunctional lacrimal gland or failure of lacrimal fluid transfer. The evaporative dry eye occurs primarily either due to dysfunction of meibomian glands or increased width of palpebral fissure. Both types of dry eye conditions can also occur simultaneously. Either of these conditions can result in abnormal tear composition and properties. The goal of treatment is to relieve symptoms, heal the ocular surface and prevent complications. Following approaches and drug classes are commonly used in the treatment of dry eye:[1]

1. Aqueous enhancement therapy
2. Anti-inflammatory therapy
3. Secretagogues
4. Hormonal therapy
5. Omega-3 fatty acids

AQUEOUS ENHANCEMENT THERAPY

The aqueous enhancement in dry eyes is achieved primarily by tear supplementation, although, methods can also be adapted for tear conservation. The tear substitutes are most commonly used for tear supplementation. Tear conservation can be achieved by reducing the evaporation or drainage of tears. Use of measures such as goggles and room humidifiers helps in reducing the evaporation. Avoiding exposure to smoke, wind, heating, air-conditioning and fans also reduces tear evaporation. Non-medicated ointments applied on the ocular surface can prevent tear evaporation. Obstruction of tear outflow pathways by surgical methods such as cautery, laser, punctal plugs and tarsorrhaphy in severe cases helps to conserve tears on ocular surface.

Tear Substitutes

Tear substitutes are the mainstay of therapy for mild to moderate aqueous tear deficiency and include artificial tear solutions, lubricant ointments, lipid emulsions and autologous serum.

Artificial Tear Solutions

The artificial tear solutions are most commonly used forms of tear substitutes. They are expected to reproduce the physical, optical and metabolic properties of natural tears as closely as possible. Currently, there are no true therapeutic tear replacements that also have biological activity. Their long residence time provides better tear film stability. Some additives in these solutions may also be of value in treating the primary or secondary ocular damage. Most artificial tears are aqueous solutions and consist of:

1. Polymers to enhance viscosity, lubrication and retention time and include polyols, polysaccharides and vinyl derivatives.
2. Electrolytes to maintain the osmolarity.
3. Buffers to maintain appropriate pH.
4. Preservative to kill or inhibit bacterial growth.
5. Nutrients as supplements for conjunctival and corneal metabolic requirements.
6. Mucolytic agents to soften the mucus and improve mucin quality

Polymers: Polymers are added to artificial tears to enhance the viscosity, lubrication and retention time. Addition of polymers allows not only the retention of added fluid for a longer time but also increases corneal surface wettability, reduces blink friction and surface tension. They may get adsorbed to corneal surface and stabilize the thicker layer of fluid adjacent to adsorbed surface. They prolong the tear break up time (TBUT). The polymers commonly used in artificial tears include polyols, polysaccharides and vinyl derivatives.

Polyols that are commonly used include glycerin, polyethylene glycol, propylene glycol and polysorbate 80. They have high water binding properties. They lubricate the ocular surface and relieve the symptoms of dry eye. Glycerin is used in 0.2–1% concentration. Polyethylene glycol is used in a concentration of 0.25–1%, propylene glycol 0.3–1% and polysorbate 80 in a concentration of 1%.

Polysaccharide polymers used in artificial tears include mucilages (substituted cellulose ethers), hydroxypropyl guar (HP guar), dextran and viscoelastic agents. Although, dextran (0.1%), a branched chain glucose polymer, is used frequently; use of substituted cellulose ethers, HP guar and viscoelastic agents is more common.

Substituted cellulose ethers used in artificial tears include methylcellulose (MC), hydroxyethylcellulose, hydroxypropyl cellulose, hydroxypropyl methylcellulose (HPMC) and carboxymethylcellulose (CMC). They dissolve in water producing solutions of varying viscosity. Optical clarity and refractive index of these solutions is close to that of cornea. They are inert substances and are, therefore, non-toxic to ocular tissue.

MC forms a viscous solution in water and is used in a concentration of 0.5–1%. At higher concentrations, the solutions are highly viscous and interfere with vision, make blinking difficult and can damage the tear film and epithelium. MC is a highly stable compound at a wide range of pH suitable for eye. During heat sterilization, it coagulates but re-dissolves on cooling. MC solutions do not support the growth of micro-organisms. Hydroxyethylcellulose and HPMC form less viscous solutions as compared to MC but consist of similar cohesive and emollient properties as MC. CMC is an anionic polymer, which has stronger bioadhesive properties than HPMC. However, due to ionic charges, CMC may form insoluble complexes with tear film components. Neutral polymers like HPMC or MC are highly water soluble and do not form such complexes.

In addition to their therapeutic use in dry eye conditions, substituted cellulose ethers are also used to moisten the contact lenses. They are also added to ophthalmic drug solutions to increase the retention time of active drug on the ocular surface. Their highly viscous solutions, such as HPMC 2.5%, are used to apply gonioscopic lens to the eye. This helps to prevent damage to corneal epithelium.

HP guar is a non-cellulose polysaccharide. It is derived from guar gum. It is used as a gelling agent along with borate and sorbitol. In the formulation, sorbitol competes with borate and reduces cross-linking of HP guar. However, when applied to ocular surface, sorbitol diffuses away due to its high water solubility. This allows borate to promote cross linking of HP guar in the presence of divalent cations normally present in the tear film. The gelling of HP guar on the ocular surface helps in stabilizing the tear film and reducing the dry eye symptoms.

Viscoelastic agents include sodium hyaluronate and chondroitin sulfate. They are mucopolysaccharides and are normally present in the extracellular matrix of connective tissue including that of ocular tissue. Although primarily used during intraocular surgery, they are also used in the treatment of severe dry eye conditions due to their lubricating properties.

Sodium hyaluronate, a hydrophilic, high molecular weight compound, is 500,000 times more viscous than normal saline. It lubricates as well as protects the ocular surface. Various investigators have described its use in concentrations ranging from 0.1 to 0.5%. In severe dry eye conditions, topical application provides quick relief of symptoms. Rose bengal staining of cornea and conjunctiva decreases, corneal luster increases and TBUT increases significantly. The effects of sodium hyaluronate in increasing the thickness of corneal tear film are better than the aqueous artificial tears. Topical application of sodium hyaluronate has also been shown to reduce fluorescein staining thus indicating improved cell-to-cell adhesions in cornea. Sodium hyaluronate is a non-toxic substance. It is available in disposable syringes. Its use in dry eye conditions is limited due to high cost.

Chondroitin sulfate is 350,000 times more viscous than saline. Frequent topical instillation in a concentration of 1% can effectively relieve the symptoms of dry eye. It is available as a mixture of sodium chonrdroitin sulfate, 40 mg/mL and sodium hyaluronate 30 mg/mL in 0.5 mL disposable syringe.

Vinyl derivatives like polyvinyl alcohol (PVA), polyvinylpyrrolidone (PVP), polyvinyl acid and polyvinyl chloride are water soluble polymers. PVA in solution is clear and transparent with refractive index approximately equal to distilled water. It is highly stable even at high temperature and, therefore, can be sterilized by autoclaving. It is compatible with most of the commonly used drugs and preservatives except sodium borate, bicarbonate and sulfate, potassium and zinc sulfate. Concomitant use of solutions containing these electrolytes and those containing PVA should be avoided. PVA is commonly used in a concentration of 1.4%. At this concentration although less viscous than MC, it significantly increases the corneal residence time. It enhances the tear film stability and increases TBUT. It is also used as wetting agent in contact lens solutions. It is non-irritant to eye and does not interfere with conjunctival and corneal epithelial integrity. PVP is a non-ionic surfactant and is used in a concentration of 3–5%. It increases the viscosity of solutions. Its ability to reduce surface tension at oil-water interface is less than that of cellulose ethers. However, it improves the wetting ability of corneal surface by forming a hydrophilic coating in the form of adsorbed layer resembling the coating formed by conjunctival mucin. It is, therefore, useful in mucin and aqueous deficient dry eyes.

Electrolytes: Electrolytes such as salts of sodium and potassium are added to artificial tear solutions to maintain osmolarity. Most of the solutions are isotonic with natural tears. Hypertonicity in tear film causes cell shrinkage due to loss of water, reduces cell viability and disrupts mucin layer. Sometimes, hypotonic solutions are used in dry eye patients to allow the tonicity of tears to drop to the levels seen in non-dry eyes. Electrolytes are also added to artificial tear solutions to provide nutrition for corneal epithelial metabolism and as a part of buffer system.

Buffers: The natural tear film components such as bicarbonates, proteins, phosphates and others maintain a pH of 7.4. Artificial tears for dry eyes have alkaline pH (~8.5) and are most comfortable at this pH. Commonly used buffer systems include phosphate, phosphate-acetate, phosphate-citrate, phosphate-citrate-bicarboante, borate and sodium hydroxide.

Preservatives: Preservatives are added to artificial tears to kill or inhibit the growth of microorganisms. Contaminated solutions are likely to cause infection in dry eyes. Commonly used preservatives include: quaternary ammonium compounds (BAK and polyquad), mercurials (thimerosal), alcohols (chlorobutanol) and esters of parahydroxybenzoic acid (methyl and propyl paraben). EDTA is added to enhance the activity of quaternary ammonium compounds. Use of preserved tears is associated with epithelial toxicity, tear film instability and hypersensitivity especially when used multiple times a day for prolonged period. Moreover, preservatives bind with contact lens polymer and prolong the residence time on corneal surface. Therefore, use of preserved tears with contact lenses further enhances the possibility of toxicity and hypersensitivity reactions. Patients requiring daily instillations of more than 3–4 times, are recommended to use unpreserved solutions, which are available as single-dose packages. Their use is inconvenient and expensive and requires additional precautions to prevent contamination and infection. Newer preservatives used in ophthalmic formulations break down on exposure to ocular surface or light. Sodium perborate preserves the solution by generating very low quantities of hydrogen peroxide. When applied to ocular surface, it breaks down to hydrogen peroxide, which further degrades to water and oxygen. Sodium chlorate used as preservative degrades to sodium chloride and water upon exposure to light.

Nutrients: Nutrients are added to support conjunctival and corneal metabolism. Water is most important component besides dextrose, sodium lactate, sodium citrate, vitamins A and B$_{12}$.

Mucolytic Agents: Mucolytic agents include bromhexine, acetylcysteine, tyloxapol, and methylcysteine. These agents soften the mucus and decrease the tear film viscosity. They stimulate the goblet cells for mucus production. The sodium salt of acetylcysteine is available as 10 or 20% solution for use in acute or chronic bronchopulmonary conditions. This solution is diluted with saline or artificial tears to 2–3% concentration for topical ocular use. The solution helps to dissolve the mucus threads but as it causes stinging sensation upon application, subjective improvement of dry eye symptoms is not significant.

Lubricant Ointments

Lubricant ointments have a longer contact time and coat the ocular surface well during sleep when aqueous tear production is normally reduced. They typically contain oily substances such as lanolin and petrolatum, which prevent tear evaporation. Preservative free ointments are now available. Daytime application causes blurred vision and sticky sensation. Non-blurring gels that dissipate rapidly are available for effective use during the day in severe dry eye.[2]

Lipid Emulsion

Lipid emulsions are available for long-lasting lubrication by fortifying the lipid component of the tear film. Lipid emulsions consist of oils like castor oil or mineral oil, viscosity enhancer like carbomer, lubricants like glycerin, polysorbate and preservative. These agents provide temporary symptomatic relief but do not reverse the ocular surface pathology. They have no direct anti-inflammatory effect although decrease inflammation indirectly by reducing tear osmolarity and diluting the concentration of inflammatory factors on the ocular surface.

Autologous Serum

Autologous serum contains growth factors such as fibronectin, vitamin A, epidermal growth factors and TGF-β that are normally present in the natural tears. It may provide anti-inflammatory effect by inhibiting the inflammatory cascades on the ocular surface. A major limitation of this therapy is that it requires special preparation and carries the risk of infection. It is useful for most severe cases of dry eye that have conjunctival metaplasia as seen in Stevens-Johnson syndrome and Sjogren's syndrome.[3]

ANTI-INFLAMMATORY THERAPY

Cyclosporin A

Cyclosporin A (CsA) is useful in the management of moderate to severe dry eye disease. It is a fungal-derived peptide that prevents the activation of transcription factors that are necessary for T-cell activation and the production of interleukin 2. The phase 2 FDA clinical trial evaluated four doses of CsA (0.05%, 0.1%, 0.2%, 0.4%). The 0.1% concentration was found to improve the objective end-points most consistently while the 0.05% concentration gave the most consistent improvement in subjective symptoms. Phase 3 clinical trials showed that the patients treated with CsA 0.1% or 0.05% had significantly greater improvement in two objective signs of dry eye disease, corneal fluorescein staining and anesthetized Schirmer test values. Both doses of CsA gave an excellent safety profile with no significant systemic or ocular adverse events except for transient burning symptoms after instillation. The clinical improvement has been accompanied by decreased expression of activation markers (HLA-DR), apoptosis markers, inflammatory cytokines and infiltrating T cells. The density of goblet cells increased on the ocular surface. No CsA was detected in the blood of patients treated with topical CsA for 12 months.

Corticosteroids

Corticosteroids act by non-specifically inhibiting many aspects of the inflammatory response. Several clinical studies have demonstrated their efficacy in improving the signs and symptoms of dry eyes. In patients with significant inflammatory disease such as Sjogren's syndrome, topical steroids may not be adequate and a short pulse of systemic corticosteroids can be more effective. Overall, topical steroids are effective for achieving a quick response. Due to many ocular complications of topical steroids, recommendation is to limit its use as pulse therapy to control exacerbations followed by substitution with low potency agents.

Tetracycline

Tetracycline is a class of antibiotic that has anti-inflammatory properties, which include reduced cytokines, nitric oxide and expression of HLA class II and inhibition of matrix metalloproteinases.

Systemic doxycycline has been reported to improve irritation symptoms, increase tear film stability and decrease the severity of ocular surface disease. It is recommended for patients with dry eyes with significant component of meibomian gland disease. Main side-effects are increased skin photosensitivity and gastrointestinal complaints. The latter side-effects diminish with lower doses.

SECRETAGOGUES

Secretagogues are therapeutic agents that stimulate tear secretion. Systemic cholinergic agents such as pilocarpine (Salagen™) have successfully been used to treat dry eyes in Sjogren's syndrome patients. Cevimeline (Evoxac™) a cholinergic agonist with high affinity to the muscarinic M_1 and M_3 receptors and long-lasting sialogenic effect has a better side effect profile.

The main limitation of these agents are their systemic cholinergic side-effects such as nausea, sweating and abdominal cramps. Although they are officially approved for mouth symptoms only, they may improve ocular symptoms in those with residual lacrimal gland function. Besides, cholinergic agents, topical UTP and other nucleotides have been shown to stimulate the P2Y2 purinergic receptors to induce secretion of mucin, chloride and fluid by conjunctival cells.

HORMONAL THERAPY

Androgenic steroids may have beneficial effect for the ocular manifestations of Sjogren's syndrome based on laboratory and epidemiologic studies that suggest the low incidence of the disease in males. Androgenic hormones such as testosterone appear to attenuate autoimmune reactions while estrogens have been implicated in the pathogenesis and progression of many autoimmune disorders. Systemic androgen has immunosuppressive effects on the lacrimal gland. It has been reported that women with primary and secondary Sjogren's syndrome are androgen deficient. Moreover, estrogens appear to contribute to the development of dry eyes. Hormone replacement therapy in postmenopausal women is associated with a significant increase in the prevalence of dry eye symptoms. The effects of sex steroids on the tear function are mediated through both meibomian and lacrimal glands. Treatment with testosterone undecanoate has been shown to provide significant improvement in Schirmer test values and ocular surface staining.

OMEGA-3 FATTY ACIDS

Tears contain essential fatty acids omega-3 and omega-6, which are only obtained through diet. Essential fatty acids are found in various foods such as flaxseed, blackcurrant seed, canola oil, walnuts, soy and cold-water fish, e.g. mackerel, tuna, salmon, sardines and herring. A higher ratio of omega-6 to omega-3 fatty acid supplement consumption may decrease incidence of dry eye syndrome.

The treatment of dry eyes has traditionally involved hydrating and lubricating the ocular surface. However, new insights into the inflammatory nature of this disease have shifted the therapeutic approach to dry eyes towards suppressing the inflammatory response on the ocular surface. Tear substitutes continue to be the first line of treatment and anti-inflammatory therapy may be considered for patients with ocular surface disease or for those who continue to be symptomatic despite copious lubrication.

REFERENCES

1. Djalilian AR, Hamarh P, Pflugfleder SC. Dry eye. In: Krachmer JH, Mannis MJ, Holland EJ, (Eds). Cornea. 2nd edn. Elsevier Mosby. 2005. pp. 521–42.
2. Davitt WF, Blooenstein M, Martin A, Christensen MT, Martin AE. Efficacy in patients with dry eye after treatment with a new lubricant eye drop formulation. J Ocul Pharmacol Ther. 2010;26(4):347–53.
3. Pensyl CD. Preparation for Dry Eye and Ocular Surface Disease. In: Bartlett JD, Jaanus SD, (eds). Clinical Ocular Pharmacology, 4th ed. Boston: Butterworth-Heinemann. 2001; pp. 315–31.

CHAPTER 19

Miscellaneous Drugs

A. Hyperosmotic Agents

Vinay Gupta, Preeti Sankaran, Sujaya Singh, Sushil Vasudevan

OVERVIEW

Hyperosmotic agents are the drugs used in the management of acute glaucomas and occasionally for reduction of corneal edema. For the glaucomas, they are administered either orally or intravenously to increase the osmotic pressure of plasma in relation to that of ocular tissues. Fluid from the ocular tissues hence moves into the plasma as a result of the osmotic gradient produced. They are used when rapid reduction of intraocular pressure is needed before definitive treatment is carried out and prior to intraocular surgeries. However, they have potentially fatal adverse effects and thus are not suitable for long-term therapy of glaucoma.

For corneal edema they are administered topically to increase the osmotic pressure of the tears. The osmotic gradient thus created allows fluid from the cornea to move into the hyperosmolar tear film (Table 19.1).

SYSTEMIC HYPEROSMOTIC AGENTS

Pharmacology of Systemic Hyperosmotic Agents

Mechanism of Action, Pharmacodynamics and Pharmacokinetics

Systemic hyperosmotic agents lower the intraocular pressure through two mechanisms.[1] Firstly they cause reduction in the volume of vitreous humour through relative increase in the osmolality of the intravascular fluid. These agents penetrate slowly in the vitreous, which results in the creation of an osmotic gradient that draws fluid out of the vitreous into the intravascular space. Hence, reduction in the total vitreous volume causes reduction of intraocular pressure. Secondly, they also have a secondary effect on the

Table 19.1 Classification of hyperosmotic agents

Systemic agents		Topical agents
Intravenous hyperosmotic agents	Oral hyperosmotic agents	
1. Mannitol 2. Urea (not in use)	1. Glycerol 2. Isosorbide (not in use)	1. Hypertonic sodium chloride 2. Glycerol

osmoreceptors in the hypothalamic center of the central nervous system. However, this secondary mechanism does not play a significant role in the reduction of intraocular pressue. Mannitol and glycerol penetrate the blood ocular barrier poorly, which is of advantage as it creates a larger osmotic gradient for water to follow.

The decrease in intraocular pressure with hyperosmotic agents depends on the osmotic gradient created, which in turn depends on the following:

1. Molecular weight: Lower the molecular weight, greater the number of milliosmoles per dose and greater the efficacy. For example, urea (molecular weight = 60) has more mOsm per gram than mannitol (molecular weight = 182).
2. Dose given and weight of the patient.
3. Rate and route of administration: More rapid and greater effect is achieved with intravenous administration than by the oral route.
4. Distribution in fluid compartments: Drugs which are confined to the extracellular compartment (e.g. mannitol, glycerol) increase the osmotic gradient to a greater extent than drugs distributed in total body water (e.g. urea, isosorbide) at the same dose in milliosmoles.
5. Ocular penetration: Drugs with poor ocular penetration (e.g. mannitol, glycerol) achieve a greater osmotic gradient than those which enter the eye rapidly (e.g. urea, isosorbide). Hyperosmotics which enter the eye, however, still enter the vitreous slowly. A blood-vitreous gradient is, therefore, created. As water leaves the eye, osmolality of the vitreous increases. However, as the drug gets cleared from the blood, the gradient may get reversed and may cause rebound increase in intraocular pressure.[2]

6. Rate of excretion: Drugs which are cleared from the circulation rapidly have less effect on blood osmolality and intraocular pressure.

Topical hyperosmotic agents are mainly used to decrease corneal edema by creating an osmotic gradient between the edematous cornea and the tear film, thereby, drawing fluid from the edematous cornea to the hyperosmolar tear film, which is then eliminated through the usual lacrimal drainage system (Table 19.2).

Therapeutic Uses

Systemic hyperosmotic agents are indicated in acute glaucomas (e.g. acute angle-closure, malignant glaucoma, post-traumatic glaucoma) for short-term and for rapid reduction of intraocular pressure prior to definitive medical or surgical management. They may also be used prior to intraocular surgery, like cataract surgery, penetrating keratoplasty, trabeculectomy, non-draining sclera buckling. Glycerol is of significant value in the management of acute angle-closure glaucoma as it not only reduces the intraocular pressure but may also cause a readjustment in the intraocular volume and pressure in the posterior and anterior chamber in such a way that the angle closure is corrected and normal aqueous humor dynamics is re-established.

Topical hyperosmotic agents are indicated for reducing corneal edema due to various causes like bullous keratopathy, acute angle closure glaucoma, corneal hydrops, and Fuch's endothelial dystrophy.

Adverse Effects

The adverse effects of systemic hyperosmotic agents include:[1,3,4]

Table 19.2 Pharmacokinetics of systemic hyperosmotics

	Distribution in body compartments	Ocular penetration	Metabolism	Excretion
Mannitol	Extracellular	Poor	Not metabolized	Renal
Urea	Total body water	Good	Not metabolized	Renal
Glycerol	Extracellular	Poor	Metabolized	Renal
Isosorbide	Total body water	Good	Not metabolized	Renal

1. Nausea and vomiting occur often with oral agents especially with glycerol. This may cause difficulties when administered preoperatively. Nausea may be avoided by administering glycerol with a flavored vehicle.
2. Diuresis, urinary retention
3. Dehydration
4. Acidemia
5. Anaphylactic shock
6. Cardiovascular overload
7. Pulmonary edema
8. Anuria
9. Backache, headache, disorientation
10. Fever, chills.

The adverse effects of topical hyperosmotic agents are mainly temporary burning, irritation and blurring of vision on instillation.

Contraindications

Systemic hyperosmotic agents are contraindicated in patients with compromised cardiac function as they may cause circulatory overload and are to be used with caution in renal disease. Glycerol is relatively contraindicated in diabetic patients as it increases the risk of hyperglycemia and ketosis.[5]

Topical hyperosmotic agents are contraindicated in patients with hypersensitivity to its contents.

Glycerol (Glycerin)

The chemical name of glycerin is 1, 2, 3-Propanetriol. Glycerin 50% and 75% is an oral osmotic agent for reducing intraocular pressure.

Indications and Usage

Glycerin 50% or 75% is indicated in the treatment of glaucoma to interrupt acute attacks and in cases where a temporary drop in pressure is required which cannot be readily obtained by other means.

Adverse Effects

Nausea, vomiting, headache, confusion and disorientation may occur. Severe dehydration, cardiac arrhythmia or hyperosmolar non-ketotic coma leading to death have been reported.

Contraindications

Use of glycerol is contraindicated in patients with anuria, frank pulmonary edema or those with severe cardiac decompensation. Diabetes is a relative contraindication for the use of glycerol.

Precautions

Caution should be exercised in patients with hypovolemia, confused mental states, congestive heart failure and dehydration such as in diabetics. Safety and effectiveness in children have not been established. Caution should be exercised while administering it before ocular surgery as it may induce nausea and vomiting. Caution is also required in the elderly senile patients especially with history of urinary retention, diabetes, cardiac problems and severe dehydration.

Dosage and Administration

Glycerol is administered orally at a dose of 1–1.5 g/kg body weight (2–3 mL of 50% glycerol/kg body weight/dose). Peak effect occurs 1 to 1.5 hours after administration and lasts for 5 hours.

Glycerol needs to be administered in a flavored vehicle such as with lemon juice or over ice to avoid severe nausea due to its unpleasantly sweet taste.[6] In elderly patients, the minimum dose (1 g/kg) required to produce the desired effect should be used to avoid side-effects.

Mannitol

Mannitol is currently the most commonly used intravenous hyperosmotic agent. It is more useful than urea as an intravenously administered osmotic agent for reducing intraocular pressure.

Mechanism of Action

The mannitol molecule is three times larger than that of urea, but it exerts a comparable osmotic effect. This is because it is concentrated in the extracellular fluid compartments, which contain only one third of the total body water. As with urea, the mannitol induced pressure lowering effect coincides with the increase in serum osmotic pressure. This ocular hypotensive effect occurs in 30–60 minutes, depending on the rate of infusion, and lasts for about 6 hours. Because of vitreous dehydration, the anterior chamber deepens with intravenous infusion of mannitol as with urea.

Indications and Usage

Same as for glycerol.

Adverse Effects

All osmotic agents may produce headache, dizziness and backache, presumably from cerebral dehydration and decreased cerebrospinal fluid volume. Dryness of mouth and increased thirst often occur. Fluid and electrolyte imbalance and acidosis may occur. Movement of potassium from intracellular to extracellular fluid may induce hyperkalemia.

Contraindications

Same as for glycerol

Precautions

Patients with impaired cardiovascular status may suddenly decompensate with congestive heart failure. By diuresis, mannitol may intensify inadequate hydration or hypovolemia. Measurements of serum electrolytes such as sodium and potassium are, therefore, important in monitoring patients on combination of oral acetazolamide, glycerol and mannitol.

Dosage and Administration

Mannitol solution tends to crystallize at cooler temperatures. The crystals will go back into solution if the container is warmed, hence bottle should be shaken well before use.

Mannitol 20% solution is given intravenously at a dose of 1–2 g/kg over a 30 minute period (7–10 mL/kg). The duration of administration may vary from 20 to 45 minutes, but it should be given slowly as rapid infusion causes a shift of intracellular water into the extracellular space, causing cellular dehydration with a high risk of hyponatremia, congestive cardiac failure) and pulmonary edema. Peak intraocular pressure reduction occurs 1–1.5 hours after administration and lasts for 2–6 hours.

Isosorbide

The chemical name of isosorbide is 1, 4:3, 6-dianhydro-D-glucitol. Isosorbide 45% w/v oral solution is a dihydric alcohol prepared in a flavored vehicle.

Isosorbide is readily absorbed after oral administration. It is not metabolized and remains in circulation until eliminated by kidneys unchanged. The physical action of isosorbide is similar to that of other osmotic agents.

Indications and Usage

Isosorbide is used for the short-term reduction of intraocular pressure to interrupt an acute attack of glaucoma. It may be used prior to and after intraocular surgery. It is used when there is less risk of nausea and vomiting than that posed by other oral hyperosmotic agents is needed.

Adverse Effects

Nausea, vomiting, headache, confusion and disorientation may occur. Very rare occurrences of syncope, gastric discomfort, lethargy, vertigo, thirst, dizziness, hiccups, irritability, rash and light headedness have been reported.

Contraindications

Same as for glycerol. However, it is relatively safer in diabetics than glycerol.

Precautions

With repeated doses, consideration should be given to maintenance of adequate fluid and electrolyte balance. If urinary output continues to decrease, the patient's clinical status should be closely reviewed. Accumulation of isosorbide may result in over-expansion of the extracellular fluid.

Repetitive doses should be used with caution particularly in patients with diseases associated with salt retention. It is important to ensure that patient's bladder has been emptied prior to surgery.

Dosage and Administration

The recommended initial dose is 1.5 g/kg body weight of isosorbide 45%. The onset of action is usually within 30 minutes while the maximum effect is expected at 1 to 1.5 hours and lasts for 3–5 hours.

TOPICAL HYPEROSMOTIC AGENTS

Topical Glycerol (Glycerin)

The chemical name of glycerol is 1, 2, 3-Propanetriol. Topical glycerol is usually available as a clear, colorless viscous solution.

Indications and Usage

Topical glycerol is usually used to temporarily clear an edematous cornea to facilitate ophthalmoscopic and gonioscopic examination of the eye in conditions like acute angle-closure glaucoma, bullous keratopathy, Fuch's endothelial dystrophy and corneal hydrops. Its action is transient and hence is used for diagnostic purposes only.

Adverse Effects

It may cause pain and irritation on instillation of the drops.

Contraindications

Use of topical glycerol is contraindicated in patients with hypersensitivity to the active ingredients or preservatives used in formulation.

Precaution

Glycerol is an irritant and hence, instillation of topical anesthetic prior to instillation of glycerol is useful.

Dosage and Administration

One or two drops of topical glycerol are administered prior to ophthalmic or gonioscopic examination.[7]

Topical Hypertonic Saline

Topical hypertonic saline (sodium chloride) is used as sodium chloride 2, 3 and 5% ophthalmic eye drops or sodium chloride 5% ophthalmic ointment.

Indications and Usage

It is usually used for the temporary relief of corneal edema caused by bullous keratopathy, Fuch's endothelial dystrophy and acute hydrops.

Adverse Effects

It may cause temporary irritation and burning on instillation of the eye drops.

Contraindications

Its use is contraindicated in patients with hypersensitivity to the active ingredient or preservatives used in formulation.

Dosage and Administration

1 or 2 drops in the affected eye(s) every 3–4 hours.[7]

SUMMARY

Systemic hyperosmotic agents are used in emergency situations where rapid reduction of intraocular pressure is required. Mannitol and glycerol are the most commonly used hyperosmotic agents administered by intravenous and oral routes respectively. Their use may be associated with serious systemic adverse effects, therefore, they should be used with caution.

Topical hyperosmotic agents are generally used for temporary relief of corneal edema.

B. Surgical Adjuncts

Puneet Agarwal

OVERVIEW

A variety of agents are used as adjuncts in various ophthalmological procedures and surgeries. In intraocular surgeries such adjuncts are the vital components. Commonly used surgical adjuncts in ophthalmic procedures include irrigating solutions, viscoelastic agents, enzymes, chelating agents, caustics and adhesives.

INTRAOCULAR IRRIGATING SOLUTIONS

Intraocular irrigating solutions serve as perfusion medium during surgery. They clean the tissue and maintain its hydration. Most importantly, they are composed in a way to meet the metabolic requirement of ocular tissue for the period of disruption of nutrient supply during surgical procedure.

The corneal epithelial cells derive energy to a great extent by anaerobic metabolism. They receive glucose supply primarily from aqueous humor and some from limbal vessels.[8] They also store glucose as glycogen. During short periods of interruption in nutrient supply as occurs during intraocular surgery, corneal epithelial cells can rely on their own glycogen stores. The keratocytes in stroma derive energy from both the aerobic and anaerobic metabolism. Their glucose supply is from aqueous humor. Their dependence on glucose contents of intraocular irrigating solutions is not well established. The corneal endothelium obtains its nutrient supply from aqueous humor and derives energy by aerobic metabolism. The cells in conjunctiva and uvea receive their oxygen and glucose supply through rich network of conjunctival and uveal vessels respectively.[9] Lens has a very low metabolic rate and depends on aqueous humor for its glucose and oxygen supply.[10] However, during short periods of interruption in nutrient supply, lens maintains its energy supply by anaerobic metabolism and is not dependent on nutrients in intraocular irrigation fluids.[11] Prolonged deprivation of glucose can, however, cause cataract development. Retinal tissue obtains nourishment from ocular vessels.

As stated above, the corneal endothelial cells obtain glucose and oxygen largely from aqueous humor. The cells in corneal endothelium contain large number of mitochondria and depend to a great extent on aerobic metabolism.[12] The endothelium is the most important component of cornea in maintaining its hydration and clarity.[13,14] Therefore, during intraocular surgery corneal endothelial cells must be supplied with glucose in irrigating solution as they are the most vulnerable to interruption in nutrient supply.

To maintain the cell viability during surgical procedure, irrigation solutions are formulated to match the physiological conditions. Accordingly, the pH of intraocular irrigation solutions is adjusted at approximately 7.4 and the osmolality at approximately 300 mOsm. A variation in pH or the osmolality is likely to damage the structure and function of the ocular tissue. The intraocular irrigating solutions also contain sodium, potassium, magnesium, calcium, chloride and bicarbonate.[15,16] These ions are required to maintain cell adhesions and cell-to-cell junctions. Due to their toxic effects on ocular tissue and doubtful efficacy against intraocular infections, preservatives are not used in intraocular irrigation solutions. Intraocular toxicities due to preservatives include damage to corneal endothelial cells, iritis and lens opacification. The three types of intraocular irrigating solutions in use include:

1. Balanced salt solution (BSS)
2. Lactated Ringer's solution
3. Balanced salt solution plus (complete)

BSS consists of chlorides of sodium, potassium, calcium and magnesium, sodium acetate and sodium citrate. It is acceptable for short-term surgery but not for surgeries lasting for more than 1 hour, because of the development of corneal edema.[17,18] Lactated Ringer's solution consists of chlorides of sodium, potassium and calcium and sodium lactate. Long-lasting intraocular surgeries require additional components in irrigating solution such as bicarbonate, glucose, glutathione and adenosine.[19] Therefore, the commercially available complete irrigation mediums contain phosphate, bicarbonate, magnesium, glucose and glutathione. Phosphate and bicarbonates act as buffers and glucose provides a source of energy. Glutathione is a peptide that acts as antioxidant and helps in maintaining the intercellular junctions. Magnesium is essential for the functions of ATPase pump in corneal endothelial cells. Adenosine is not added to the complete irrigating solutions as it makes the medium unstable.

In a prospective randomized double-blind trial, comparison of Ringer's lactate with BSS plus was done in patients undergoing phacoemulsification surgery for cataract. It was observed that the two solutions were comparable if the time of surgery was short and limited volume of solution was used.[20] Dextrose bicarbonate Ringer's lactate was also shown to provide similar results as BSS plus for short duration surgeries. As the Ringer's lactate and Dextrose bicarbonate Ringer's lactate are many times cheaper than BSS plus, they are considered preferred choice for short surgeries, especially in developing countries.[20,21] However, in patients that required longer surgery time and use of large volumes of solution, the reduction in corneal endothelial cell density was significantly higher with Ringer's lactate.[20] The complete irrigation mediums like BSS plus are also required for patients with compromised corneal endothelium even if the surgery lasts for less than 1 hour.[22,23] Similarly,

if the intraocular surgery is to be done without the use of a viscoelastic agent, a complete irrigation solution is required to adequately protect corneal endothelium even if the surgery lasts for less than 1 hour.[24] Diabetic patients have high polyol contents in lens fibers, which exert a high osmotic pressure. Therefore, for diabetic patients a higher osmolarity irrigation solution is used to prevent osmotic movement of water into the lens and subsequent development of posterior subcapsular cataract.[25] For vitreoretinal surgeries, use of oxygenated intraocular irrigation fluid by using an in-line oxygenator has been described.[26] Oxygenated intraocular irrigation fluid facilitates significantly earlier return of electroretinogram voltage to baseline after vitreoretinal surgery as compared to unoxygenated BSS plus.[27]

The complete irrigation solutions are available in two parts, which are mixed together just before use and remain stable for the period of surgery. The composition of two commercially available complete and incomplete intraocular solutions is given in Table 19.3.

EXTRAOCULAR IRRIGATING SOLUTIONS

Extraocular irrigating solutions are used to remove unwanted substances from the ocular surface. As mostly they are used for short period they do not require nutrients or specific ion as is the case with intraocular irrigating solutions. However, their pH and osmolality is physiologically maintained. Prolonged exposure to these solutions can cause cellular swelling and damage.[28] Composition of different commercially available extraocular irrigation solutions is shown in Table 19.4.

Extraocular irrigating solutions are used to wash out debris, mucus, purulent discharge and other unwanted material from the ocular surface, removal of foreign body, after tonometry to remove the dye, after gonioscopy to remove methycellulose and for diagnostic nasolacrimal duct irrigation in patients with epiphora. These solutions can be used to wash eyes after wearing

Table 19.3 Composition of various commercially available intraocular irrigating solutions

Components (mmol/L)	BSS (Alcon)	AMO endosol (Akron)	BSS plus (Alcon)	AMO endosol extra (Akron)
Sodium chloride	109.5	109.5	122.2	109.4
Potassium chloride	10.1	10.1	5.1	4.6
Calcium chloride	4.3	4.3	1.1	1.2
Magnesium chloride	1.5	1.5	1.0	1.9
Sodium bicarbonate			25	22.4
Sodium phosphate			2.8	2.7
Sodium citrate	5.8	5.8		
Sodium lactate				
Sodium acetate	28.6	28.6		
Sodium gluconate				
Glutathione disulfide			0.3	0.3
Glucose			5.1	4.6

Table 19.4 Composition of various commercially available extraocular irrigating solutions

Components (%)	Eye-stream (Alcon)	Eye wash (Levoptik)	Eye irrigating wash (Roberts Hauck)
Sodium chloride	0.64	0.49	
Potassium chloride	0.75		0.38
Magnesium chloride	0.03		
Calcium chloride	0.048		
Sodium acetate	0.39		
Sodium citrate	0.17		
Sodium biphosphate		0.4	
Sodium phosphate		0.45	
Sodium carbonate			0.014
Boric acid			1.2
EDTA			0.05
Benzalkonium chloride	0.013	0.005	0.01

contact lens but cannot be used with contact lens in place. They cause irritation and can alter the lens surface. Preservatives in the solution can get absorbed in the hydrogel lens and then will be delivered to corneal surface over a prolonged period causing corneal toxicity.

VISCOELASTIC AGENTS

Viscoelastic substances are widely used in intraocular surgery. They are viscous solutions of high molecular weight substances. Due to the viscosity of solution, they protect and lubricate the ocular tissue during surgery. Their elasticity provides protection against the mechanical damage caused by vibrating instruments. Their pseudoplasticity allows safe manipulation of the tissue. During surgery they have been shown to reduce the endothelial cell loss.[29,30] Use of viscoelastic agents during surgery helps to maintain the depth of anterior chamber and protect the newly formed and exposed surfaces. They are routinely used as adjuncts in cataract surgery, intraocular lens implantation, keratoplasty, glaucoma filtration surgery and vitreoretinal surgery. These agents are tissue-protective, non-antigenic and do not interfere with wound healing. The use of sodium hyaluronate as a component of vitreous substitute needed to replace vitreous humor after vitrectomy has also been described.[31] Küçükerdönmez et al. reported that intraocular injection of hyaluronic acid may be useful for stabilizing IOP and vision in patients with previous vitreoretinal surgery.[32]

The viscoelastic agents can largely be classified into two classes: cohesive and dispersive. Cohesive agents are high molecular weight substances with highly entangled molecular structure whereas dispersive agents are smaller molecular weight with more straight chain structure. Cohesive viscoelastics such as Healon® (sodium hyaluronate 1%, 4×10^6 daltons) and Healon GV® (sodium hyaluronate 1.4%, 5×10^6 daltons) are useful in maintaining the depth of anterior chamber and are easy to remove after surgery whereas dispersive agents such as Viscoat® (sodium hyaluronate 3%, 5×10^5 daltons—chondroitin sulfate 4%) provide effective coating over corneal endothelium and are difficult to remove. DisCoVisc® (sodium hyaluronate 1.6%, 1.7×10^6 daltons—chondroitin sulfate 4%) is a new viscoelastic agent that does not fit into either category as it has viscosity similar to Healon®, but is dispersive like Viscoat®.[33] Sodium hyaluronate is also available in combination with lidocaine as VisThesia topical (sodium hyaluronate 0.3%, lidocaine 2%), for corneal hydration and topical anesthesia, and VisThesia intracameral (sodium hyaluronate 1.5% and lidocaine 1%), for cohesive viscoelastic use and intracameral anesthesia.

Sodium hyaluronate (hyaluronic acid) is composed of two monosaccharide units and is a main component of vitreous humor. It has been shown to play an important role in inflammation by stimulating neutrophil migration, aggregation and proliferation and promoting wound healing.[34,35] Healon® was first introduced to clinical practice in 1979 and since has become an important component in ocular surgery. Healon®5 (sodium hyaluronate 2.3%, 4×10^6 daltons) was used in 1998. It has a higher viscosity but its injection and removal after surgery is more difficult. In a randomized multicenter clinical trial comparing Healon®5 and Healon®, it was observed that retention during phacoemulsification, anterior chamber maintenance during continuous curvilinear capsulorhexis (CCC), and facilitation of intraocular lens (IOL) implantation was better achieved with Healon®5 as compared to Healon®, however, Healon®5 was more difficult to inject and remove than Healon®.[36] DisCoVisc® due to its dual nature has been shown to provide corneal endothelial cell protection comparable to Viscoat® during phacoemulsification and at the same time is better retained with shorter removal time as compared to Viscoat® or Healon®5.[37,38]

While clearing from the anterior chamber, sodium hyaluronate can block the outflow channels in trabecular meshwork due to its large molecular size and causes post-operative rise in intraocular pressure. Therefore, after completion of surgery, sodium hyaluronate is removed from the anterior chamber.[39,40] The residual amount can cause postoperative inflammation and allergy. Corneal haze sometimes may occur due to altered water balance in the cornea causing change in its refractive index.[41] Sodium hyaluronate can also cause crystalline deposits on intraocular lenses.[42]

Hydroxypropyl methylcellulose (HPMC), ***chondritin sulfate*** and ***type IV collagen*** are the other viscoelastic substances used during intraocular surgery. HPMC is a derivative of cellulose, chondroitin sulfate is similar to hyaluronic acid in its chemical structure and collagen is a protein found in the connective tissue. The uses and adverse effects of these agents are similar to those of sodium hyaluronate. Combinations of viscoelastic agents are also available for use.

SURGICAL MIOTICS

Acetylcholine (ACh) chloride solution (1:100) is applied directly to exposed iris to induce miosis during surgical procedures such as cataract extraction, keratoplastry, iredectomy. ACh is ineffective if applied topically but is safe and effective for intraocular use. However, its effect is short-lasting as it is quickly destroyed by acetylcholinesterase.

Carbachol, a direct-acting cholinomimetic agent, produces long-lasting miosis. Its 0.01% solution is applied by gentle irrigation in a dose of 0.5 mL. Longer acting and topically effective miotics like pilocarpine can be used to produce miosis immediately after surgery but they cause increased postoperative pain and inflammation.

SURGICAL ENZYMES

Hyaluronidase, an enzyme often added to local anesthetic solutions to produce enhanced anesthesia and akinesia. The enzyme depolymerizes the hyaluronic acid, which is a component of connective tissue and acts as tissue cement. Break down of hyaluronic acid allows easy and rapid spread of anesthetic solution through the tissue. It is added to local anesthetic solutions for retrobulbar and peribulbar block in a dose of 75 units per 10 mL of solution.

Urokinase is used to irrigate hyphema and in cases of retinal artery and vein occlusion. The conversion of plasminogen to plasmin by urokinase causes degradation of plasma proteins, fibrinogen and fibrin clots.

BOTULINUM TOXIN

Botulinum toxin is derived from bacterium *Clostridium botulinum*. Its serotype A is used in therapeutics. The botulinum toxin interferes with the release of acetylcholine from nerve fibers, blocks neuromuscular transmission and relieves localized muscle spasm. The effect is dose-dependent and lasts for up to 9 months. Once injected into the muscles it is not absorbed systemically. The dose needs to be individualized and sometimes multiple injections are necessary. Response also depends upon the type and severity of disorder. Botulinum toxin is used in the treatment of blepharospasm, strabismus, nystagmus, hemifacial spasm, lower lid entropion and corneal ulcer resulting from exposure. Use of botulinum toxin is associated with several adverse effects such as diplopia, ptosis, scleral perforation, reduced accommodation, hemorrhage, pupillary dilation, dry eye and local tissue reactions.

TRYPAN BLUE

Trypan blue is a dye that selectively stains the connective tissue structures such as anterior lens capsule. It can be used as an aid in ophthalmic surgery as it stains only the anterior capsule, which can be visualized against unstained interior of the lens. The dye is immediately removed from the anterior chamber and its use is contraindicated if non-hydrated hydrophilic acrylic lens is planned to be inserted as it stains the lens. During small incision cataract surgery, trypan blue has been shown not to affect the IOP in immediate and early post-operative period.[43]

GROWTH FACTORS

Growth factors are endogenous polypeptides that are known to promote wound healing. Growth factors regulate normal turnover of a variety of cells including corneal epithelium. They play a role in ocular healing by stimulating cell division and migration of corneal cells, synthesis of extracellular matrix in cornea and chemotaxis.[44-46]

Epidermal growth factor (EGF) has been shown to promote corneal wound healing following mechanical and chemical injury. This effect of EGF is mediated by cyclic adenosine monophosphate (cAMP)-dependent cell proliferation and differentiation. It is a dose-dependent effect and has been observed in corneal epithelium and endothelium.[47,48] EGF has not been used widely in clinical practice as the mitogenic properties of EGF that promote wound healing are non-specific and, therefore, may also promote undesired growth of other tissues. Moreover, EGF also has angiogenic properties and has been found to be elevated in patients with neovascular glaucoma.[49]

Fibroblast growth factor (FGF), like EGF is known to promote corneal wound healing after mechanical or chemical injury by stimulating cell division, migration, differentiation and chemotaxis.[50] The exact mechanism of action of FGF is not known but it seems to be associated with specific receptors linked to diacylglycerol-inositol phosphate second messenger system. FGF is also associated with neovascular glaucoma due to its angiogenic properties.[51]

Transforming growth factors (TGFs) α and β have been isolated from various parts of ocular tissue. They promote wound healing by promoting cell division, migration and differentiation in corneal epithelium, endothelium and stroma.[50] TGF β_2 may also enhance the closure of macular holes. TGFs have not been widely used so far in clinical practice due to their non-specific action and TGF β_2 also seems to play a role in the development of proliferative diabetic retinopathy.[52]

Other growth factors that can promote ocular wound healing include ***Insulin-like growth factor*** (IGF), ***fibronectin*** and ***keratinocyte growth factors*** (KGF). IGF has been shown to promote neovascularization and fibronectin promotes cataract development.[53]

MITOMYCIN C

Mitomycin C is an antineoplastic antibiotic agent, which is now used widely in ophthalmic practice. It is isolated from the soil bacterium *Streptomyces caespitosus*. It affects rapidly dividing cells such as fibroblasts in a healing wound by interfering with DNA synthesis, RNA transcription and protein synthesis. The cell cycle is most affected at late G-I and early S-phase. It is available as 2 mg/mL solution and is further diluted for use in sterile water at neutral pH. It is inactivated at acidic pH. Due to its hydrophobic nature, it penetrates tissue easily.

Subconjunctival or scleral application of mitomycin C at a concentration of 0.2–0.4 mg/mL is used intraoperatively during glaucoma filtration surgery to prevent scarring of filtering bleb as it inhibits fibroblast growth. After pterygium excision also it is applied at the same concentration to prevent recurrence. In patients undergoing dacryocystorhinostomy, mitomycin C is used to suppress fibrous proliferation and scar formation under the flaps near osteotomy sites. Topical mitomycin C has been shown to reduce post-operative adhesions following squint surgery. It has also been used to prevent development of corneal haze after laser surface ablation in refractive surgeries. It prevents recurrence of localized conjunctival-corneal intraepithelial neoplasia.

Complications associated with the use of mitomycin C include necrotizing scleritis, scleral ulceration, perforation, uveitis, cataract, glaucoma, symblephron formation, photophobia, lid edema and ocular pain. Its use is contraindicated in one-eyed and very elderly patients.

C. Sterilization, Disinfection and Antiseptics in Ophthalmology

Lwin Lwin Nyein

OVERVIEW

Medical equipments and surgical instruments are devices that are essential for the care of patients and their use in preventive medicine is inseparable from diagnostic procedures and therapeutic practices. Aseptic techniques in hospitals involve systematic, appropriate and continued effort to eliminate pathogenic microorganisms from the patient's environment to prevent infection. The basis for aseptic procedures rests on fundamental concepts related to the mode of transmission, virulence, and destruction of microbes and the resistance or susceptibility of the host. These basic concepts are firmly established in microbiology, epidemiology and general surgery: specialized considerations determine their application to ophthalmology.[54]

Decontamination, disinfection and sterilization are basic components of eye care services. Lack of knowledge or negligence in standard practices would result in hazardous effects, as sterile instruments and environment are essential for successful eye care services. In ophthalmic practice, major hospital associated infectious diseases are minimal as the hospital stay of a patient rarely exceeds 48 hours. Moreover, such infections are preventable.

Currently, the concept of sterilization in ophthalmology is focused towards safe aseptic practices and the range of techniques and compounds used to achieve a clean surgical environment has greatly increased.

DEFINITIONS

Sterilization is defined as the method that destroys all viable microorganisms including bacterial spores. The objective of sterilization is to remove or destroy microorganisms, since they cause contamination, infection and decay. The purpose for sterilization, the material to be sterilized and the nature of the microorganisms that are to be removed or destroyed determines the choice of methods of sterilization.[55] Sterilization processes involve chemical and biological methods such as pressure, temperature and others.

Disinfection is a process, chemical or physical, that destroys viable microorganisms excluding bacterial spores. The most important factor in using disinfectant is its concentration, time of contact with the disinfectant and precautions advised by the manufacturer. Several methods of disinfection are available, but standardization and uniformity throughout a hospital setting is essential. Disinfection is not a substitute for sterilization.

High-level disinfection (HDL) is a process that eliminates all microorganisms except some bacterial endospores from inanimate objects by boiling, steaming or the use of chemical disinfectants.[56]

The compounds commonly used in the opthalmic practice are listed in Table 19.5

METHODS OF STERILIZATION

The most common methods used for sterilization are:

1. ***Dry Heat:*** It kills microorganisms by destructive oxidation of cell constituents. It is effective for sterilizing metal instruments as by conduction, the heat reaches all surfaces of the instrument to be sterilized. It cannot be used for plastic and rubber items as temperature used in hot air oven (160–170° C) is too high and penetrates materials slowly and unevenly.

Table 19.5 Compounds commonly used for antisepsis, disinfection and sterilization in ophthalmic practice

Compounds	Mechanism of action	Properties	Antiseptic action	Disinfection	Sterilization	Uses in ophthalmic practice
Alcohols Ethyl alcohol and Isopropyl alcohol	Precise mechanism unknown but act by causing membrane damage and protein denaturation	Rapid broad spectrum antimicrobial activity but not sporicidal	+	+		Hand washing and as antiseptic before surgery To clean skin or surfaces
Aldehydes Glutaraldehyde and Formaldehyde	Affect enzyme systems	High antimicrobial activity including mycobacteria, viruses and spores Less active at an acidic pH		+	+	To sterilize ophthalmic instruments
Anilides Triclocarbon	Destroys the cytoplasmic membrane	Active against Gram-negative bacteria	+			Used mainly in soaps and deodorants but rarely clinically
Biguanides Chlorhexidine **PHMB** (Polyhexamethylene Biguanide)	At higher concentrations, increases membrane permeability and coagulates intracellular contents	Broad spectrum but not sporicidal, poor effect on mycobacteria and variable antiviral effect Activity is pH dependent and reduced in the presence of organic matter. The most widely used biocide	+			Used for preoperative hand washing or for preoperative skin preparation in patients with iodine allergies. Used in a specialized formulation (PHMB) for the treatment of Acanthamoeba keratitis

Contd...

Contd...

	Mechanism of action	Properties			Uses
Halogen Releasing Agents Sodium hypochlorite	Highly active oxidizing agents. Inhibit DNA synthesis	Disinfect blood spillages containing HBV and HIV and sporicidal at high concentrations	+	+	Most widely used to disinfect tonometer heads
Iodine		Wide scope of antimicrobial activity including spores	+	+	
Iodophors, e.g. povidine-iodine		Better tolerated than iodine and leaves a depot of active iodine, therefore, leading to a persistent effect			Surgical skin preparation and preoperative handwashing Rarely used now
Silver Compounds Silver sulfadiazine and silver nitrate	Bind to membrane bound enzymes via thiol groups	Broad spectrum of activity	+		Rarely used now Traditionally used as prophylaxis and for the treatment of ophthalmia neonatorum
Peroxygens Hydrogen peroxide	Oxidizing agent and breaks DNA strands	Good antifungal and antiviral properties. Need higher concentrations and longer exposure for sporicidal activity. Environment friendly as it breaks down to water and oxygen but needs a stabilizer to prevent decomposition	+	+	Commonly used in contact lens disinfectant solutions
Phenols and Bisphenols e.g. tricloscan	Affects microbial membranes	Broad spectrum of activity and good sporostatic agent. Most commonly used as a preservative or as an antiseptic towel. Inactivated by anionic surfactants, e.g. soap	+	+	Used as preoperative hand antisepsis and cleansing Used in treating MRSA carriers preoperatively
Quaternary Ammonium Compounds e.g. benzalkonium chloride	Affects microbial cytoplasmic membranes	Broad spectrum of activity and good sporostatic agent. Most commonly used as a preservative or as an antiseptic towel. Inactivated by anionic surfactants, e.g. soap	+		Most widely used as a preservative in eyedrops An active ingredient in some contact lens soaking solutions

2. ***Moist Heat:*** It kills microorganisms by coagulation and denaturation of the enzymes and structural proteins. It is most commonly used and an effective method of sterilization.

   Steam under increased pressure is more efficient sterilizing agent than hot air oven as it provides greater lethal action, shorter sterilization time and penetrates porous material effectively.

3. ***Chemical Method:*** Glutaraldehyde and formaldehyde are examples of chemical sterilant. Both are used for instruments that will not tolerate heat sterilization such as laparoscopes. They are irritant to skin, eyes and respiratory tract.

Compounds that are commonly used in ophthalmic practice are summarized in Table 19.5.

While ensuring safe sterilization systems, ophthalmologists should be more concerned about properly preparing the surface of the eye, where the majority of flora is found and which commonly is the biggest source of infection.

Proper sterilization, coupled with appropriate cleaning of eye instruments; use of well-designed trays, packaging, and sterilization indicators; meeting manufacturer's recommendations with regard to time, temperature, and pressure; and effective transfer to the site of use, is a highly effective means of sterilization in ophthalmic surgery.[57,58]

METHODS OF PREVENTING CONTAMINATION IN OUTPATIENT SERVICES

Sources of infection to outpatients are mainly due to contamination on the surgeon's and paramedic's hands, tonometer, slit lamp and opened old medication bottles. Patients in contact with contaminated ophthalmic diagnostic instruments like the tonometer and slit lamp are at high risk of getting ocular infections due to bacteria and viruses.

Hand Hygiene

Failure to achieve appropriate hand hygiene is considered to be the leading cause of nosocomial (hospital-acquired) infections and spread of multi-drug resistant microorganisms, and has been recognized as a significant contributor to outbreaks.[56] The most important procedures for preventing such infections include the following:

1. Hand washing should be done before:
   - Examining (direct contact with) a patient; and
   - Putting on sterile or high-level disinfected surgical gloves prior to an operation, or examination for routine procedures.
2. Hand washing should be done after:
   - Any situation in which hands may become contaminated, such as:
   - Handling soiled instruments and other items;
   - Touching mucous membranes, blood or other body fluids (secretions or excretions);
   - Having prolonged and intense contact with a patient; and
   - Removing gloves.
3. In high-risk areas, an antiseptic liquid hand-washing agent (such as an iodophor or chlorhexidine gluconate) should be used, both before and after direct contact with patient. High-risk areas include cornea clinic and minor operation theater.
4. General patient care areas, outpatient clinics and clinical laboratories require only a general liquid hand-washing agent.
5. Bar soap and towels should not be used for multipatient purpose.[55]

Needle Stick/Splash Policy

Splash policy is to be strictly adhered to avoid transmission of infection through accidental splash of a needle stick with blood contamination, body fluids, mucous membranes or non-intact skin. The needle stick injuries should be thoroughly cleaned, and the affected area rinsed with soap and water.[55]

Disinfecting Tonometers

1. Dry heat
2. Mechanical cleaning with disposable wipe/ sterile gauze.

3. Wipe with gauze soaked in alcohol or chemicals like hydrogen peroxide and merthiolate.
4. Soaking in chemicals like 70% isopropyl alcohol, 1:1000 merthiolate, 3% hydrogen peroxide and 1:10 diluted house hold bleach (sodium hypochlorite).[55]

Disinfecting Slit Lamp

1. Mechanical cleaning with disposable wipe/sterile gauze.
2. Wipe with gauze soaked in alcohol or chemicals like hydrogen peroxide and merthiolate.[55]

PREVENTIVE METHODS IN THE OPERATION THEATER

Post-operative infection remains a major cause of morbidity among patients undergoing surgery. Maintenance of strict asepsis is essential if post-operative infections and their consequences are to be minimized. Such infections can be either endogenous or exogenous. Factors associated with transmission of infective material exogenously in a hospital are: use of unsterile equipment, presence of shedders of pathogenic microorganisms amongst hospital personnel, contaminated environment and contaminated surfaces.[55]

The ophthalmic operating room (OR) is a highly specialized unit where strict asepsis needs to be maintained because of the fear of post-operative infections including endophthalmitis. The incidence of post-operative endophthalmitis sporadically or as mini-outbreaks especially in ophthalmic camps has increased. It is possible and feasible to prevent such infective complications with proper disinfection and sterilization routines.

Post-operative endophthalmitis, external ocular infections such as conjunctivitis, infections transmissible through corneal transplantation, hepatitis and HIV are major hospital-borne infection and preventive measures should be taken in order to avoid them.

Preventing infections following an operation is a complex process. Surgical aseptic techniques are designed to create such environment by controlling four main sources of infection: the patient, surgical staff, equipment and the operating room environment. Specific techniques are established through following procedures:

- Patient considerations: skin cleaning pre-operatively, skin antisepsis and wound covering
- Surgical staff considerations: hand hygiene (hand washing and/or hand rub with waterless, alcohol-based antiseptic agents); use and removal of gloves and gowns
- Equipment and room preparation considerations: traffic flow and activity pattern as well as housekeeping practices and decontamination, cleaning and either sterilization or high-level disinfection of instruments, gloves and other items
- Environmental considerations: maintaining an aseptic operating field and using safe operating practices and techniques.[44]

PREVENTION IN HIGH-RISK AREAS/STAFF

Healthcare professionals are at high risk of infection: anesthetists, surgeons, laboratory personnel, operating-room staff and places that are exposed to contaminated blood and body fluids. Preventing accidents (needle sticks) and other blood and body fluid exposures are the primary means of preventing transmission of HIV or HCV/HBV.

Hepatitis

Hepatitis is a hospital-acquired-infection in health care workers and hence prevention against it is essential. The major sources of infections are needle sticks and blood spills.

For HBV, an effective vaccine has been available for nearly 20 years. Personnel working in high risk areas should be given information about hepatitis B and the risk of developing the disease. The decision to have hepatitis B vaccine administered shall be left to the employee.

Priorities for the administration of hepatitis B vaccine to employees shall be developed by the infection control committee.[44]

Human Immunodeficiency Virus (HIV)

The plan for assessing the risk of accidental exposure to HIV is similar to that for HBV. Since there is no vaccine against HIV, post-exposure prophylaxis is much more complicated; therefore, the decision to recommend it needs to be based on a careful assessment of the injury.

The suggested steps for managing an injury are as follows:

- Direct contact of skin and mucous membranes with blood, blood products, secretions, wastes and tissues of patients should be avoided
- Regardless of the use of gloves, hands should be washed routinely
- Gloves should be worn for contact with moist body substances
- If soiling of cloths with moist body substances is anticipated, gowns or aprons should be used
- Masks or goggles should be worn
- If infection requiring a private room is mandated, then it should be arranged
- Care should be taken to avoid needle splash, while handling needle sticks on patients
- Reusable items should be reprocessed and kept in the soiled utility room.[55,56]

Infective Waste Disposal

Infective waste should be incinerated or should be autoclaved prior to disposal. Sharp items like needles, scalpel blades that could cause injury, should be placed intact into puncture-resistant containers. Needles should not be recapped, bent, broken or manipulated by hand, in order to avoid needle-stick injuries.

Strict rules should be followed for waste disposal in a hospital. The paramedics should be aware of the specific color codes of bags used for disposal of infective waste.[55]

STERILIZATION IN OPHTHALMIC PRACTICE: CURRENT STATUS

Health and safety measures should be well informed to the personnel in the operation theater, staff in direct contact with patients or those involved with disposal of infective waste materials, so that they can protect themselves and others from infection. Since there are substantial epidemiological evidences of diseases caused by hospital borne infection, there should be regular monitoring of disinfectant and sterility procedures by "Infection Control Committee (ICC)" with an Infection Control Nurse and adequate surveillance. Since patient care is a priority, infections due to negligence should not occur. It is highly essential to take preventive measures to maintain hygienic and sterile environment for eye care service.[54]

One of the commonly used methods of sterilization by the ophthalmologist is the "flash sterilization". The Center for Disease Control and Prevention (CDC) guideline are used as a guide for disinfection and sterilization. In 1999, this guideline described flash sterilization as having very limited applicability for sterilizing instruments. At that time, flash sterilization was commonly used when an instrument was dropped. It was then 'flashed' for immediate re-use. Some of the ophthalmologists used this method not as an exception but often as the sole method. Such process appeared to violate (CDC) guidelines and triggered a closer look into ophthalmologist's use of steam sterilization and the entire process of cleaning, disinfecting, and sterilizing surgical instruments.

In 2008, the CDC updated its stance in its "Guideline for Disinfection and Sterilization in Healthcare Facilities", stating: "Correctly performed flash sterilization is an effective process for the sterilization of critical medical devices."

The flash method also called steam sterilization is the most common form of sterilization used by ophthalmologists, and the infection rate it carries in ophthalmic surgeries is very low. In fact, while ensuring safe sterilization systems, ophthalmologists should be more concerned about properly preparing the surface of the eye, where the majority of flora is found and which commonly is the biggest source of infection.[58,59]

It is critical that hospitals and surgical centers keep and follow the policies and procedures regarding the sterilization and disinfection. In addition, other ancillary procedures are also necessary to control nosocomial infection. It is important that administrative controls should be implemented; policies and instructions for correct sterilization methods should be followed; a sufficient number of instrument sets should be available to allow adequate time for cleaning and sterilizing between procedures and all employees should be trained uniformly regarding the handling and cleaning of the surgical instruments. Under these circumstances there can be no justification for the use of method which does not achieve absolute sterility of instruments, materials, and solutions. Whatever may be the method of sterilization in ophthalmology, the objective is to stress the indispensable nature of aseptic technique in ocular surgery.

D. Contact Lens Care Systems

Puneet Agarwal

OVERVIEW

All types of contact lenses except the daily disposable and extended wear lenses require careful maintenance with disinfectant and cleaning solutions. Commercial development of solutions for contact lens care started emerging in 1940s with increasing usage of rigid contact lenses (polymethylmethacrylate, PMMA lenses). Initially two types of solutions, i.e. "wetting" and "soaking" solutions were used. In 1970s, hydrogel lenses became popular and it was observed that they had greater affinity for surface deposits. Therefore, several newer forms of contact lens care systems such as dual, triple and multipurpose solutions were developed. Moreover, the enzymatic cleaners were introduced for more effective cleaning of lenses and efforts were made to develop soft hydrogel lenses that are resistant to surface deposits. As a result in 1990s very high oxygen permeability soft silicone hydrogel lenses were developed that adsorbed less proteins.

Wearing contact lenses renders eye at a greater risk of acquiring infections as compared to non-contact lens wearers. According to Brennan and Coles, the risk of bacterial keratitis is 60 times higher in contact lens wearers as compared to non-wearers.[60] According to a survey done over a period of 2 years in public hospitals of Singapore, infective keratitis secondary to soft contact lens wear was found to be the most common complication. Other complications included epithelial keratitis and allergic conjunctivitis.[61] The reason for higher risk of infection is primarily due to interference with the normal defense mechanisms on the ocular surface such as flow of tears, blinking, antibacterial enzymes, immunoglobulins in tear film and presence of ocular surface mucus as a physical barrier. Interference with the normal defense mechanisms impairs clearance of debris and microorganisms from the ocular surface and predisposes to infections. The occurrence of contact lens related adverse effects has also been partly attributed to hypoxia. Currently available high oxygen permeability lenses have reduced the incidence of adverse effects.[62-64] Microbial keratitis is the most serious contact lens related complication.[65-67]

Besides facilitating the contact lens wear and preserving the optical and physical properties of lenses, one of the most important objectives of using contact lens solutions is to reduce the risk of infection. Cleaning contact lenses before disinfection is extremely important because the adhered debris can cause lens distortion, discoloration, discomfort and damage to ocular surface. Prior cleaning also enhances disinfection by reducing the contamination. The efficacy of disinfectant solutions is regulated by the International Organization for Standardization–ISO. All solutions must pass the recommended tests prior to commercialization. In practice, the efficacy of disinfectant solutions is related more to the user's compliance rather than the type of solution used. Rewetting and saline solutions are used to enhance ocular comfort and reduce contamination.

Daily enzymatic cleaning is not required for disposable soft hydrogel and soft silicone hydrogel lenses but is optional for rigid lenses (Tables 19.6 and 19.7).

CLEANING SYSTEMS

All contact lens users are advised to clean the lenses after each use. During wear, lenses get contaminated by lipid, proteins and mucus in tears, pollutants and cosmetics. The cleaning systems that are in use include:

Table 19.6 Desirable properties and usage of contact lens solutions

	Rigid lenses	Soft hydrogel lenses	Soft silicone hydrogel lenses
Daily cleaning	Required	Required*	Required
Daily disinfection	Required	Required*	Required
Desirable properties in all contact lens care solutions	1. Be sterile and not a source of infection 2. Should not interact with the material of lens and cause changes in optical and physical properties of lens 3. Should not discolor the lens 4. Should be nonirritant and nontoxic to eyes 5. Easy and user-friendly application		

*Daily disposable types of lenses do not require daily cleaning and disinfection.

1. Surfactant cleaners
2. Enzymatic cleaners

Surfactant cleaners help to remove loose proteins and debris from the lens surface. They act as detergents, form micelles with the lipid droplets and clean the lenses by solubilizing the debris. Some cleaning preparations also contain substances like isopropyl alcohol as a lipid solvent and preservative. Other surfactant solutions contain preservatives like sorbic acid and potassium sorbate to prevent microbial contamination of the solution. Thimerosal and chlorhexidine are not in use now because of the hypersensitivity reaction that they can cause. Besides a preservative, many cleaning solutions also contain a chelating agent like EDTA, which helps to chelate calcium ions. Calcium ions facilitate adhering of proteins to lens surface. To obtain a stable pH, phosphate or borate buffers are also added to the cleaning solutions.

Enzymatic cleaners help in removing closely adherent proteins from the lens surface that cannot be removed by surfactant solutions. Cleaning of soft lenses with enzymatic cleaners helps in removing the mucin coating, which plays a significant role in the pathogenesis of contact lens-associated *Pseudomonas* corneal ulceration.[68] Enzymatic cleaning solutions contain enzymes like papain, pancreatin or subtilisin-A. Lenses cleaned weekly with pancreatin containing enzymatic cleaners in addition to daily cleaning showed less deposits, more comfort and less complications as compared to daily cleaning alone.[69] Sugihara, et al. described a cholesterol esterase from *Pseudomonas aeruginosa* that can be utilized for cleaning lipid-stained contact lenses.[70] Methyltrypsin loaded poly (D, L-lactide-coglycolide) nanoparticles have been shown to provide effective lens cleaning and acceptable ocular tolerance.[71] The cleaning systems are available as tablets, which can be dissolved in either a multipurpose solution or hydrogen peroxide. Liquid formulations are also available that can be added to the disinfectants. The use of enzymatic preparations has declined due to increased popularity of frequently replaced soft lenses.

DISINFECTION SYSTEMS

Disinfection is the primary objective of contact lens care. The earliest methods for disinfecting the lens relied on the use of heat. Heating as a method of disinfection required exposure to a temperature of 80°C for 10 minutes. Although the method was very effective, it carried a number of disadvantages like altered lens parameters and denaturation of proteins leading to reduced visual acuity and ocular surface reactions such as giant papillary conjunctivitis. The method used unpreserved saline, which increased the chances of microbial contamination and, moreover, the method was inconvenient to users. Subsequently, microwave irradiation was used. The method was cheap and effective, provided clinically insignificant parameter changes but

Table 19.7 Commonly used contact lens solutions: constituents and properties

| | Hydrogen peroxide | | Single disinfectants | | | Dual disinfectants | | |
	Clear Care	Oxysept	Complete easy rub	Renu fresh	Renu sensitive	Biotrue	Opti-free express	Opti-free replenish
Maker	CIBA Vision	AMO	AMO	Bausch and Lomb	Bausch and Lomb	Bausch and Lomb	Alcon	Alcon
Preservatives and concentration	3% H_2O_2	3% H_2O_2	PHMB 0.0001%	PHMB 0.0001%	PHMB 0.00005%	PHMB 0.00013% PQ-1 0.0001%	PQ-1 0.001% MAPD 0.0005%	PQ-1 0.001% MAPD 0.0005%
Chelators	None	None	EDTA	EDTA	EDTA	EDTA	EDTA	None
Surfactant	Pluronic 17R4	HPMC	Poloxamer 237	Poloxamine hydranate	poloxamine	Hyaluronan, poloxamine	Tetronic 1304	Tear Glyde
Buffer	Phosphate	Phosphate	Sodium phosphate	Boric acid, sodium borate	Boric acid, sodium borate	Boric acid, sodium citrate	Boric acid, sodium citrate	Sodium borate, sodium citrate
pH	6.7	Not tested	7.2	7.3	7.3	7.5	7.8	7.8
Regimen	Rinse only	Rinse only	Rub/rinse	Rub/rinse	Rub/rinse	Rub/rinse	Rinse only	Rinse only
Minimum soak time	6 hours	6 hours	6 hours	4 hours	4 hours	4 hours	6 hours	6 hours
Minimum storage	7 days	7 days	30 days	30 days	30 days	30 days	30 days	30 days

required availability of a microwave oven. Use of ultraviolet rays and ultrasonic systems was also suggested but the efficacy of these systems was limited. Because of the problems associated with these systems, newer methods were introduced that can disinfect the lens without altering its physical or chemical structure and are suitable to eye. The early disinfectant solutions consisted of a combination of chlorhexidine gluconate and thimerosal. Chlorhexidine kills bacteria and yeast by attacking their cell wall. Thimerosal is more effective than chlorhexidine against fungi. Although, the use of these agents was convenient but they were adsorbed on the lens surface and caused hypersensitivity reaction. After repeated use of these agents the lens becomes uncomfortable to eye. These solutions are now superseded by others that provide similar convenience and efficacy with less adverse effects. The newer systems require overnight storage of lenses in the disinfectant solution. In 1980s, chlorine releasing systems were very popular but later on were found to be associated with microbial keratitis. Currently, available disinfection systems are required to pass ISO/DIS 14729 standard for antimicrobial efficacy. The regulation requires 1 million organisms/mL challenge (6 log units) and the solution must be efficacious in reducing the growth of:

1. The following bacteria by 99.9% (3 log) in stated soaking time
   a. *Staphylococcus aureus*
   b. *Pseudomonas aeruginosa*
   c. *Serratia marcescens*.

2. The growth of following fungi by 90% (1 log) in stated soaking time
   a. *Candida albicans*
   b. *Fusarium solani*

The current standards do not include testing against *Acanthamoeba* and, therefore, thorough cleaning seems to be the best protection against this organism. Two types of disinfecting/cleaning solutions are in use:

1. Hydrogen peroxide (H_2O_2) solutions
2. Multipurpose disinfecting solutions (MPDS)

Hydrogen peroxide is a strong oxidizing agent and has a broad-spectrum antimicrobial action against bacteria, fungi and yeast. It produces hydroxyl free radicals, which damage the essential cell proteins and lipids. A solution of 3% H_2O_2 can kill the trophozoites of *Acanthamoeba* within 3 minutes and cysts after 9 hours of storage. Hydrogen peroxide based solutions also help in removing protein deposits on the soft lenses.[72] It is stabilized with phosphates because it breaks down on storage. H_2O_2 is toxic to eyes and, therefore, after overnight disinfection/cleaning, it must be neutralized before putting the lens in the eye. Failure to neutralize before insertion into the eye causes ocular pain and trauma. Thus, this disinfection system is a two step process and is highly effective. One step H_2O_2 disinfection systems are also available now, which do not require the second step of neutralization. They contain an in-built neutralizing agent capable of converting H_2O_2 into water. The one step systems are less efficacious than two step systems and allow regrowth of microbes upon prolonged storage due to decomposition of H_2O_2. Tablet-based one step disinfection systems neutralize at a slower rate compared to disc-based peroxide systems.[73] Although the two step H_2O_2 disinfection systems are highly effective in terms of disinfecting lenses, their popularity is much less due to the inconvenience of using extra procedures.

Multipurpose disinfecting solutions (MPDS) are most popular as they eliminate the need for the use of multiple care systems. They can be used for cleaning, disinfection, rinsing and storage.[74] Several antimicrobial agents have been used in MPDS. Polyhexanide or polyhexamethylene biguianide (PHMB) was one of the first preservatives used. It is used in a concentration range of 0.5–5 ppm. PHMB acts by causing disruption of bacterial cell membrane. It is chemically similar to chlorhexidine but has a large molecular weight. Because of the larger size it fails to penetrate into the lens matrix, thereby reducing the chances of toxic hypersensitivity reactions. The ocular comfort depends upon the formulation and concentration of PHMB used.[75] Staining by PHMB is much higher especially with group II lenses as compared to another antimicrobial - polyquad.[76-78]

Polyquad is the largest molecule used as preservative with molecular weight of 5000. The incidence of toxic hypersensitivity is minimal but it has higher affinity for methacrylic acid and less efficacy against *Acanthamoeba.*

One of the newer disinfectants used is sodium chlorite $(NaClO_2)$/peroxide (H_2O_2) system. Sodium chlorite generates chlorine dioxide which effectively kills Gram-positive and negative bacteria, yeast and fungi and subsequently breaks down into salt, water and oxygen. The solution is safe and non-toxic to corneal epithelium.[79]

Alexidine is another newly introduced antimicrobial agent for MPDS. It is a bis-biguianide and acts by disrupting the microbial cell membrane like polyhexanide. It has shown efficacy against *Acanthamoeba* and is non-irritant to the eyes.[80,81]

In addition to antimicrobial agents, MPDS also contain a surfactant. Some of the surfactants used in MPDS include poloxamine, poloxamer-237 and pluronic F-127. Other ingredients in MPDS may include EDTA as a chelating agent and buffers to stabilize the pH. Some studies have shown that MPDS containing boric acid buffers downregulate expression of membrane associated mucins and enhance cytotoxicity [82,83] whereas others have shown that cytotoxic effects of solutions containing boric acid cannot be attributed to boric acid but are an outcome of the unique combination of all ingredients.[84] Some of the newer solutions also contain a viscosity enhancer like hydroxypropyl methylcellulose for improved ocular comfort or a sequestering agent to reduce protein deposition. MPDS do not decompose and, therefore, provide continued disinfection. The efficacy of MPDS is much higher than the one-step H_2O_2 disinfection systems.

REWETTING SOLUTIONS

Rewetting solutions also known as 'lubricants' or 'comfort drops' have been used to reduce ocular discomfort, which is the primary cause of discontinuation of contact lens wear. They provide comfort for about 6 hours. Their mechanism of providing ocular comfort is uncertain as they have been shown not to enhance the pre-lens tear film. The single-dose forms are free of preservatives but multiple-dose forms contain preservatives to prevent microbial contamination of the solution. Some of the rewetting solutions contain viscosity enhancers to increase the ocular residence time of the solution and, therefore, to provide prolonged ocular comfort. Other components of rewetting solutions include sodium chloride and buffering agents.

SALINE SOLUTIONS

Saline solutions are used to rinse the lenses before insertion. The user of H_2O_2 disinfection systems require saline solution to avoid stinging at insertion. These solutions are especially of use for beginners as they need to handle the lenses more for insertion and can contaminate lenses by fingers. Rinsing helps to remove microbes from the surface of lenses and, therefore, reduces chances of infections. Unpreserved saline solutions are not recommended as they are likely to be associated with higher incidence of infection. These solutions are buffered to maintain a stable pH. Single-dose forms are free of preservatives but multi-dose forms contain preservatives to prevent contamination of the solution.

THE LENS STORAGE CASE

The lens storage case is an important component of contact lens care system, which stores the lens and the disinfecting solution. Significantly high proportion of contact lens cases show microbial contamination, which has not been found to be related to the type of solution used. Microbial contamination of contact lens cases reduces the efficacy of disinfectant solution. Long-term use of a particular solution allows build-up of naturally-resistant microbes that can survive in the presence of that disinfectant. Use of H_2O_2 disinfection systems allows the growth of bacteria capable of producing catalase. This catalase hydrolyses the H_2O_2 and facilitates bacterial growth. Lack of compliance in keeping the lens cases clean predisposes to ocular infections. Rinsing the lens cases with disinfecting solution and leaving it open to air dry may help in reducing the contamination. Rubbing and rinsing with a disinfecting solution followed by wiping the silver-impregnated cases has been shown to be effective in removing biofilms. Resoaking the cases in hydrogen peroxide between uses also effectively removes the biofilm, reducing the risk of infection.[85]

Increasing use of daily disposable and extended wear lenses has reduced the requirement of contact lens solutions but still a large number of contact lens users require these solutions. Unfortunately, the compliance with their use is poor and, therefore, physicians need to emphasize the proper use of these solutions in accordance with the instructions provided by the manufacturer. Regular replacement of old cases with the new ones is the best alternative.

E. Nutritional Supplements

Sushma Srivastava, Igor N Iezhitsa, Srikant Gaur

OVERVIEW

Nutrition plays an important role in keeping the eyes healthy and in maintaining clear vision. A balanced quantity of both macro and micronutrients is needed for general and visual health. Macronutrients like carbohydrates, fat and proteins build the body and provide it energy for all physiological functioning. Micronutrients that include trace elements and vitamins aid in carrying out various enzymatic processes and prevent and treat several pathological conditions.

Vitamins are the organic compounds, required by the body in small amounts whereas trace elements are required in very minute quantity. The amount of these nutritional agents required for normal physiological functioning is called as Recommended Dietary Allowance (RDA).

Certain eye diseases are the consequences of improper and inadequate quantities of nutrients in diet. These diseases can be treated by supplementation with these nutrients or can be prevented by consuming balanced diet. This chapter gives a brief account of some of the vitamins and minerals required for the maintenance of healthy eyes.

MINERALS AND TRACE ELEMENTS

The trace elements are elements required in very minute quantities by the body. These elements act as catalysts in several enzymatic processes. In minute quantities they are beneficial but can cause toxicity in excess amounts. Some of the elements, which affect the normal functioning of the eye, are described here.

Zinc

Zinc is the most abundantly found trace metal in the human body. It is a constituent of about 25 enzymes involved in digestion and metabolism and aids to release vitamin A from liver so that it can be used in ocular tissues. It affects the cell metabolism through various mechanisms and maintains normal functioning of the eye. It occurs in high concentrations in ocular tissue, particularly in retina and choroid.[86] The essentiality of this element has been well established in the retina, choroid, cornea and lens.[86] Zinc is required for the structure and activity of many ocular metalloenzymes. Zinc interacts with taurine and vitamin A in the retina, modifies plasma membranes in the photoreceptors, regulates the light-rhodopsin reaction within the photoreceptors, modulates synaptic transmission and serves as an antioxidant in both the retinal pigment epithelium and retina.[86]

Deficiency: Zinc deficiency has been suggested to occur in Parkinson's disease and may be specifically related to the vision, olfactory and taste loss in these patients.[87] It also affects immune system, vision, fertility, protein synthesis and other metabolic activities. It is also well known that zinc deficiency causes functional impairment in various parts of the eye and dramatically affects the ocular development during early prenatal period.[88] Zinc deficiency is also being linked to aging and age-related degenerative diseases, which manifest with an increase in the copper/zinc ratio and systemic oxidative stress in general.[89] Zinc and antioxidants delay the progression of age-related macular degeneration (AMD) and vision loss, possibly by preventing cellular damage in the retina.[90-93] Zn-deficiency induce a decrease of myelinated nerve fibers, and it is thought that optic neuropathy in patients treated with some drugs such as ethambutol may be a secondary change due to Zn-deficiency following drug administration.[94]

Toxicity: Zinc related toxicities have been shown in human and animal eyes.[88] An excessive intake of zinc can cause secondary copper deficiency because of the interaction between these two trace elements. [86]

Sources: Zinc rich food are oysters, shell fish, red meat, poultry and eggs, pork, dairy products, nuts, fresh fruits, potatoes, beans, canned vegetables, pumpkin seeds and seafood.

RDA is 11 milligrams of zinc per day for men and 8 mg/day for women.[95]

Copper

Copper is a naturally occurring element in the human body and is associated with collagen production. It is a constituent of several metalloenzymes such as superoxide dismutase. Copper along with zinc and vitamin C has an important role in oxidative defense mechanism of the body. Copper actively participates in the formation of hemoglobin in the blood. Copper with several other antioxidants has been shown to prevent the progression of AMD in clinical trials. It is stored in the liver and is excreted in bile.

Deficiency: Copper deficiency is rarely seen, however, anemia, poor collagen levels, arthritis, mental deterioration, etc. are some of the deficiency symptoms of copper. It causes premature graying and discoloration of skin. Zinc depletes copper, therefore, too much of zinc intake can result in deficiency of copper.

Toxicity: Copper toxicity affects many systems in the body. In the nervous system, high levels of copper produce an abundance of neurotransmitters like dopamine and epinephrine. These neurotransmitters can cause an overstimulation of the occipital lobe, the visual processing center,

which being overstimulated, cannot interpret the signals it receives from the eyes. It focuses on the function of one eye while neglecting the other causing amblyopia.[96] High levels of copper can cause nausea, diarrhea, hepatitis, cirrhosis, renal dysfunction, sunflower cataract, coma and even death (more than 15 mg). Copper levels are increased due to abnormal metabolism in Wilson's disease.

Sources: Rich sources of copper are beans, mushrooms, barley, tomato juice, potato, cooked turnip, beef, chicken, liver, eggs, fish and nuts.[97] RDA is 2 mg.[98]

Magnesium

Magnesium is an essential mineral, which has an important role in human as well as animal physiology. Its role in systemic diseases such as hypertension, heart diseases, and neurological disorders is known but in ocular tissues the role is not very clear. Magnesium plays significant role as a cofactor for more than 350 enzymes in the body, regulates neuroexcitability and several ion channels. Membrane associated ATPase functions that are crucial in regulating the intracellular ionic environment, are magnesium-dependent.[99] Moreover, the enzymes involved in ATP production and hydrolysis are also magnesium-dependent.

Deficiency: Magnesium deficiency by interfering with ATPase functions causes increased intracellular calcium and sodium and decreases intracellular potassium concentration. Such ionic imbalances in turn alter the other cellular enzymatic reactions and form the basis of the association of magnesium deficiency with ophthalmic diseases such as cataract.[100-101] In the presence of magnesium deficiency, an imbalance between mediators of vasoconstriction and vasorelaxation may underlie the vasospasm, which is one of the pathogenic factors in primary open angle glaucoma. Furthermore, magnesium deficiency is also a contributing factor in increased oxidative stress and stimulation of inducible nitric oxide synthase (iNOS) that can further contribute to the initiation and progression of ocular pathologies such as cataract, glaucoma and diabetic retinopathy. Researchers have shown its role in the development and maintenance of corneal structures and cataractogenesis.[102] Magnesium relaxes smooth muscles, therefore, regulates the outflow of aqueous humor from the eye. Its role has been suggested in glaucoma, diabetic retinopathy, macular degeneration and keratoconus.

Source: Nuts, wheat germ, leafy vegetables.

RDA of magnesium is 320 mg for adult women and 420 mg for adult man.

Manganese

It functions as a component of the antioxidant enzyme super oxide dismutase (SOD) that prevents the damaging effect of superoxide radicals from destroying the cellular components.[103] Implication of altered SOD activity in various ocular diseases have been reported by numerous researchers.

Deficiency: In ocular tissues, a deficiency of manganese may result in decreased contact between photoreceptor outer segments and retinal pigment epithelium. This is probably related with the role of manganese in mucopolysaccharide synthesis, because acid mucopolysaccharides are present between the photoreceptor outer segments and retinal pigment epithelium.[104-105] Another effect of manganese deficiency is a decrease of SOD activity resulting in the accumulation of free radicals in the cell with consequent lipid peroxidation in biomembranes.[105] Excess manganese affects the adsorption of iron.

Source: Found in nuts spinach and pineapples. RDA for males 19 years and older is 2.3 mg of manganese per day and for females 19 years and older, 1.8 mg of manganese per day.

Selenium

The benefits and risks of selenium are not fully understood. Its low levels have been associated with number of diseases such as cardiovascular diseases, cataract, cancer and autoimmune diseases. It is a mineral and a component of glutathione peroxidase and thioredoxin, which recycle glutathione and vitamin C respectively. Glutathione is important in various age-related diseases such as cataract and diabetic retinopathy. It increases the immunity and reduces age-related effects. Selenium helps in the absorption of vitamin E and converts it to antioxidants that are vital for ocular health.[106] Selenium is used as a cataract inducing agent in experimental rats.[107] However, deficient alimentary supply of the essential trace element is also implicated in the development of cataracts. Several studies have been done on its relevance to age-related ocular diseases. Selenium has a physiological role as selenocysteine residue in at least 25 distinct selenoenzymes in mammals. Flohé reported that clinical evidence for a protective role of selenium in the development of cataract, macula degeneration, retinitis pigmentosa or any other ocular disease is not available.[108]

Sources: High levels of selenium is found in egg yolk, poultry, sea food, whole grains, wheat bran, brewer's yeast, and moderate levels are found in onions, garlic, broccoli, etc.

RDA is 55 μg for teens and adults.

VITAMINS

Vitamins are essential for various physiological processes. They can not be synthesized in the body or the quantity synthesized is not sufficient to meet the requirement, therefore, these are obtained from the diet. Body vitamin requirement is usually fulfilled by the diet consumed but some people need vitamin supplements according to their health regimen. There are 13 vitamins that include vitamins A, C, D, E, K, and vitamins B (thiamine, riboflavin, niacin, pantothenic acid, biotin, vitamin B_6, vitamin B_{12} and folate). Each vitamin has a special role to play. The low levels of any of these may lead to deficiency states. Vitamins can be water soluble or fat soluble. Following vitamins are important in maintaining good vision. Their role in preventing ophthalmic diseases is described here.

Fat Soluble Vitamins

Vitamin A

In general, there are two categories of vitamin A, depending on whether the food source is an animal or a plant. vitamin A obtained from animal source is the preformed vitamin A. The body absorbs vitamin A in the form of retinol, which is one of the most active form and gets converted to retinal and retinoic acid, which are other forms of vitamin A. Preformed vitamin A can be obtained from liver, whole milk, cheese, eggs, fish, fortified food products.

Vitamin A obtained from plant sources is called provitamin A, carotenoids. These can be converted into retinol (Fig. 19.1) in the body. Out of the several carotenoids, commonly found is beta-carotene (Fig. 19.2), alpha carotene and beta cryptoxanthin. Among these, beta carotene can be most easily converted into retinol in the body.[109] Lycopene, lutein, and zeaxanthin are carotenoids without vitamin A activity but possess other health promoting properties. Consumption of carotenoid-rich fruits and vegetables should be encouraged for their health-promoting benefits.

Some provitamin A carotenoids have been shown to function as antioxidants in laboratory studies; however, this role has not been consistently demonstrated in humans. Antioxidants protect cells from free radicals, which are potentially damaging by-products of oxygen metabolism that may contribute to the development of some chronic diseases.[110-113]

Out of several important roles in the body vitamin A has an important function of the maintenance of vision. It maintains the healthy surface lining of the eye forming a barrier to the bacteria and viruses and preventing infections. Its deficiency results into dry eyes also known as xerophthalmia. It is important for the night vision. Some carotenoids are reported to have antioxidant activity.

Deficiency of vitamin A may lead to dryness of the conjunctiva and cornea; Sjogren's and night blindness, poor growth and dryness of skin and hair. Severe deficiency can lead to corneal ulcers which might progress to permanent blindness.[114] RDA of vitamin A is 800 micrograms.

Lycopene

Lycopene, (Fig. 19.3) a carotenoid, is a potent antioxidant and scavenges free radicals especially derived from oxygen. It imparts red color to the fruits like, tomatoes, strawberries, watermelon, guava, apricots, etc. Its absorption in the body improves when ingested with good quality oil, such as olive oil.[115] Studies have indicated that the absorption of lycopene is more from processed fruits in comparison to raw fruits and vegetables. It protects important cellular biomolecules like lipids, proteins, DNA, etc. from the effects of oxidative stress, thereby preventing diseases like cancer, atherosclerosis, AMD and various other age related diseases. Studies have shown its efficacy in preventing cataract in experimental models.[116,117]

In a cross-sectional study, investigating relationships between plasma concentrations of

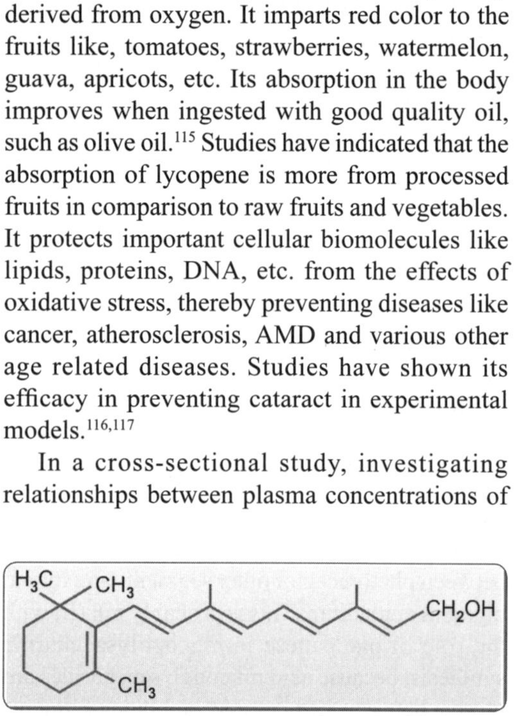

Figure 19.1 Chemical structure of retinol

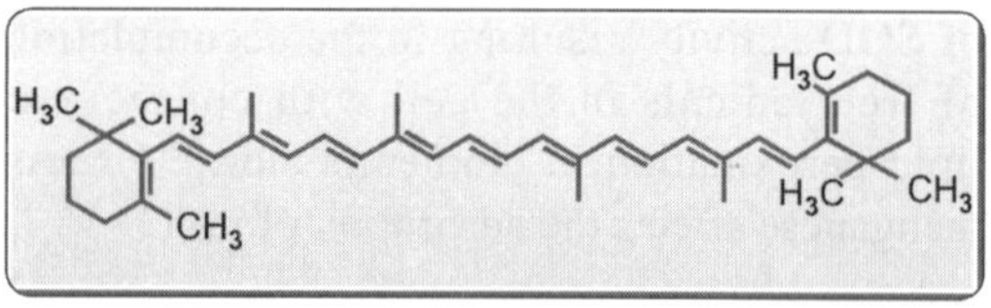

Figure 19.2 Structure of beta-carotene

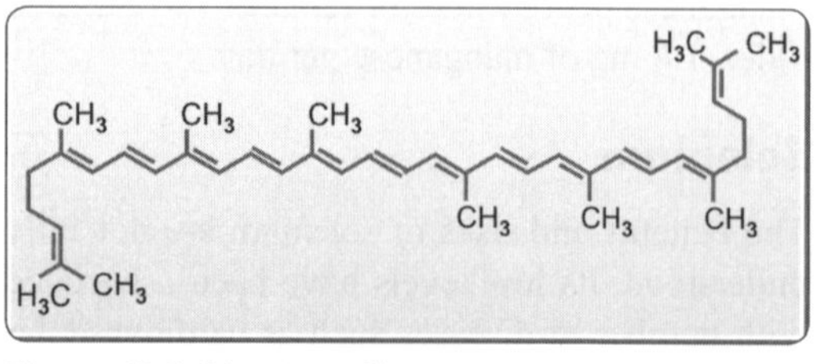

Figure 19.3 Structure of lycopene

antioxidant vitamins and carotenoids and cataract in elderly men and women, risk of cortical cataract was lowest in those with the highest plasma concentrations of lycopene.[118]

Important dietary sources of lycopene include apricots, strawberries and tomatoes.

Lutein

Lutein is a xanthophyll from the carotenoid group having antioxidant properties. It is highly concentrated in the macular region responsible for central vision and high visual acuity. Lutein protects the macula against photo-oxidative damage by functioning as antioxidant and/or optical filter.[119,120] It is found in dark green leafy vegetables such as spinach, broccoli, fruits, corn, egg yolk, etc. Lutein's role in reducing the risk of AMD has been reported by several researchers.[110-113] It has also been shown that people consuming high quantities of lutein have 25 to 50% less risk for having cataract than the people consuming lesser amounts of lutein. No RDA has been specified for lutein, however, a minimum of 6–10 mg of lutein per day provides necessary health benefit.[111]

Zeazanthin

An isomer of lutein, zeazanthin is also found in the retina of eye. It predominates in the central macula. High dietary intake of zeazanthin rich food is associated with lower incidence of AMD.[121,122]

Several carotenoids are present in the human body as a result of consumption of food or dietary supplements. These are not synthesized by the human body. Among all the carotenoids present, lutein and its isomer zeazanthin are present in the eye where the light is focused by the lens, the macula lutea. Cornea and the lens of the eye are the two structures, which protect the eye from the ill effects of the ultraviolet light acting as a filter to remove the UV light. The light thus filtered falls on the retina. The lens due to the exposure to light gradually loses its transparency because of the changes in the protein structure and

becomes cataractous.[123] The visible light entering the eye also produces free radicals and focuses on the macula lutea of the retina. This area has highest concentration of photoreceptors and is responsible for central vision and high resolution visual acuity. Lutein and zeazanthin present in this area act as antioxidants to prevent the area from damage due to free radicals and act as filters to protect the retina from the ill effects of light.[124]

Both lutein and zeazanthin delay age-related cataract development. In a 12-year-prospective study of carotenoid intakes and risk of cataract extraction in women, those with the highest intake of lutein and zeazanthin had a 22% reduced risk of cataract extraction when other potential risk factors were controlled. These researchers also found that increasing intake of spinach and kale, foods rich in both lutein and zeazanthin, was associated with a moderate decrease in the risk of cataract.[125] Results from another large prospective study, with eight years of follow-up, showed that men with the highest lutein and zeazanthin intake had a 19% lower risk of cataract than those with the lowest intake.[126]

Vitamin D

Vitamin D is synthesized in the body upon exposure to UV light. It increases the absorption of calcium and phosphate and maintains healthy immune system. The common naturally occurring form of vitamin D is cholecalciferol. Sunlight is the best source of vitamin D. Codliver oil, eggs and milk are some of the other sources of vitamin D.

An ophthalmic composition containing ergocalciferol or cholecalciferol, i.e. a vitamin D, has been shown to be effective in normalizing the transparency and refraction of the eye by restoring the disturbed metabolism in eye tissue. By protecting the eyes against UV radiation, the ophthalmic composition of vitamin D has been shown to prevent corneal diseases such as photokeratitis, corneal ulceration and corneal dystrophy, which may be caused by UV radiation. Moreover, it reduces opacity of the lenticular capsule after cataract surgery.[127] An ophthalmic composition of vitamin D, active vitamin D, and active vitamin D analogues has been shown to be effective for prophylaxis and treatment of keratoconjunctivitis sicca.[128]

Animal experiments have shown that vitamin D plays an important role in treating retinoblastoma.[129]

Recommended Daily Allowance (RDA) for vitamin D is 5 micrograms per day (200 IU).

Vitamin E

Vitamin E (Fig. 19.4) is a fat soluble vitamin which occurs in several chemical forms such as α-tocopherol, β-tocopherol, γ-tocopherol and δ-tocopherol. Alpha tocopherol is predominantly present in retina and plasma[130,131] and is the most potent free radical scavenger. It protects against various ocular diseases such as glaucoma, cataract and macular degeneration. It also inhibits the toxic effects of fat oxidation on the retina.

Sources of vitamin E are wheat germ oil, margarine, egg yolk, nuts, spinach, etc. Daily requirement of vitamin E is 10 mg.

Water Soluble Vitamins

Vitamins B

Group of eight distinct vitamins including vitamins B_1 (Thiamine), B_2 (Riboflavin), B_3 (Niacin or niacinamide), B_5 (Pantothenic acid), B_6 (Pyridoxine), B_7 (Biotin), B_9 (Folic acid), B_{12} (Various cobalamins, commonly cyanocobalamins) is called as vitamin B complex.

Thiamine (B_1): It is a water soluble B complex vitamin, earlier known as aneurine. It is essential for growth and development (Fig. 19.5). Vitamin B_1 imparts anti-stress action like other B vitamins. It helps in the synthesis of a neurotransmitter, acetylcholine, which is an essential neurotransmitter. Any abnormality in acetylcholine metabolism compromises the formation of new memories and the ability of cells to send messages to each other is lost. Thiamine is involved in several body functions such as nervous system and muscle functioning; flow of electrolytes in and out of nerve and muscle cells; multiple enzyme processes; carbohydrate metabolism and production of hydrochloric acid in the stomach.[132] It preserves the muscle tone along the digestive tract and maintains the general health of eye, skin, hair and mouth. Researchers have shown its involvement in heart failure, Alzheimer's and eye diseases such as cataract.[133-135]

It is found in lean meat, unpolished grains, cereals, dried beans, bran, soyabeans, wheat germ etc. Deficiency causes Beri-beri, Wernicke's encephalopathy and Wernicke-Korsakoff syndrome. RDA is 0.3 to 1.6 mg/day.

Riboflavin (B_2): Riboflavin or vitamin B_2 is the central component of cofactors FAD and flavin mononucleotide (FMN) or Flavin 5 phosphate required by all flavoproteins (Fig. 19.6). It has an important role in energy production from fat, carbohydrate and protein metabolism and activation of vitamin B_6 and folic acid. It is found in milk, liver, kidneys, legumes, leafy vegetables,

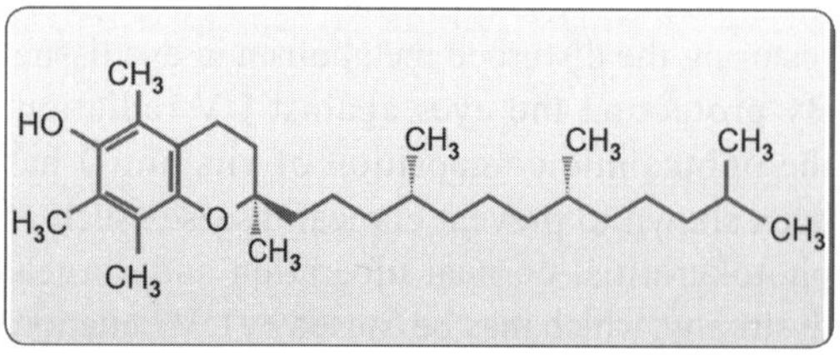

Figure 19.4 Structure of vitamin E

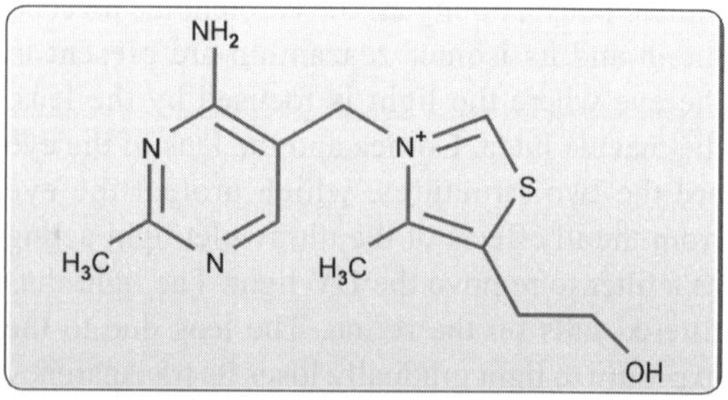

Figure 19.5 Structure of thiamine

yeast, tomatoes, and nuts. The food containing riboflavin should not be kept in light as it gets destroyed by exposure to light. It is water soluble and excess quantity is excreted in urine. Excess riboflavin excreted in the urine gives the typical yellow color to the urine. Sore throat, bloodshot eyes, abnormal skin sensitivity, itching and burning of the eyes, cracked lips and corners of mouth, swelling of mucous membranes and skin are some of the symptoms of deficiency of riboflavin. Its use in the prevention and treatment of cataracts and glaucoma has been described.[136]

Corneal vascularization, corneal opacity and cataracts have been described in animals fed diets low in riboflavin. However, the importance of riboflavin deficiency in the etiology of cataracts in elderly humans is not fully understood. Riboflavin deficiency may be associated with night blindness in some communities and that improving riboflavin status might enhance the improvement in night blindness evoked by vitamin A.[137]

RDA for riboflavin is 1.7 mg/day for an adult man and 1.3 mg/day for an adult woman.[138]

Niacin or Niacinamide (Vitamin B$_3$): Niacin (Fig. 19.7) refers to both nicotinic acid and its amide derivative, nicotinamide (niacinamide).

Both form the coenzymes nicotinamide adenine dinucleotide (NAD) and nicotinamide adenine dinucleotide phosphate (NADP), which are used for a number of biological oxidation reduction reactions.[139] Like all other B vitamins, it plays a role in lowering the blood pressure and blood cholesterol. It also dilates the blood vessels. Because of this property it might help in improving the blood flow to the optic nerve. It has been shown to produce retinal arterial vasodilation.[140]

Yeast, fish, sunflower, legumes, liver, kidney, poultry and lean meat are some of the best dietary sources of vitamin B$_3$. The deficiency of B$_3$ causes pellagra, which is characterized by cracked scaly skin, dementia and diarrhea.

RDA is 16 mg (RDA) for males 19 years and older and 14 mg for females 19 years and older.

Pantothenic acid (Vitamin B$_5$): This vitamin aids in the metabolism of fat, protein and carbohydrate and production of neurotransmitters, hormones and antibodies.

Deficiency leads to neuromuscular degeneration and adrenocortical insufficiency.

Mostly found in meat, vegetables, cereal grains, legumes, eggs, and milk. RDA is 6 mg.

Pyridoxine (Vitamin B$_6$): Pyridoxin (Fig. 19.8) is one of the B vitamins that helps in maintaining the healthy nerves and muscles and the production of DNA and RNA. It activates several enzymes, helps in absorption of vitamin B$_{12}$, fats and proteins, boosts immune functions and antibody production. It may be useful for people with eye infections, bladder infections, prevention of cancer, AMD and kidney stones.

Pyridoxine deficiency is characterized by the development of a greasy and scaling dermatitis involving the skin around the eyes, ears, nose

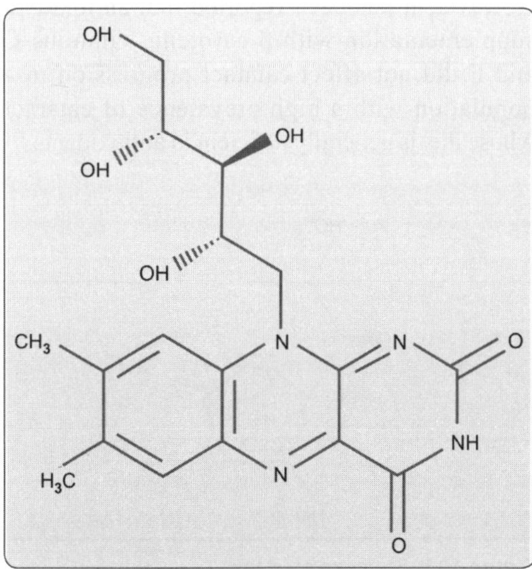

Figure 19.6 Structure of riboflavin

Figure 19.7 Structure of niacin

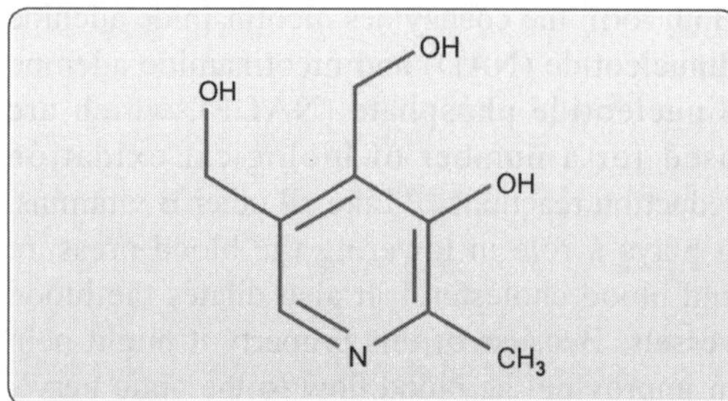

Figure 19.8 Structure of pyridoxin

and the mouth, and the areas of the body that are frequently rubbed together, like the skin around the inner thighs. In rare cases, the deficiency of vitamin B_6 can induce impaired immunity and retardation of the immune response, skin lesions and mental confusion.[141]

Rich sources of B_6 are poultry, fish, whole grains, soybeans, bananas, cabbage, spinach, peas, carrots, avocados, etc.; 10–25 mg per person a day is recommended.

Cyanocobalamin or hydroxocobalamin (Vitamin B_{12}): This vitamin is not synthesized in human body but can be obtained from yeast, liver, meat, fish, and eggs. The vitamin is important in production of red blood cells, lipids and amino acids.

The deficiency is characterized by pale skin, shortness of breath, headache, dizziness, cold palms and feet. Pernicious anemia is a serious complication of reduced production of RBCs. Deficiency can also lead to permanent nerve damage. Daily requirement is 2–3 µg/day.

Folic acid (Vitamin B_9): Folic acid is another water-soluble vitamin B which is useful in maintaining overall health. Children and adults require folic acid for healthy red blood cells. Its deficiency may result in fetal abnormalities.

Absence of folic acid and a handful of other micronutrients causes preventable deformities and diseases, especially in fetal development. It is useful in Alzheimer's disease, depression, anemia, and certain types of cancer. Studies indicated that women on supplementation of folic acid with B_6 and B_{12} had lower risk of AMD compared to other women.[142] Green vegetables, fruits, milk, eggs, liver, kidney, yeast are good sources of folic acid. Deficiency causes megaloblastic anemia and teratogenic effects.

Vitamin C (L-ascorbic acid or L-ascorbate)

Vitamin C (Fig.19.9) is an essential nutrient for humans and animals. It is an antioxidant and protects against oxidative stress.[143] It is synthesized by most of the animals in sufficient amount but not in humans.

It acts as a cofactor in a number of enzymatic reactions. Its antioxidant property helps in reducing the effect of free radicals in the eye. Studies have indicated that the vitamin C intake has resulted in lowering of intraocular pressure in patients with elevated pressure.[144] Higher intake of vitamin C, alone or in combination with other antioxidants, had a protective association with the long-term (10 years) incidence of nuclear cataract in one of the population-based cohort study. These findings support the hypothesis that diet and supplement intakes of vitamin C and other antioxidants may exert age-related ocular benefits, as well as beneficial effects on aging itself.[145] However, it has been reported that antioxidant supplementation with β carotene, vitamins C and E did not affect cataract progression in a population with a high prevalence of cataract whose diet is generally deficient in antioxidants.[146]

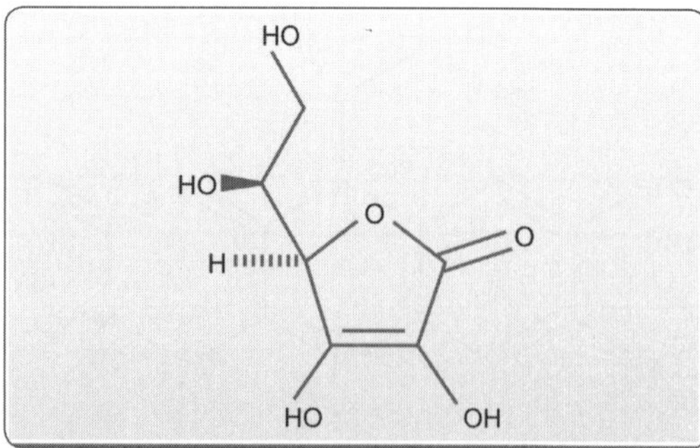

Figure 19.9 Structure of vitamin C

High doses of vitamin C have also been reported to be associated with higher risk of age related cataracts in women.[147] Vitamin C as eyewash is used for quick healing of conjunctivitis. It also alleviates dry eyes.

Plants are the main source of vitamin C for humans. Rich sources of vitamin C are broccoli, green cabbage, kale, cauliflower, tomatoes, kiwi fruit, oranges, lemons, papayas.

The RDA for vitamin C is 60 mg for both men and women.

AMINO ACIDS

Not only vitamins and minerals affect the normal vision, but some amino acids like cysteine and taurine are reported to have a significant role in maintaining the normal vision and repairing the damaged ocular tissues.

Cysteine is an important amino acid that helps to maintain a healthy retina. It helps in increasing the production of glutathione. It has an important role in macular degeneration, glaucoma and cataract.[148] It can be obtained from eggs. Recommended dose is 500–1000 mg daily as N-acetyl cysteine.

Taurine is a free amino acid that acts as an antioxidant, conjugates biliary acids, detoxifies some xenobiotics, modulates intracellular calcium levels and aids in osmoregulation, neuromodulation and stabilization of membranes.[149] It has been established that visual dysfunction in both human and animal subjects results from taurine deficiency. Moreover, the deficiency is reversed with simple nutritional supplementation with taurine. The data suggest that taurine is an important neurochemical factor in the visual system.

High concentrations of taurine have been found in the retina.[150] It maintains the vision and regenerates the damaged ocular tissues. Several studies have suggested that taurine can be used as nutritional supplement to protect against oxidative stress, neurodegenerative diseases and atherosclerosis. Clinical trials are being done to investigate its effects on various diseases.[151]

Low levels of taurine are related with macular degeneration and glaucoma. Animal products such as meat, eggs, and fish are good source of taurine.

In some countries (Russia, Armenia, Georgia, Ukraine, Kazakhstan and Belarus) taurine 4% solution (Taufon Eye Drops) is prescribed to adults with hereditary tapetoretinal degeneration, corneal dystrophy, senile, diabetic and traumatic cataract. Taufon reduces intraocular pressure in patients with glaucoma.[152,153]

SUMMARY

Nutritional agents have a remarkable role in maintaining the clarity of vision and this has been proved by a number of studies. The diet consumed should contain green leafy vegetables, fruits, nuts, milk, milk products, meat, egg, etc. It should be rich in antioxidants, vitamins, minerals, and omega-3-fatty acids and deficient in saturated fat. This can ameliorate the age related changes occurring in eye and provide protection from the harmful effects of chemicals, radiations and various pathological conditions.

REFERENCES

1. Allingham RR, Damji K, Freedman S, et al. Hyperosmotics. In: Shields Textbook of Glaucoma. 5th edn. Lippincot Williams and Wilkins, Philadelphia, 2005.
2. Kolker AE. Symposium on glaucoma. Invest Ophthalmol Vis Sci. 1970;9(6):418.
3. O'Keefe M, Nabil M. The use of mannitol in intraocular surgery. Ophthalmic Surg. 1983; 14(1):55.
4. Grabie MT, Gipstein RM, Adams DA, Hepner GW. Contraindications for mannitol in aphakic glaucoma. Am J Ophthalmol. 1981;91(2):265.
5. Oakley DE, Ellis PP. Glycerol and hyperosmolar nonketotic coma. Am J Ophthalmol. 1976; 81(40):469.
6. Maris PJ, Mandal AK, Netland PA. Medical therapy of pediatric glaucoma and glaucoma in pregnancy. Opthalmol Clin North Am. 2005;18(3):461–8.

7. Bartlett JD: Ophthalmic Drug Facts. St Louis, Facts and Comparisons, Wolters Kluwer Health, 2006; pp. 252–8.

8. Friend J. Biochemistry of ocular surface epithelium. Int Ophthalmol Clin. 1979;19(2):73–91.

9. Records RE. Conjunctiva and lacrimal system. In: Records RE. ed. Physiology of human eye and visual system. Hagerstown, MD: Harper & Row. 1979; pp. 25–46.

10. Zagord ME, Whikehart DR. Cyclic neucleotides in anatomical subdivisions of the bovine lens. Curr Eye Res. 1981;1(1):49–52.

11. Kinoshita JH, Kern HL, Merola LO. Factors affecting the cation transport of calf lens. Biochem Biophys Acta. 1961;47:458.

12. Maurice D. The location of the fluid pump in cornea. J Physiol. 1972;221(1):43–54.

13. Hogan MJ, Alvarado JA, Weddel JE. Histology of the human eye. Philadelphia: WB Saunders. 1971; pp. 102–9.

14. Green K. Ion transport in the isolated cornea of rabbit. Am J Physiol. 1965;209:1311–6.

15. Edelhauser HF, VanHorn DL, Schultz RO, Hyndick RA. Comparative toxicity of intraocular irrigating solutions on the corneal endothelium. Am J Ophthalmol. 1976;81(4):473–81.

16. Winkler BS, Simson V, Benner J. Importance of bicarbonate in retinal function. Invest Ophthalmol Vis Sci. 1977;16(8):766–8.

17. Rosenfeld SI, Waltman SR, Olk RJ, Gordon M. Comparison of intraocular irrigating solutions in pars plana vitrectomy. Ophthalmology 1986;93(1):109–15.

18. Kramer KK, Thomassen T, Evoul J. Intraocular irrigating solution: a clinical study of BSS plus and dextrose bicarbonate lactated Ringer's solution. Ann Ophthalmol. 1991;23(3):101–5.

19. Li J, Akiyama R, Kuang K, Fischborg J. Effects of BSS and BSS + irrigation solutions on rabbit corneal transendothelial electrical potential difference. Cornea. 1993;12:199–203.

20. Lucena DR, Ribeiro MS, Messias A, Bicas HE, Scott IU, Jorge R. Comparison of corneal changes after phacoemulsification using BSS Plus versus Lactated Ringer's irrigating solution: a prospective randomised trial. Br J Ophthalmol. 2011;95(4):485–9.

21. Puckett TR, Peele KA, Howard RS, Kramer KK. Intraocular irrigating solutions. A randomized \ clinical trial of balanced salt solution plus and dextrose bicarbonate lactated Ringer's solution. Ophthalmology. 1995;102(2):291–6.

22. Rao GN, Aquavella JV, Goldberg SH, Berk SL. Psudophakic bullous keratopathy: relationship to preoperative corneal endothelial status. Ophthalmology. 1984;91(10):1135–40.

23. Joussen AM, Barth U, Cubuk H, Koch H. Effect of irrigating solution and irrigation temperature on the cornea and pupil during phacoemulsification. J Cataract Refract Surg. 2000;26(3):392–7.

24. Kline OR, Symes DJ, Lorenzetti OJ, de faller JM. Effect of BSS plus on the corneal endothelium with intraocular lens implantation. J Toxicol-Cut Ocul Toxicol. 1983;2:243–7.

25. Haiman MH, Abrams GW, Edelhauser HF, Hatchell DL. The effect of intraocular irrigating solutions on lens clarity in normal and diabetic rabbits. Am J Opthalmol. 1982;94(5):594–605.

26. Khurana RN, Chang YH, Barnes AC, Fujii GY, De Juan E Jr, Humayun MS. A novel method to oxygenate intraocular irrigation fluids with an in-line oxygenator. Retina. 2007;27(1):83–6.

27. Javaheri M, Fujii GY, Rossi JV, Panzan CQ, Yanai D, Lakhanpal RR, et al. Effect of oxygenated intraocular irrigation solutions on the electroretinogram after vitrectomy. Retina. 2007;27(1):87–94.

28. Zand LM. The effect of non-therapeutic ophthalmic preparations on the cornea and tear film (review). Aust J Optom. 1981;64(2):44.

29. Balazs EA. Sodium hyaluronate and viscosurgery. In Miller D, Stegmen R, (eds). Healon: a guide to its use in ophthalmic surgery. New York: John Wiley & Sons, 1983; pp. 259.

30. Fechner PU, Fechner MU. Methylcellulose and lens implantation. Br J Ophthalmol. 1983;67(4):259.

31. Su WY, Chen KH, Chen YC, Lee YH, Tseng CL, Lin FH. An injectable oxidated hyaluronic acid/adipic acid dihydrazide hydrogel as a vitreous substitute. J Biomater Sci Polym. 2011;22(13):1777–97.

32. Küçükerdönmez C, Beutel J, Bartz-Schmidt KU, Gelisken F. Treatment of chronic ocular hypotony with intraocular application of sodium hyaluronate. Br J Ophthalmol. 2009;93(2):235–9.

33. Arshinoff SA, Jafari M. New classification of ophthalmic viscosurgical devices. J Cataract Refract Surg. 2005;31(11):2167–71.

34. Hakansson L, Venge P. The molecular basis of hyaluronic acid-mediated stimulation of granulocyte function. J Immunol. 1987;138(12):4347.

35. Inoue M, Katakami C. The effect of hyaluronic acid on corneal epithelial cell proliferation. Invest Ophthalmol Vis Sci. 1993;34(7):2313–6.

36. Oshika T, Eguchi S, Oki K, Yaguchi S, Bissen-Miyajima H, Ota I, et al. Clinical comparison of Healon5 and Healon in phacoemulsification and intraocular lens implantation; Randomized multicenter study. J Cataract Refract Surg. 2004;30(2):357–62.

37. Bissen-Miyajima H. In vitro behavior of ophthalmic viscosurgical devices during phacoemulsification. J Cataract Refract Surg. 2006;32(6):1026–31.

38. Oshika T, Okamoto F, Kaji Y, Hiraoka T, Kiuchi T, Sato M, et al. K. Retention and removal of a new viscous dispersive ophthalmic viscosurgical device during cataract surgery in animal eyes. Br J Ophthalmol. 2006;90(4):485–7.

39. Silver FH, LiBrizzi J. Use of viscoelastic solutions in ophthalmology: a review of physical properties and long term effects. J Long Term Eff Med Implants. 1992;2(1):49–66.

40. Agapitos PJ. Cataract surgical techniques and adjuncts. Curr Opin Ophthalmol. 1992;3:13–28.

41. Hessell J, Cintorn C, Kublin C, Newsome D. Proteoglycan changes during restoration of transparency in corneal scars. Arch Biochem Biophys. 1983;222(2):362.

42. Jensen MK, Crandall AS, Mamalis N, et al. Crystallization intraocular lens surfaces associated with use of Healon GV. Arch Ophthalmol. 1994;112(8):1037–42.

43. Ziakas NG, Boboridis K, Nakos E, Mikropoulos D, Margaritis V, Konstas AG. Does the use of trypan blue during phacoemulsification affect the intraocular pressure? Can J Ophthalmol. 2009;44(3):293–6.

44. Leschey KH, Hackett SF, Singer JH, Campochiaro PA. Growth factor responsiveness of human retinal pigment epithelial cells. Invest Ophthalmol. Vis Sci. 1990;31(5):839–46.

45. Lynch SE, Noxon JC, Colvin RB, Antoniades HN. Role of platelet-derived growth factor in wound healing: synergistic effect with other growth factors. Proc Natl Acd Sci USA. 1987;84(21):7696.

46. Sporn MB, Roberts AB. Peptide growth factors and inflammation, tissue repair and cancer. J Clin Invest. 1986;78(2):329.

47. Schultz GS, Davis JB, Eiferman RA. Growth factors and corneal epithelium. Cornea. 1988;7(2):96.

48. Nayak SK, Samples JR, Deg JK, Binder PS. Growth characteristics of primate (baboon) corneal endothelium in vitro. Invest Ophthalmol. Vis Sci. 1986;27(4):607.

49. Schultz GS, Grant MB. Neovascular growth factors. Eye. 1991;5(Pt 2):170–80.

50. Roberts AB, McCune BK, Sporn MB. Kidney Int. 1992;41(3):557–9.

51. Postlewaite AE, Koski-Oja J, Moses HL, Kang AH. Stimulation of the chemotactic migration of human fibroblasts by transforming growth factor beta. J Exp Med. 1987;165(1):251–6.

52. Hirase K, Ikeda T, Sotozono C, Nishida K, Sawa H, Kinoshita S. transforming growth factor beta2 in the vitreous in proliferative diabetic retinopathy. Arch Ophthalmol. 1998;116(6):738–41.

53. Olivero DK, Furcht LT. Type IV collagen, laminin and fibronectin promote the adhesion and migration of rabbit lens epithelial cells in vitro. Invest Ophthalmol. Vis Sci. 1993;34(10):2825–33.

54. Roman F. Antiseptics in ophthalmology. Br J Ophthalmol. 1994;74:697.

55. Prajnam L. Priya CR, Noor S. Sterilization is ophthalmic practice. Illumination. 2003;3(1):29–32.

56. Abelson MB, Howe A, Capriotti J, Shapiro A. Get to know your antiseptic options: The most efficient way to eradicate microorganisms from the surgical field and the patient's eye. Rev Ophthalmol. 2008;15:1211.

57. Shanmuganathan V, Pease R, Horgan S. Antiseptics and Disinfectants: An update for ophthalmologists, Ophthalmology at the Royal Eye Unit, Kingston Hospital article. www.pinpointmedical.com.

58. Rutula WA, Weber DJ. The Healthcare Infection Control Practices Advisory Committee (HICPAC). Guideline for Disinfection and sterilization in Healthcare Facilities, 2008.

59. Webb JA. Ophthalmology Times: Permitted sterilization techniques for surgical instruments clarified by Joint commission, Jul 15, 2009.

60. Brennan NA, Coles ML. Extended wear in perspective. Optom Vis Sci. 1997;74(8):609–23.

61. Teo L, Lim L, Tan DT, Chan TK, Jap A, Ming LH. A survey of contact lens complications in Singapore. Eye Cont Lens. 2011;37(1):16–9.

62. Fonn D, MacDonald KE, Richter D, Pritchard N. The ocular response to extended wear of high Dk silicone hydrogel contact lens. Clin Exp Optom. 2002;85:176–82.

63. Gleason W, Tanaka H, Albright RA, Cavanagh HD. A 1-year prospective clinical trial of Menicon Z (tisifilcon) rigid gas-permeable contact lenses worn on a 30-days continuous wear schedule. Eye Contact Lens. 2003;29:2–9.

64. Morgan PB, Efron N, Hill EA, Raynor MK, Whiting MA, Tullo AB. Incidence of keratitis of varying severity among contact lens wearers. Br J Ophthalmol. 2005;89(4):430–6.

65. Dart JK, Stapleton F, Minassian D. Contact lenses and other risk factors in microbial keratitis. Lancet. 1991;338:650–3.

66. Cheng KH, Leugh SL, Hoekman H W, Beekhuis WH, Mulder PGH, Geerards AJM, Kijlstra A. Incidence of contact-lens-associated microbial keratitis and its related morbidity. Lancet. 1999;354(9174):181–5.

67. Bourcier T, Thomas F, Borderie V, Chaumeil C, Laroche L. Bacterial keratitis: predisposing factors, clinical and microbiological review of 300 cases. Br J Ophthalmol. 2003;87(7):834–8.

68. Stern GA, Zam ZS. The effect of enzymatic contact lens cleaning on adherence of Pseudomonas aeruginosa to soft contact lenses. Ophthalmology. 1987;94(2):115–9.

69. Nilsson SE, Lindh H. Hydrogel contact lens cleaning with or without multi-enzymes. A prospective study. Acta Ophthalmol (Copenh). 1988;66(1):15–8.

70. Sugihara A, Shimada Y, Nomura A, Terai T, Imayasu M, Nagai Y, et al. Purification and characterization of a novel cholesterol esterase from Pseudomonas aeruginosa, with its application to cleaning lipid-stained contact lenses. Biosci Biotechnol Biochem. 2002; 66(11):2347–55.

71. Jimenez N, Galan J, Vallet A, Egea MA, Garcia ML. Methyl trypsin loaded poly(D,L-lactide-coglycolide) nanoparticles for contact lens care. J Pharm Sci. 2010;99(3):1414–26.

72. Kiel JS. Protein removal from soft contact lens using disinfection/neutralization with hydrogen peroxide/catalytic disc. Clin Ther. 1993;15(1):30–5.

73. Ngo W, Heynen M, Joyce E, Jones L. Impact of protein and lipid on neutralization times of hydrogen peroxide care regimens. Eye Cont Lens. 2009;35(6):282–6.

74. McLaughlin R. Rub vs. no rub: looking at MPS care solutions. Contact Lens Spectr. 2001;16:40–5.

75. Bois A, Brazeau D, Goldberg S et al. Performance of two single-solution contact lens care systems. Optician. 1996;211(5533):37–42.

76. Jones L, Jones D, Houlford M. Clinical comparison of three polyhexinide-preserved multipurpose solutions. Cont Lens Ant Eye. 1997;20:23–30.

77. Pritchard N, Young G, Coleman S. Subjective and objective measures of corneal staining related to multipurpose care systems. Cont Lens Ant Eye. 2003;26:3–9.

78. Lebow KA, Schachet JL. Evaluation of corneal staining and patient preference with use of three multipurpose solutions and two brands of soft contact lenses. Eye Cont Lens. 2003. 29(4):213–20.

79. Karageozian HL, Gates BW. Novel soft contact lens disinfection with sodium chlorite and hydrogen peroxide, 1993. Poster, BCLA Annual Clinical Conference.

80. Borazjani RN, Kilvington S. Efficacy of multipurpose solutions against Acanthamoeba species. Cont Lens Ant Eye. 2005;28(4):169–75.

81. Wolffsohn J, Borazjani R, Groeminger S. ReNu with Moisture Loc: A literature Review. Optician. 2005;229(6004):16–8.

82. Imayasu M, Hori Y, Cavanagh HD. Effects of multipurpose contact lens care solutions and their ingredients on membrane-associated mucins of human corneal epithelial cells. Eye Cont Lens. 2010;36(6):361–6.

83. Tanti NC, Jones L, Gorbet MB. Impact of multipurpose solutions released from contact lenses on corneal cells. Optom Vis Sci. 2011;88(4):483–92.

84. Lehmann DM, Cavet ME, Richardson ME. Nonclinical safety evaluation of boric acid and a novel borate-buffered contact lens multi-purpose solution, Biotrue™ multi-purpose solution. Cont Lens Anterior Eye. 2010;33 Suppl 1:S24–32.

85. Wu YT, Zhu H, Willcox M, Stapleton F. Impact of cleaning regimens in silver-impregnated and

hydrogen peroxide lens cases. Eye Cont Lens. 2011;37(6):365–9.

86. Grahn BH, Paterson PG, Gottschall-Pass KT, and Zhang Z. Zinc and the Eye. J Am Coll Nutr. 2001;20(2 Suppl):106–18.

87. Forsleff L, Schauss AG, Bier ID, Stuart S. Evidence of functional zinc deficiency in Parkinson's disease. J Alt Comp Med. 1999;5(1):57–64.

88. Karcioglu ZA. Zinc in the eye. Surv Ophthalmol. 1982;27(2):114–22.

89. Mezzetti A, Pierdomenico SD, Costantini F, Romano F, De Cesare D, Cuccurullo F, et al. Copper/zinc ratio and systemic oxidant load: Effect of aging and aging-related degenerative diseases. Free Radic Biol Med. 1998;25(6):676–81.

90. http://ods.od.nih.gov/factsheets/Zinc-Health Professional.

91. Eugenio M, Marco M, Fiorella M, Graham P. Zinc, oxidative stress, genetic background and immunosenescence: implications for healthy ageing. Immun Aging. 2006;3:6 doi:10.1186/1742-4933-3-6.

92. ARED Study Research Group. A randomized, placebo-controlled, clinical trial of high-dose supplementation with vitamins C and E, beta carotene, and zinc for age-related macular degeneration and vision loss: AREDS report no. 8. Arch Ophthalmol. 2001;119(10):1417–36.

93. Haase H, Rink L. The immune system and the impact of zinc during aging. Immun Ageing 2009;12:6–9.

94. Gong H, Amemiya T. Optic nerve changes in zinc-deficient rats. Exp Eye Res. 2001;72(4):363–36.

95. Maret W, Sandstead HH. Zinc requirements and the risks and benefits of zinc supplementation. J Trace Elem Med Biol. 2006;20(1):3–18.

96. http://www. ehow.com/ how-does_5542003_amblyopia-caused-copper-toxicity.html.

97. http://www.protect-your-eyesight.com/dietary-antioxidants-for-eye-health.html.

98. http://www.nutrientfacts.com/AlmanacPages/Copper_Recommended_Daily_Allowance_RDA.htm.

99. Spasov AA. Magnesium in clinical practice (monograph). Publisher OOO "Otrok", Volgograd, 2000. p. 272. (in Russian).

100. Agarwal R, Iezhitsa I, Agarwal P, Spasov A. Magnesium deficiency: does it have a role to play in cataractogenesis? Exp Eye Res. 2012;101:82–9.

101. Agarwal R, Iezhitsa I, Awaludin NA, Ahmad Fisol NF, Bakar NS, Agarwal P, et al. Effects of magnesium taurate on the onset and progression of galactose induced experimental cataract: In vivo and in vitro evaluation. Exp Eye Res. 2013;110:35-43.

102. Gong H, Takami Y, Kitaoka T, Amemiya T. Corneal changes in magnesium-deficient rats. Cornea. 2003;22(5):448–56.

103. Frank Eperjesi, Stephen Beatty. Nutrition and the eye: a practical approach. Elsevier Health Sciences, 2006.

104. Cohen AI. The Retina. In: Hart WM Jr. (eds). Adler's Physiology of the Eye, Mosby Year Book St. Louis, MO.1992; 6th ed. pp. 592.

105. Gong H, Amemiya T. Ultrastructure of retina of manganese-deficient rats. Invest Ophthalmol. Vis Sci. 1996 Sep;37(10):1967–74.

106. http://vitamins.ygoy.com/2010/06/15/ eye-health-vitamins.

107. Gupta SK, Kalaiselvan V, Srivastava S, Agrawal SS, Saxena R. Evaluation of anticataract potential of Triphala in selenite-induced cataract: In vitro and in vivo studies. J Ayurveda Integr Med. 2010; 1(4):280–6.

108. Flohé L. Selenium, Selenoproteins and Vision. In: Augustin A (ed): Nutrition and the Eye. Dev Ophthalmol. Volume 38. Basel, Karger, 2005; pp. 89–102.

109. http://ods.od.nih.gov/factsheets/vitamina/#en9#en9.

110. Eye Disease Case-Control Study Group. Antioxidant status and neovascular age-related macular degeneration. Arch Ophthalmol. 1993;111(1):104-9.

111. Seddon JM, Ajani UA, Sperduto RD, Hiller R, Blair N, Burton TC, et al. Dietary carotenoids, vitamins A, C, and E, and advanced age-related macular degeneration. Eye Disease Case-Control Study Group. JAMA. 1994;272(18):1413–20.

112. Bernstein PS, Zhao DY, Wintch SW, Ermakov IV, McClane RW, Gellermann W. Resonance Raman measurement of macular carotenoids in normal subjects and in age-related macular degeneration patients. Ophthalmology. 2002;109(10):1780–7.

113. Snellen EL, Verbeek AL, Van Den Hoogen GW, Cruysberg JR, Hoyng CB. Neovascular age-related macular degeneration and its relationship

to antioxidant intake. Acta Ophthalmol Scand. 2002;80(4):368–71.

114. http://www.anyvitamins.com/vitamin-a-info.htm

115. http://www.protect-your-eyesight.com/dietary-antioxidants-for-eye-health.html.

116. Gupta SK, Trivedi D, Srivastava S, Joshi S, Halder N, Verma SD. 2002, Lycopene attenuates oxidative stress induced experimental cataract development: an in vitro and in vivo study. Nutrition. 2003;19(9):794–9.

117. Mohanty I, Joshi S, Trivedi D, Srivastava S, Gupta SK. Lycopene prevents sugar-induced morphological changes and modulates antioxidant status of human lens epithelial cells. Br J Nutr. 2002;88(4):347–54.

118. Gale C, Hall N, Phillips D, Martyn C. Plasma antioxidant vitamins and carotenoids and age-related cataract. Ophthalmology. 2001; 108(11):1992–8.

119. Schalch W. Carotenoids in the retina, a review of their possible role in preventing or limiting damage caused by light and oxygen. Emerit I Chance B (eds). Free Radicals and Ageing. 1992;62:280–98.

120. Snodderly DM. Evidence for protection against age-related macular degeneration by carotenoids and antioxidant vitamins. Am J Clin Nutr. 1995;62(suppl)1448S–1461S.

121. Krishnadev N, Meleth AD, Chew EY. Nutritional supplements for age-related macular degeneration. Curr Opi Ophthalmol. 2010; 21(3):184–9.

122. SanGiovanni JP, Chew EY, Clemons TE, Ferris FL 3rd, Gensler G, Lindblad AS, et al. The relationship of dietary carotenoid and vitamin A, E, and C intake with age-related macular degeneration in a case-control study: AREDS Report No. 22. Arch Ophthalmol. 2007;125(9):1225–32.

123. Roberts RL., Green J, Lewis B. Lutein and zeaxanthin in eye and skin health. Clinics in Dermatology. 2009;27(2):195–201.

124. Krinsky N, Landrum J and Bone R. Biologic mechanisms of the protective role of lutein and zeaxanthin in the eye. Annu Rev Nutr. 2003;23:171–201.

125. Chasan-Taber L, Willett W, Seddon J, et al. A prospective study of carotenoid and vitamin A intakes and risk of cataract extraction in US women. Am Clin Nutr. 1999;70(4):509–16.

126. Brown L, Rimm E, Seddon J, et al. A prospective study of carotenoid intake and risk of cataract extraction in US men. Am J Clin Nutr. 1999;70(4):517–24.

127. Kita K., European Patent EP0862916. Topical use of vitamin D for the treatment of eye disorders, Filing Date: 22 April 1996, Publication Date: 05 March 2003, http://www.freepatentsonline.com/EP0862916B1.html.

128. Itoh S, Ishii Y, Mukai K, Kita K. United States Patent 6,187,331. Composition for prophylaxis and/or treatment of dry syndrome comprising vitamin D. Filing date: 23 May 2000, Issue date: 13 Feb 2001.

129. Albert DM, Kumar A, Strugnell SA, Darjatmoko SR, Lokken JM, Lindstrom MJ, et al. Effectiveness of vitamin D analogues in treating large tumors and during prolonged use in murine retinoblastoma models. Arch Ophthalmol. 2004;122(9):1357–62.

130. Alvarez RA, Liou GI, Fong SL, Bridges CD. Levels of alpha-and gamma-tocopherol in human eyes: evaluation of the possible role of IRBP in intraocular alpha-tocopherol transport. Am J Clin Nutr. 1987;46(3):481–7.

131. Friedrichson T, Kalbach HL, Buck P, van Kuijk FJ: Vitamin E in macular and peripheral tissues of the human eye. Curr Eye Res. 1995;14(8):693–701.

132. http://www.enotalone.com/article/9412.html.

133. Leslie D, Gheorghiade M. Is there a role for thiamine supplementation in the management of heart failure? Am Heart J. 1996;131(6):1248–50.

134. Ott BR, Owens NJ. Complementary and alternative medicines for Alzheimer's disease. J Geriatr Psychiatry Neurol. 1998;11(4):163–73.

135. Kuzniarz M, Mitchell P, Cumming RG, Flood VM. Use of vitamin supplements and cataract: the Blue Mountains Eye Study. Am J Ophthalmol. 2001;132(1):19–26.

136. http://www.nlm.nih.gov/medlineplus/druginfo/natural/957.html.

137. Powers HJ. Riboflavin (vitamin B-2) and health. Am J Clin Nutr. 2003;77(6):1352–60.

138. http://www.vitamins-supplements.org/vitamin-B2-riboflavin.php.

139. http://www.vitamin-basics.com/index.php?id=49).

140. Barakat MR, Metelitsina TI, Dupont JC, Grunwald JE. Effect of niacin on retinal vascular

diameter in patients with age-related macular degeneration. Curr Eye Res. 2006; 31(7-8):629-634.

141. http://www.herbs2000.com/vitamins/v_b6.htm.

142. http://www.boston.com/news/health/blog/2009/02/vitamin_b_folic.html.

143. Padayatty SJ, Katz A, Wang Y, Eck P, Kwon O, Lee, JH, et al. Vitamin C as an antioxidant: evaluation of its role in disease prevention. J Am Coll Nutr. 2003;22(1):18–35.

144. Herschell H Boyd. Eye Pressure Lowering Effect of Vitamin C. J Orthomol Med. 1995;10(3-4): 165–8.

145. Tan AG, Mitchell P, Flood VM, Burlutsky G, Rochtchina E, Cumming RG, et al. Antioxidant nutrient intake and the long-term incidence of age-related cataract: the Blue Mountains Eye Study. American J Clinl Nutr. 2008;87(6):1899–905.

146. Gritz DC, Srinivasan M, Smith SD, Kim U, Lietman TM, Wilkins JH, et al. The antioxidants in prevention of cataracts study: effects of antioxidant supplements on cataract progression in South India. Br J Ophthalmol. 2006;90(7):847–51.

147. Rautiainen S, Lindblad BE, Morgenstern R, Wolk A. Vitamin C supplements and the risk of age-related cataract: a population-based prospective cohort study in women. Am J Clin Nutr. 2010;91(2):487–93.

148. http://www.naturaleyecare.com/prev-food.asp#minerals.

149. Bidri M, Choay P. Taurine: a particular aminoacid with multiple functions. Ann Pharm Fr. 2003;61(6):385–91.

150. Militante JD, Lombardini JB. Taurine: evidence of physiological function in the retina. Nutr Neurosci. 2002;5(2):75–90.

151. Bouckenooghe T, Remacle C, Reusens B. Is taurine a functional nutrient? Curr Opin Clin Nutr Metab Care. 2006;9(6):728–33.

152. Vodovozov AM, Glotova NM, Iartsev EI, Varnovotskiĭ AM, Boriskina LN. Use of taufon in pigmented dystrophy of the retina. Vestn Oftalmol. 1986; 102(6):38–39. (Article in Russian);

153. Shpak NI, Naritsyna NI, Konovalova NV. Taufon and emoksipin in the combined treatment of sclerotic macular dystrophies. Oftalmol Zh. 1989; (8):463–5 (Article in Russian).

CHAPTER 20

Gene Delivery and Disease Modulation in the Eye

OVERVIEW

Blindness resulting from trauma, injury or disease is a notable health care concern worldwide.[1] Limitations of currently available management options for prevalent ocular impairments such as glaucoma, corneal damage and disease, and age-related macular degeneration, etc. result in treatments that are ineffective, costly to patients and healthcare systems, and toxic to application sites due to various adverse effects.[2, 3] Therefore, much work has been done to develop effective, affordable, and practical treatments for patients.

Gene therapy is a promising therapeutic approach for many ocular pathologies. The concept of using this strategy to alleviate blindness in humans was supported by the first successful ocular gene therapy studies in 2008 in which vision was restored to patients with Leber's congenital amaurosis, a congenital disease characterized by severe retinal dystrophy.[4-8] With gene therapy, specific cell types can be targeted and converted into pharmacological factories able to continuously generate therapeutic agents.[9] Consequently, with a single dose, gene therapy has the capability to correct the underlying disease mechanisms, contrasting conventional methods that mask symptoms.[9]

CONVENTIONAL OCULAR DELIVERY METHODS AND BARRIERS

The unique protective structures of the eye prevent the entrance of foreign molecules, including therapeutic molecules. Thus ocular drug delivery has been a major challenge plaguing pharmaceutical scientists. The most common and preferred method employed is topical treatment (Fig. 20.1) (e.g. eye drops, and ointments), because of low cost and ease of treatment application.[10, 11] Unfortunately, low bioavailability results from reflex blinking, lacrimation, and nasolacrimal drainage that cause the loss of a major fraction of the topically applied treatment. Additionally the corneal epithelium is a restrictive barrier compromising drug permeability into target ocular tissues. As a result, less than 5% of the applied treatment reaches intraocular regions.[12] This approach may be useful in treating disorders in the anterior segment of the eye, however in order to maintain therapeutic concentrations, frequent application is required which may cause adverse effects.[13, 14]

Delivery methods used to bypass the protective barriers of the ocular anterior surface include systemic and microinjection administration (Fig. 20.1). Systemic administration is beneficial in the management of diseases involving posterior eye regions. However, tight junctions of the blood retinal barrier may restrict therapeutic molecule entry into the retina. Like with topical applications, this limitation results in frequent administration and potential toxic side effects.[15, 16] Another drawback is that only a small fraction (1–2%) of systemically dispensed therapeutic agents will reach the vitreous.[15] This issue can be resolved by direct injections into the vitreous. Intravitreal injections supply the retina and the

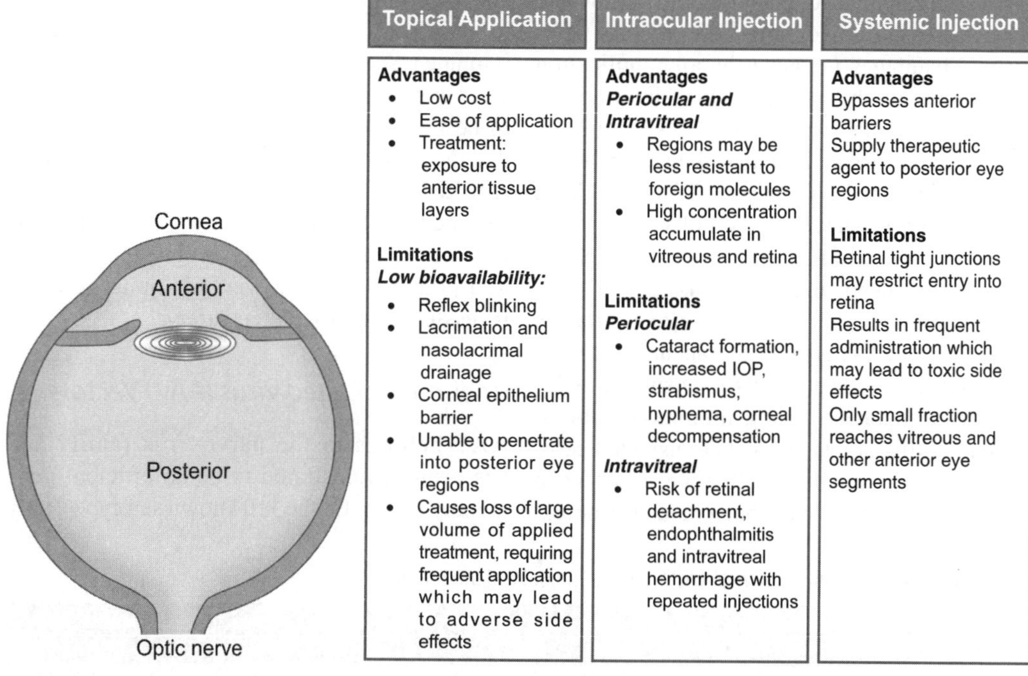

Figure 20.1 Advantages and limitations of conventional ocular therapeutic delivery methods

vitreous with adequate concentrations of the treatment.[17] However, although this technique bypasses physical barriers, repeated injections of treatments with shorter half-lives increase the risk of retinal detachment, endophthalmitis, and intravitreal hemorrhage.[11,18] Periocular injections, injections into areas neighboring the eye, have also been considered an efficient delivery method for administering therapeutic agents to posterior segments of the eye. Periocular is a broad term that indicates peribulbar, retrobulbar, subconjunctival, and posterior juxtascleral delivery routes.[10] The sclera, for example, is less resistant to foreign molecule permeability due to its fibrous tissue make up. Therapeutic molecules applied near this region lead to high concentrations within the vitreous and retina.[19] Complications associated with periocular injections include cataract formation, increased intraocular pressure, strabismus, hyphema, and corneal decompensation.[20]

TYPES OF GENE THERAPY VECTORS

There are two major types of gene therapy delivery vectors, viral (Table 20.1) and non-viral. An ideal vector is able to target dividing and non-dividing cells, deliver beneficial levels of therapeutic genes at desired ocular tissue or location, and does not induce an immunological response or cause toxic side effects.[9]

Viral Vectors

Adenovirus (AV) Vectors

AV is a virus with double stranded DNA and over 50 known human serotypes. Serotypes 2 and 5 are most commonly used in gene therapy.[21] AVs deliver foreign genes into host cells via receptor-mediated endocytosis. To gain entry into the cell, the AV binds to a cell surface receptor (coxsackie-adenovirus receptor), and assembles a clathrin-coated pit. Upon entry, the viral genome is released and transported into the nucleus where it is expressed episomally.[3] AV vectors offer many advantages for gene therapy application including their ability to transduce dividing and non-dividing cells, carry genes ~30 kb, naturally infect human tissue, and also their inability to integrate into the host genome. AV vectors have been shown to successfully deliver genes *in vivo* and *in vitro* to specific cornea cell types in rodents and sheep, and *ex vivo* in humans.[3, 22-29] High immunogenicity is one major limitation to the use of AV-mediated therapeutic delivery. Also patients with previous exposure to wild-type AV generate a strong immune response, which rapidly targets and kills transfected cells. To improve the suitability of AV vector usage in gene therapy, efforts have been made to address and overcome this challenge.[25,30] However, in addition to being associated with a severe immune response and subsequent inflammation, gene expression of AV vectors has been noted to be transient. Previous studies demonstrated that the short-term transgene expression requires repeated dose administrations, and consequently repeated treatments were toxic.[22] In summary, AV vectors are promising ocular gene therapy tool (Table 20.1), however, additional research is needed to improve their safety.

Adeno-associated Virus (AAV) Vectors

AAV belongs to the parvovirus family and has been demonstrated to be an efficient gene therapy vector. Of the 110 known serotypes, only

Table 20.1 Characteristics of viral vectors used in ocular gene therapy

	Adenovirus	Adeno-associated virus	Retrovirus	Lentivirus
Vector size (nm)	70–90	18–26	80–130	80–130
Viral genome size (kb)	38–39	4–7	3–9	3–9
Genome type	dsDNA	ssDNA	ssRNA	ssRNA
Payload size capacity (kb)	~7.5	~1.8	~8	~8
Tropism	Mitotic cells	Mitotic and post-mitotic cells	Mitotic cells	Mitotic and post-mitotic cells
Integration into host genome	No	No	Yes	No, Yes if impaired
Transduction efficiency	Low-high	Mid-high	Mid-high	High
Transgene expression duration	Transient (days-weeks)	Potentially extended (months-years)	Extended (months-years)	Extended (months-years)
Immunogenicity level	High	Low-mid	Mid-high	Mid-high
Pros	High titer, able to infect most cell types, non-mutagenic	Very effective for all cell types, stable transduction, site-specific integration	Very effective, allows sustained gene expression	Very effective for all cell types, allows sustained gene expression
Cons	Immunogenic, common virus in humans that reduces potency	Small size of insert, low immunogenicity, potential for HSV or adenovirus contamination	Requires dividing cells, low titer, oncogenic, random integration	Immunogenic, HIV origin, random integration potential

serotypes 1-10 have been tested for gene therapy. This small virus has an icosahedral capsid, and a single-stranded DNA genome spanning 4.7 kb. The AAV genome has two open reading frames (ORFs) encoding for *Rep* and *Cap*. These ORFs are found between inverted terminal repeats that are comprised of 145 bases and located at the 5' and 3' ends. The Cap genes encode for capsid proteins VP1, VP2, and VP3. The Rep ORF encodes four proteins: Rep40, Rep52, Rep68, and Rep78. Rep68 and Rep78 are responsible for replication and translation of the AAV genome, while Rep40 and Rep52 orchestrate the packaging of the genome within the capsid.

Once assembled, the virus binds to the appropriate cell surface receptor. This serotype-specific event is determined by capsid sequence, and is responsible for tissue trophism variability between serotypes. After binding of the viral capsid to its primary receptor, the viral particle enters the cell via receptor-mediated endocytosis and through endosomal lysis the genome is released into the cytoplasm. The genome then anneals to a complementary DNA strand provided either by host machinery or another infecting virus. After reaching the nucleus, the AAV genome either remains episomal, or is integrated into chromosome 19 of the host genome by Rep68 and 78. Translation of the viral genome is conducted by host cell machinery.[3]

The first recombinant AAV (rAAV) vectors were generated by replacing the two ORFs with a gene of interest. This process required both E1 expressing HEK293 cells that contained a helper plasmid expressing Rep and Cap, and E1 deficient AV. Initially, helper virus contamination impeded vector production, however, this problem was resolved in the second-generation rAAV vectors, by replacing the E1 deficient AV with an AV-helper-plasmid expressing E4 and E2A. To eliminate the need for dual transduction, further modifications were instituted, including the combination of the AAV-helper and AV-helper genes into one plasmid.[31]

AAV2 was the first serotype to demonstrate significant gene delivery in the cornea using a rabbit model *in vivo*.[32] After creating a lamellar flap using a microkeratome, this vector was applied topically onto the stromal bed and caused considerable gene transfer, supporting the hypothesis that successful keratocyte gene delivery is dependent on a breached epithelial barrier. Because AAV2 is naturally found in humans, AAV2 may induce a humoral immune response or inflammation, and consequently diminish the AAV2 potency. To circumvent this problem, hybrid AAV vectors were developed using the genome from AAV2, and the capsid from different serotypes. These hybrids were capable of efficiently transducing several ocular tissues in several species.[33-38] Significant tissue-specific delivery of AAV2/5 to the stroma of rabbit and rodent cornea was observed, and transgene expression lasted up to 12 months.[25, 38] Serotype AAV2/6, 2/8, and 2/9 hybrid vectors have also shown promising results in the transfer of genes to human corneal fibroblasts *in vitro*, human corneas *ex vivo*, and in rodent corneas *in vivo*.[37-39]

The delayed initial appearance of transgene expression was another limitation in the development of efficient AAV vectors. The delayed initial expression occurs due to the complementary DNA annealing step where the single-stranded viral genome is converted into double-stranded DNA. To resolve this problem, double-stranded self-complementary AAV (scAAV) vectors were developed. Hairpin-forming terminal repeat segments are necessary for AAV replication and packaging, and the encouragement of the formation of dimeric inverted repeat genomes is possible. If small enough, dimers can be packaged into the viral envelope, and upon release into the host cell, they can spontaneously self-anneal. This process results in double-stranded DNA that is available for quicker gene expression.[40-42]

Although many of the limitations encountered with initial AAV vectors have been resolved, there are several inherent drawbacks of these vectors, which have been proven challenging to overcome. Because of their small size, therapeutic genes greater than 1.8 kb are difficult to package. Also generating high viral titers is time consuming and technically demanding, and immunological concerns exist in cases where humans have been previously exposed to serotypes 1–6.

Retrovirus Vectors

Retroviruses are composed of two identical, linear single-stranded RNAs located in a cylindrical nuclear core. With a genome size of ~7–11 kb, retroviruses consist of three subfamilies including oncovirinae, lentivirinae and spumavirinae, with oncoretroviruses being the first viruses used in gene therapy. Retroviruses contain three vital genes: *Gag*, *pol*, and *env*. *Gag* encodes for structural proteins of the virus, *pol* for reverse transcriptase/intergrase, and *env* for long terminal repeat (LTR) flanked viral envelope glycoproteins. To deliver foreign DNA to a cell, viral envelope proteins bind host cell surface receptors.[3] Prior to membrane fusion, the viral core enters the cell where the viral genome is released. Reverse transcriptase converts the viral genome into double stranded proviral DNA. The genome is then translocated to the nucleus and integrated into the host genome, via viral intergrase, where LTR-associated transcription factors in the viral genome initiate transcription of new viral particles.[3]

Retroviral vectors are very valuable tools for *in vitro* studies. They are commonly used to immortalize ocular cells that characteristically do not grow in culture; including corneal epithelial and endothelial cells and donor corneas from normal and Fuchs' dystrophy patients.[43-46] Retroviral vectors can hold large therapeutic genes (~8 kb) and are capable of providing long-term expression of therapeutic genes in dividing cells.[9] However, because random integration into the host genome increases the risk of insertional mutagenesis, retroviral vectors may be oncogenic and, therefore, limit their application in human therapies.[9] They are also not capable of transducing non-dividing cells, and similar to AV vectors,

retroviral vectors are also highly immunogenic.[9] Therefore, while there are many advantageous characteristics of viral vector usage for gene delivery, major safety and toxicity concerns have been noted. [9]

Lentivirus Vectors

Lentiviruses, like the commonly used HIV1 vector, are a type of retrovirus that can be modified for gene therapy use. Similar to other retroviruses, lentiviruses are enveloped viruses containing a single-stranded RNA genome within its cylindrical core. Approximately100 nm in size, each particle has two copies of its genome containing characteristic retroviral genes (e.g. *p7*, *gag*, *pol*, and *env*). Encoding for several additional gene products, they also have six ORFs.[47-49] The mode of gene delivery is essentially the same as other retroviruses, except that the lentiviral genome is expressed episomally.[3]

HIV-derived vectors used in gene therapy undergo several modification steps in order to develop a vector without infectious and replication capabilities. For example, removal of integration capabilities has been achieved by the replacement of LTRs with self-inactivating LTR hybrids. The subsequent construct has a small fraction of the original viral genome[50], and reduced potential of integrating into the host genome. Lentiviral vectors are capable of penetrating intact nuclear membranes allowing them to transduce non-dividing cells. Also, compared to other retroviral vectors, they appear less toxic to the host genome. Lentiviruses have been demonstrated to target and efficiently transduce many corneal cell types (e.g. epithelium, endothelium and keratocytes) *in vitro*, *in vivo* and *ex vivo* with high transgene expression.[51-55] These integration-deficient vectors appear promising for ocular gene therapy over other retroviral systems, however, the risk of integration still remains a major translational obstacle.[49]

Development of nonviral gene delivery vectors was initiated in the early 1970's after Graham and colleagues utilized chemical methods to successfully transform cells.[56] This early success led to the development of many other nonviral vectors including plasmids, lipids, and nanoparticles. Nanoparticles are promising tools in ophthalmology because they have low immunogenicity, high gene-carrying capacity, and an affordable cost of commercial production.[57] One of the biggest limitations of non-viral vectors has been low transfection efficacy and short gene expression duration.[58] Working at the subcellular level, the ultimate goal of nanomedicine is to achieve therapeutic benefit through the comprehensive defense, repair, and control of biological systems using nanostructures.[59]

Nonviral Vectors: Nanoparticles

Nanoparticles are particles ranging between 1–100 nm in size. Because living cells generally have a diameter between 10,000 nm and 20,000 nm, the small magnitude of nanoparticles gives them the ability to access intracellular compartments with little impact on cell membranes.[38] The smallness also provides a large surface area to volume ratio; therefore, a myriad of ligands (e.g. antibodies, peptides, DNA, and probes) can be incorporated giving rise to a multitude of therapeutic treatment options.[30] Nanoparticles can also be tagged with molecular sensors and fluorescent markers to enhance uptake into specific target cells, and to track *in vivo*.[9] Additionally, the high specificity and small size may reduce the amount of therapeutic agent administered and side effects.

There are three major categories of nanoparticles that have been investigated for therapeutic delivery into ocular tissue including polymeric, metallic, and hybrid metal-polymeric nanoparticles. Polymeric particles are composed of organic polymers such as polyethylene glycol (PEG), chitosan, albumin and polyethyleneimine (PEI).[10] PEG is the most commonly studied polymer in ocular application due to low immunogenicity.[60] It has also been used to successfully deliver plasmids to the retina, lens, cornea, and trabecular meshwork *invivo*.[58] Chitosan is a deacetylated chitin, which is biocompatible, biodegradable and non-

toxic.[61, 62] It has also been shown to transiently increase corneal permeability, enhance ocular bioavailability, and penetrate conjunctival epithelia cells via paracellular and transcellular pathways.[62-64] Due to its electrostatic interaction with negative charges in the mucus layer, polycationic chitosan has been identified as a promising ophthalmic treatment vector.[62] Additionally in rodent keratocytes, successful marker gene expression was reported following intrastromal injection of chitosan nanoparticles.[65] Albumin facilitates its role as a vector for drugs and oligonucleotides because of its highly charged amino acid composition.[66] Albumin nanoparticles have been documented to effectively deliver a gene encoding a soluble vascular endothelium growth factor into the cornea, and to decrease neovascularization without major adverse effects.[67] Polymers and copolymers like PLA (poly lactic acid) and (poly D,L-lactide-co-glycolide) PLGA, are also biocompatible and biodegradable resulting in their common use as building blocks for nanocarriers. PLGA has shown some capability to transport genetic material to rabbit conjunctival epithelium.[68]

Gold nanoparticles (GNPs) are appealing gene therapy vectors because they have minimal toxicity, can efficiently condense DNA, and are easy to synthesize.[69] It has also been demonstrated that GNPs successfully transported marker genes in various mammalian cells.[70-74] Recently our group was one of the first to investigate the applications of hybrid GNPs as therapeutic delivery vectors in the cornea. A study was conducted to assess the safety and efficiency of PEI2-GNPs (2 kDa PEI conjugated to GNPs) *in vivo* using a rabbit model.[75] With and without the removal of corneal epithelium, PEI2-GNPs were applied topically using a cloning cylinder (to enhance target tissue delivery specificity). Corneal tissue exhibited marked PEI2-GNP uptake with slow clearance over time. Additionally, GNPs were detected in the extracellular matrix and keratocytes, and slit-lamp biomicroscopy revealed no signs of inflammation or edema.[75] The results from this study indicated that PEI2-GNPs are attractive candidate vectors for safe and effective gene therapy in corneal tissue.[75]

GENE THERAPY APPLICATIONS IN OPHTHALMOLOGY

Anterior Eye

Applications of gene therapy have been investigated in diseases of anterior segment, particularly those affecting the cornea. A summary of gene therapy vectors and genes tested for anterior eye disorders is presented in Table 20.2.

Corneal Graft Rejection

Keratoplasty is a commonly used treatment for various corneal pathologies. While this procedure is generally effective, allograft immunological rejection and consequent failure are major concerns.[76] Attempts to enhance graft survival by gene therapy have focused on modulating wound healing, angiogenesis, apoptosis, and cellular

Table 20.2 Gene therapy vectors and genes tested for anterior eye disorders

Corneal Graft Rejection	Corneal Wound Healing	Corneal Alkali Burns	Conjunctiva and lacrimal glad dysfunctions
Adenovirus vector • CTLA-4 • CE2F2 *Lentivirus vector* • bcl-xl • bcl-2 • p35 • IDO	*Adenovirus vector* • Soluble Type II transforming growth factor (TGFb) receptor *Adeno-associated virus vector* • Decorin *Plasmid* • Tissue plasminogen activator	*Adenovirus vector* • SMAD 7 • BMP 7 • Peroxisome proliferator-activated receptor (PPAR) λ *Gold nanoparticle* • BMP 7	*Adenovirus vector* • IL 10 • p38 activated protein kinase • SMAD 9 • (PPAR) λ
Corneal neovascularization: *Plasmid* • Kringle 5 plasminogen • IL12 • IL10 • Vascular endothelial growth factor receptor FLT-1 • FLT24K • FLT23K *Albumin-derived nanoparticle* • FLT23K *Adenovirus vector* • Vascular endothelial growth factor receptor FLT-1 *Adeno-associated virus vector* • Vascular endothelial growth factor receptor FLT-1 • Angiostatin • Pigment epithelium-derived factor (PEDF) • Decorin *Lentivirus vector* • Endostatin/kringle-5 domain of plasminogen fusion protein		**Corneal scarring:** *Retrovirus vector* • Herpes simplex virus (HSV) thymidine kinase • Dominant-negative cyclin G1 *Nanoparticle* • Bone morphogenic protein 7 • Soluble type II transforming growth factor (TGFβ) receptor *Adeno-associated virus vector* • SMAD 7 • Decorin	**Herpes simplex virus type-1** *Plasmid* • HSV-1 glycoprotein's (G, D, and gB1) • Interferon • TNFα • IL2 • IL4 • IL10
		Corneal neuropathy and epithelopathy, and dystrophies *Adenovirus vector* • cmet • β-glucuronidase	

transport.[76] Lentiviral transport of anti-apoptotic genes (Bcl-xL, Bcl-2, surviving, and p35) was shown to extend graft survival in a rodent model.[77] Similarly enhanced endothelial cell survival was observed after delivery of anti-apoptotic genes into human corneas and primary endothelial cells using lentiviral vectors.[78] Adenoviral vectors have also been shown to extend endothelial cell survival and amplify cell counts in human and rabbit corneas.[79] McAlister and colleagues demonstrated that the delivery of transcription factor E2F2 *ex vivo* protected endothelial cells via modulation of cell cycle phases.[79]

Modulation of T cell activation in and around the graft site has also been tested in efforts to decrease the odds of immune rejection. Encouraging immune tolerance, indoleamine 2, 3-dioxygenase (IDO) is believed to prevent activated T cell division by halting T cells in the G1 phase. Lentivirus-mediated delivery of IDO significantly prolonged graft survival in rodent full-thickness corneal grafts and corneal endothelium.[80] These studies emphasize the promising potentials of gene therapy applications in enhancing corneal allograft survival.

Corneal Scarring and Wound Healing

Injury, infection or trauma of the cornea often results in corneal opacification and vision loss. This opacification is believed to result from a fibrotic response, regulated by numerous chemokines and cytokines. In a rabbit fibrosis model, corneal retroviral-mediated delivery of dominant-negative mutant cyclin G1 was used to block cyclins and cyclin-dependent kinases involved in the control of cell division.[81] Corneas expressing the construct displayed decrease corneal haze, likely because of activated keratocytes apoptosis.[81] An alternative tactic to modulate fibrosis would be to limit keratocyte proliferation. In a laser-induced corneal haze model, haze was reduced by retroviral delivery of the thymidine kinase gene following keratectomy.[81]

Another cytokine believed to play a large role in the fibrotic cascade is transforming growth factor beta (TGFβ). TGFβ's increased release and hyperactivity following injury has been shown to be involved in profibrotic myofibroblast generation. Because TGFβ can transmit signals through the Smad pathway, it has been demonstrated that modulating Smad protein expression (Smad 2, 3, and 7) may potentially inhibit corneal scarring.[82] Additionally, inhibition of the fibrotic function of TGFβ has been accomplished utilizing a natural inhibitor of TGFβ, decorin (a small leucine-rich proteoglycan). Decorin significantly inhibited myofibroblast induction when delivered into human corneal fibroblasts, without affecting cell viability.[83, 84] Furthermore, tissue specific delivery of decorin significantly decreased corneal fibrosis when administered via AAV2/5 vector *in vivo* without apparent side effects.[85]

Corneal Neovascularization

Corneal neovascularization (CNV) results in increased risk of anti-inflammatory response, loss of corneal transparency and blindness. Targeting the vascular endothelial growth factor (VEGF) pathway may be a promising approach to treating this disorder. Inhibition of injury-induced neovascularization was seen after albumin-derived nanoparticles were used to deliver constructs containing *Flt32K*, a VEGF receptor gene, to keratocytes.[67] Similarly Flt-1 and Flk-1 also inhibited CNV in rodent eyes when delivered via adenoviral vectors.[86, 87] Inhibition of CNV was also demonstrated by the coupling of Flt23K or Flt24K peptides with an endoplasmic reticulum-retaining peptide, which led to the intracellular sequestering of VEGF following intrastromal injection into rodent eyes.[88, 89] Genes involved in regulating vascular endothelial cell adhesion, proliferation, migration, and apoptosis have also shown reduction of CNV in rodents.[90-92] Additionally, epithelium derived factor, CD26, GA-binding protein, IL18, and decorin are other genes showing promise for CNV treatment. Decorin, for example, significantly reduced CNV in rabbit eyes *in vivo* when delivered with an AAV5 vector, and showed no apparent adverse side effects.[93]

Corneal Dystrophies

Patients suffering from various corneal dystrophies may benefit from gene therapy treatment. Mucopolysaccharidosis is a group of metabolic disorders characterized by the absence of altered activity of lysosomal enzyme. In this condition, AV-mediated ocular delivery of human beta-glucuronidase resulted in rapid clearance of lysosomal storage in keratocytes. Additionally in congenital stromal corneal dystrophy, stromal accumulation of mutant decorin can be treated by siRNA-based gene therapy whereby mutant decorin formation can be prevented (Mohan et al, unpublished data). Gene therapy could also be used for the development of treatments for Fuch's corneal endothelial dystrophy (FD), which is the third most common cause of blindness in Americans.[2] FD is characterized by the formation of bumps along the endothelium, called "guttae", which disrupt this corneal layer and cause corneal swelling, corneal haze, pain, and eventually blindness as the cornea thickens and loses its transparency.[94] TGFβ signaling pathway has been identified to play a prominent role in the formation of guttae[94-96], and gene therapy approaches are currently underway in efforts to modulate this pathway to eliminate the formation of guttae (Mohan et al., unpublished data). One major roadblock for successful gene therapy development for corneal dystrophies is the lack of experimental models; however, it has recently been reported that a rodent disease model of congenital stromal corneal dystrophy has been identified.[97] While this is an important milestone for the field, much work is needed before potential treatments can be translated to clinical application.

Corneal Alkali Burn

Ocular alkali injuries result in corneal ulceration, scarring, neovascularization, and opacification, and gene therapy approaches have been tested for the treatment of these complications through modifications of the TGFβ pathway. When Smad7 gene was topically administered, Cre-adenovirus-mediated Smad7 expression antagonized corneal scarring. Bone morphogenic protein-7 (BMP7) also demonstrated antagonistic effects against TGFβ-mediated pathology. In alkali-injured rodent corneas, adenoviral delivery of BMP7 into the cornea was shown to suppress formation of myofibroblasts and infiltration of monocytes and macrophages. It was also shown to decrease the expression of collagens, TGFβ and macrophage chemo-attractant protein-1 and accelerate re-epithelization.[98] Hybrid gold nanoparticle-mediated BMP7 delivery *in vivo* significantly reduced corneal haze in an alkali and laser-induced rabbit model. Additionally, reduction of the inflammatory and fibrogenic responses *in vivo* was accomplished in alkali-burn mouse corneas via adenoviral-mediated corneal delivery of peroxisome proliferator-activated receptor-gamma.

Ocular Surface Disorders

Herpes simplex virus type-1 (HSV-1) is a widespread human pathogen that can cause HSV keratitis, the leading cause of corneal blindness and corneal graft rejection.[99, 100] Recent progress has been made using gene therapy to disrupt the HSV-1 genome.[101-103] Following intramuscular injection of plasmids expressing HSV-1 glycoproteins (G, D, and gB1), marked protection against keratitis pathology was observed. Topical application of naked plasmids encoding for interferon, tumor necrosis factor α (TNFα), or interleukin (IL) 2, IL4, and IL10 have been shown to relieve HSV keratitis and prevent scarring.

Gene therapy has also been implicated for the treatment of corneal ailments caused by type 1 and 2 diabetes, including corneal neuropathy and epitheliopathy. *In vitro* adenovirus-mediated transfer of *cmet*, a hepatocyte growth factor (HGF) receptor gene, improved HGF signaling, restored wild type protein expression and improved wound healing.[104] Research has also been conducted to evaluate gene-based treatments for conjunctiva and lacrimal gland dysfunctions (e.g. dry eye, and Sjogren's syndrome).[105-109] Rabbit lacrimal glands were protected from immunopathology, and tear production was not increased following virus-mediated delivery of IL10. Additionally inhibition of TNFα resulted in reduced immune cell infiltration and increased tear production.[105,106] In conjunctival gene delivery investigations, prevention of scarring has been the main focus. Suppression of the fibrogenic response was reported in cultured human subconjunctival fibroblasts and in an *in vivo* model of conjunctival scarring, subsequent to adenovirus-mediated transfer of p38 mitogen-activated protein kinase, Smad7, and peroxisome proliferator-activated receptor gamma.[107-109]

Glaucoma

Glaucoma is characterized by the death of retinal ganglion cells (RGCs), which are believed to be vulnerable to an increase in intraocular pressure (IOP). IOP is generally regulated within the anterior eye segment, and the primary cause of this increase in pressure is an increase in fluid outflow resistance through the trabecular meshwork. The first-line in glaucoma treatment is the topical application of ophthalmic solution or ointment that lowers IOP via suppression of aqueous humor generation at the ciliary body, or enhancement of aqueous humor outflow through the trabecular meshwork.[110] However, physiologic ocular barriers significantly limit the long-term benefits of topical glaucoma therapeutics.[111]

Studies have identified genetic risk factors associated with glaucoma development, and gene therapy approaches may achieve a more permanent solution for patients.[112] Trabecular meshwork cell function has been reported to be affected by mutations in *myocilin*.[113] Research has also demonstrated that mutations in *optineurin* increased RGC susceptibility to cellular damage and death.[114] While the genetic basis of glaucoma is not entirely understood, potential target genes have been identified.[115] For example, AAV-mediated delivery of neuroprotective genes successfully transduced RGCs in glaucoma

models.[116] Unfortunately, clinical translation of these results was limited due to safety concerns, gene size, and cost of production of the viral vectors. Nanoparticles, on the other hand, may represent an alternative to viral vector gene transfer. Utilization of nanoparticles to efficiently reduce IOP may potentially decrease dosing frequency and adverse effects and improve compliance.[111]

Posterior Eye

Retina

Mutations in some retinal pigment epithelium (RPE) genes (e.g. lecithin retinol acyltransferase [LRAT], RPE65, and bestrophin) have been associated with several blinding disorders including Leber's congenital amaurosis (LCA), and retinitis pigmentosa (RP).[117] Other retinal diseases associated with RPE-related changes include age-related macular degeneration (AMD) and choroidal neovascularization.[118] Secondary to RPE pathology, blindness typically is a result of photoreceptor degeneration and loss. There is no cure for RPE-associated diseases; however, major advancements have been made in the field of gene therapy for these particular ocular conditions.

Viral vectors (e.g. lentivirus, AV, and AAV) are capable of efficiently transferring therapeutic genes to the retina and RPE.[119] AAV-mediated delivery of p581PK, a 58 kD protein kinase inhibitor, was performed in a rat diabetic model to test this approach in the treatment of diabetic retinopathy.[120] Intravitreal injection of p58IPK resulted in decreased expression of VEGF, and TNFα, and marked decrease in vascularization. Additionally, based on positive results of extensive preclinical studies, several clinical trials are underway for the testing of AAV-mediated therapies for LCA.[118,121-123] From a drug development point of view, AAV vectors have limitation in the treatment of retinal diseases because of their small carrying capacity.[124] For instance, AAV vectors are unable to accommodate large genes involved in diseases like Stargardt's macular degeneration (ABCA4)[125] and Usher's syndrome type 2 (USH2A),[126] nor can they carry large regulatory elements like LRAT.[127] Thus non-viral gene therapy is a major focus in the development of retinal disease therapies.

In RPE cell transfection, PEI-based nanoparticles have mainly been studied *in vitro*,[128-131] however, the efficacy of these vectors in RPE disease models has not yet been determined. Similarly, chitosan-based gene transfer has been shown to transfect retinal cells,[132] yet therapeutic rescue of normal phenotype in disease models has not been demonstrated[117]. PLGA nanoparticles have also been reported to safely and efficiently deliver genes to RPE cells *in vitro* and *in vivo*.[133] Compacted DNA nanoparticles can be targeted to many ocular tissues including the various retinal layers.[134] In an animal model of retinitis pigmentosa (rds +/-), partial rescue of photoreceptor structure and function was achieved using DNA nanoparticles to deliver the wild-type retinal degeneration slow gene (Rds).[135] These studies support the potential usage of gene therapy in the treatment of retinal disease.

NANOPARTICLE PHARMACOKINETICS: CONSIDERATIONS FOR GENE THERAPY DEVELOPMENT AND CLINICAL USE

As described above, there are several different types of nanoparticles. Consequently, each type has a unique pharmacokinetic (PK) profile. To better understand and predict efficacy and toxicity before clinical utilization of any given nanoparticle system, it is necessary to understand the PK and biodistribution. This involves longitudinal monitoring of particle concentration in critical tissues until the elimination phase, and includes parameters like: Half-life, mean resident time, maximum concentration, and clearance.[136] Optimization of the nanoparticle PK profile can enhance tissue-specific delivery to maximize therapeutic effect while reducing non-specific delivery to minimize adverse effects.

The physical and chemical features (e.g. size, charge, and surface chemistry) of nanoparticles determine the PK profile and consequently how the particle will react within the body.[136-138] Take for example cellular internalization. Size is a key player regarding cellular uptake because it affects internalization mechanisms. In mammalian cells, nanoparticles are internalized via phagocytosis, macropinocytosis, or endocytosis pathways [139-141]. Nanoparticles ~60 nm in size undergo caveolae-mediated endocytosis, those ~90 nm undergo clathrin-independent or caveolin-independent endocytosis, and those ~120 nm undergo clathrin-mediated endocytosis.[142] This is important because the mode of entry determines the path of trafficking through subcellular compartments.[137]

Shape and charge of nanoparticles have also been shown to affect cell internalization. A previous study reported that non-spherical nanoparticles were easily taken up by HeLa cells.[143] Likewise, it was also reported that rod-like mesoporous silica nanoparticles [144] and iron oxide nanoworms [145] displayed enhanced cellular uptake compared to spherical counterparts. However, other studies have demonstrated that spherical gold[146] and polymeric nanoparticles[147] were internalized more efficiently than non-spherical counterparts. Additionally in contrast to anionic particles, cationic nanoparticles typically have increased cellular uptake.[148-150] Polarity of a particle (hydrophobic vs. hydrophilic) also plays a role in the cellular uptake, as well as the mean residence time and clearance.[136]

As with most novel technologies, there are rising concerns about the potential side effects associated with the use of nanoparticles to deliver therapeutic molecules. Therefore, to better grasp the risks associated with nanoparticle exposure, routes of entry and cytotoxicity, extensive studies should be conducted. Unfortunately the same features that make nanoparticles attractive for nanodelivery, could also lead to cytotoxicity. The small magnitude of nanoparticles, for example, could make them very reactive within the cell.[151] Small size may also allow nanoparticles to enter and deposit in major organs (i.e. the skin, intestines, blood and lungs), which could result in severe adverse reactions.[152-154] Consequently, nanoparticle toxicity is also dependent on the body's ability to properly clear deposited particles from different organs. It is therefore necessary to take into consideration the risks/benefits ratio in nanomedicine applications.

CONCLUSIONS

Nano-ophthalmology is a translational field and its earliest impact will likely include areas like biopharmaceuticals (e.g. therapeutic molecule discovery and delivery).[155] Consequently, gene therapy is a very promising innovative tool that could aid in the development of preventative care/treatments for currently incurable ocular impairments that often lead to blindness. In order to address deficiencies of current treatments and resolve these incurable problems, steps should be taken to generate efficient techniques for cellular delivery of genetic material, identify novel therapeutic targets, and enhance target tissue specificity. Although there are numerous reports on the efficiency of viral and non-viral vectors to successfully deliver gene constructs to target tissues/cell and alleviate clinical symptoms, several obstacles must still be addressed in order to optimize translational success rates. To ensure patient safety, these current obstacles include improvement of current vectors, safe vector production methods, detailed PK, biodistribution, and cytotoxicity investigations. Several of these impediments have already been partly overcome, highlighting the promise of the use of gene therapy in the treatment of ophthalmic diseases and disorders.

REFERENCES

1. Roodhooft JM. Leading causes of blindness worldwide. Bull Soc Belge Ophtalmol. 2002(283):19-25.

2. Frick KD, Gower EW, Kempen JH, Wolff JL. Economic impact of visual impairment and blindness in the United States. Arch Ophthalmol. 2007;125(4):544-50.

3. Mohan RR, Rodier JT, Sharma A. Corneal gene therapy: Basic science and translational perspective. Ocul Surf. 2013;11(3):150-64.

4. Bainbridge JW, Smith AJ, Barker SS, Robbie S, Henderson R, Balaggan K, et al. Effect of gene therapy on visual function in Leber's congenital amaurosis. N Engl J Med. 2008;358(21):2231-9.

5. Hauswirth WW, Aleman TS, Kaushal S, Cideciyan AV, Schwartz SB, Wang L, et al. Treatment of Leber congenital amaurosis due to RPE65 mutations by ocular subretinal injection of adeno-associated virus gene vector: Short-term results of a phase I trial. Hum Gene Ther. 2008;19(10):979-90.

6. Maguire AM, High KA, Auricchio A, Wright JF, Pierce EA, Testa F, et al. Age-dependent effects of RPE65 gene therapy for Leber's congenital amaurosis: A phase 1 dose-escalation trial. Lancet. 2009;374(9701):1597-605.

7. Maguire AM, Simonelli F, Pierce EA, Pugh EN, Jr, Mingozzi F, Bennicelli J, et al. Safety and efficacy of gene transfer for Leber's congenital amaurosis. N Engl J Med. 2008;358(21):2240-8.

8. Simonelli F, Maguire AM, Testa F, Pierce EA, Mingozzi F, Bennicelli JL, et al. Gene therapy for Leber's congenital amaurosis is safe and effective through 1.5 years after vector administration. Mol Ther. 2010;18(3):643-50.

9. Mohan RR, Rodier JT. Gene Therapy in the Cornea: Principles and Promise. Copeland and Afshari's Principles and Practice of Cornea (Volume 1 and Volume 2): Jaypee Brothers Medical Publishers (P) Ltd; 2013; pp. 863-86.

10. Gaudana R, Jwala J, Boddu SHS, Mitra AK. Recent perspectives in ocular drug delivery. Pharmaceutical Research. 2009;26(5):1197-216.

11. Vandervoort J, Ludwig A. Ocular drug delivery: Nanomedicine applications. Nanomedicine (Lond). 2007;2(1):11-21.

12. Lee VH, Robinson JR. Topical ocular drug delivery: Recent developments and future challenges. J Ocul Pharmacol. 1986;2(1):67-108.

13. Baudouin C. Side effects of antiglaucomatous drugs on the ocular surface. Curr Opin Ophthalmol. 1996;7(2):80-6.

14. Salminen L. Review: Systemic absorption of topically applied ocular drugs in humans. J Ocul Pharmacol. 1990;6(3):243-9.

15. Duvvuri S, Majumdar S, Mitra AK. Drug delivery to the retina: Challenges and opportunities. Expert Opin Biol Ther. 2003;3(1):45-56.

16. Janoria KG, Gunda S, Boddu SH, Mitra AK. Novel approaches to retinal drug delivery. Expert Opin Drug Deliv. 2007;4(4):371-88.

17. Marmor MF, Negi A, Maurice DM. Kinetics of macromolecules injected into the subretinal space. Exp Eye Res. 1985;40(5):687-96.

18. Ausayakhun S, Yuvaves P, Ngamtiphakom S, Prasitsilp J. Treatment of cytomegalovirus retinitis in AIDS patients with intravitreal ganciclovir. J Med Assoc Thai. 2005;88 Suppl 9:S15-20.

19. Raghava S, Hammond M, Kompella UB. Periocular routes for retinal drug delivery. Expert Opin Drug Deliv. 2004;1(1):99-114.

20. Castellarin A, Pieramici DJ. Anterior segment complications following periocular and intraocular injections. Ophthalmol Clin North Am. 2004;17(4):583-90, vii.

21. Volpers C, Kochanek S. Adenoviral vectors for gene transfer and therapy. J Gene Med. 2004;6 Suppl 1:S164-71.

22. Borras T, Gabelt BT, Klintworth GK, Peterson JC, Kaufman PL. Non-invasive observation of repeated adenoviral GFP gene delivery to the anterior segment of the monkey eye in vivo. J Gene Med. 2001;3(5):437-49.

23. Budenz DL, Bennett J, Alonso L, Maguire A. In vivo gene transfer into murine corneal endothelial and trabecular meshwork cells. Invest Ophthalmol Vis Sci. 1995;36(11):2211-5.

24. Carlson EC, Liu CY, Yang X, Gregory M, Ksander B, Drazba J, et al. In vivo gene delivery and visualization of corneal stromal cells using an adenoviral vector and keratocyte-specific promoter. Invest Ophthalmol Vis Sci. 2004;45(7):2194-200.

25. Fehervari Z, Rayner SA, Oral HB, George AJ, Larkin DF. Gene transfer to ex vivo stored corneas. Cornea. 1997;16(4):459-64.

26. Klebe S, Sykes P, Coster D, Krishnan, Williams K. Prolongation of sheep corneal allograft survival by ex vivo transfer of the gene encoding interleukin-10. Transplantation. 2001; 71:1214-20.

27. Larkin DF, Oral HB, Ring CJ, Lemoine NR, George AJ. Adenovirus-mediated gene delivery to the corneal endothelium. Transplantation. 1996;61(3):363-70.

28. Mashhour B, Couton D, Perricaudet M, Briand P. In vivo adenovirus-mediated gene transfer into ocular tissues. Gene Ther. 1994;1(2):122-6.

29. Tsubota K, Inoue H, Ando K, Ono M, Yoshino K, Saito I. Adenovirus-mediated gene transfer to the ocular surface epithelium. Exp Eye Res. 1998;67(5):531-8.

30. Mohan RR, Tovey JC, Sharma A, Tandon A. Gene therapy in the cornea: 2005--present. Prog Retin Eye Res. 2012;31(1):43-64.

31. Grimm D, Kay MA, Kleinschmidt JA. Helper virus-free, optically controllable, and two-plasmid-based production of adeno-associated virus vectors of serotypes 1 to 6. Mol Ther. 2003;7(6):839-50.

32. Mohan RR, Schultz GS, Hong JW, Wilson SE. Gene transfer into rabbit keratocytes using AAV and lipid-mediated plasmid DNA vectors with a lamellar flap for stromal access. Exp Eye Res. 2003;76(3):373-83.

33. Stieger K, Cronin T, Bennett J, Rolling F. Adeno-associated virus mediated gene therapy for retinal degenerative diseases. Methods Mol Biol. 2011;807:179-218.

34. Buss DG, Giuliano E, Sharma A, Mohan RR. Gene delivery in the equine cornea: a novel therapeutic strategy. Vet Ophthalmol. 2010;13(5):301-6.

35. Lebherz C, Maguire A, Tang W, Bennett J, Wilson JM. Novel AAV serotypes for improved ocular gene transfer. J Gene Med. 2008;10(4):375-82.

36. Mohan RR, Sinha S, Tandon A, Gupta R, Tovey JC, Sharma A. Efficacious and safe tissue-selective controlled gene therapy approaches for the cornea. PLoS One. 2011;6(4):e18771.

37. Sharma A, Ghosh A, Hansen ET, Newman JM, Mohan RR. Transduction efficiency of AAV 2/6, 2/8 and 2/9 vectors for delivering genes in human corneal fibroblasts. Brain Res Bull. 2010;81(2-3):273-8.

38. Sharma A, Ghosh A, Siddappa C, Mohan RR. Ocular surface: Gene therapy. In: Besharse JC, Dartt DA, editors. Encyclopedia of the Eye: Elsevier; 2010; pp. 185-94.

39. Sharma A, Tovey JC, Ghosh A, Mohan RR. AAV serotype influences gene transfer in corneal stroma in vivo. Exp Eye Res. 2010;91(3):440-8.

40. Buie LK, Rasmussen CA, Porterfield EC, Ramgolam VS, Choi VW, Markovic-Plese S, et al. Self-complementary AAV virus (scAAV)

safe and long-term gene transfer in the trabecular meshwork of living rats and monkeys. Invest Ophthalmol Vis Sci. 2010;51(1):236-48.

41. Kong F, Li W, Li X, Zheng Q, Dai X, Zhou X, et al. Self-complementary AAV5 vector facilitates quicker transgene expression in photoreceptor and retinal pigment epithelial cells of normal mouse. Exp Eye Res. 2010;90(5):546-54.

42. Yokoi K, Kachi S, Zhang HS, Gregory PD, Spratt SK, Samulski RJ, et al. Ocular gene transfer with self-complementary AAV vectors. Invest Ophthalmol Vis Sci. 2007;48(7):3324-8.

43. Mohan RR, Possin DE, Sinha S, Wilson SE. Development of genetically engineered tet HPV16-E6/E7 transduced human corneal epithelial clones having tight regulation of proliferation and normal differentiation. Exp Eye Res. 2003;77(4):395-407.

44. Jester JV, Huang J, Fisher S, Spiekerman J, Chang JH, Wright WE, et al. Myofibroblast differentiation of normal human keratocytes and hTERT, extended-life human corneal fibroblasts. Invest Ophthalmol Vis Sci. 2003;44(5):1850-8.

45. Wilson SE, Weng J, Blair S, He YG, Lloyd S. Expression of E6/E7 or SV40 large T antigen-coding oncogenes in human corneal endothelial cells indicate regulated high-proliferative capacity. Invest Ophthalmol Vis Sci. 1995;36(1):32-40.

46. He Y, Weng J, Li Q, Knauf HP, Wilson SE. Fuchs' corneal endothelial cells transduced with the human papilloma virus E6/E7 oncogenes. Exp Eye Res. 1997;65(1):135-42.

47. Clements JE, Zink MC. Molecular biology and pathogenesis of animal lentivirus infections. Clin Microbiol Rev. 1996;9(1):100-17.

48. Durand S, Cimarelli A. The inside out of lentiviral vectors. Viruses. 2011;3(2):132-59.

49. Sakuma T, Barry MA, Ikeda Y. Lentiviral vectors: Basic to translational. Biochem J. 2012;443(3):603-18.

50. Miyoshi H, Blomer U, Takahashi M, Gage FH, Verma IM. Development of a self-inactivating lentivirus vector. J Virol. 1998;72(10):8150-7.

51. Bainbridge JW, Stephens C, Parsley K, Demaison C, Halfyard A, Thrasher AJ, et al. In vivo gene transfer to the mouse eye using an HIV-based lentiviral vector; efficient long-term transduction of corneal endothelium and retinal pigment epithelium. Gene Ther. 2001;8(21):1665-8.

52. Beutelspacher SC, Ardjomand N, Tan PH, Patton GS, Larkin DF, George AJ, et al. Comparison of HIV-1 and EIAV-based lentiviral vectors in corneal transduction. Exp Eye Res. 2005;80(6):787-94.

53. Challa P, Luna C, Liton PB, Chamblin B, Wakefield J, Ramabhadran R, et al. Lentiviral mediated gene delivery to the anterior chamber of rodent eyes. Mol Vis. 2005;11:425-30.

54. Parker DG, Kaufmann C, Brereton HM, Anson DS, Francis-Staite L, Jessup CF, et al. Lentivirus-mediated gene transfer to the rat, ovine and human cornea. Gene Ther. 2007;14(9):760-7.

55. Takahashi K, Luo T, Saishin Y, Sung J, Hackett S, Brazzell RK, et al. Sustained transduction of ocular cells with a bovine immunodeficiency viral vector. Hum Gene Ther. 2002;13(11):1305-16.

56. Graham FL, van der Eb AJ. A new technique for the assay of infectivity of human adenovirus 5 DNA. Virology. 1973;52(2):456-67.

57. Glover DJ, Lipps HJ, Jans DA. Towards safe, non-viral therapeutic gene expression in humans. Nat Rev Genet. 2005;6(4):299-310.

58. Cai X, Conley S, Naash M. Nanoparticle applications in ocular gene therapy. Vision Res. 2008;48(3):319-24.

59. Freitas RA Jr. What is nanomedicine? Dis Mon. 2005;51(6):325-41.

60. Petros RA, DeSimone JM. Strategies in the design of nanoparticles for therapeutic applications. Nat Rev Drug Discov. 2010;9(8):615-27.

61. Rabinovich-Guilatt L, Couvreur P, Lambert G, Dubernet C. Cationic vectors in ocular drug delivery. J Drug Target. 2004;12(9-10):623-33.

62. Alonso MJ, Sanchez A. The potential of chitosan in ocular drug delivery. J Pharm Pharmacol. 2003;55(11):1451-63.

63. Calvo P, Vila-Jato JL, Alonso MJ. Comparative in vitro evaluation of several colloidal systems, nanoparticles, nanocapsules, and nanoemulsions, as ocular drug carriers. J Pharm Sci. 1996;85(5):530-6.

64. Enriquez de Salamanca A, Diebold Y, Calonge M, Garcia-Vazquez C, Callejo S, Vila A, et al. Chitosan nanoparticles as a potential drug delivery system for the ocular surface: toxicity, uptake mechanism and in vivo tolerance. Invest Ophthalmol Vis Sci. 2006;47(4):1416-25.

65. Klausner EA, Zhang Z, Chapman RL, Multack RF, Volin MV. Ultrapure chitosan oligomers as carriers for corneal gene transfer. Biomaterials. 2010;31(7):1814-20.

66. Zarbin MA, Montemagno C, Leary JF, Ritch R. Nanotechnology in ophthalmology. Can J Ophthalmol. 2010;45(5):457-76.

67. Jani PD, Singh N, Jenkins C, Raghava S, Mo Y, Amin S, et al. Nanoparticles sustain expression of Flt intraceptors in the cornea and inhibit injury-induced corneal angiogenesis. Invest Ophthalmol Vis Sci. 2007;48(5):2030-6.

68. Qaddoumi MG, Ueda H, Yang J, Davda J, Labhasetwar V, Lee VH. The characteristics and mechanisms of uptake of PLGA nanoparticles in rabbit conjunctival epithelial cell layers. Pharm Res. 2004;21(4):641-8.

69. Pissuwan D, Niidome T, Cortie MB. The forthcoming applications of gold nanoparticles in drug and gene delivery systems. J Control Release. 2011;149(1):65-71.

70. Ghosh PS, Kim CK, Han G, Forbes NS, Rotello VM. Efficient gene delivery vectors by tuning the surface charge density of amino acid-functionalized gold nanoparticles. ACS Nano. 2008;2(11):2213-8.

71. Li D, Li P, Li G, Wang J, Wang E. The effect of nocodazole on the transfection efficiency of lipid-bilayer coated gold nanoparticles. Biomaterials. 2009;30(7):1382-8.

72. Li HL, Zheng XZ, Wang HP, Li F, Wu Y, Du LF. Ultrasound-targeted microbubble destruction enhances AAV-mediated gene transfection in human RPE cells in vitro and rat retina in vivo. Gene Ther. 2009;16(9):1146-53.

73. Zhou X, Zhang X, Yu X, Zha X, Fu Q, Liu B, et al. The effect of conjugation to gold nanoparticles on the ability of low molecular weight chitosan to transfer DNA vaccine. Biomaterials. 2008;29(1):111-7.

74. Thomas M, Klibanov AM. Conjugation to gold nanoparticles enhances polyethylenimine's transfer of plasmid DNA into mammalian cells. Proc Natl Acad Sci USA. 2003;100(16):9138-43.

75. Sharma A, Tandon A, Tovey JC, Gupta R, Robertson JD, Fortune JA, et al. Polyethylenimine-conjugated gold nanoparticles: Gene transfer potential and low toxicity in the cornea. Nanomedicine. 2011;7(4):505-13.

76. Williams KA, Coster DJ. Gene therapy for diseases of the cornea: A review. Clin Experiment Ophthalmol. 2010;38(2):93-103.

77. Barcia RN, Dana MR, Kazlauskas A. Corneal graft rejection is accompanied by apoptosis of the endothelium and is prevented by gene therapy with Bcl-xL. Am J Transplant. 2007;7(9):2082-9.

78. Fuchsluger TA, Jurkunas U, Kazlauskas A, Dana R. Corneal endothelial cells are protected from apoptosis by gene therapy. Hum Gene Ther. 2011;22(5):549-58.

79. McAlister JC, Joyce NC, Harris DL, Ali RR, Larkin DF. Induction of replication in human corneal endothelial cells by E2F2 transcription factor cDNA transfer. Invest Ophthalmol Vis Sci. 2005;46(10):3597-603.

80. Beutelspacher SC, Pillai R, Watson MP, Tan PH, Tsang J, McClure MO, et al. Function of indoleamine 2,3-dioxygenase in corneal allograft rejection and prolongation of allograft survival by over-expression. Eur J Immunol. 2006;36(3):690-700.

81. Seitz B, Moreira L, Baktanian E, Sanchez D, Gray B, Gordon EM, et al. Retroviral vector-mediated gene transfer into keratocytes in vitro and in vivo. Am J Ophthalmol. 1998;126(5):630-9.

82. Tandon A, Tovey JC, Sharma A, Gupta R, Mohan RR. Role of transforming growth factor Beta in corneal function, biology and pathology. Curr Mol Med. 2010;10(6):565-78.

83. Mohan RR, Gupta R, Mehan MK, Cowden JW, Sinha S. Decorin transfection suppresses profibrogenic genes and myofibroblast formation in human corneal fibroblasts. Exp Eye Res. 2010;91(2):238-45.

84. Mohan RR, Tovey JC, Gupta R, Sharma A, Tandon A. Decorin biology, expression, function and therapy in the cornea. Curr Mol Med. 2011;11(2):110-28.

85. Mohan RR, Tandon A, Sharma A, Cowden JW, Tovey JC. Significant inhibition of corneal scarring in vivo with tissue-selective, targeted AAV5 decorin gene therapy. Invest Ophthalmol Vis Sci. 2011;52(7):4833-41.

86. Lai CM, Brankov M, Zaknich T, Lai YK, Shen WY, Constable IJ, et al. Inhibition of angiogenesis by adenovirus-mediated sFlt-1 expression in a rat model of corneal neovascularization. Hum Gene Ther. 2001;12(10):1299-310.

87. Yu H, Wu J, Li H, Wang Z, Chen X, Tian Y, et al. Inhibition of corneal neovascularization by recombinant adenovirus-mediated sFlk-1 expression. Biochem Biophys Res Commun. 2007;361(4):946-52.

88. Cho YK, Uehara H, Young JR, Tyagi P, Kompella UB, Zhang X, et al. Flt23k nanoparticles offer additive benefit in graft survival and anti-angiogenic effects when combined with

triamcinolone. Invest Ophthalmol Vis Sci. 2012;53(4):2328-36.

89. Singh N, Amin S, Richter E, Rashid S, Scoglietti V, Jani PD, et al. Flt-1 intraceptors inhibit hypoxia-induced VEGF expression in vitro and corneal neovascularization in vivo. Invest Ophthalmol Vis Sci. 2005;46(5):1647-52.

90. Lai LJ, Xiao X, Wu JH. Inhibition of corneal neovascularization with endostatin delivered by adeno-associated viral (AAV) vector in a mouse corneal injury model. J Biomed Sci. 2007;14(3):313-22.

91. Cheng HC, Yeh SI, Tsao YP, Kuo PC. Subconjunctival injection of recombinant AAV-angiostatin ameliorates alkali burn induced corneal angiogenesis. Mol Vis. 2007;13:2344-52.

92. Zhou SY, Xie ZL, Xiao O, Yang XR, Heng BC, Sato Y. Inhibition of mouse alkali burn induced-corneal neovascularization by recombinant adenovirus encoding human vasohibin-1. Mol Vis. 2010;16:1389-98.

93. Mohan RR, Tovey JC, Sharma A, Schultz GS, Cowden JW, Tandon A. Targeted decorin gene therapy delivered with adeno-associated virus effectively retards corneal neovascularization in vivo. PLoS One. 2011;6(10):e26432.

94. Elhalis H, Azizi B, Jurkunas UV. Fuchs endothelial corneal dystrophy. Ocul Surf. 2010;8(4):173-84.

95. Jurkunas UV, Bitar M, Rawe I. Colocalization of increased transforming growth factor-beta-induced protein (TGFBIp) and Clusterin in Fuchs endothelial corneal dystrophy. Invest Ophthalmol Vis Sci. 2009;50(3):1129-36.

96. Jurkunas UV, Bitar MS, Rawe I, Harris DL, Colby K, Joyce NC. Increased clusterin expression in Fuchs' endothelial dystrophy. Invest Ophthalmol Vis Sci. 2008;49(7):2946-55.

97. Chen S, Sun M, Meng X, Iozzo RV, Kao WW, Birk DE. Pathophysiological mechanisms of autosomal dominant congenital stromal corneal dystrophy: C-terminal-truncated decorin results in abnormal matrix assembly and altered expression of small leucine-rich proteoglycans. Am J Pathol. 2011;179(5):2409-19.

98. Saika S, Ikeda K, Yamanaka O, Flanders KC, Nakajima Y, Miyamoto T, et al. Therapeutic effects of adenoviral gene transfer of bone morphogenic protein-7 on a corneal alkali injury model in mice. Lab Invest. 2005;85(4):474-86.

99. Kaye S, Choudhary A. Herpes simplex keratitis. Prog Retin Eye Res. 2006;25(4):355-80.

100. Shtein RM, Garcia DD, Musch DC, Elner VM. Herpes simplex virus keratitis: Histopathologic inflammation and corneal allograft rejection. Ophthalmology. 2009;116(7):1301-5.

101. Arnould S, Delenda C, Grizot S, Desseaux C, Paques F, Silva GH, et al. The I-CreI meganuclease and its engineered derivatives: Applications from cell modification to gene therapy. Protein Eng Des Sel. 2011;24(1-2):27-31.

102. Galetto R, Duchateau P, Paques F. Targeted approaches for gene therapy and the emergence of engineered meganucleases. Expert Opin Biol Ther. 2009;9(10):1289-303.

103. EI Badawy HM, Gailledrat M, Desseaux C, Ponzin D, Ferrari S. Targeting herpetic keratitis by gene therapy. J Ophthalmol. 2012;2012:594869.

104. Saghizadeh M, Kramerov AA, Yu FS, Castro MG, Ljubimov AV. Normalization of wound healing and diabetic markers in organ cultured human diabetic corneas by adenoviral delivery of c-Met gene. Invest Ophthalmol Vis Sci. 2010;51(4):1970-80.

105. Selvam S, Thomas PB, Hamm-Alvarez SF, Schechter JE, Stevenson D, Mircheff AK, et al. Current status of gene delivery and gene therapy in lacrimal gland using viral vectors. Adv Drug Deliv Rev. 2006;58(11):1243-57.

106. Thomas PB, Samant DM, Selvam S, Wei RH, Wang Y, Stevenson D, et al. Adeno-associated virus-mediated IL-10 gene transfer suppresses lacrimal gland immunopathology in a rabbit model of autoimmune dacryoadenitis. Invest Ophthalmol Vis Sci. 2010;51(10):5137-44.

107. Yamanaka O, Ikeda K, Saika S, Miyazaki K, Ooshima A, Ohnishi Y. Gene transfer of Smad7 modulates injury-induced conjunctival wound healing in mice. Mol Vis. 2006;12:841-51.

108. Yamanaka O, Miyazaki K, Kitano A, Saika S, Nakajima Y, Ikeda K. Suppression of injury-induced conjunctiva scarring by peroxisome proliferator-activated receptor gamma gene transfer in mice. Invest Ophthalmol Vis Sci. 2009;50(1):187-93.

109. Yamanaka O, Saika S, Ohnishi Y, Kim-Mitsuyama S, Kamaraju AK, Ikeda K. Inhibition of p38MAP kinase suppresses fibrogenic reaction in conjunctiva in mice. Mol Vis. 2007;13:1730-9.

110. Weinreb RN, Khaw PT. Primary open-angle glaucoma. Lancet. 2004;363(9422):1711-20.

111. Pita-Thomas DW, Goldberg JL. Nanotechnology and glaucoma: Little particles for a big disease. Curr Opin Ophthalmol. 2013;24(2):130-5.

112. Fingert JH. Primary open-angle glaucoma genes. Eye (Lond). 2011;25(5):587-95.

113. Resch ZT, Fautsch MP. Glaucoma-associated myocilin: a better understanding but much more to learn. Exp Eye Res. 2009;88(4):704-12.

114. Chi ZL, Akahori M, Obazawa M, Minami M, Noda T, Nakaya N, et al. Overexpression of optineurin E50K disrupts Rab8 interaction and leads to a progressive retinal degeneration in mice. Hum Mol Genet. 2010;19(13):2606-15.

115. Borras T, Brandt CR, Nickells R, Ritch R. Gene therapy for glaucoma: Treating a multifaceted, chronic disease. Invest Ophthalmol Vis Sci. 2002;43(8):2513-8.

116. Borras T. Advances in glaucoma treatment and management: Gene therapy. Invest Ophthalmol Vis Sci. 2012;53(5):2506-10.

117. Koirala A, Conley SM, Naash MI. A review of therapeutic prospects of non-viral gene therapy in the retinal pigment epithelium. Biomaterials. 2013;34(29):7158-67.

118. Strauss O. The retinal pigment epithelium in visual function. Physiol Rev. 2005;85(3):845-81.

119. Rossmiller B, Mao H, Lewin AS. Gene therapy in animal models of autosomal dominant retinitis pigmentosa. Mol Vis. 2012;18:2479-96.

120. Yang H, Liu R, Cui Z, Chen ZQ, Yan S, Pei H, et al. Functional characterization of 58-kilodalton inhibitor of protein kinase in protecting against diabetic retinopathy via the endoplasmic reticulum stress pathway. Mol Vis. 2011;17:78-84.

121. Van Hooser JP, Liang Y, Maeda T, Kuksa V, Jang GF, He YG, et al. Recovery of visual functions in a mouse model of Leber congenital amaurosis. J Biol Chem. 2002;277(21):19173-82.

122. Bennicelli J, Wright JF, Komaromy A, Jacobs JB, Hauck B, Zelenaia O, et al. Reversal of blindness in animal models of Leber congenital amaurosis using optimized AAV2-mediated gene transfer. Mol Ther. 2008;16(3):458-65.

123. Le Meur G, Stieger K, Smith AJ, Weber M, Deschamps JY, Nivard D, et al. Restoration of vision in RPE65-deficient Briard dogs using an AAV serotype 4 vector that specifically targets the retinal pigmented epithelium. Gene Ther. 2007;14(4):292-303.

124. Wu Z, Yang H, Colosi P. Effect of genome size on AAV vector packaging. Mol Ther. 2010;18(1):80-6. PMCID: 2839202.

125. Allikmets R, Singh N, Sun H, Shroyer NF, Hutchinson A, Chidambaram A, et al. A photoreceptor cell-specific ATP-binding transporter gene (ABCR) is mutated in recessive Stargardt macular dystrophy. Nat Genet. 1997;15(3):236-46.

126. Liu X, Bulgakov OV, Darrow KN, Pawlyk B, Adamian M, Liberman MC, et al. Usherin is required for maintenance of retinal photoreceptors and normal development of cochlear hair cells. Proc Natl Acad Sci USA. 2007;104(11):4413-8.

127. den Hollander AI, Roepman R, Koenekoop RK, Cremers FP. Leber congenital amaurosis: Genes, proteins and disease mechanisms. Prog Retin Eye Res. 2008;27(4):391-419.

128. Sunshine JC, Sunshine SB, Bhutto I, Handa JT, Green JJ. Poly(beta-amino ester)-nanoparticle mediated transfection of retinal pigment epithelial cells in vitro and in vivo. PLoS One. 2012;7(5):e37543.

129. Peng CH, Cherng JY, Chiou GY, Chen YC, Chien CH, Kao CL, et al. Delivery of Oct4 and SirT1 with cationic polyurethanes-short branch PEI to aged retinal pigment epithelium. Biomaterials. 2011;32(34):9077-88.

130. Jayaraman MS, Bharali DJ, Sudha T, Mousa SA. Nano chitosan peptide as a potential therapeutic carrier for retinal delivery to treat age-related macular degeneration. Mol Vis. 2012;18:2300-8.

131. Lai JY, Li YT, Wang TP. In vitro response of retinal pigment epithelial cells exposed to chitosan materials prepared with different cross-linkers. Int J Mol Sci. 2010;11(12):5256-72.

132. Jin J, Zhou KK, Park K, Hu Y, Xu X, Zheng Z, et al. Anti-inflammatory and antiangiogenic effects of nanoparticle-mediated delivery of a natural angiogenic inhibitor. Invest Ophthalmol Vis Sci. 2011;52(9):6230-7.

133. Bejjani RA, BenEzra D, Cohen H, Rieger J, Andrieu C, Jeanny JC, et al. Nanoparticles for gene delivery to retinal pigment epithelial cells. Mol Vis. 2005;11:124-32.

134. Farjo R, Skaggs J, Quiambao AB, Cooper MJ, Naash MI. Efficient non-viral ocular gene transfer with compacted DNA nanoparticles. PLoS One. 2006;1:e38.

135. Cai X, Nash Z, Conley SM, Fliesler SJ, Cooper MJ, Naash MI. A partial structural and functional rescue of a retinitis pigmentosa model with

compacted DNA nanoparticles. PLoS One. 2009;4(4):e5290.

136. Li SD, Huang L. Pharmacokinetics and biodistribution of nanoparticles. Mol Pharm. 2008;5(4):496-504.

137. Ernsting MJ, Murakami M, Roy A, Li SD. Factors controlling the pharmacokinetics, biodistribution and intratumoral penetration of nanoparticles. J Control Release. 2013;172(3):782-94.

138. Moghimi SM, Hunter AC, Andresen TL. Factors controlling nanoparticle pharmacokinetics: An integrated analysis and perspective. Annu Rev Pharmacol Toxicol. 2012;52:481-503.

139. Ragusa A, Garcia I, Penades S. Nanoparticles as nonviral gene delivery vectors. IEEE Trans Nanobioscience. 2007;6(4):319-30.

140. Hillaireau H, Couvreur P. Nanocarriers' entry into the cell: Relevance to drug delivery. Cell Mol Life Sci. 2009;66(17):2873-96.

141. Wang J, Byrne JD, Napier ME, DeSimone JM. More effective nanomedicines through particle design. Small. 2011;7(14):1919-31.

142. Zhao F, Zhao Y, Liu Y, Chang X, Chen C. Cellular uptake, intracellular trafficking, and cytotoxicity of nanomaterials. Small. 2011;7(10):1322-37.

143. Gratton SE, Ropp PA, Pohlhaus PD, Luft JC, Madden VJ, Napier ME, et al. The effect of particle design on cellular internalization pathways. Proc Natl Acad Sci USA. 2008;105(33):11613-8.

144. Huang X, Teng X, Chen D, Tang F, He J. The effect of the shape of mesoporous silica nanoparticles on cellular uptake and cell function. Biomaterials. 2010;31(3):438-48.

145. Park JH, von Maltzahn G, Zhang L, Schwartz MP, Ruoslahti E, Bhatia SN, et al. Magnetic Iron Oxide Nanoworms for Tumor Targeting and Imaging. Adv Mater. 2008;20(9):1630-5.

146. Chithrani BD, Ghazani AA, Chan WC. Determining the size and shape dependence of gold nanoparticle uptake into mammalian cells. Nano Lett. 2006;6(4):662-8.

147. Zhang K, Fang H, Chen Z, Taylor JS, Wooley KL. Shape effects of nanoparticles conjugated with cell-penetrating peptides (HIV Tat PTD) on CHO cell uptake. Bioconjug Chem. 2008;19(9):1880-7.

148. Osaka T, Nakanishi T, Shanmugam S, Takahama S, Zhang H. Effect of surface charge of magnetite nanoparticles on their internalization into breast cancer and umbilical vein endothelial cells. Colloids Surf B Biointerfaces. 2009;71(2):325-30.

149. Santel A, Aleku M, Keil O, Endruschat J, Esche V, Fisch G, et al. A novel siRNA-lipoplex technology for RNA interference in the mouse vascular endothelium. Gene Ther. 2006;13(16):1222-34.

150. Chung TH, Wu SH, Yao M, Lu CW, Lin YS, Hung Y, et al. The effect of surface charge on the uptake and biological function of mesoporous silica nanoparticles in 3T3-L1 cells and human mesenchymal stem cells. Biomaterials. 2007;28(19):2959-66.

151. Donaldson K, Aitken R, Tran L, Stone V, Duffin R, Forrest G, et al. Carbon nanotubes: A review of their properties in relation to pulmonary toxicology and workplace safety. Toxicol Sci. 2006;92(1):5-22.

152. Oberdorster G, Maynard A, Donaldson K, Castranova V, Fitzpatrick J, Ausman K, et al. Principles for characterizing the potential human health effects from exposure to nanomaterials: Elements of a screening strategy. Part Fibre Toxicol. 2005;2:8.

153. Oberdorster G, Oberdorster E, Oberdorster J. Nanotoxicology: An emerging discipline evolving from studies of ultrafine particles. Environ Health Perspect. 2005;113(7):823-39.

154. Medina C, Santos-Martinez MJ, Radomski A, Corrigan OI, Radomski MW. Nanoparticles: Pharmacological and toxicological significance. Br J Pharmacol. 2007;150(5):552-8.

155. Wei C, Wei W, Morris M, Kondo E, Gorbounov M, Tomalia DA. Nanomedicine and drug delivery. Med Clin North Am. 2007;91(5):863-70.

CHAPTER 21

Ocular Adverse Effects of Systemically Administered Drugs

OVERVIEW

A number of common eye diseases ranging from simple corneal infections to retinoblastoma are currently being targeted by medications delivered either systemically or through topical ophthalmic preparations. The adverse effects associated with the drugs used for diagnostic and therapeutic purposes in ophthalmology have already been discussed in preceding chapters.

Ironically, drugs prescribed for several systemic diseases are known to precipitate ocular toxicity upon chronic use.[1] Some of these adverse effects include acuity changes, dry eye complication, disturbances in color vision, alteration of lens proteins, changes in aqueous humor dynamics and damage to nervous tissue, viz. retina.[2] This means that these molecules not only cross the transport barriers, but also have the propensity to interfere with the normal physiological functions in the eye such as retinal neurotransmitters, which reflects in the alteration of vision perception.[3] However, these adverse effects could also be due to some unknown action on the cerebral cortex, which needs to be ascertained. Clearly, these drugs are capable of crossing the blood-brain/ blood-ocular barriers through their unknown effects on the transporters.

Interaction between co-administered drugs further complicates the scenario. Drugs could interact at the site of their absorption or at the binding site. While the drug interactions at the systemic level are widely recognized and interpreted, effects of drug interactions at the blood-ocular site still need to be determined and this could possibly throw light on the failure or unusual responses to various therapeutic regimens. This chapter summarises available literature on the ocular side effects of some commonly prescribed medications for the treatment of systemic diseases with an attempt to understand the pharmacology behind their unusual effects.

OCULAR ADVERSE EFFECTS OF DRUGS ACTING ON AUTONOMIC NERVOUS SYSTEM

Drugs acting on autonomic nervous system are used to treat a myriad of symptoms ranging from appetite disorders, urinary incontinence, motion sickness and glaucoma. Amphetamine used in the treatment of Attention Deficit Hyperactivity Disorder is known to precipitate angle-closure glaucoma due to its propensity to cause pupillary dilation.[4] Benztropine is widely used as a second-line treatment of Parkinsonism. Though there is no widely available information about the prevalence of this disease in developing countries, certain populations show high prevalence. This drug has also been used to reverse symptoms of oculogyric crisis (ocular pain and sustained upward gaze) caused by the combination therapy of imipramine, methylphenidate and valproic acid in the treatment of depression and epilepsy.[5] Benztropine when given in combination with phenothazine or a butyrophenone results in difficulty in near vision and reduced accommodation, the extent of impairment ranges from 40–100%.[5-6] Mydriasis, decreased vision, loss or paralysis of accommodation, diplopia, angle-closure glaucoma, decreased tolerance to contact lenses, subconjunctival/retinal hemorrhages secondary to drug induced anemia have also been reported with the use of this drug.[7] Benzhexol, an antimuscarinic drug, also used in the treatment of Parkinsonism, is known to cause rise in intraocular pressure.[5] Beta-blockers are one of the firstline treatment approaches for hypertension. Patients on treatment with metoprolol and pindolol develop eye discomfort resulting in poor patient compliance.[8]

Anticholinergic or adrenergic agents most commonly induce "pupillary block" angle-closure glaucoma.[9] Nebulized ipratropium bromide and salbutamol routinely prescribed for chronic obstructive airways disease are also known to precipitate angle-closure glaucoma.[10]

Antimuscarinic agents are used in the treatment of overactive bladder.[11,12] Oxybutynin is one of the commonly prescribed drugs for overactive bladder in elderly. This drug is reported to reduce accommodation amplitude and precipitate acute angle-closure glaucoma. In children, this drug is frequently (56%) prescribed for the treatment of enuresis.[13] Esotropia has been reported in a 5 year old girl (with no previous history) while being treated for enuresis. Oxybutynin also produces dose-dependent effect on near vision.[1,13-21] Solifenacin is another routinely prescribed drug for overactive bladder, which is reported to cause dry eye and blurred vision.[22,23]

To summarize, most of the drugs acting on the autonomic nervous system seem to precipitate adverse effects on the anterior segment of the eye, particularly the ciliary body, iris and lens. The most common adverse effect associated with these medications is angle-closure glaucoma and decrease in accommodation (Table 21.1).

OCULAR ADVERSE EFFECTS OF DRUGS ACTING ON CENTRAL NERVOUS SYSTEM

The drugs acting on the CNS cross the blood-brain barrier and are associated with neural adverse effects. Retina, the neurosensory part of the eye, originates as a direct projection of the optic stalk during early development. It is protected from the adverse effects of most of the drugs as they are prevented from entering the ocular compartment due to the presence of transporter molecules both at the posterior and anterior sides. However, many psychotropic medications are reported to overcome the transporter barriers and produce numerous diverse and unwanted ocular adverse effects.

Phenothiazines are one of the widely prescribed centrally active drugs. They are used as preanesthetic medication, to alleviate anxiety and to provide additional sedation by synergistic action with co-administered sedatives or analgesics. Eyelid and kerato-conjunctival disorders are widely reported as adverse effects.[24] Chlorpromazine, one of the phenothiazines, is known to cause abnormal pigmentation of eyelids, cornea and conjunctiva. It also results in corneal edema leading to visual impairment. Chronic use of high doses of chlorpromazine and thioridazine is reported to cause lenticular opacification and retinopathy.[24,25] Carbamazepine has been associated with deficiency in color vision and reduced contrast sensitivity.[26-28] Nystagmus, diplopia, and extraocular muscle palsies have also been reported when this drug was used in the treatment of epilepsy.[1] In-utero exposure to this drug has resulted in congenital ocular malformations in the fetus.[1]

Depression is one of the most common disorders of the central nervous system which affects approximately 1 in 18 (5%) of the world population in general. It is estimated that an individual suffers depression at least once in a lifetime and there is a lifetime risk of 7% of depressive episode in men and about 20% in women. On an average, at least 10% of the

Table 21.1 Ocular adverse effects of drugs acting on autonomic nervous system

Drug/class	Therapeutic uses	Ocular adverse effects
Amphetamine, Hydroxy amphetamine	Appetite suppression	Pupillary-block glaucoma
Benzatropine	Muscular cramps Parkinson disease	Mydriasis, decreased vision, loss or paralysis of accommodation, diplopia, pupillary-block glaucoma, decreased tolerance to contact lenses, subconjunctival/retinal hemorrhages secondary to drug-induced anemia
Beta-blockers	Hypertension, angina, arrhythmia, myocardial infarction	Dry eye, diplopia, decreased intraocular pressure, visual hallucination, reduced perfusion of the optic nerve head resulting in glaucoma progression
Demecarium Echothiophate	Glaucoma	Anterior subcapsular granular cataract
Oxybutynin chloride	Urinary incontinence	Dry eye, blurred vision, increased risk of angle-closure glaucoma
Pralidoxime	Organophosphate poisoning	Iritis
Prazosin	Hypertension	Blurred vision, reddened sclera
Salbutamol	Asthma	Mydriasis, decreased vision, conjunctival hyperemia and chemosis due to blood vessel dilation, petechial conjunctival hemorrhages
Scopolamine	Motion sickness	Relative pupillary-block glaucoma
Solifenacin succinate	Urinary incontinence	Dry eye, blurred vision
Tamsulosin	Benign hypertrophy of prostate	Intraoperative floppy iris syndrome during cataract surgery
Tolterodine tartrate	Urinary incontinence	Blurred vision, xerophthalmia

affected population of depressed individuals is prescribed medications. Lithium is one of the principle drugs used as a mood stabilizer.[29] This drug is associated with keratin deposits in the cornea.[24,30] It affects sodium transport and causes eye irritation.[24] Some cases of exophthalmos and papilledema have also been reported.[25] Corneal deposits and keratitis has been observed with amantadine and amiodarone.[31] Diffuse and fine keratin deposits were observed in the central part of corneal endothelium. Monocyclic amines were shown to accumulate in the eyes of animals even after acute administration.[32] Tricyclic antidepressants (TCAs) may affect the uveal tract and in some cases transient mydriasis has been reported with the use of these drugs.[25] TCAs also interfere with accommodation and cause blurred vision in up to one-third of the patients. Patients with narrow irido-corneal angles may get an acute attack of glaucoma with TCA treatment.[26]

Epilepsy is another major class of disorder treated with centrally-acting medications. Drugs frequently prescribed under this category include phenytoin, vigabatrin and valproic acid. Diplopia, blurred vision, nystagmus, extraocular muscle palsies, disturbances in eye movement and color disturbances are frequently reported side-effects with antiepileptic drugs. Vigabatrin is a well-known drug extensively employed for the treatment of childhood epilepsy and partial seizures.[26] However, this drug is known to cause visual field defect in approximately one-third of the patients as a result of retinal toxicity. ERG changes with vigabatrin have been observed in humans reflecting bilateral concentric visual field loss, including contrast sensitivity and abnormal color perception.[33] Peripheral defects are more prominent than central.[3,26] Visual field defects have also been reported with other antiepileptic drugs such as phenytoin and carbamazepine.[1,27,28] Bilateral concentric visual field loss and color vision defects have also been reported with valproic acid.[34] Sodium valproate, phenytoin and carbamazepine possess the propensity to cause congenital ocular malformations in fetus and thus should be avoided during pregnancy.[1] Lorazepam, a classical benzodiazepine co-prescribed as an anti-anxiety treatment to epileptic patients, is also reported to influence visual perception. An analog molecule, alprazolam, may cause glaucoma. Benzodiazepines are also known to cause disturbance in eye movements.[24, 35,36]

Antipsychotics are known to produce several ocular adverse effects such as mydriasis, ocular dystonia, angle-closure glaucoma, uveal tract disorders, hypersensitivity of unknown origin, eye movement disorders and abnormality in color perception.[24] In this regards, particular mention needs to be given to a low-potency antipsychotic, topiramate. Topiramate originally used to treat epilepsy in children was later known to enhance GABAergic transmission and cure cases of bipolar disorder.[26] Though the exact mechanism of action of this drug remains unknown, psychiatrists and neurologists believe that the drug has additional mood stabilizing properties which precede its classical anticonvulsant action. This drug may have GABAergic effect on the visual field. Mydriasis induced angle-closure glaucoma is a serious dose-dependent adverse effect also noted with this drug. Unusually, glaucoma occurs due to an allergic-type of reaction wherein the structures of the lens and ciliary body are displaced. Additional adverse effects include ocular dystonia, uveal tract disorders, myopia, eye movement disorders, color abnormalities and reduced contrast discrimination.[1]

Angle-closure glaucoma and uveal tract disorders are one of the most frequent adverse effects seen with many typical anti-psychotics and selective serotonin reuptake inhibitors (SSRIs).[24] Almost all the drugs belonging to this class are known to cause transient mydriasis leading to glaucoma in predisposed patients. While low-potency antipsychotics could lead to problems with accommodation, ocular dystonias have been observed with high-potency drugs.

This reaffirms that these drugs have potential to cross the blood-ocular barrier and interfere with the physiological activities of the ocular tissue. Several of the adverse effects such as glaucoma are vision-threatening but often patients fail to recognize or describe the symptoms appropriately. Therefore, neurologists must make adequate observations while prescribing these drugs (Table 21.2).

Table 21.2 Ocular adverse effects of drugs acting on central nervous system

Drug/class	Therapeutic uses	Ocular adverse effects
Alprazolam, clonazepam, midazolam	Epilepsy, anxiety and panic	Blurred vision, diplopia, burning, tearing, allergic conjunctivitis, angle-closure glaucoma, decreased corneal reflex and accommodation
Amitriptyline	Depression	Cycloplegia, dry eye, diplopia, increased intraocular pressure, toxic amblyopia, pupillary-block glaucoma
Codeine	Cough	Miosis, decreased vision, myopia, lid dermatitis, iritis
Dexmethylphenidate	Attention deficit hyperactivity disorder	Blurred vision, visual changes

Count...

Count...

Diazepam	Anxiety	Allergic conjunctivitis, blurred vision, dry eye, diplopia, decreased accommodation, mydriasis, retinal hemorrhages, pupillary-block glaucoma
Ethanol	Methanol poisoning	Toxic neuropathy, diplopia
Ethosuximide	Epilepsy	Dyskinesia, photophobia, myopia
Felbamate	Epilepsy	Diplopia, nystagmus
Gabapentin, lamotrigine, topiramate	Epilepsy, migraine, bipolar affective disorder	Allergic conjunctivitis, mydriasis, visual disturbances, secondary angle-closure glaucoma, nystagmus, ocular hyperemia, macular edema, uveitis
Isocarboxazid	Depression	Photophobia
Levetiracetam	Epilepsy	Diplopia
Lithium	Acute mania	Contact lens intolerance, downbeat jerk nystagmus, diplopia, decreased accommodation, cycloplegia, blurred vision, papilledema
LSD, mescaline, marijuana, hashish, psilocybin	To alter mood and behavior (hallucinogen)	Diplopia, cycloplegia, miosis
Morphine, opium, heroin	Cancer pain	Miosis, iritis
Methadone	Cough	Decreased vision, pupillary changes, talc retinopathy
Methylphenidate	Concentration and attention deficits	Mydriasis, decreased accommodation, blurred vision, visual hallucination
Oxcarbazepine	Epilepsy	Diplopia, blurred vision
Phenobarbitone	Insomnia Anxiety	Ptosis, nystagmus, mydriasis, cycloplegia, disturbances of color vision, glare, extraocular palsies
Phenothiazines	Schizophrenia	Dry eye, blue conjunctiva, diplopia, endothelial pigmentation, mydriasis, cycloplegia, anterior subcapsular cataract, exacerbation of open-angle glaucoma, blurred vision, blue-yellow color vision
Phenytoin Carbamazepine	Epilepsy	Allergic conjunctivitis, cataract, color vision disturbances, blurred vision, secondary angle-closure glaucoma, downbeat nystagmus, ocular hyperemia, macular edema
Primidone	Epilepsy	Diplopia, nystagmus
Selective serotonin reuptake inhibitors (SSRIs)	Obsessive compulsive disorder, panic disorder, premenstrual syndrome	Keratitis sicca, conjunctivitis, diplopia, blurred vision, photophobia, angle-closure glaucoma, eyelid changes, increased extraocular movements during sleep
Tiagabine	Epilepsy	Abnormal color perception, blurred vision, nystagmus, diplopia
Topiramate	Epilepsy	Diplopia, acute myopia and angle-closure glaucoma
Valproic acid	Epilepsy	Oculomotor disturbances
Venlafaxine	Depression	Blurred vision
Vigabatrin	Epilepsy	Diplopia, nystagmus, peripheral visual field loss, color perception abnormalities, retinal abnormalities, optic nerve pallor, visual electrophysiological changes, reduced contrast sensitivity, reduced ocular blood flow

OCULAR ADVERSE EFFECTS OF DRUGS ACTING ON CARDIOVASCULAR SYSTEM

Cardiovascular diseases are considered world's largest killers. Over 80% of deaths related to these diseases are known to occur in the developing nations. According to disease estimate taken in year 2000, approximately 29 million people were suffering from CVS diseases in India.[37] Angiotensin Converting Enzyme (ACE) inhibitors, calcium channel blockers, diuretics, cardiotonics, nitrates and quinidine are the most frequently prescribed drugs for the treatment of hypertension, ischemic heart disease, arrhythmia and cardiac failure.

Of the various classes, ACE inhibitors are considered by far the safest category of drugs for the treatment of hypertension and maintain a high popularity among physicians. The only ACE inhibitor with reported ocular side effect is fosinopril. Hydrochlorothiazide, a diuretic also used in the treatment of hypertension, is associated with visual changes and yellowing of the eyes. However, it needs to be ascertained whether the side effect is due to the drug or its salt form.

Digitalis, a cardiotonic, used for the treatment for congestive heart failure is now the last resort for treatment. It has a tendency to cause photopsia and color vision abnormalities. Approximately, 11–25% of the patients treated with this drug have expressed ocular symptoms such as abnormal visual sensations or flickering vision in addition to abnormal color vision. High concentrations of the drug accumulate in the retina and choroid indicating its easy entry through the retinal transport processes. Digitalis also inhibits the sodium potassium (Na^+, K^+) transporter in the ciliary epithelium resulting in alteration in aqueous humor dynamics.[38]

Increase in intraocular pressure is also observed with the use of calcium channel blockers and most notably with ditliazem.[39] Topical instillation of verapamil, diltiazem and nifedipine has also been demonstrated to reduce the outflow facility in experimental rabbits.[39] Amlodipine is known to cause conjunctival chemosis while chronic use of nifedipine for the treatment of hypertension is associated with substantial reduction in visual function.[40,42] Both nifedipine and captopril are believed to cause ocular vasodilatation, which could lead to glaucoma although sufficient clinical reports are lacking.[43] Another category of drugs widely used in the treatment of hypertension are beta-blockers. They tend to reduce tear lysozyme levels along with total amount of tear secretion. Patients generally complain of ocular irritation and exhibit dry eye symptoms. Contact lens intolerance may also develop.

Amiodarone is one of the frequently prescribed drugs for the treatment of arrhythmia. Since the drug seems to have a dual action (beta-blocker and calcium channel blocker), it is generally the drug of choice when all other treatment modalities fail. However, this drug is known to be a photosensitizer. Keratopathy of the entire cornea, including the endothelium and lens, is observed in patients because of its tendency to increase lipid storage. Corneal deposits are seen in most of the patients who receive amiodarone treatment for more than 6 months. Some of the other abnormalities reported are maculopathy, optic neuropathy (high incidence of 1.3% to 1.8%), and optic neuritis. Optic neuropathy is, however, reversible with the discontinuation of drug.[31,44,45]

Diuretics are another drug class used for the treatment of hypertension as well as congestive heart failure. Most of the drugs are generally considered safe. However, few rare reports on the side-effects are noted. One of the rare reports is association of furosemide with blurred vision and xanthopsia.

Angle-closure glaucoma in predisposed patients generally develops upon treatment with nitrates due to their vasodilating action. Nitroglycerines are known to cause color vision disturbances, changes in intraocular pressure and eyelid dandruff. Some of the other adverse effects, which require mention are blurred vision, eyelid swelling, cataract with losartan; allergy of lids and conjunctiva, decreased vision, decreased IOP, subconjunctival/ retinal hemorrhages with methyldopa; optic neuritis, visual field loss, abnormal retinal pigmentation and vision disturbances with quinidine (Table 21.3).

OCULAR ADVERSE EFFECTS OF LIPID LOWERING AGENTS

HMG-CoA reductase inhibitors, also referred to as "statins", act by blocking the rate-limiting step in cholesterol biosynthesis and are, therefore,

Table 21.3 Ocular adverse effects of drugs acting on cardiovascular system

Drug/class	Therapeutic uses	Ocular adverse effects
ACE inhibitors	Hypertension, congestive heart failure, diabetic nephropathy	Conjunctivitis, photosensitivity, loss of vision, decrease in intraocular pressure, amblyopia, diplopia, myopia
Amiodarone	Arrhythmias	Anterior subcapsular cataract, yellow or brown deposits in conjunctiva, blurred vision, colored halos, dry eye, nystagmus, whorl-like corneal deposits, optic neuropathy, photophobia
Amlodipine	Hypertension	Abnormal vision, conjunctivitis
Diltiazem	Systemic hypertension, angina pectoris	Amblyopia, photosensitivity, hallucinations, irritation periorbital edema, lacrimation, subconjunctival and retinal hemorrhage
Digoxin	Congestive heart failure	Corneal edema, diplopia, mydriasis, decreased intraocular pressure, yellow vision, flickering vision
Diuretics	Congestive heart failure, hypertension	Dry eye, myopia, color vision disturbances, allergy of lids and conjunctiva, decreased intraocular pressure, subconjunctival or retinal hemorrhages
Doxazosin, Terazosin	Hypertension	Abnormal vision, photophobia, conjunctivitis
Hydralazine	Hypertension	Rarely cause appearance of inflammatory cells in the vitreous and macular edema
Nitrates Isosorbide	Angina pectoris	Transient blurred vision
Losartan	Hypertension	Blurred vision, eyelid swelling, cataract
Methyl dopa	Acute or severe hypertension	Allergy of lids and conjunctiva, decreased vision, decreased intraocular pressure, subconjunctival or retinal hemorrhages
Nifedipine, verapamil	Hypertension, angina, heart failure	Vision changes, ocular irritation, periorbital and angioneurotic edema, lacrimation, pain, lid edema, conjunctival chemosis, erythema, conjunctivitis, rotary nystagmus, photosensitivity
Nitroglycerine	Angina pectoris	Yellow/ blue halos, alteration of intraocular pressure, eyelid dandruff
Quinidine	Arrhythmias	Color vision distortions, scotoma, optic neuritis, visual field loss, abnormal retinal pigmentation

effective in lowering the plasma cholesterol levels.[46] The Physicians Desk Reference in the USA mentions ocular hemorrhages as a possible side effect for some of the statins.[47] Lovastatin, a cholesterol lowering agent isolated from a strain of *Aspergillus terreus,* is associated with a high rate of lens opacities.[48] Evidences suggest that statins reduce platelet aggregation and decrease thrombin formation and, therefore, could contribute to ocular hemorrhages.[49] Atorvastatin is found to be associated with several ocular adverse effects such as blurred vision, dry eye, increase in intraocular pressure and development of intraocular hemorrhage.[50] Studies have reported reversal of ptosis in patients upon discontinuation of drug. Incidences of diplopia, ptosis and ophthalmoplegia have also been reported with fluvastatin, rosuvastatin, pravastatin, and simvastatin.[51] Niacin is another antihyperlipidemic drug associated with ocular adversities such as dry eye and cystoid macular edema in addition to the symptoms of lid edema and blurred vision.[52]

OCULAR ADVERSE EFFECTS OF ANTI-HYPERGLYCEMIC AGENTS

Diabetic macular edema is associated with glitazones.[53] Insulin and sulfonylureas may give rise to crystalline lens changes and refractive error shifts in the absence of blood glucose variation. Other adverse effects may include diplopia, optic neuritis, decreased vision, toxic amblyopia, photophobia, extraocular muscle paresis and myopia.[54, 55]

OCULAR ADVERSE EFFECTS OF THERAPEUTIC HORMONES

Bisphosphonates are mainly used in treatment of osteoporosis and inhibition of bone resorption in postmenopausal woman as well as management of hypocalcaemia of malignancy. Alendronate was shown to cause inferonasal nodular scleritis after five weeks of treatment.[56] After intravenous administration of pamidronate disodium, cases of unilateral and bilateral scleritis have been reported. Repeated drug exposure may lead to blurred vision, non-specific conjunctivitis, ocular pain, episcleritis and bilateral anterior uveitis.[57,58] Combination of esterified estrogen and methyl testosterone produces significant increase in intraocular pressure in postmenopausal women.[59] Tamoxifen treatment is reported to lead to perifoveal white refractile deposits associated with pigmentary changes, cystoid macular edema and changes in cornea. Patients receiving high dose of tamoxifen develop extensive retinal lesions and macular edema with visual impairment whereas low doses of drug for prolonged periods may lead to extensive retinal changes. Authors have observed isolated retinal crystals in patients treated with this drug. (Table 21.4)[60,62]

Table 21.4 Ocular adverse effects of therapeutic hormones

Drug/class	Therapeutic uses	Ocular adverse effects
Alendronate	Osteoporosis, metastatic bone pain	Anterior uveitis, retinitis, vision changes, lacrimation, photophobia, episcleritis, scleritis, non-specific conjunctivitis
Dextrothyroxine Levothyroxine	Hypothyroidism	Conjunctival hyperemia, pseudotumor cerebri, visual hallucination
Estradiol	Estrogen replacement	Contact lens intolerance
Estrogen, progestogens, medroxyprogesterone	Premenstrual tension, postmenopausal hormone replacement	Dry eye, loss of vision, retinal vascular disorders, pseudotumor cerebri, decreased tolerance to contact lenses, papilledema
Levonorgestrel Ethinyl estradiol	Conception (Oral contraceptive)	Diplopia, dry eye, mydriasis, macular edema, vascular occlusion, pseudotumor cerebri, papilledema, myopia
Tamoxifen	Breast cancer	Posterior subcapsular cataract, deposits in cornea, crystalline dot like yellowish deposits in surrounding area of macula

OCULAR ADVERSE EFFECTS OF ANALGESIC AND ANTI-INFLAMMATORY AGENTS

Ocular toxicity is associated with widely used non-steroidal anti-inflammatory drugs (NSAIDs). Aspirin therapy is known to cause dry eye, blurred vision and subconjunctival hemorrhages. Aspirin, in combination with warfarin therapy may lead to hyphema and retinal detachment.[63] Ibuprofen, another routine over the counter medicine, is known to cause centrocecal field defects, reduced visual acuity, and in some cases optic neuritis with defects in visual field.[64,65] COX-2 inhibitors such as celecoxib and rofecoxib may lead to temporary blindness, visual field defects, scotoma, teichopsia, blurred vision, decreased vision and abnormal vision.[66] Allopurinol, an anti-hyperuricemic drug used in treatment of gouty arthritis, is associated with cataract.[67] Gold administered for the treatment of rheumatoid arthritis causes ocular and corneal chrysiasis (deposition of gold particles in ocular tissue).[68,69]

Indomethacin prescribed for rheumatoid arthritis is also found to cause severe ocular toxicity leading to decreased vision, diplopia, blue-yellow color vision, lid or conjunctival erythema, toxic amblyopia, corneal toxicity and optic neuritis.[70] Dexamethasone used for rheumatoid arthritis, may cause blue conjunctivitis, diplopia, stromal opacities, mydriasis, posterior subcapsular cataract, increased intraocular pressure, myopia, retinopathy, impaired colour vision, reduced visual acuity, visual field loss and blurred vision.[71] Beclomethasone, hydrocortisone, methylprednisolone and prednisone are widely used glucocorticoids, which cause mydriasis, posterior subcapsular cataract, increased intraocular pressure, delayed corneal wound healing, central serous chorioretinopathy and ocular hypertension.[72-74] Along with these optic nerve related disorders, retrobulbar neuritis or papilledema secondary to pseudotumor cerebri are found to be associated with different NSAIDs such as ibuprofen, indomethacin, diflunisal (Table 21.5).[75]

Table 21.5 Ocular adverse effects of analgesic and anti-inflammatory agents

Drug/class	Therapeutic uses	Ocular adverse effects
Allopurinol	Gout	Cataracts, macular changes
Aspirin	Post-myocardial infarction, rheumatoid arthritis	Dry eye, transient blurred vision, subconjunctival hemorrhages, post-surgical retinal bleeds
Beclomethasone, hydrocortisone, methyl predinosolone, prednisone	Inflammation allergic disorders	Mydriasis, posterior subcapsular cataract, increased intraocular pressure, delayed corneal wound healing, papilledema secondary to pseudotumor cerebri
Dexamethasone	Rheumatoid arthritis	Blue conjunctivitis, diplopia, stromal opacities, mydriasis, posterior subcapsular cataract, increase in intraocular pressure (secondary open-angle glaucoma), myopia, retinopathy, impaired color vision, pseudotumor cerebri, visual acuity/ visual field loss, blurred vision
Gold	Rheumatoid arthritis	Ocular chrysiasis, nystagmus, gold deposits in conjunctiva, anterior subcapsular cataract, retinal hemolysis, blurred vision
Ibuprofen	Rheumatoid arthritis, osteoarthritis	Decreased vision, scotomata, lid or conjunctival erythema, photophobia
Indomethacin	Rheumatoid arthritis	Decreased vision, diplopia, blue-yellow color vision, lid or conjunctival erythema, toxic amblyopia, corneal toxicity, optic neuritis
Mometasone	Bronchial asthma	Increased intraocular pressure, progressing glaucoma, tearing
Valdecoxib, Rofecoxib	Arthritis	Vision changes, conjunctivitis, yellowish eyes, temporary blindness

OCULAR ADVERSE EFFECTS OF ANTIHISTAMINES

Systemic loratidine and cetrizine have been associated with ocular dryness, decreased tear film breakup time and conjunctival staining.[76] Dry eye, decreased accommodation, increase in intraocular pressure and even the pupillary-block glaucoma have been reported with diphenhydramine and chlorpheniramine (Table 21.6).[77]

OCULAR ADVERSE EFFECT OF ANTIULCER DRUGS

Omeprazole, a proton pump inhibitor, is a commonly used drug for the treatment of peptic ulcer. Intravenous use of omeprazole can cause loss of vision.[78] Pirenzepine is an anticholinergic agent with selective M_1 receptor antagonist action. The clinically effective doses of this drug can cause dry mouth and blurred vision.[79] Ranitidine may cause impaired color vision, angioneurotic edema, hyperemia and urticaria of lids and conjunctivitis.

OCULAR ADVERSE EFFECTS OF ANTIMICROBIAL AGENTS

Aminoglycosides, especially gentamicin, has been associated with cases of retinal toxicity and initial loss of function.[80] There are reported cases of diplopia with fluoroquinolone therapy.[81] Phototoxicity and neurotoxicity have been reported with the use of ciprofloxacin, ofloxacin, trovafloxacin, moxifloxacin and pefloxacin.[82]

Cephaloridine therapy has been associated with unilateral retinal pigmentosa leading to extinction of ERG and total irreversible blindness after subconjunctival and intracameral injection in few cases.[83] Intravitreal injection of cefotetan resulted in mild degeneration of photoreceptor outer segments and sporadically in cataract formation.[84] There are some evidences of retrobulbar neuritis with chloramphenicol therapy.[85] In experimental models, antifungal agent amphotericin-B causes inflammatory changes in the anterior chamber and corneal epithelial defects when given intravitreally or topically.[86] Oral voriconazole, an antifungal agent, leads to photopsia and color changes in some patients.[87] Quinine is known to produce acute visual loss.[88] Antimalarial drugs like systemic hydroxychloroquine and chloroquine related retinal toxicity is well documented. Hydroxychloroquine causes irreversible retinopathy.[89-92] Optic neuropathy has been reported with isoniazid and ethambutol.[93] Ethambutol may produce optic neuropathy if the daily dosage exceeds 15 mg/kg.[94] Rifampin is associated with blepharoconjunctivitis and optic neuritis.[95] Cystoid macular edema is seen in HIV patients who are receiving highly active antiretroviral therapy (HAART). Intravenous cidofovir precipitates anterior uveitis (Table 21.7).[96,97]

OCULAR ADVERSE EFFECTS OF ANTICANCER AGENTS

Treatment with anticancer drugs is also associated with several ocular adverse effects. Methotrexate causes ocular irritation and cataracts.[98] Tamoxifen and interferons cause

Table 21.6 Ocular adverse effects of antihistaminics

Drug/class	Therapeutic uses	Ocular adverse effects
Diphenhydramine Chlorpheniramine	Seasonal allergies	Dry eye, anisocoria, decreased accommodation, increased intraocular pressure, pupillary-block glaucoma, retinal hemorrhages, blurred vision, mydriasis, diplopia
Orphenadrine	Parkinsonism	Decreased vision, diplopia, decreased accommodation, mydriasis, subconjunctival/retinal hemorrhages secondary to drug-induced anemia

Table 21.7 Ocular adverse effects of antimicrobial agents

Drug/class	Therapeutic uses	Ocular adverse effects
Acyclovir	Genital herpes simplex, chicken pox	Visual hallucinations, periocular edema
Amphotericin-B	Oral and cutaneous candidiasis	Greenish discoloration of cornea, retinal necrosis
Ampicillin	UTI, gonorrhea, meningitis	Eyelid erythema multiforme, conjunctivitis
Cephalosporins	Respiratory, urinary and soft tissue infection	Nystagmus, decreased vision, allergy of lids and conjunctivitis
Chloramphenicol	Typhoid fever, influenza	Toxic amblyopia, retrobulbar neuritis
Chloroquine, hydroxy chloroquine	Malaria, rheumatoid arthritis	Bull's eye maculopathy, blue-yellow color vision, optic atrophy, ptosis, nystagmus, whorl-like epithelial deposits in cornea, cycloplegia, whitening of lashes
Didanosine	HIV	Retinal changes, night blindness, optic neuritis
Enfuvirtide	HIV	Conjunctivitis
Erythromycin	Respiratory infection	Colour vision, allergy of lids and conjunctivitis
Ethambutol	Tuberculosis	Retrobulbar optic neuritis, green-red color vision, diplopia, mydriasis
Fluoroquinolones	Urinary tract infections (UTI), gonorrhea, typhoid, respiratory infections, soft tissue and bone infections	Photosensitivity
Gentamicin	UTI, pneumonia	Intraretinal hemorrhage, cotton wool spots, opaque retina, superficially edematous retina
Isoniazid	Tuberculosis	Optic neuritis, green-red color vision, accommodation impairment
Linezolid	Hospital acquired pneumonia, Febrile neutropenia	Dyschromatopsia, ecocentral scotomas, decreased visual acuity
Quinine	Malaria, Nocturnal leg cramps	Decreased vision, optic nerve damage, venous congestion, retinal changes and arteriolar constriction
Rifampin	Tuberculosis	Blepharoconjunctivitis, optic neuritis
Sulfonamides	Bacterial infection	Eye lid edema, conjunctivitis, myopia, retinal hemorrhages, optic neuritis
Tetracyclines	Venereal disease, plague	Retinal hemorrhages, pseudotumor cerebri, dark deposits, paresis, diplopia
Zidovudine, lamivudin, abacavir	HIV	Colour vision, diplopia, nystagmus, cystoid macular edema, hypertrichosis, urticaria, eyelid rashes, eyelid and conjunctival hyperpigmentation

considerable ocular morbidity, visual losses even in therapeutic doses.[99] Taxanes cause capillary leak syndrome and hydroxyurea causes ulceration and pseudodermatomyositis.[100] High doses of systemic chemotherapy such as carmustine and mitomycin can cause qualitative changes in the tear film indicating damage to the corneal and conjunctival epithelium (Table 21.8).[101]

OCULAR ADVERSE EFFECTS OF DRUGS USED IN DERMATOLOGICAL DISORDERS

Acitretin is an active metabolite of etretinate used for systemic treatment of psoriasis. It has largely replaced etretinate because of its acceptable pharmacokinetics. However, it causes blepharoconjunctivitis with lymphocyte infiltration and involves keratinized epithelial cells.[102] Isotretinoin is an isomer of tretinoin (all Trans vitamin-A acid). Several ocular adverse effects have been reported with the use of isotretinoin and include abnormal meibomian gland secretion, blepharoconjunctivitis, corneal opacities, decreased dark adaptation, keratitis, increased tear osmolarity, photophobia and teratogenic ocular abnormalities. Decreased color vision is a reversible adverse effect. Few cases of persistent dry eye syndrome have also reported (Table 21.9).[103,104]

OCULAR ADVERSE EFFECTS OF ANTICOAGULANTS

Warfarin is the most commonly used oral anticoagulant. Its ocular side effects include ocular bleeding like hyphema, hemorrhagic tears, subconjunctival, vitreal, retinal or choroidal hemorrhages.[105,106] Angle closure glaucoma has also been reported as a complication of warfarin treatment.[107] Spontaneous anterior chamber hyphema can occur in any patient on anticoagulant treatment. Cases have been reported for nontraumatic retrobulbar hematoma due to warfarin toxicity.[108]

OCULAR ADVERSE EFFECTS OF VITAMINS

Isotretinoin (13-cis-retinoic acid) is associated with ocular complications like dryness of eye, blepharitis, conjunctivitis, decreased tear break-up time (BUT) and alterations in lid margins. Increased *Staphylococcus aureus* in conjunctival flora has also been reported.[109,110] Ocular adverse effects associated with other vitamins are presented in Table 21.10.

Table 21.8 Ocular adverse effects of anticancer drugs

Drug/class	Therapeutic uses	Ocular adverse effects
Busulphan	Chronic myeloid leukemia	Anterior subcapsular cataract
Docetaxel, paclitaxel	Breast cancer	Open-angle glaucoma
Methotrexate	Psoriasis, rheumatoid arthritis	Conjunctival hyperemia, photophobia, blepharitis, periorbital edema, ocular irritation

Table 21.9 Ocular adverse effects of drugs used in dermatological disorders

Drug/class	Therapeutic uses	Ocular adverse effects
Etretinate	Cystic acne, severe refractive psoriasis	Blepharoconjunctivitis
Isotretinoin	Acne, psoriasis	Cataract, night blindness, retinal toxicity, optic neuritis, dry eye, blepharoconjunctivitis, keratitis, corneal neovascularization, myopia

Table 21.10 Ocular adverse effects of vitamins

Drug/class	Therapeutic uses	Ocular adverse effects
Vitamin A	Acne, psoriasis	Loss of brows and lashes, ocular palsies, nystagmus, exophthalmos, papilledema, retinal hemorrhage
Retinoic acid	Xerophthalmia, acne, psoriasis	Dry eye, corneal infection
Vitamin D	Rickets, osteomalacia	Band shaped corneal degeneration
Paricalcitol	Secondary hyperparathyroidism associated chronic renal failure	Redness or discharge, increased light sensitivity

OCULAR ADVERSE EFFECTS OF OTHER MEDICATIONS

Dexmethylphenidate, a drug for attention deficit hyperactivity disorder, has been reported to cause blurred vision and visual changes.[111] FDA released an alert stating that a small number of men had unilateral complete vision loss following a course of sildenafil, tadalafil or vardenafil. Blue haze, change in color perception and blurred vision are associated with sildenafil citrate.[112,113] Budesonide used for bronchial asthma, can cause ocular side-effects such as increased risk of ocular hypertension, subcapsular cataract and elevated intraocular pressure. Drugs like cyclosporine, diphenoxylate, dornase alfa, iopamidol, leuprolide acetate, talc can also cause ocular side-effects such as severe ocular pain, optic disc edema, eyelid irritation, hyperemia, reversible cortical blindness, eyelash proliferation, pupillary-block glaucoma, conjunctivitis, unilateral and bilateral loss of vision, blurred vision, pseudotumor cerebri, refractive bodies and changes in posterior pole.[114]

Other adverse effects to remember with some of the infrequently prescribed medications are *in-utero* retinal hemorrhagic lesions due to cocaine, decrease in vision due to desferoxamine, ocular allergy to bovine-derived collagen, uveitis due to rifabutin, transient refractive error changes and dry eye due to acetazolamide.[115,116]

REFERENCES

1. Hadjikoutis S, Morgan JE, Wild JM, Smith PE. Ocular complications of neurological therapy. Eur J Neurol. 2005;12(7):499-507.
2. Hermans G. Harmful effects of common drugs on the visual apparatus. Psychotropic drugs. Bull Soc Belge Ophthalmol. 1972;160(1):15-85.
3. Hosking SL, Hilton EJ. Neurotoxic effects of GABA-transaminase inhibitors in the treatment of epilepsy: ocular perfusion and visual performance. Ophthalmic Physiol Opt. 2002;22(5):440-7.
4. Fechtner RD, KA, Figueroa E, Ramirez M, Federico M, Dewey SL, Brodie JD. Short-term treatment of cocaine and/or methamphetamine abuse with vigabatrin: ocular safety pilot results. Arch Ophthalmol. 2006;124(9):1257-62.
5. Tahiroglu AY. Polypharmacy and EPS in a child; a case report. Psychopharmacol Bull. 2007;40(2):129-33.
6. Thaler J. Effects of benztropine mesylate (Cogentin) on accommodation in normal volunteers. Am J Optom Physiol Opt. 1982;59(11):918-9.
7. Arthurs B, FM, Codère F, Gauthier S, Dresner S, Stone L. Treatment of blepharospasm with medication, surgery and type A botulinum toxin. Can J Ophthalmol. 1987;22(1):24-8.
8. Sakai H, Shinjyo S, Nakamura Y, Nakamura Y, Ishikawa S, Sawaguchi S. Comparison of latanoprost monotherapy and combined therapy of 0.5% timolol and 1% dorzolamide in chronic primary angle-closure glaucoma (CACG) in Japanese patients. J Ocul Pharmacol Ther. 2005;21(6):483-9.

9. Razeghinejad MR, Myers JS, Katz LJ. Iatrogenic glaucoma secondary to medications. Am J Med. 2011;124(1):20-5.

10. Watson WT, Shuckett EP, Becker AB, Simons FE. Effect of nebulized ipratropium bromide on intraocular pressures in children. Chest. 1994;105(5):1439-41.

11. Yoshida A, Fujino T, Maruyama S, Ito Y, Taki Y, Yamada S. The forefront for novel therapeutic agents based on the pathophysiology of lower urinary tract dysfunction: bladder selectivity based on in vivo drug-receptor binding characteristics of antimuscarinic agents for treatment of overactive bladder. J Pharmacol Sci. 2010;112(2):142-50.

12. MacDiarmid SA. Maximizing anticholinergic therapy for overactive bladder: has the ceiling been reached? BJU Int. 2007;99 Suppl 3:8-12.

13. Wong EY, Harding A, Kowal L. Oxybutynin-associated esotropia. J AAPOS. 2007;11(6):624-25.

14. Sung VC, Corridan PG. Acute-angle closure glaucoma as a side-effect of oxybutynin. Br J Urol. 1998;81(4):634-5.

15. Diefenbach K, Arold G, Wollny A, Schwantes U, Haselmann J, Roots I. Effects on sleep of anticholinergics used for overactive bladder treatment in healthy volunteers aged > or = 50 years. BJU Int. 2005;95(3):346-9.

16. Leung DY, Kwong YY, Lam DS. Ocular side-effects of tolterodine and oxybutynin, a single-blind prospective randomized trial. Br J Clin Pharmacol. 2005;60(6):668.

17. Altan-Yaycioglu R, Yaycioglu O, Aydin Akova Y, Guvel S, Ozkardes H. Ocular side-effects of tolterodine and oxybutynin, a single-blind prospective randomized trial. Br J Clin Pharmacol. 2005;59(5):588-92.

18. Kerrebroeck PV. Clinical study results of tolterodine in patients with overactive bladder. Expert Rev Neurother. 2003;3(2):155-63.

19. Choppin A, Eglen RM, Hegde SS. Pharmacological characterization of muscarinic receptors in rabbit isolated iris sphincter muscle and urinary bladder smooth muscle. Br J Pharmacol. 1998;124(5):883-8.

20. Pietzko A, Dimpfel W, Schwantes U, Topfmeier P. Influences of trospium chloride and oxybutynin on quantitative EEG in healthy volunteers. Eur J Clin Pharmacol. 1994;47(4):337-43.

21. Jonville AP, Dutertre JP, Autret E, Barbellion M. Adverse effects of oxybutynin chloride (Ditropan). Evaluation of the official survey of Regional Pharmacovigilance Centers. Therapie. 1992;47(5):389-92.

22. Vardy MD, Mitcheson HD, Samuels TA, Wegenke JD, Forero-Schwanhaeuser S, Marshall TS, He W. Effects of solifenacin on overactive bladder symptoms, symptom bother and other patient-reported outcomes: results from VIBRANT - a double-blind, placebo-controlled trial. Int J Clin Pract. 2009;63(12):1702-14.

23. Garely AD, Kaufman JM, Sand PK, Smith N, Andoh M. Symptom bother and health-related quality of life outcomes following solifenacin treatment for overactive bladder: the VESIcare Open-Label Trial. VOLT). Clin Ther. 2006;28(11):1935-46.

24. Richa S, Yazbek JC. Ocular adverse effects of common psychotropic agents: a review. CNS Drugs. 2010;24(6):501-26.

25. Oshika T. Ocular adverse effects of neuropsychiatric agents. Incidence and management. Drug Saf. 1995;12(4):256-63.

26. Hilton EJ, Hosking SL, Betts T. The effect of antiepileptic drugs on visual performance. Seizure. 2004;13(2):113-28.

27. López L, Thomson A, Rabinowicz AL. Assessment of colour vision in epileptic patients exposed to single-drug therapy Eur Neurol. 1999;41(4):201-5.

28. Arndt CF, Salle M, Derambure PH, Defoort-Dhellemmes S, Hache JC. The effect on vision of associated treatments in patients taking vigabatrin: carbamazepine versus valproate. Epilepsia. 2002;43(8):812-7.

29. Bourgeois JA. Ocular side effects of lithium--a review. J Am Optom Assoc. 1991;62(7):548-51.

30. Hiroz CA., Assimacopoulos T, Cuendet JF, Calanca A, Carron R. Ophthalmological side effects of lithium. Encephale. 1981;7(2):23-8.

31. Erdurmus M, Selcoki Y, Yagci R, Hepsen IF. Amiodarone-induced keratopathy: full-thickness corneal involvement. Eye Contact Lens. 2008;34(2):131-2.

32. Mason CG. Ocular accumulation and toxicity of certain systemically administered drugs. J Toxicol Environ Health. 1977;2:977-95.

33. Harding GF, Robertson K, Spencer EL, Holliday I. Vigabatrin; its effect on the electrophysiology of vision. Doc Ophthalmol. 2002;104(2):213-29.

34. Jung P, Doussard-Lefaucheux S. Visual field defect in a patient given sodium valporate then carbamazepine: possible effect of aminotransferase inhibition. Rev Neurol (Paris). 2002;158(4): 477-79.

35. Speeg-Schatz C, Giersch A, Boucart M, Gottenkiene S, Tondre M, Kauffmann-Muller F, et al. Effects of lorazepam on vision and oculomotor balance. Binocul Vis Strabismus Q. 2001;16(2):99-104.

36. Giersch A, Boucart M, Speeg-Schatz C, Muller-Kauffmann F, Danion JM. Lorazepam impairs perceptual integration of visual forms: a central effect. Psychopharmacology (Berl). 1996;126(3):260-70.

37. Melena J, Zalduegui A, Arcocha P, Santafé J, Segarra J. Topical verapamil lowers outflow facility in the rabbit eye. J Ocul Pharmacol Ther. 1999;15:199-205.

38. Honrubia A, Andrés JM, Alcaine F, Bonasa E, Fernández J, Luján B. Visual disorders induced by therapeutic levels of digoxin. Arch Soc Esp Oftalmol. 2000;75(1):55-6.

39. Beatty JF, Krupin T, Nichols PF, Becker B. Elevation of intraocular pressure by calcium channel blockers. Arch Ophthalmol. 1984;102(7):1072-6.

40. Say EA, Shields CL, Bianciotto C, Shields JA. Chronic Conjunctival Chemosis from Amlodipine Besylate (Norvasc). Cornea. 2011; 30(5):604-7.

41. Gasser P, Flammer J. Short- and long-term effect of nifedipine on the visual field in patients with presumed vasospasm. J Int Med Res. 1990;18(4):334-9.

42. Harris A, Evans DW, Cantor LB, Martin B. Hemodynamic and visual function effects of oral nifedipine in patients with normal-tension glaucoma. Am J Ophthalmol. 1997;124(3):296-302.

43. Coulter DM. Eye Pain with Nifedipine and Disturbance of Taste with Captopril: A Mutually Controlled Study Showing a Method of Postmarketing Surveillance. Br Med J. 1988;296(6629):1086-8.

44. Lloyd MJ, Fraunfelder FW. Drug-induced optic neuropathies. Drugs Today (Barc). 2007;43(11):827-36.

45. Bratulescu M, Zemba M, Gheorghieva V, Andrei S, Cucu,B, Dobrescu N. Ocular manifestation in amiodarone toxicity--case report. Oftalmologia. 2005;49(4):18-23.

46. Hardman JG, Limbird L, Gilman AG. The Pharmacological Basis of Therapeutics, 10th edn. New York: McGraw-Hill; 2001.

47. Montvale NJ. Physicians' Desk Reference. 2002; Vol.56; Thomson Medical Economics; pp. 2642.

48. Moorthy RS, Valluri S. Ocular toxicity associated with systemic drug therapy. Curr Opin Ophthalmol. 1999;10(6):438-6.

49. Hussein O, et al. Reduced platelet aggregation after fluvastatin therapy is associated with altered platelet lipid composition and drug binding to the platelets. Br J Clin Pharmacol. 1997;44(1):77-84.

50. Fraunfelder FW. Ocular hemorrhage possibly the result of HMG-CoA reductase inhibitors. J Ocul Pharmacol Ther. 2004;20(2):179-82.

51. Fraunfelder FW, Richards AB. Diplopia, blepharoptosis, and ophthalmoplegia and 3-hydroxy-3-methyl-glutaryl-CoA reductase inhibitor use. Ophthalmology. 2008;115(12): 2282-5.

52. Fraunfelder FW, Fraunfelder FT, Illingworth DR. Adverse ocular effects associated with niacin therapy. Br J Ophthalmol. 1995;79(1):54-6.

53. Fong DS, Contreras R. Glitazone use is associated with diabetic macular edema. Am J Ophthalmol. 2009;147(4):583-6.

54. Lightman JM, Townsend JC, Selvin GJ. Ocular effects of second generation oral hypoglycemic agents. J Am Optom Assoc. 1989;60(11):849-53.

55. Hampson JP, Harvey JN. A systematic review of drug induced ocular reactions in diabetes. Br J Opthalmol. 2000;84(2):144-9.

56. Tabbara KF. Nodular scleritis following alendronate therapy. Ocul Immunol Inflamm. 2008;16(3):99-101.

57. Fraunfelder FW, Fraunfelder FT, Jensvold B. Scleritis and other ocular side effects associated with pamidronate disodium. Am J Ophthalmol. 2003;135(2):219-22.

58. Fraunfelder FW. Ocular side effects associated with bisphosphonates. Drugs Today (Barc). 2003;39(11):829-35.

59. Khurana RN, LaBree LD, Scott G, Smith RE, Yiu SC. Esterified estrogens combined with methyltestosterone raise intraocular pressure in postmenopausal women. Am J Ophthalmol. 2006;142(3):494-5.

60. Hui-Bon-Hoa AA, Defoort-Dhellemmes S, Tran TH. Atrophic tamoxifen maculopathy. J Fr Ophtalmol. 2011;34:35.e1 e5.

61. Hager T, Hoffmann S, Seitz B. Unusual symptoms for tamoxifen-associated maculopathy. Ophthalmologie. 2010;107(8):750-2.

62. Nayfield SG, Gorin MB. Tamoxifen-associated eye disease. J Clin Oncol. 1996;14(3):1018-26.

63. Trivedi D, Newton JD, Mitra A, Puri P. A serious drug interaction leading to spontaneous total hyphema. J Postgrad Med. 2010;56(1):46-7.

64. Collum L, Bowen D. Ocular side effects of Ibuprofen. Br J Ophthalmol. 1971;55:472.

65. Gamulescu M, Schalke B. Optic neuritis with visual field defect-possible Ibuprofen-related toxicity. Ann Pharmacother. 2006;40(3):571-3.

66. Coulter DM, Clark DW. Disturbance of vision by COX-2 inhibitors. Expert Opin Drug Saf. 2004;3(6):607-14.

67. Fraunfelder FT, Hanna C, Dreis MW, Cosgrove KW Jr. Cataracts associated with allopurinol therapy. Am J Ophthalmol. 1982;94(2):137-40.

68. Singh AD, Puri P, Amos RS. Deposition of gold in ocular structures, although known, is rare. A case of ocular chrysiasis in a patient of rheumatoid arthritis on gold treatment is presented. Eye. 2004;18(4):443-4.

69. Prouse PJ, Kanski JJ, Gumpel JM. Corneal chrysiasis and clinical improvement with chryso-therapy in rheumatoid arthritis. Ann Rheum Dis. 1981;40(6):564-6.

70. Burns CA. Indomethacin induced ocular toxicity. Am J Oph. 1973;76(2).312-3.

71. Whitlock NA, McKnight B, Corcoran KN, Rodriguez LA, Rice DS. Increased intraocular pressure in mice treated with dexamethasone. IOVS. 2010;51(12):6496-503.

72. Opatowsky I, Feldman RM, Gross R, Feldman ST. Intraocular pressure elevation associated with inhalation and nasal corticosteroids. Ophthalmology. 1995;102(2):177-9.

73. Haimovici R, Gragoudas ES, Duker JS, Sjaarda RN, Eliott D. Central serous chorioretinopathy associated with inhaled or intranasal corticoster-oids. Ophthalmology. 1997;104(10):1653-60.

74. Behbehani AH, Owayed AF, Hijazi ZM, Eslah EA, Al-Jazzaf AM. Cataract and ocular hyper-tension in children on inhaled corticosteroid therapy. J Pediatr Ophthalmol Strabismus. 2005; 42(1):23-7.

75 Fraunfelder F, Samples J. Possible Optic nerve side effects associated with Nonsteroidal anti inflammatory drugs. J Toxicol. 1994;13:311-6.

76. Ousler GW, Wilcox KA, Gupta G, Abelson MB. An evaluation of the ocular drying effects of 2 systemic antihistamines: loratadine and cetirizine hydrochloride. Ann Allergy Asthma Immunol. 2004;93(5):460-4.

77. Farber AS. Ocular side effects of antihistamine-decongestant combinations. Am J Ophthalmol. 1982;94(4):565.

78. Lessell S. Omeprazole (correction of omepraxole) and ocular damage. Concerns on safety of drug are unwarranted. BMJ.1997;316(7124):67.

79. García Rodríguez LA, Mannino S, Wallander MA, Lindblom B. A cohort study of the ocular safety of anti-ulcer drugs. Br J Clin Pharmacol. 1996; 42(2):213-6.

80. Hancock HA, Guidry C, Read RW, Ready EL, Kraft TW. Acute aminoglycoside retinal toxicity in vivo and in vitro. Invest Ophthalmol Vis Sci. 2005;46(12):4804-8.

81. Fraunfelder FW, Fraunfelder FT. Diplopia and fluoroquinolones. Ophthalmology. 2009; 116(9):1814-7.

82. Thompson AM. Ocular toxicity of fluoro-quinolones. Clin Experiment Ophthalmol. 2007;35(6):566-77.

83. Turut P, Malthieu D. The ocular toxicity of cephaloridine-A clinical and experimental study. J Fr Ophtalmol. 1980;3(6-7):401-8.

84. Philipp W, Schmid K, Steiner HJ, Pümpel B, Allerberger F, Aichberger HP, et al. Toxicity and clearance of intravitreal cefotetan. Graefes Arch Clin Exp Ophthalmol. 1990;228(5):475-80.

85. Kairys D, Smith MB. Topical ocular chloramphenicol: Clinical pharmacology and toxicity in optometric practice. J Am Optom Assoc. 1990;61(1):14-7.

86. Barza M, Baum J, Tremblay C, Szoka F, D'Amico DJ. Ocular toxicity of intravitreally injected liposomal Amphotericin-B in rhesus monkeys. Am Ophthalmol. 1985;100(2):259-63.

87. Kadikoy H, Barkmeier A, Peck B, Carvounis PE. Persistent photopsia following course of oral voriconazole. J Ocul Pharmacol Ther. 2010;26(4):387-8.

88. Brinton GS, Norton EW, Zahn JR, Knighton RW. Ocular quinine toxicity. Am J Ophthalmol. 1980;90(3):403-10.

89. Pluta JP, Rüther K. Retinal damage by (hydroxy) chloroquine intake: published evidence for an

efficient ophthalmological follow-up. Klin Monbl Augenheilkd. 2009;226(11):891-6.

90. Gouveia EB, Morales MS, Gouveia GB, Lourenzi VP. Ocular toxicity due to 4-aminoquinoline derivatives. Arq Bras Oftalmol. 2007;70(6):1046-51.

91. Yam JC, Kwok AK. Ocular toxicity of hydroxychloroquine. Hong Kong Med J. 2006;12(9):294-304.

92. Weiner A, Sandberg MA, Gaudio AR, Kini MM, Berson EL. Hydroxychloroquine retinopathy. Am J Ophthalmol. 1991;112(5):528-34.

93. Jimenez-Lucho VE, del Busto R, Odel J. Isoniazid and ethambutol as a cause of optic neuropathy. Eur J Respir Dis. 1987;71(1):42-5.

94. Rennie IG. Clinically important ocular reactions to systemic drug therapy. Drug Saf. 1993;9(3):196-211.

95. Cayley FE, Majumdar SK. Ocular toxicity due to rifampicin. Br Med J. 1976; 24supp.1 (6003):199-200.

96. Ambati J, Wynne KB, Angerame MC, Robinson MR. Anterior uveitis associated with intravenous cidofovir use in patients with cytomegalovirus retinitis. Br J Ophthalmol. 1999;83(10):1153-8.

97. Cassoux N, Lumbroso L, Bodaghi B, Zazoun L, Katlama C, LeHoang P. Cystoid macular oedema and cytomegalovirus retinitis in patients with HIV disease treated with highly active antiretroviral therapy. Br J Ophthalmol. 1999;83(1):47-9.

98. Guillot B, Bessis D, Dereure O. Mucocutaneous side effects of antineoplastic chemotherapy. Expert Opin Drug Saf. 2004;3(6):579-87.

99. Noureddin BN, Seoud M, Bashshur Z, Salem Z, Shamseddin A, Khalil A. Ocular toxicity in low-dose tamoxifen: a prospective study. Eye. 1999;13(6):729-33.

100. Fraunfelder FT, Meyer SM. Ocular toxicity of antineoplastic agents. Ophthalmol. 1983;90(1):1-3.

101. Schmid KE, Kornek GV, Scheithauer W, Binder S. Update on ocular complications of systemic cancer chemotherapy. Surv Ophthalmol. 2006;51(1):19-40.

102. Denis P, Nordmann JP, Saiag P, Liotet S, Laroche L, Saraux H. Chronic blepharoconjunctivitis during a treatment with acitretin (soriatane). J Fr Ophthalmol. 1993;16(3):191-4.

103. Fraunfelder FT, Fraunfelder FW, Edwards R. Ocular side effects possibly associated with isotretinoin usage. Am J Ophthalmol. 2001; 132(3):299-305.

104. Lerman S. Ocular side effects of accutane therapy. Lens Eye Toxic Res. 1992;9(3-4):429-38.

105. Marie I, Bodack OD. A warfarin-induced subconjunctival hemorrhage. Optometry. 2007; 78(3):113-8.

106. Valerie Q, Wren OD. Ocular and visual side effects of systemic drugs. J Behav Optomet. 2000;11(6):149-57.

107. Caronia RM, Sturm RT, Fastenberg DM, et al. Bilateral secondary angle-closure glaucoma as a complication of anticoagulation in a nanophthalmic patient. Am J Ophthalmol. 1998;126(2):307-9.

108. Thompson D, Stanescu C, Pryor P, Laselle B. Retrobulbar hematoma from warfarin toxicity and the limitations of bedside ocular sonography. West J Emerg Med. 2010;11(2):208-10.

109. Bozkurt B, Irkeç MT, Atakan N, Orhan M, Geyik PO. Lacrimal function and ocular complications in patients treated with systemic isotretinoin. Eur J Ophthalmol. 2002;12(3):173-6.

110. Egger SF, Huber-Spitzy V, Böhler K, Scholda C. Isotretinoin administration in treatment of acne vulgaris. A prospective study of the kind and extent of ocular complications. Ophthalmologie. 1995;92(1):17-20.

111. Santaella RM, Fraunfelder FW. Ocular adverse effects associated with systemic medications: recognition and management. Drugs. 2007;67(1):75-93.

112. Jerrod SK, Shefalee Shukla. Drug induced ocular disorders. Drug Saf. 2008;31:127-41.

113. Laties A, Sharlip I. Ocular safety in patients using Sildenafil citrate therapy for erectile dysfunction. J Sex Med. 2006;3(1):12-27.

114. Jannus SD. Ocular side effects of selected systemic drugs. Optom Clin. 1992;2:73-96.

115. Rulo AH, Greve EL, Hoyng PF. Additive ocular hypotensive effect of latanoprost and acetazolamide. A short-term study in patients with elevated intraocular pressure. Ophthalmology. 1997; 104(9):1503-7.

116. Duperré J, Grenier B, Lemire J, Mihalovits H, Sebag M, Lambert J. Effect of timolol vs. acetazolamide on sodium hyaluronate-induced rise in intraocular pressure after cataract surgery. Can J Ophthalmol. 1994; 29(4):182-6.

Index

Page numbers followed by *f* refer to figure and *t* refer to table.

topical 250
    glycerol (glycerin) 250
    hypertonic saline 250
Hyphema 199
Hypopyon 199

I

K

L

M